W9-BBZ-258

Contemporary Classics in Clinical Medicine

Contemporary Classics in Science

EUGENE GARFIELD, *Editor-in-Chief*

This volume is one of a series published by ISI Press®. The series is designed to bring together analyses of papers that have been designated Citation Classics because they are influential and widely quoted.

Books published in this series:

Contemporary Classics in the Life Sciences
Volume 1: Cell Biology
Volume 2: The Molecules of Life

Contemporary Classics in Clinical Medicine

Books to be published in this series:

Contemporary Classics in Plant, Animal, and Environmental Sciences

Contemporary Classics in Physical, Chemical, and Earth Sciences

Contemporary Classics in Engineering and Applied Science

Contemporary Classics in the Social and Behavioral Sciences

Contemporary Classics in Science

Contemporary Classics in Clinical Medicine

Edited by
James T. Barrett

Foreword by
Edward J. Huth

Preface by
Eugene Garfield

ISI PRESS®

Philadelphia

Published by
ISI PRESS® A Subsidiary of the Institute for Scientific Information®
3501 Market Street, Philadelphia, Pennsylvania 19104 U.S.A.

Library of Congress Cataloging in Publication Data

Contemporary classics in clinical medicine.

(Contemporary classics in science)
Selected articles originally appearing in *Current Contents.*
Includes index.
1. Medicine, Clinical—Research. I. Barrett, James T., 1927– . II. Series. [DNLM: 1. Medicine—collected works. WB 100 C7586]
R850.C66 1986 610'.72 86-7103

ISBN 0-89495-054-1

Printed in the United States of America
92 91 90 89 88 87 86 7 6 5 4 3 2 1

Contents

Foreword

Today's scientific literature possibly relevant to the immediate interests of a clinical investigator is itself so large and the effort for its surveillance so great as to preclude attention to literature more remote. Just keeping up with today's clearly relevant literature can be a burden. Why, then, should anyone look back at those papers that so refreshingly informed and influenced clinical research as to become Citation Classics, the papers cited far more frequently than others of their times? If we have the chance or bent for such a look backwards, we do risk seeing Citation Classics as stale rather than nascent. For it is true that what they had to say that was then fresh, even unsettling, in the orthodoxies of their time now looks like firmly cemented stones in the conceptual foundation for today's clinical science. But there may be some conceptual gain in looking back at Citation Classics; we may come to see more clearly what is truly central in the base of today's science. And we may come to see in their due proportions the greater premises, and the lesser, for the problems that are the subjects of today's research. In essence these are the values in history.

Those who know well their own field of science will necessarily know today's central concepts, which were built at least in part on the key papers that became Citation Classics. But will they remember the setting into which a now classic paper emerged, the orthodoxies of that time, the older frame of ideas? Very likely the younger of today's scientists will not know what that setting was and hence how the classic paper struck the contemporaries of its author before it changed a view of the world. Even older scientists who were already at work when Citation Classics were published may have forgotten such moments. Here lies some of the value of the short commentaries first published in *Current Contents* as "This Week's Citation Classic" and collected within these covers: the authors of some of the classic papers remind us in their commentaries of the state of science at the time they were published and hence make clear how today's classics became the classics they are.

Some of these little essays do more than sketch by retrospect the conceptual landscape the classic papers entered. When we read scientific papers, classics or not, we are likely to see a picture of the hypothesis conceived, an experiment designed, that experiment carried out to clear findings, and firm conclusions drawn from those findings. Scientific papers are, however, something of a fiction. Their neat structure and forward narrative imply that the research started with a clear hypothesis and proceeded with no wasted motion, no technical difficulties, to unequivocal findings. They rarely tell us of the false starts, the needs to refine methods. In this collection we find out that science does not move with steady and unwavering progress. And we see that scientists are not emotionless robots, free of human frailties, passions, conflicts. They do have real lives. Some of these commentaries remind us that scientific publishing is far from a perfect system. Some authors struggled to get papers published in the face of disbelieving referees and timid editors. Some faced contemporaries' misjudgments and their inability to see past the dogmas of their time. We get the colors, the sounds, the motions that show us and will show future historians what really happened, what touched off research, the picture so hard to repaint when the principals are long off the scene.

Scientists of our time should be grateful to the Institute for Scientific Information for having invited these commentaries for publication in *Current Contents.* They should be grateful to the ISI Press for gathering them in this collection. The full value of these commentaries may not be seen, however, until the histories of the science of our time are written. Very likely tomorrow's historians will be even more grateful than we could have been.

Edward J. Huth
Annals of Internal Medicine

Preface

For almost 20 years I've been writing about Citation Classics, my term for highly cited papers and books that are classics in their fields. In 1977 we began publishing in *Current Contents*® (*CC*®) the feature "This Week's Citation Classic"—an invited 500-word commentary by the author of a Citation Classic. Over 2,100 autobiographical commentaries have appeared so far. In requesting these commentaries, we asked authors of Citation Classics to describe their research, its genesis, and circumstances that affected its progress and publication. We encouraged them to include the type of personal details that are rarely found in formal scientific publication, such as obstacles encountered and by-ways taken. We also asked that they mention the contributions of co-authors, any awards or honors they received for their research, and any new terminology arising from their work. Finally, we asked them to speculate on the reasons for their paper or book having been cited so often.

With Volume One and Two we inaugurated the series "Contemporary Classics in Science." These two volumes contain the commentaries published in *CC/Life Sciences* from the beginning of 1977 to the end of 1984. The first volume, *Cell Biology,* includes Citation Classics from research on the cellular level, while the second volume, *The Molecules of Life,* includes those from research on the molecular level. This third volume in the series, *Contemporary Classics in Clinical Medicine,* collects all the commentaries published in *CC/Clinical Practice* from 1979 to 1984. Subsequent volumes will cover the physical sciences and applied sciences, as well as plant, animal, and environmental sciences.

Although I have previously described how we choose a paper or book as a Citation Classic,[1,2,3] it is useful to review these procedures in order to make the purpose of this monographic series clear. Not every scientific publication that deserves the designation "classic" is included in this series, which is limited to *Citation* Classics. There are other types of classics, including those that are rarely or only occasionally cited. More about these later. Our primary criterion for inviting a researcher to contribute a commentary is the number of citations that a particular work has accumulated.

We begin the selection process in gross terms by singling out the 300,000 papers and books most cited in our *Science Citation Index*® (*SCI*®) and *Social Sciences Citation Index*® (*SSCI*®) files (which presently span the years 1955 to 1985 and 1966 to 1985, respectively). We do not, however, rely solely on the highest number of citations in the entire population of publications, but make our selections by fields, in some of which, such as ecology, engineering, or mathematics, 100 citations or even fewer may qualify a work as a Citation Classic.

Searching for Citation Classics, therefore, is like fishing with nets. We seine the waters of the scientific literature in search of the biggest fish in a school. The big fish are the relatively few papers and books with the highest number of citations *in their field.* Now it's plain that the biggest fish in one school will be dwarfed by even the smallest fish in another school. So, too, the number of citations necessary to make a work a Citation Classic in radio astronomy, with its much smaller population of researchers and papers, is smaller than the number giving a work status as a Citation Classic in biochemistry. Realizing that one discipline is more populated than another, we have used different nets when searching different waters. In the Sea of Biochemistry we expect to encounter many giant fish, since in these waters the population of published papers is so great. The net we select has a wide mesh that captures only the big fish and allows the little ones to swim through. But the net we drop into the Bay of Radio Astronomy has a much smaller mesh and is designed to catch the largest of the relatively small fish found there. The mesh of the nets corresponds to the different thresholds of citation frequency we set depending on the fields in which we are searching for Citation Classics.

Along with the initial search for Citation Classics in terms of absolute and relative frequency of citation, we extend the search by creating a separate file for each journal to identify the most-cited papers published in that journal. If one assumes that a journal uniquely defines a field or specialty, then the list of most-cited papers for that journal will include many of the classics for that field. We have found that many classics were published in the first volumes of a specialty journal associated with the emergence of the then new field. But we have also found that the classic paper for a new field was sometimes published in a multidisciplinary journal such as *Nature* or *Science.* Thus, the most-cited paper published in a specialty journal may have been cited only 50 times, whereas the primordial paper for the same field may have appeared in *Nature* and received 100 citations. In cases such as these, we ask both the author of the paper published in the multidisciplinary journal and the author of the paper published in the specialty journal for commentaries. Not surprisingly, we often find that both papers were written by the same author(s).

We are further refining our selection process by relying increasingly on research-front data derived from co-citation analysis.[4] An analysis of most-cited, or core, papers in a research front provides a more sensitive classification of subjects than does citation analysis by journal.

Furthermore, and as a supplement to analytical methods, we ask for nominations from *CC* readers of works which they believe may qualify as Citation Classics.

* * * * *

We emphasize that this collection represents only a sample from the larger group we have identified as Citation Classics. About half of the authors invited to write commentaries actually do so. It follows, then, that the omission of a paper in this volume in no way signifies that it is not a Citation Classic. In the recent series of essays in *CC* devoted to the 1,000 most-cited papers in the *SCI* from 1961 to 1982, I identified papers for which we have received and published a *Citation Classics®* commentary.[5] In Appendix A of Volume One I provided a sampling of 100 most-cited works for which we have not yet received a commentary. I hope that some of the authors of these Citation Classics will put pen to paper to reminisce and interpret the citation impact of their research. Still, a remarkable number of Nobel laureates and other scientists I have described as *of Nobel class* have contributed commentaries. These are balanced by many from hundreds of other scientists who have received rather little formal recognition for their contributions.

* * * * *

Finally, a word about those classics I have reported as rarely or only occasionally cited. I have taken to describing these papers and books as uncited classics, and there are many reasons for a classic work having few or no citations. I have already described how a relatively low citation count can qualify a work as a classic when weighed against its companions in other fields, and how we use a flexible, composite, and, we hope, intelligent algorithm to compensate for this problem. It is most difficult, however, to compensate for the lifetime citation counts of papers and books published as long as 50 years ago or even more recently than that. We know that most older works receive fewer citations since typically most citations are received in the first decade after publication. Moreover, the exponential growth of the literature has changed the significance of any fixed threshold. In 1955 we processed 80,000 papers in about 600 journals in the *SCI,* whereas in 1985 we indexed about 600,000 from 3,000 journals in the natural and physical sciences. These numbers reflect the rapid expansion of modern science, which in turn affects the size of bibliographies and the potential for citation impact.

Furthermore, a recognized classic work may fail to be a Citation Classic because it has suffered what Robert K. Merton terms "obliteration by incorporation": "the obliteration of the source of ideas, methods, or findings, by their incorporation in currently accepted knowledge."[6,7] Thus, some works are no longer cited because their substance has been absorbed in the literature.[8] Just as neologisms and eponyms become part of scientific language, obliterated works become the common knowledge within a field, and explicit citation to them is viewed as unnecessary or pedantic. Quite often, a classic work is cited for a few years, excites rapid advances in its subject, and is then superseded by reviews or other papers containing new information. For a variety of reasons including little understood citation behavior, the primordial work is not mentioned; it nevertheless remains classic. On such matters I urge the reader to examine Joshua Lederberg's pithy remarks on obliteration in connection with the discovery that DNA is involved in the genetic transformation in bacteria.[9] The commentary published by Maclyn McCarty[10] on that milestone paper will be included in a future volume in this series for the life sciences.

* * * * *

I have always believed that these commentaries contribute to future historiography by preserving important biographical and behind-the-scenes information, otherwise generally unavailable. Working scientists reading this book will learn about unfamiliar aspects of otherwise familiar and classic research. These commentaries provide grist for the mill of historians and sociologists of science. They also help sensitize students and the public to the diverse nature and methods of science. The publication of these commentaries in this collected form adds to their value. Perhaps, too, the appearance of this book will stimulate other scientists to write *Citation Classics* commentaries. Since this is a continuing monographic series, their contributions will always be welcome.

Eugene Garfield
Institute for Scientific Information

REFERENCES

1. **Garfield E.** *Citation Classics*—four years of the human side of science. *Essays of an information scientist.* Philadelphia: ISI Press, 1982. Vol. 5. p. 123–34.
2. ———. The 100 most-cited papers ever and how we select *Citation Classics. Ibid.,* 1985. Vol. 7. p. 175–81.
3. ———. *Contemporary Classics in the Life Sciences:* an autobiographical feast. *Current Contents* (44):3–8, 4 November 1985.
4. ———. ABCs of cluster mapping. Parts 1 & 2. Most active fields in the life and physical sciences in 1978. *Essays of an information scientist.* Philadelphia: ISI Press, 1981. Vol. 4. p. 634–49.
5. ———. The articles most-cited in the *SCI*, 1961–1982. Pts. 1–5. *Ibid.,* 1985. Vol. 7. p. 175–81; 218–27; 270–6; 306–12; 325–35. Pts. 6–8. *Current Contents* (14): 3–10; (20):3–12; (33):3–11, 1985. Pts. 9–10. *Ibid.* (8):3–12; (16):3–14, 1986.
6. **Merton R K.** *Social theory and social structure.* New York: Free Press, 1968. pp. 27–9, 35–8.
7. ———. Foreword. (Garfield E) *Citation indexing—its theory and application in science, technology, and humanities.* New York: John Wiley & Sons, 1979. p. vii–xi.

8. **Garfield E.** The "obliteration phenomenon" in science—and the advantage of being obliterated. *Essays of an information scientist.* Philadelphia: ISI Press, 1977. Vol. 2. p. 396–8.
9. **Lederberg J.** Foreword. (Garfield E) *Ibid.,* 1977. Vol. 1. p. xiv.
10. **McCarty M.** *Citation Classic.* Commentary on Avery O T, MacLeod C M & McCarty M. Studies on the chemical nature of the substance inducing transformation of pneumococcal types. Induction of transformation by a desoxyribonucleic acid fraction isolated from pneumococcus Type III. *J. Exp. Med.* 79:139–58, 1944. *Current Contents/Life Sciences* 28(50):26, 16 December 1985.

Introduction

Biographies and autobiographies of scientists have proliferated in recent years. Few of these, however, supply detailed information on a specific experiment or publication. Exceptional, therefore, is the paper published by the Nobel Prize-winning British physiologist Sir Alan L. Hodgkin entitled "Chance and Design in Electrophysiology: An Informal Account of Certain Experiments on Nerve Carried Out between 1934 and 1952." Hodgkin recalls the books, papers, people, and environments that determined his choice of research. He attempts to estimate the portion of his results obtained by planning and the portion obtained by accident. At the outset he explains why such an account is needed:

> I believe that the record of published papers conveys an impression of directness and planning which does not at all coincide with the actual sequence of events. The stated object of a piece of research often agrees more closely with the reason for continuing or finishing the work than it does with the idea which led to the original experiments. In writing papers, authors are encouraged to be logical, and, even if they wished to admit that some experiment was done for a perfectly dotty reason, they would not be encouraged to "clutter-up" the literature with irrelevant personal reminiscences. But over a long period I have developed a feeling of guilt about suppressing the part which chance and good fortune played in what now seems to be a rather logical development.[1]

The biologist Sir Peter B. Medawar, another British Nobel Prize winner, puts it rather more directly by asking if the scientific paper is not a fraud. His question is not meant to cast suspicion on the facts that are published in a scientific paper; rather, he asks if the universally accepted format of the scientific article, generally presented in terms of a fictional inductive method, does not systematically misrepresent the thought processes that led to scientific discoveries.[2] Medawar believes it does.

The sociologist Robert K. Merton notes that

> Typically, the scientific paper or monograph presents an immaculate appearance which reproduces little or nothing of the intuitive leaps, false starts, mistakes, loose ends, and happy accidents that actually cluttered up the inquiry. The public record of science therefore fails to provide many of the source materials needed to reconstruct the actual course of scientific developments. . . . This practice of glossing over the actual course of inquiry results largely from the mores of scientific publication which call for a passive idiom and format of reporting which imply that ideas develop without benefit of human brain and that investigations are conducted without benefit of human hand.[3]

He then goes on to observe that Bacon, Leibniz, and Mach all took note of the difference between logical casuistry, based on the Euclidean and Cartesian ideals, and the often nonrational, nearly always circuitous course of discovery. Since the scientific article was invented 300 years ago there has evolved a format embracing these ideals and leading to typically immaculate, linear, and flawed accounts of discovery. There is room, therefore, for accounts, however brief, of the actual paths of inquiry.

The feature "This Week's Citation Classic" published in each weekly issue of *Current Contents*® (*CC*®) since 1977 has provided scientists with a forum in which they are permitted to describe their discoveries as they recall their having happened. In this way, *Citation Classics* commentaries continue to fill a lacuna in the history of science.

REFERENCES

1. **Hodgkin A L.** Chance and design in electrophysiology: an informal account of certain experiments on nerve carried out between 1934 and 1952. *The pursuit of nature: informal essays on the history of physiology.* Cambridge: Cambridge University Press, 1977. p. 1.
2. **Medawar P B.** Is the scientific paper a fraud? (Edge D, ed.) *Experiment.* London: BBC, 1964. p. 7–12.
3. **Merton R K.** On the history and systematics of sociological theory. *Social theory and social structure.* New York: Free Press, 1968. p. 4–6.

Chapter

1

Microbiology and Infectious Disease

Of the 26 Citation Classics represented in this chapter, only seven are based on studies that deal exclusively with viral disease. This was unexpected for an era when broad-spectrum antibacterial agents were in such widespread use. However, a contributing factor is the inclusion of more than a dozen studies on viruses in the first volume of this series, *Contemporary Classics in the Life Sciences, volume 1, Cell Biology.* Virtually all the 19 remaining Classics are founded on studies in bacteriology. In future volumes we can expect to see a greater representation from parasitology, a field that has been gaining momentum as a research area.

Periodontal disease of some degree is virtually inescapable by the time adulthood is reached. The promise that new dentifrices will limit both plaque and tartar formation is yet to be realized, except perhaps in the volunteers who participated in the early clinical trials. The ultimate proof of efficacy of these products will be evaluated partially through a classification and scoring system for periodontitis similar to that advanced by Russell. To such a system it may be possible to add data about the microbial flora of the gingiva since over 30 years ago it was determined that an increase in the density of this population is directly associated with gingival inflammation (p. 7). Two organisms often isolated from oral tissues and dental plaque are *Streptococcus mutans* and *Streptococcus sanguis.* The former was proved to be the cause of infectious dental caries in hamsters in a study conducted at the National Institute for Dental Research. A streptomycin-resistant mutant of *S. mutans* was used in this study (p. 8), and this genetic marker enabled the bacterium to be traced easily and identified in new carious foci. These two streptococci are also present in the human oral flora, and their numbers increase significantly when oral hygiene is not practiced. Another factor contributing to an increased population of these microorganisms is a diet high in sucrose. These bacteria convert sucrose, but not other sugars, into a capsular slime that facilitates their adhesion to the tooth surface (p. 9).

Streptococci unrelated to those causing caries or periodontal disease and placed in serological group B have been a significant cause of infections in very young infants. This was not fully appreciated until 1973 when an extensive study of vaginal flora, infections of newborn infants, autopsy records, etc., indicated that as many as 12,000 to 15,000 cases of "strep B" infection were occurring annually in the United States in newborn children (p. 10), though these may be on the wane at the present time. Since the immune defense system of very young infants is not fully developed, microbial infections are an expected part of infant life. The logical practice of prophylactic antibiotic and chemotherapeutic treatment of those infants believed to be most at risk for infection, for example, premature infants, resulted in an unexpected higher mortality and a ninefold greater incidence of kernicterus (p. 11) than was seen in other infants. Later it was discovered that many drugs release bilirubin from its nontoxic, albumin-bound state. When free from its protein carrier, bilirubin, if not removed as a diglucuronic acid conjugate, causes bilirubin encephalopathy or kernicterus.

The next four Classics focus on intestinal infections. The incidence of diarrhea, colitis, and other intestinal disorders with a microbial etiology continues to exceed that of other infectious diseases. In the example of clindamycin-associated colitis, a novel pathogenic opportunity is provided to *Clostridium difficile.* Clindamycin and structurally related derivatives sharply curtail the normal bacterial flora that usually compete efficiently with *C. difficile.* When this competition is reduced by the selective action of these antibiotics, the clostridial organism is able to cause a novel iatrogenic disease. The fragile status of drug company stocks is indicated in Tedesco's "This Week's Citation Classic" (TWCC) on antibiotic-associated colitis. Bartlett's TWCC on the same subject reveals that the paper that was the first to identify *C. difficile* as the causative organism was rejected by the editors of the first journal to which it was submitted. The second journal then misplaced the paper. Since the data in the paper had been described at an earlier national meeting, the authors were anxious to achieve formal publication. Finally, the article was published and became a Citation Classic.

Enterotoxin-producing strains of *Escherichia coli* can be identified by several means. The feeding of culture filtrates to baby mice is one method and has two advantages over other methods. It is rapid: within a few hours the mouse intestinal lumen becomes filled with fluid elicited by the heat-stable toxin. This assay is also more convenient than the rabbit intestinal loop assay since it does not require laparotomy (p. 14). The TWCC by Barlow on neonatal enterocolitis emphasizes how ridiculous contemporary science can be. In her study in which human breast milk was fed to human babies, prior *approval of the human experimentation committee was required!* How far will protectionist policies disenfranchise us from our normal activities? Will we soon be required to have walking permits rather than, or in addition to, driver's licenses?

A review of more than 100 pages on pyelonephritis and a 35-page summary of techniques to distinguish bladder infections from renal infections are the only two Citation Classics on urinary tract infections. The last paragraph of the second TWCC (p. 17) reveals how changes in the scientific scene result from the slow but incessant increase in our knowledge. In this instance, a 100 percent reversal from an earlier opinion of the authors occurred.

The effective chemotherapy of patients with acute leukemia is one of the most significant accomplishments in oncology. Because of the general cytotoxicity of the agents used, it is necessary to monitor the immune system very closely. One portion of this system that is easily examined on a routine basis is the neutrophil count. It is possible to adjust leukemia therapy to prevent a severe neutropenia and maintain a near-normal level of immunity. Bodey and his colleagues observed that neutrophil counts as low as, but not lower than, 1,000/mm^3 still permitted good protection against infections. Their data were so convincing that biostatisticians advised them against inserting those "sacred p values." Active neutrophils consume oxygen during metabolism, as opposed to the use of the glycolytic pathway when at rest. During aerobic metabolism these cells will transfer hydrogen to acceptor molecules other than oxygen. The dye nitroblue tetrazolium (NBT) is an excellent hydrogen acceptor and assumes a dark-blue color in its reduced state, hence the basis for the NBT reductase test. In freshly drawn blood, a large number of neutrophils with an NBT reducing capability signifies an earlier *in vivo* activation of these cells, usually because of an infection. The NBT reductase test is currently used to identify reductase-deficient cells, as in chronic granulomatous disease, rather than to identify infections.

Two reviews by Weinstein, one co-authored with Lerner and the other with Rubin, on the same subject, infective endocarditis, became Citation Classics. The first, a four-part article in the *New England Journal of Medicine,* has been cited more than 1,025 times. As late as 1982, the authors lamented that the correct dose, combination, and duration of antibiotic treatment for bacterial endocarditis was still not known.

The classification of leprosy according to the immune status of the leper has proved valuable in determining the potential outcome of this disease. An imbalance of the T-cell system in leprosy is the more recent cellular explanation for the changes in the immune system seen in lepers. A final paper on medical bacteriology targeted the physician or other hospital personnel as instrumental in initiating bacteremia through a failure to follow aseptic techniques when starting intravenous drips. A second cause of these infections was contaminated intravenous fluid itself. Both problems persist, but Maki and his co-workers did write a short supplementary article at the editor's request that contained their recommendations for prophylaxis against infection from this source.

Aspergillosis, like many diseases of immunosuppressed patients, is one which can be expected to increase in incidence as more victims of cancer and transplant recipients are exposed to cytotoxic and immunosuppressive drugs. Aspergillosis in otherwise healthy persons is a rare disease. The paper referred to here described the broad manifestations of aspergillosis.

The Citation Classics on viral disease cover only two virologic phenomena—the description of a virus as the etiologic agent of a familiar disease and the unexpected association of a well-known virus with a second, unexpected disease.

The hepatitis B virus was discovered through studies of the Australia antigen, and this history is well known to medical scientists. The prevalence of hepatitis in dialysis patients led to a new understanding of this disease, since these patients often had a mild form of the illness. This contrasts to the more serious disease in otherwise healthy persons. Consequently, a strong or normal immune response contributes to a more fulminant form of the disease, strange as this may seem. The Australia antigen exists as the surface protein of the hepatitis B virus (HBsAg). The intact virus is the larger Dane particle, whose discovery is described by Dane in his TWCC. Both the 42-nm whole virus (Dane particle) and the HBsAg at 22 nm were first observed physically in the blood of a hemophiliac. These two TWCCs on hepatitis B virus seem to be little more than glimpses of an exciting past, but several TWCCs on hepatitis virus are included in the first volume of this series. The future of hepatitis B research includes the exciting possibility of constructing a hepatitis vaccine through genetic engineering by placing the virus genome in a second cell which will then produce the desired HBsAg.

Weller is the author of the next two TWCCs, both of which deal with studies of cytomegalovirus (CMV). The first article, published in 1962, described the clinical features of CMV infection in newborn children and its etiologic role in the congenital malformations that follow intrauterine infections. Nine years later, the knowledge and interest in CMV helped popularize a review article on the clinical and virological events in CMV disease. Even today, the rubella virus is a better known associate of fetal malformations than CMV, although the latter is responsible for far more such events. Readers will remember Weller, Robbins, and Enders for their Nobel Prize winning labors in tissue culturing the poliomyelitis virus.

The discovery of adenoviruses as the cause of pneumonia in children was made because Chany was not satisfied by the axiom of his time that it was simply a "virus infection when we were not able to find any other explanation for the diseases." He began a study of childhood pneumonia in a foundling home and identified the viral etiology that was expected. The relationship of measles virus to subacute sclerosing panencephalitis described by Connolly apparently depends upon an antenatal infection of the fetus when it is unable to muster the essential immunity needed to protect itself against this virus. The resulting proliferation of the virus in the host that has become tolerant to the infection allows a slow destruction of neural tissue and encephalitis. Because of the limited number of cases of subacute sclerosing panencephalitis, it is not responsible for nearly as many infant or childhood deaths as CMV infection.

The association of Epstein-Barr virus (EBV) with infectious mononucleosis reported in the final TWCC is also woven into the story of Burkitt's lymphoma. Much of this history is presented in the first Life Sciences volume. EBV is apparently the etiologic agent of mononucleosis and possibly lymphoma. Evans' group focused on the role of the EBV agent in infectious mononucleosis and established the essential information for this association. From Evans' first interest in infectious mononucleosis until his Classic was published, 20 years elapsed.

This chapter contains a number of topics—hepatitis B virus, cytomegalovirus, *Clostridium difficile* enterocolitis, and streptococcal diseases—that were of emerging interest when the research articles became Citation Classics. In the interim, many of these retained their importance and popularity. Naturally, there has been a shift in emphasis, usually from a description of these agents and their associated diseases to the development of vaccines or other preventive measures, the molecular biology of the pathogens, and their relationship to other human ailments (cancer). Some of these changes are indicated in the recent references listed here.

George W L. Antimicrobial agent-associated colitis and diarrhea: historical background and clinical aspects. *Rev. Infect. Dis.* **6**(Suppl. 1):S208–S213, 1984.

Gerber M A & Thung S N. Molecular and cellular pathology of hepatitis B. *Lab. Invest.* **52:**572–90, 1985.

Griffiths P D. Diagnostic techniques for cytomegalovirus infection. *Clin. Haematol.* **13:**631–44, 1984.

Jacobson I M & Dienstag J L. Viral hepatitis vaccines. *Annu. Rev. Med.* **36:**241–61, 1985.

Kirchner H. Immunobiology of infection with human cytomegalovirus. *Adv. Cancer Res.* **40:**31–105, 1983.

Kliegman R M & Fanaroff A A. Necrotizing enterocolitis. *New Engl. J. Med.* **310:**1093–1103, 1984.

Rapp F & Robbins D. Cytomegalovirus and human cancer. *Birth Defects* **20:**175–92, 1984.

Rice P A & Dale P A. Infections of the genitourinary tract in women: selected aspects. *Adv. Intern. Med.* **30:**53–78, 1984.

Ross P W. Group B streptococcus—profile of an organism. *J. Med. Microbiol.* **18:**139–66, 1984.

Sherman M & Shafritz D A. Hepatitis B virus and hepatocellular carcinoma: molecular biology and mechanistic considerations. *Semin. Liver Dis.* **4:**98–112, 1984.

Stamm W E & Turck M. Urinary tract infection. *Adv. Intern. Med.* **28:**141–59, 1983.

Trnka Y M & LaMont J T. *Clostridium difficile* colitis. *Adv. Intern. Med.* **29:**85–107, 1984.

This Week's Citation Classic

NUMBER 45
NOVEMBER 5, 1979

Russell A L. A system of classification and scoring for prevalence surveys of periodontal disease. *J. Dental Res.* **35**:350-9, 1956.
[National Inst. Dental Res., National Institutes of Health, Bethesda, MD]

A scoring method is proposed for the study of chronic destructive periodontal disease in human populations. Individual scores are increased as the disease progresses through a syndrome ending with loss of function of the dentition. Few instruments or adjuncts are required. Emphasis is on examiner comparability. [The *SCI*® indicates that this paper has been cited over 235 times since 1961.]

A.L. Russell
1720 Palomar Drive
Ann Arbor, MI 48103

August 9, 1979

"The classic epidemiological approach to a disease of unknown etiology involves the division of a population into groups with and without the disease so that the determining factors in their ways of life can be identified. But, some degree of chronic destructive periodontal disease affects virtually every adult. Hence, it was necessary to develop a strategy of separating groups with the greater from groups with the lesser degree of involvement before the disease could be studied epidemiologically. The Periodontal Index was devised for this purpose. It was developed over a period of ten years prior to publication.

"During its gestation it was trimmed from a 30-minute procedure requiring an extensive armamentarium to a one-minute inspection conducted mostly with a dental mirror. This was done through elimination of items which proved to be extraneous, or were irreversible, and by elimination or deemphasis of items on which examiners found it difficult to agree.

"There were difficulties with statistical management. Distribution of Index values is a function of the ages of the persons studied. At younger ages right skewness is severe, evolving into a roughly square pattern in the middle ages, and finally into extreme left skewness in persons over the age of 40 or 50 years. No one transformation seemed appropriate over the entire range. Average scores for small groups were normally distributed, and some of my later findings were reported on this basis. Weighting of scores was manipulated experimentally to reflect the gravity of the condition as judged by clinical periodontologists, and to yield straight-line curves with age for some scores of thousands of persons aged up through 84 years. This last permitted comparison of the status of two or more groups differing in mean age.

"The Index has since been recommended for epidemiological research by the World Health Organization and other evaluatory bodies.

"In 1956 there were as many concepts of the etiology of chronic destructive periodontal disease as there were professors of periodontics. Since that time the consensus has developed that the disease is due basically to bacterial activity as modified by host defensive factors. This is consistent with my findings in a series of nutrition surveys in world areas where dental care was virtually nonexistent and oral hygiene practices were ineffective[1]—in short, where there was little interference with the natural progression of the disease. My data, since corroborated,[2] showed no consistent association with diet, or nutrition, or ethnicity, or a host of other factors once considered etiologic. The factors that emerged invariably as important were chronological age and evidence of past or present oral infection."

1. **Russell A L.** World epidemiology and oral health. *Environmental variables in oral disease.* (Kreshover S J & McClure F J, eds.) Washington, DC: American Association for the Advancement of Science, 1966. p. 21-39.
2. **Ramfjord S P, Emslie R D, Greene J C, Held A J & Waerhaug J.** Epidemiological studies of periodontal diseases. *Amer. J. Pub. Health* **58**:1713-22, 1968.

This Week's Citation Classic

Löe H, Theilade E & Jensen S B. Experimental gingivitis in man.
J. Periodontology **36**:177-87, 1965.
[Depts. Periodontol., Microbiol., and Oral Diagnosis, Royal Dental College, Aarhus, Denmark]

The paper provided evidence for the role of dental plaque bacteria in the initiation of human periodontal disease. Complete withdrawal of oral hygiene for three weeks invariably caused gingivitis. The number of bacteria colonizing the teeth increased dramatically and distinct changes in bacterial ecology occurred over time. Reinstitution of plaque control resulted in reestablishment of healthy gingiva. [The *SCI*® indicates that this paper has been cited in over 455 publications since 1965.]

Harald Löe
Office of the Dean
School of Dental Medicine
University of Connecticut Health Center
Farmington, CT 06032

June 11, 1982

"In a crude sense, the notion that debris on teeth plays a role in the destruction of the tissues supporting the teeth is centuries old. On the other hand, the scientific evidence to accept or reject the idea had been lacking; the etiology of periodontal disease was poorly understood and, consequently, the clinical management of this disease was generally confused and ineffective. More teeth were lost in adult life due to periodontal disease than to any other condition.

"In 1952, Jens Waerhaug of the University of Oslo had published his thesis, *The Gingival Pocket*,[1] which constituted a comprehensive study of the dynamics of the gingiva in health and disease. As a recent graduate, I was afforded the opportunity to work with Waerhaug on various clinical aspects of periodontal disease for some ten years prior to assuming the chair in periodontology at the Royal Dental College in Aarhus, Denmark, in 1962. By that time, there was a fair amount of clinical experience as well as epidemiological data to indicate that a close relationship existed between deposits on teeth and destruction of the periodontal tissue and the loosening and eventual loss of teeth. The time and mind were ripe for a definitive test of the hypothesis that it was the dental plaque component of oral accumulations that is responsible for the initiation of periodontal disease.

"In the study to follow, we asked 12 healthy, young individuals with clean dentitions and normal gingiva to refrain from any measure of oral hygiene for a period of three weeks. By assessing the gradual buildup of deposits on the dentition and the response of the gingival tissues, it appeared that in all individuals the rapid accumulation of bacterial plaque elicited an inflammatory reaction in the gingival tissues, which clinically was characterized as gingivitis. The time necessary to develop gingivitis varied between ten and 21 days. Concurrent microbiological examinations showed that the number of bacteria colonizing the tooth surfaces increased dramatically with time and that distinct changes in the composition of the flora occurred as well. When good oral hygiene was reinstituted, the original sparse microflora was reestablished and the inflamed gingiva reverted back to normal.

"Since this first experimental gingivitis study, we and others have reproduced the results in different age groups and in different racial groups in various geographical locations. It was soon apparent that this constituted a reproducible, low cost human experimental model[2] for the study of the detailed microbiology of dental plaque, the immunological and other host responses to the bacterial attack, and the cytological characteristics of the lesion. Over the years a substantial amount of data has been accumulated and continues to emanate from such studies. However, beyond the scientific utility and potential of this experimental system, the study has had major clinical impact as a basic reference to the bacterial etiology of periodontal disease, its infectious nature, and the importance of oral hygiene in the control of this major dental disease.[3]

"Personally, I find the simplicity of the model aesthetically satisfying and its lack of compromise calls for the objective truth. There is, perhaps, some intrinsic heroism in the execution of this model, but there is no permanent damage to the participant."

1. **Waerhaug J.** The gingival pocket. *Odontol. Tidskrift* **60**(Suppl. 1):1-186, 1952.
2. **Löe H.** A human research model for the production and prevention of gingivitis. *J. Dent. Res.* **50**:256-64, 1971.
3. --------. The role of bacteria in periodontal diseases. *Bull. WHO* **59**:821-5, 1981.

CC/NUMBER 38
SEPTEMBER 22, 1980

This Week's Citation Classic

Fitzgerald R J & Keyes P H. Demonstration of the etiologic role of streptococci in experimental caries in the hamster.
J. Amer. Dent. Ass. **61**:9-19, 1960.
[National Institute of Dental Research, National Institutes of Health, Bethesda, MD]

Dental caries was induced in 'caries-inactive' albino hamsters by oral inoculation of pure cultures of a streptococcus isolated from a caries lesion of a caries-active hamster. A streptomycin-resistant mutant of this organism was used to demonstrate its presence in caries lesions and to trace the transmission of the 'labeled' organisms between animals. [The *SCI*® indicates that this paper has been cited over 265 times since 1961.]

Robert J. Fitzgerald
Dental Research Unit
Veterans Administration Hospital
Miami, FL 33125

August 14, 1980

"It was surprising to learn how popular this paper has been since it was aimed primarily at dental researchers. The frequency with which it has been cited is probably due to several 'firsts' which it reported. It was the first demonstration of caries induction by the organism we now know as *Streptococcus mutans* and which is now highly suspect as a cause of caries in humans; it was the first report of caries induction by a single organism in an animal harboring a 'conventional' microflora, as distinguished from the germfree animal model; and it was the first time antibiotic-resistant labeled organisms had been utilized to trace the transmission of an oral disease.

"As in the case of a number of studies which have become *'Citation Classics'* serendipity played a prominent part in this research. Paul Keyes had obtained a strain of albino hamsters from the National Institutes of Health's Animal Production Unit which appeared to be virtually immune to caries when fed the high sucrose diet that resulted in high caries activity in golden hamsters. At first, thinking that this was a genetically mediated phenomenon, he soon discovered that when albino and golden hamsters were caged together both strains developed caries.[1] This indicated that the albinos did not harbor a cariogenic microflora but could acquire the infection on contact with the golden hamsters.

"At the time, I had been using germfree rats to test the potential cariogenicity of pure cultures of microorganisms isolated from caries in rats and humans. Recognizing that the albino hamster would be simpler and more convenient as a test animal for these studies, Keyes and I joined forces. I isolated a series of organisms from caries lesions in golden hamsters and we began to infect the albinos with them. Within a few months we showed that only a single type of streptococcus was cariogenic. By making this organism resistant to streptomycin and using selective media containing streptomycin to re-isolate it, we had a convenient way to show that it fulfilled Koch's postulates as the cause of caries in these animals.

"It was not until several years later that we learned that a similar organism had been isolated from human caries by Clarke[2] in 1924 and named *Streptococcus mutans*. Unfortunately, Clarke had no way to demonstrate that his organism actually caused caries. Ironically, the success of our study depended on the advent of antibiotics, for it turned out that the albino hamster breeding colony had been treated with a number of antibiotics to eliminate intercurrent infections. This treatment apparently also eliminated any cariogenic organisms they may have harbored."

1. **Keyes P H.** Infections and transmissible nature of experimental dental caries. *Arch. Oral Biol.* **1**:304-20, 1960.
2. **Clarke J K.** On the bacterial factor in the etiology of dental caries. *Brit. J. Exp. Pathol.* **5**:141-7, 1924.

This Week's Citation Classic

Carlsson J. Presence of various types of non-haemolytic streptococci in dental plaque and in other sites of the oral cavity in man. *Odontol. Revy* **18**:55-74, 1967. [Depts. Oral Microbiology and Periodontology, Sch. Dentistry, Univ. Lund, Malmö, Sweden]

The paper describes the streptococcal flora in various sites of the oral cavity of four subjects. In all, 243 streptococcal isolates are studied. The tooth surface is shown to be a most favorable habitat of the extracellular polysaccharide-producing streptococci, *Streptococcus sanguis* **and** *Streptococcus mutans*. **[The** *SCI®* **indicates that this paper has been cited over 185 times since 1967.]**

Jan Carlsson
Department of Oral Microbiology
School of Dentistry
University of Umeå
S-901 87 Umeå
Sweden

November 10, 1981

"In the early-1960s it was generally recognized that periodontal disease was caused by the bacteria accumulating along the gingival margin of the teeth. At that time Hilding Björn, department of periodontology, School of Dentistry, University of Lund, initiated my studies on dietary components which may influence the amount of bacteria accumulating on the teeth. Methods of evaluating the bacterial accumulation were developed and in cooperation with Jan Egelberg it was demonstrated that sucrose was a key component of diet in facilitating accumulation of bacteria on the teeth.[1] My attention was then focused on the capabilities of the bacteria on the teeth in utilizing sucrose. It was found that *S. sanguis* was among the predominant bacteria on the teeth.[2] This organism was known to produce copious amounts of extracellular polysaccharides from sucrose, but not from other sugars, and it was suggested that these polysaccharides may serve as a glue for the accumulation of bacteria on the teeth.

"At that time, Bo Krasse, department of cariology, School of Dentistry, University of Lund, had spent a sabbatical year at the laboratory of R.J. Fitzgerald and P.H. Keyes, National Institute of Dental Research, National Institutes of Health, Bethesda, Maryland. In 1960, Fitzgerald and Keyes had demonstrated that certain streptococci induce caries in hamsters[3] and Krasse, during his stay in their laboratory, had shown that sucrose was much more potent than glucose in inducing caries in hamsters infected with the 'caries-inducing streptococci.'[4] These findings indicated a significant role for streptococci and sucrose in the microbial ecology of the oral cavity and in the publication cited above the characteristics of streptococci from various sites of the human oral cavity were studied.

"The reason why this publication has been cited may be that it demonstrated the tooth surface as the most favorable habitat of *S. sanguis* and *S. mutans*. It also showed that streptococci with the characteristics of the 'caries-inducing streptococci' were similar to *S. mutans*. A review of this field was recently published in *Microbiological Reviews*.[5]

"It is worth noticing that the studies aimed at elucidation mechanisms in the pathogenesis of periodontal disease did not give any clue, but they appear to have contributed to the understanding of the other major disease of the oral cavity, dental caries. Sucrose and streptococci have in numerous studies since then been shown to play a role in the accumulation of bacteria on the teeth and in the initiation of dental caries, while there is no evidence whatsoever that streptococci or sucrose have any effect on the development of periodontal disease in man.

"In recognition of my work in this area I received the G.V. Black Prize, 1970 (Swedish Dental Association) and the Science Award, 1972 (International Association for Dental Research)."

1. **Carlsson J & Egelberg J.** Effect of diet on early plaque formation in man. *Odontol. Revy* **16**:112-25, 1965.
2. **Carlsson J.** Zooglea-forming streptococci, resembling *Streptococcus sanguis*, isolated from dental plaque in man. *Odontol. Revy* **16**:348-58, 1965.
3. **Fitzgerald R J & Keyes P H.** Demonstration of the etiologic role of streptococci in experimental caries in the hamster. *J. Amer. Dent. Ass.* **61**:9-19, 1960. [Citation Classic. *Current Contents/Clinical Practice* **8**(38):16, 22 September 1980.]
4. **Krasse B.** The effect of caries-inducing streptococci in hamsters fed diets of sucrose or glucose. *Arch. Oral Biol.* **10**:223-6, 1965.
5. **Hamada S & Slade H D.** Biology, immunology, and cariogenicity of *Streptococcus mutans*. *Microbiol. Rev.* **44**:331-84, 1980.

CC/NUMBER 25
JUNE 20, 1983

This Week's Citation Classic

Franciosi R A, Knostman J D & Zimmerman R A. Group B streptococcal neonatal and infant infections. *J. Pediatrics* **82**:707-18, 1973.
[Streptococcal Dis. Sect., Ecol. Invest. Program, Ctr. for Dis. Control, Hlth. Serv. and Mental Hlth. Admin., Public Hlth. Serv., US Dept. HEW, Fort Collins, CO and Dept. Pathol., Children's Hosp., Minneapolis, MN]

Epidemiologic studies of group B streptococcal (GBS) infection revealed an incidence of three per 1,000 live births and a mortality of one per 1,000 live births. Vaginal cultures for GBS were positive in 4.6 percent of women at delivery, and 1.2 percent of their infants. Two distinct types of sepsis occurred; one type presented within hours of birth with respiratory distress and the second presented as meningitis in the later neonatal. [The *SCI*® indicates that this paper has been cited in over 305 publications since 1973.]

Ralph A. Franciosi
Minneapolis Children's Health Center
2525 Chicago Avenue
Minneapolis, MN 55404

April 26, 1983

"My experience with group B streptococcal (GBS) infection began in July 1969 when I joined the pathology staff at the Children's Hospital in Denver, Colorado. My curiosity was aroused quickly by observing in the first eight months of work five newborns who died of GBS infection. This experience caused me to review the problem of neonatal sepsis at Children's Hospital.[1] These five cases accounted for 45 percent of the neonatal septic mortality that year.

"Robert A. Zimmerman, chief of the Ecological Investigation Program of the Streptococcal Disease Section of the Center for Disease Control in Fort Collins, Colorado, directed the reference laboratory for streptococcal identification. He confirmed the isolates from our cases as group B streptococcus. When asked if his laboratory would support a study of this potential problem, he readily agreed. Zimmerman's work in the area of streptococcal research was well known and he was able to enlist the aid of Rebecca Lancefield. James D. Knostman was an internist with a special interest in renal disease assigned as a public health officer to Zimmerman. He was very interested in helping with the epidemiologic aspects of this study.

"Our study of GBS was designed to address these questions: What is the prevalence of GBS in maternal vagina at delivery and the incidence of neonatal infection? What is the prevalence of GBS in newborns at delivery and discharge from the hospital? What is the prevalence of GBS vaginally positive nonpregnant women? What is the prevalence of GBS in the male urethra? Is antepartum prevention possible? What are the clinical, laboratory, and pathologic findings in GBS infection?

"Three months were needed to recruit the necessary cooperation, i.e., four obstetrical units, one private obstetric and gynecology clinic, three neighborhood health centers, and one state penal institution. During the two and a half years of study, cultures were collected from over 1,200 deliveries, 350 nonpregnant women, 100 nursery staff, and 130 men; 43 clinical and autopsy records of GBS cases were abstracted; 500 placentas were examined; and 800 paired maternal and infant serums were collected.

"We were able to conclude that GBS sepsis was a significantly underestimated problem. Clinically there were two distinct presentations of GBS sepsis, one defined as acute onset occurring within 48 hours of birth and the other delayed onset usually occurring a week or more after birth. The pathogenesis of acute onset GBS infection was colonization of the newborn *in utero* or in transit through the birth canal of a vaginally colonized mother.

"In 1979, I reviewed the published cases of acute onset GBS infection.[2] It was clear that the morbidity and mortality could be reduced by earlier diagnosis and treatment. In 1980, I proposed a hypothesis to explain the rising incidence of acute onset GBS infection.[3]

"A recent review on GBS infection indicates that this is a worldwide problem.[4] With so many talented researchers working on this problem, the next decade should see a marked reduction in the 12,000-15,000 GBS cases per year in the US. I feel that our original paper illustrated the epidemiology and pathogenesis of GBS infection in newborns. For this reason, it is often quoted as a reference. In addition, the paper is referred to as a model for approaching the problem of neonatal bacterial infection."

1. **Franciosi R A, Zimmerman R A, Favara B E & Butterfield J.** Neonatal infection due to group B streptococcus. *Rocky Mt. Med. J.* **68**:48-52, 1971.
2. **Franciosi R A.** Infant at risk for early onset group B streptococcal infection. *Minn. Med.* **62**:801-4, 1979.
3. ------------------. Hypothesis to explain the emergence of early onset group B streptococcal infection in newborns. *Minn. Med.* **63**:267-9, 1980.
4. **Christensen K K, Christensen P, Hägerstrand I, Lindén V, Nordbring F & Svenningsen N.** The clinical significance of group B streptococci. *J. Perinatal Med.* **10**:133-46, 1982.

CC/NUMBER 3
JANUARY 21, 1980

This Week's Citation Classic

Silverman W A, Andersen D H, Blanc W A & Crozier D N. A difference in mortality rate and incidence of kernicterus among premature infants allotted to two prophylactic antibacterial regimens. *Pediatrics* **18**:614-25, 1956.
[Babies Hosp., and Dept. Pediat., Columbia Univ., Coll. Physicians & Surgeons, New York, NY]

A controlled clinical trial to evaluate the relative effectiveness of two prophylactic antibacterial regimens in premature infants resulted in an unexpected and inexplicable outcome: kernicterus (and death) occurred significantly more often among infants who received penicillin/sulfisoxazole. [The *SCI*® indicates that this paper has been cited over 240 times since 1961.]

William A. Silverman
90 La Cuesta Drive
Greenbrae, CA 94904

January 7, 1980

"In 1949, a logical, but unevaluated, practice began in American premature infant nurseries: administration of antibacterial drugs to all small newborn infants. Previous results of treating identified infections had been poor; the principal difficulty was the vague nature of early signs of invasion. Improved survival rates were attributed to the new practice and the approach spread rapidly. In 1954, it was learned that routine oxygen treatment, begun 12 years earlier, had been responsible for blinding 10,000 premature infants. This led all to wonder about other bombs which might be ticking away in American nurseries.

"When, in the same year, a new recommendation for antibacterial prophylaxis was made, we, at Columbia University, seized upon the opportunity to begin a long-delayed examination of this element of care. The grounds for using preventive treatment were reasonable; only the ideal agent(s) seemed in doubt. Consequently, we decided to make a formal comparison between the new proposal and the 'established' regimen (used for 1½ years with no recognizable hint of difficulty). We anticipated this would be the first in a plodding series to find an ideal regimen. Much to our amazement, the first controlled trial gave a definitive result. Much to our horror, the mortality rate was higher in infants who received the 'established' treatment (penicillin plus sulfisoxazole). Moreover, kernicterus occurred nine times more often in this group. It was clear that this unexpected (and, at the time, completely inexplicable) complication accounted for the increased fatalities. We took no comfort in the knowledge that the formal trial saved half of the infants from exposure to the unsuspected hazards of a treatment which had been used so confidently in our institution and others throughout the country. If a controlled trial had been carried out at the time of the original shift in practice, the saving in lives would have been truly impressive. It was not until 1959 that the mechanism underlying the disaster was uncovered by Odell who conducted *in vitro* studies demonstrating that sulfonamides uncouple protein-bound bilirubin permitting extravascular diffusion of the neurotoxic pigment.[1] In the same year Johnson and co-workers demonstrated the effect in newborn Gunn rats.[2]

"I found it interesting, in the years which followed our report, that it was cited because of the startling finding—the first demonstration that bilirubin-related kernicterus could be produced by a potentiating factor—rather than as a striking demonstration of the inherent safety of the hedging strategy of controlled trials in clinical studies. I can recall the initial skepticism about our bizarre findings—'mere statistics.' Naively, I thought the antipathy toward use of controlled trials would surely change. The methodology had been so well validated by R.A. Fisher[3] in agricultural research and was so well accepted in pre-clinical studies, I was certain a double standard could not last for long. I can see how wrong I was to be so optimistic."

1. **Odell G B.** Studies in kernicterus: I. The protein binding of bilirubin. *J. Clin. Invest.* **38**:823-33, 1959.
2. **Johnson L, Sarmiento F, Blanc W A & Day R.** Kernicterus in rats with an inherited deficiency of glucuronyl transferase. *Amer. J. Dis. Child.* **97**:591-608, 1959.
3. **Fisher R A.** *The design of experiments.* Edinburgh: Oliver and Boyd, 1935. 252 p.

CC/NUMBER 25
JUNE 18, 1984

This Week's Citation Classic™

Tedesco F J, Barton R W & Alpers D H. Clindamycin-associated colitis: a prospective study. *Ann. Intern. Med.* **81**:429-33, 1974.
[Dept. Internal Medicine, Washington Univ. Sch. Medicine, St. Louis, MO]

A prospective study of patients receiving clindamycin showed a 21 percent incidence of diarrhea and a ten percent incidence of pseudomembranous colitis. If the diagnosis is made early after the onset of diarrhea and the antibiotic is stopped, the pseudomembranous colitis seems to be self-limited. [The *SCI*® indicates that this paper has been cited in over 325 publications since 1974.]

Francis J. Tedesco
Section of Gastroenterology
School of Medicine
Medical College of Georgia
Augusta, GA 30912

May 16, 1984

"In 1973, while I was a gastroenterology fellow, Burton Shatz and I were performing colonoscopy on a patient with diarrhea and a colonic polyp noted on barium enema. During this examination, we noted multiple raised plaque-like lesions studding the colonic mucosa. We proceeded to remove the colonic polyp as well as taking multiple biopsies of these unusual lesions. The biopsies of these lesions were interpreted as 'pseudomembranous colitis.' Over the next several months, I saw several other patients with these peculiar lesions, and I reviewed their clinical course and hospital charts to see if a common feature was present. During this same period, Cohen, McNeill, and Wells published an interesting report[1] of several patients who had classic pseudomembranes on proctoscopic examination, yet their biopsies showed nonspecific inflammation. The common feature in their patients was that they were receiving an antibiotic, clindamycin.

"The patients I had examined also had been receiving clindamycin. My early experience with clindamycin-associated pseudomembranous colitis led me to believe that the association between clindamycin and pseudomembranous colitis was valid, but the natural history and mortality of antibiotic-associated pseudomembranous colitis was different than the reported 50 to 75 percent mortality figure usually associated with pseudomembranous colitis. I, in collaboration with Barton and Alpers, devised a prospective study of all in-hospital patients receiving clindamycin to determine the actual incidence of diarrhea, colitis, or both, and to uncover the natural history of clindamycin-associated colitis.

"The report of this study had immediate reactions including a flurry of other reports of this condition as well as an early reluctance by some people in industry to accept the scope of the problem. An article in the *Wall Street Journal*,[2] which quoted from the *Medical Letter*[3] and utilized information from our article, intimated that these reports led stock analysts to modify their opinion of Upjohn Company stocks. In fact, the Upjohn Company stocks dropped nearly 27 percent in three days. Shortly thereafter, an invitation was extended to me by Senator Gaylord Nelson to testify before his subcommittee concerning clindamycin-associated pseudomembranous colitis.

"This paper appears to be highly cited because it focused on a rarely recognized problem and led investigators in fields other than gastroenterology to aggressively investigate this problem. This paper led to further publications on the etiology,[4-6] stool toxin assays,[4] and treatment.[7] Our knowledge concerning antibiotic-associated colitis has rapidly expanded since this publication in 1974."

1. **Cohen L E, McNeill C J & Wells R F.** Clindamycin-associated colitis. *J. Amer. Med. Assn.* **223**:1379-80, 1973. (Cited 155 times.)
2. **Elia C J.** Heard on the street. *Wall Street J.* 12 September 1974, p. 35.
3. Colitis associated with clindamycin. *Med. Letter Drugs Ther.* **16**:73-4, 1974.
4. **Bartlett J G, Chang T W, Gurwith M, Gorbach S L & Onderdonk A B.** Antibiotic-associated pseudomembranous colitis due to toxin-producing clostridia. *N. Engl. J. Med.* **298**:531-4, 1978. (Cited 270 times.)
5. **Larson H E, Price A B, Honour P & Borriello S P.** Clostridium difficile and the aetiology of pseudomembranous colitis. *Lancet* **1**:1063-6, 1978. (Cited 195 times.)
6. **Kappas A, Shinagawa N, Arabi Y, Thompson H, Burdon D W, Dimock F, George R H, Alexander-Williams J & Keighley M R B.** Diagnosis of pseudomembranous colitis. *Brit. Med. J.* **1**:675-8, 1978. (Cited 80 times.)
7. **Tedesco F, Markham R, Gurwith M, Christie D & Bartlett J G.** Oral vancomycin for antibiotic-associated pseudomembranous colitis. *Lancet* **2**:226-8, 1978. (Cited 115 times.)

This Week's Citation Classic™

Bartlett J G, Chang T W, Gurwith M, Gorbach S L & Onderdonk A B. Antibiotic-associated pseudomembranous colitis due to toxin-producing clostridia. *N. Engl. J. Med.* **298**:531-4, 1978.

[VA Hosp.; New England Med. Ctr. Hosp.; Tufts Univ. Sch. Med., Boston, MA; and Univ. Manitoba, Winnipeg, Canada]

Stools from four patients with antibiotic-associated pseudomembranous colitis contained a cytotoxin that is neutralized by gas-gangrene antitoxin. These specimens caused colitis when injected intracecally into hamsters. The toxicity in tissue cultures and hamsters could be reproduced with broth cultures of *Clostridium difficile* strains recovered from three of the four specimens. [The *SCI*® indicates that this paper has been cited in over 280 publications since 1978.]

John G. Bartlett
Johns Hopkins Hospital
600 N. Wolfe Street
Baltimore, MD 21205

August 20, 1984

"In the early 1970s, there were three interrelated observations that prompted our interest in antibiotic-associated pseudomembranous colitis (PMC). First, a prior *Citation Classic* by Francis Tedesco showed an extraordinarily high incidence of this complication among clindamycin recipients at Barnes Hospital.[1,2] Second, *Staphylococcus aureus* was the traditionally accepted pathogen, but this organism could not be recovered from these patients. Third, multiple other antimicrobial agents caused a lethal colitis when given to hamsters, and the etiology of this lesion was also enigmatic.

"In 1975, our investigative group of 12 moved from the UCLA-Sepulveda VA Hospital program in Los Angeles to Tufts-New England Medical Center. Andy Onderdonk and I decided to take on antibiotic-induced colitis in hamsters as a major new project despite skepticism that this mechanism had anything to do with the disease in patients. Under the advice of Sherwood Gorbach, it was decided that stool cultures would be futile, since this traditional approach had failed in extensive studies, presumably reflecting the complexity of normal stool flora. The alternative study plan we used was a number of indirect tests to demonstrate a transferable agent via intracecal injections in hamsters and then to characterize the substances responsible for disease transmission. The work eventually led to the detection of *C. difficile* and its toxin.[3] We collaborated with Te Wen Chang, the virologist at Tufts, who failed to find the virus he anticipated but discovered the tissue-culture assay with clostridial antitoxin neutralization that has subsequently become the standard method used to detect *C. difficile* toxin. These studies were far less simple than they may appear. Experimental groups were labeled sequentially starting with 1HA through 1HZ, then 2HA, and so forth. The original appellation applied to the putative agent in the hamster project was 'Clostridium 17HF 1-9' indicating it was the ninth stool isolate picked from the first hamster in the 422nd experimental group!

"Once this work was completed, it was then rather easy to utilize the techniques developed in hamsters to show that the mechanism applied to patients with antibiotic-associated PMC. The major problem encountered at this juncture was simply finding appropriate patients to study, since the experience with clindamycin in Boston was far different from that reported by Tedesco. After six months, our first stool specimen was finally obtained in March 1977 from a patient with lethal PMC at our prior institution, the Sepulveda VA. Additional specimens were added by Marc Gurwith, who had the foresight to save stools during a study of antibiotic-associated diarrhea in Canada.[4] The *Citation Classic* detailing this work in patients was rejected by the first journal we sent it to, although the editor subsequently wrote me an apology, noting that he had 'overlooked an important observation.' The *New England Journal of Medicine* also caused us considerable anxiety, since one reviewer lost the paper, causing an extraordinary delay in the review process. The fact that we had reported these data at the annual meeting of the American Society for Microbiology five months earlier threatened our pride of place in the publication scheme.

"The paper cited was one of several that identified *C. difficile* as the agent of antibiotic-associated colitis. We think it has been frequently cited because the disease was topical, it was the first to identify *C. difficile* as the responsible agent, and most importantly, it provided convincing evidence based on the Koch-Henle postulates using the hamster model. This initiated the anticipated cascade of events that have subsequently led to efficient methods for both disease detection and effective therapy."[5]

1. **Tedesco F J, Barton R W & Alpers D H.** Clindamycin-associated colitis: a prospective study. *Ann. Intern. Med.* **81**:429-33, 1974.
2. **Tedesco F J.** Citation Classic. Commentary on *Ann. Intern. Med.* **81**:429-33, 1974. *Current Contents/Clinical Practice* **12**(25):16, 18 June 1984.
3. **Bartlett J G, Onderdonk A B, Cisneros R L & Kasper D L.** Clindamycin-associated colitis due to a toxin-producing species of *Clostridium* in hamsters. *J. Infec. Dis.* **136**:701-5, 1977. (Cited 105 times.)
4. **Gurwith M J, Rabin H R & Love K.** Diarrhea associated with clindamycin and ampicillin therapy: preliminary results of a cooperative study. *J. Infec. Dis.* **135**:S104-S110, 1977. (Cited 50 times.)
5. **Bartlett J G, Taylor N S, Chang T W & Dzink J A.** Clinical and laboratory observations in *Clostridium difficile*-induced colitis. *Amer. J. Clin. Nutr.* **33**:2521-6, 1980. (Cited 45 times.)

CC/NUMBER 45
NOVEMBER 7, 1983

This Week's Citation Classic

Dean A G, Ching Y-C, Williams R G & Harden L B. Test for *Escherichia coli* enterotoxin using infant mice: application in a study of diarrhea in children in Honolulu. *J. Infec. Dis.* **125**:407-11, 1972.

[Pacific Res. Sect., Natl. Inst. Allergy and Infectious Dis., Natl. Insts. Health; Dept. Pediat., Kaiser Med. Ctr.; and Dept. Pediat., US Army Tripler Gen. Hosp., Honolulu, HI]

This paper described a new test for *Escherichia coli* enterotoxin, based on intragastric inoculation of infant mice with culture supernates. Fluid accumulation in the gut was used as an index of toxin production. The toxin was found to be heat stable. A study of 37 Honolulu children with diarrheal disease disclosed no heat-stable enterotoxin (ST)-producing *E. coli*, in contrast to reported studies in India.[1] [The *SCI*® indicates that this paper has been cited in over 455 publications since 1972.]

Andrew G. Dean
Division of Disease Prevention and Control
Minnesota Department of Health
Minneapolis, MN 55440

August 4, 1983

"The rabbit loop test for cholera and *E. coli* enterotoxin (heat labile or LT toxin), described by De *et al.* in 1956,[2] was a useful test. But it required anesthesia, laparotomy, tying off intestinal segments, and an overnight wait. At times, only half the rabbits responded properly and the test had to be repeated.

"In 1970, I was using the rabbit test to search for causative agents of diarrhea in specimens from seasonal diarrhea outbreaks in the Philippines. The screening of adequate numbers of specimens for enterotoxigenic *E. coli* with the rabbit test was a severe drain on available resources, and, while continuing the daily rabbit surgery, I began experiments to develop a better method. Baby chicks were cheaper than rabbits, but the gut was too short for more than a few tests, and the surgery no easier. Frogs, adult rats, and mice had the same drawbacks. Mosquito larvae swam happily in the toxin without swelling or shrinking. *In vivo* segments of extirpated mouse intestine failed to react to the toxin.

"Baby mice, on the other hand, responded nicely to culture supernates given by polyethylene esophageal tube, but getting the tube down without ripping the esophagus required delicate handling. The milk-filled stomach, visible through the translucent body wall of neonatal mice, offered a convenient target for direct intragastric inoculation.

"Feeling sure that the ensuing peritonitis would negate the results, I ventured a few mice to find out. Peritonitis aside, the results at four hours were beautiful, and the toxin turned the intestine into a tiny glistening bicycle tire full of fluid. It was obvious that the mouse intestine was responding to something different from cholera toxin, which is heat stable, since brief boiling failed to inactivate culture filtrates, and cholera toxin gave only a very weak response. Refinements were added over the next several months, such as weighing the gut, calculating the gut-to-carcass ratio, adding dye to the inoculum to document success of the injection, and experimenting with timing and various culture media. The result was a much more convenient test than the rabbit intestinal segment method.

"In collaboration with the clinical coauthors of the paper, Ching, Williams, and Harden, the stools of 37 Honolulu children with diarrheal disease were analyzed for ST-producing *E. coli*, with negative results. Subsequent studies have confirmed that ST strains are rare in the US, but relatively common in developing countries.

"In 1971, it seemed likely that someone would develop a simpler, more convenient test, based on biochemical or immunologic techniques, within months. This was not the case, however, and it has taken a decade of effort by many investigators to discover that human ST is a small molecule composed of 18 amino acid residues with important disulfide linkages.[3]

"The test has been used for detection of ST in clinical, epidemiologic, and laboratory research and is therefore cited frequently. By attaching ST to a carrier molecule, specific neutralizing antibody has been prepared, and a radioimmunoassay for ST has now been described.[4] Recently, Klipstein *et al.*[5] have reported synthesizing a molecule which has almost identical biological activity to ST. The production of ST by *E. coli* is under plasmid control,[6] and it seems that all the crucial facts are in place for further remarkable advances in understanding the exact mechanisms of production and action of ST and for development of a vaccine and/or effective method of treatment for ST-related diarrheal disease."

1. **Sack R B, Gorbach S L, Banwell J G, Jacobs B, Chatterjee B D & Mitra R C.** Enterotoxigenic *Escherichia coli* isolated from patients with severe cholera-like disease. *J. Infec. Dis.* **123**:378-85, 1971. (Cited 185 times.)
2. **De S N, Bhattacharya K & Sarkar J K.** A study of the pathogenicity of strains of *Bacterium coli* from acute and chronic enteritis. *J. Pathol. Bacteriol.* **71**:201-9, 1956. (Cited 105 times.)
3. **Staples S J, Asher S E & Giannella R A.** Purification and characterization of heat-stable enterotoxin produced by a strain of *E. coli* pathogenic for man. *J. Biol. Chem.* **255**:4716-21, 1980.
4. **Frantz J C & Robertson D C.** Immunological properties of *Escherichia coli* heat-stable enterotoxins: development of a radioimmunoassay specific for heat-stable enterotoxins with suckling mouse activity. *Infec. Immunity* **33**:193-8, 1981.
5. **Klipstein F A, Engert R F & Houghten R A.** Properties of synthetically produced *Escherichia coli* heat-stable enterotoxin. *Infec. Immunity* **39**:117-21, 1983.
6. **Willshaw G A, Smith H R & Rowe B.** Cloning of regions encoding colonisation factor antigen 1 and heat-stable enterotoxin in *Escherichia coli*. *FEMS Microbiol. Lett.* **16**:101-6, 1983.

CC/NUMBER 52
DECEMBER 28, 1981

This Week's Citation Classic

Barlow B, Santulli T V, Heird W C, Pitt J, Blanc W A & Schullinger J N. An experimental study of acute neonatal enterocolitis—the importance of breast milk. *J. Pediat. Surg.* 9:587-95, 1974. [Depts. Surg., Pediat., and Pathol., Coll. Physicians & Surgeons, Columbia Univ., and Surg. Serv., Babies Hosp., Children's Med. and Surg. Ctr., Columbia-Presbyterian Med. Ctr., New York, NY]

An animal model demonstrated that formula feeding in conjunction with hypoxia produced enterocolitis in newborn rats. Breast-feeding under the same circumstances was completely protective. Enteric overgrowth of potentially pathogenic bacteria in only the formula-fed rats indicated that the gut flora played an important role in the pathogenesis of enterocolitis. [The *SCI*® indicates that this paper has been cited over 125 times since 1974.]

Barbara Barlow
Department of Pediatric Surgery
Harlem Hospital Center
College of Physicians & Surgeons
Columbia University
New York, NY 10037

August 27, 1981

"Necrotizing enterocolitis of the newborn with its high mortality and morbidity has been a topic of great clinical and research interest since the 1960s. In addition, research in enteric immunity and in breast milk components was increasing during this period. As the number of neonatal units multiplied and more sick premature infants were kept alive, the number of infants developing necrotizing enterocolitis also increased. In this milieu, this study of necrotizing enterocolitis and breast milk protection was received with great interest.

"Research training at Vassar College and in the department of experimental psychology at Columbia University Graduate School made me a great friend of the laboratory rat. The career change to medicine and then long surgical training had kept me from research for many years, so when T.V. Santulli and J.N. Schullinger offered me the time, laboratory space, and financial support during my pediatric surgical residency I eagerly embarked on this study of enterocolitis and breast-feeding.

"W.C. Heird developed an artificial formula suitable for the newborn rat and J. Pitt suggested isolation of the cellular component of the rat milk which later proved to be the most protective factor in the model.[1] W.A. Blanc, an expert in the pathology of human enterocolitis, reviewed the pathologic material from the study.

"Although the laboratory rat was an old friend, I found that tame female rats accustomed to human handling were needed in order to obtain rat breast milk without anesthetizing the rat. I raised female rats at home and then returned them to the laboratory to be impregnated for milk production. The New York telephone company believed that I had a dog who chewed telephone wires because I was too embarrassed to tell them that I was raising female rats in my apartment who liked to run free and enjoyed eating telephone wires.

"Translating findings from animal models to human disease is always difficult. In fact, at our hospital, feeding breast milk to premature infants was considered an experimental feeding practice which needed the approval of the human experimentation committee. Breast milk banks have disappeared from hospitals in this country and expensive reorganization is required to change newborn feeding practices. Breast milk trials in this country have been hampered by bacterial contamination of the milk during collection or storage. The protection offered by any biologic system can be overwhelmed, in this case by heavy bacterial contamination of the milk or the infant. Many European neonatal centers use only breast milk feeding or predominately breast milk feeding for their premature units and rarely see necrotizing enterocolitis. If breast milk banks were reestablished in this country for feeding of neonates I am convinced that necrotizing enterocolitis would rarely occur and then only in the most severely stressed infants or in infants inappropriately fed enterally when significant bowel injury had already occurred.

"An excellent collective review was published by A. Kosloske in *Surgery, Gynecology and Obstetrics*."[2]

1. **Pitt J, Barlow B & Heird W C.** Protection against experimental enterocolitis by maternal milk. Role of milk leukocytes. *Pediat. Res.* **11**:906-9, 1977.
2. **Kosloske A.** Necrotizing enterocolitis in the neonate. *Surg. Gynecol. Obstet.* **148**:259-69, 1979.

CC/NUMBER 49
DECEMBER 7, 1981

This Week's Citation Classic

Kleeman C R, Hewitt W L & Guze L B. Pyelonephritis. *Medicine* **39**:3-116, 1960. [Wadsworth Hosp., Veterans Admin. Ctr., and Dept. Medicine, Univ. California Medical Sch., Los Angeles, CA]

Pyelonephritis may be defined as the pathologic alterations which occur subsequent to the multiplication of pathogenic bacteria in the renal parenchyma and pelvocalyceal system. Quantitative investigations of the normal and pathogenic bacteriology of the genito-urinary tract have brought to the attention of the medical world the prevalence and insidious character of significant infection of the urinary tract. [The *SCI*® indicates that this paper has been cited over 255 times since 1961.]

Lucien B. Guze
Research Service
Veterans Administration
Wadsworth Hospital Center
Los Angeles, CA 90073

October 27, 1981

"We are very pleased to know that our article written in 1960 has been cited frequently. We wrote this article with the intention of reviewing most of the pertinent literature published up to that time. Interest and research activity in the field of urinary tract infections were becoming markedly accelerated due to the establishment of the validity of quantitative urinary culture as an epidemiological tool. In 1939, Soma Weiss and Frederic Parker, Jr., of the Harvard Medical School, had published their classic contribution, 'Pyelonephritis: its relationship to vascular lesions and to arterial hypertension.'[1] That review presented now widely used histologic criteria for the diagnosis of pyelonephritis, as well as pointed out the clinical variability of this disease and its possible association with hypertension. With the advent of diagnostic quantitative urinary cultures, it was possible to study large segments of the population to determine the occurrence and natural history of this disease. All of us had been interested in urinary tract infections and had conducted research in this area. Kleeman, who is a clinician primarily interested in renal physiology, had studied many of the functional aberrations associated with renal infection. Hewitt was interested in treatment experiences as well as selected clinical aspects of the disease. My laboratory had been conducting experiments dealing with the pathogenesis of pyelonephritis, with particular emphasis on the host-parasite relationship. It was, therefore, natural for the three of us to review this disease, including the literature as well as our own personal clinical and laboratory experiences.

"The resulting publication made available to other investigators and interested scientists a fairly complete update of the information that they might need to build on past observations, thus accounting for its frequent citation. We are pleased that our intentions have been realized and that the manuscript served as a valuable resource upon which other useful studies were conducted."[2-4]

1. **Weiss S & Parker F, Jr.** Pyelonephritis: its relationship to vascular lesions and to arterial hypertension. *Medicine* **18**:221-315, 1939.
2. **Bhathena D B, Weiss J H, Holland N H, McMorrow R G, Curtis J J, Lucas B A & Luke R G.** Focal and segmental glomerular sclerosis in reflux nephropathy. *Amer. J. Med.* **68**:886-92, 1980.
3. **Olsson P J, Black J R, Gaffney E, Alexander R W, Mars D R & Fuller T J.** Reversible acute renal failure secondary to acute pyelonephritis. *Southern Med. J.* **73**:374-6, 1980.
4. **Vivaldi E, Gonzalez E, Conejeros M, Bergeret I & Zemelamn R.** Bacteriuria, urinary infection and pyelonephritis. 4. *Rev. Med. Chile* **107**:1128-34, 1979.

This Week's Citation Classic

CC/NUMBER 48
NOVEMBER 26, 1979

Stamey T A, Govan D E & Palmer J M. The localization and treatment of urinary tract infections: the role of bactericidal urine levels as opposed to serum levels. *Medicine* **44**:1-36, 1965.
[Div. Urology, Stanford Univ. Sch. Med., Palo Alto, CA]

Techniques are presented for accurately localizing the specific site of urinary tract infections, especially the separation of bladder from renal infection and the identification of the urethra or prostate as the tissue site of bacterial persistence in the male. Additional data demonstrate that the cure of kidney infections is dependent upon the urinary concentrations of antimicrobial agents and not the serum levels. [The *SCI*® indicates that this paper has been cited over 300 times since 1965.]

Thomas A. Stamey
Department of Surgery
Division of Urology, S287
Stanford University School of Medicine
Stanford, CA 94305

August 9, 1979

"These data were collected between the years 1961 and 1964, less than 10 years after the diagnosis of bacteriuria was statistically established on a firm basis by counting the number of bacteria in voided urine.[1] At that time, there was a general feeling that most patients with bacteriuria had pyelonephritis, but there were no techniques available to distinguish renal from bladder infection. By using the cystoscope and ureteral catheter, and by measuring the magnitude of renal contamination from bladder bacteria, we developed a technique which showed that only 50% of bacteriuric patients had renal bacteriuria and that these were equally distributed between unilateral and bilateral involvement. Several studies from different parts of the world have confirmed these results in diverse population groups.[2]

"Other localization techniques were presented in this paper, including suprapubic needle aspiration of the bladder to avoid perineal bacteria. Prostatic fluid cultures were shown to be meaningless unless bacterial contamination by urethral organisms was measured and accounted for. These latter studies placed the diagnosis of bacterial prostatitis on an objective microbiologic basis for the first time, even though we were incorrect in believing that urethral persistence of Enterobacteriaceae was more common than prostatic persistence as the cause of recurrent bacteriuria.

"I think most of the above observations were easily accepted by the medical community, but the other half of this paper—that the cure of urinary infections was determined by urinary levels rather than serum concentrations of antimicrobial agents—met with substantial and often emotional resistance, especially by infectious disease physicians. The evidence, however, was clear. We localized urinary infections to the kidneys and then treated these patients with antimicrobial agents that were bactericidal at urinary concentrations (penicillin-G, nitrofurantoin, and tetracycline hydrochloride), but non-inhibitory at concentrations achieved in the serum: the patients, of course, were cured of their infection. I am glad to note that this thesis is widely accepted in 1979, although an occasional microbiologist who never treats infections still espouses the traditional dictum that serum levels are the determinant factor.

"It is humbling to read in the discussion section of this paper, 'It is unlikely that the problem of reinfection in the female is an immunological one...' and to realize that exactly 13 years later to the very month (January) and in the *same* journal, we have just published our most recent work entitled, 'The immunologic basis of recurrent bacteriuria: role of cervicovaginal antibody in enterobacterial colonization of the introital mucosa.'"[3]

1. **Kass E H.** Asymptomatic infections of the urinary tract. *Trans. Assoc. Amer. Phys.* **69**:56-64, 1956.
2. **Stamey T A, Fair W R, Timothy M M, Millar M A, Mihara G & Lowery Y C.** Serum versus urinary antimicrobial concentrations in cure of urinary-tract infections. *New Eng. J. Med.* **291**:1159-63, 1974.
3. **Stamey T A, Wehner N, Mihara G & Condy M.** The immunologic basis of recurrent bacteriuria: role of cervicovaginal antibody in enterobacterial colonization of the introital mucosa. *Medicine* **57**:47-56, 1978.

This Week's Citation Classic

CC/NUMBER 36
SEPTEMBER 7, 1981

Bodey G P, Buckley M, Sathe Y S & Freireich E J. Quantitative relationships between circulating leukocytes and infection in patients with acute leukemia. *Ann. Intern. Med.* **64**:328-40, 1966.
[Med. Branch, Leukemia Serv., and Math. and Statist. and Appl. Math. Sect., Natl. Cancer Inst., NIH, Bethesda, MD]

The frequency of infectious complications correlates inversely with the absolute number of neutrophils and lymphocytes circulating in the blood of leukemic patients. Both the degree and duration of neutropenia determine the risk of infection. Furthermore, recovery from infection in neutropenic patients depends upon whether or not the neutrophil count returns toward normal. [The *SCI*® indicates that this paper has been cited over 365 times since 1966.]

Gerald P. Bodey
M.D. Anderson Hospital and
Tumor Institute
Texas Medical Center
University of Texas System Cancer Center
Houston, TX 77030

July 17, 1981

"The mid-1960s was an exciting period for those of us working on the Leukemia Service of the National Cancer Institute under the leadership of Emil J. Freireich. This is the second *Citation Classic* that was written during those years.[1] With the advent of effective treatment for childhood leukemia, attention was focused on complications which interfered with this therapy. Infection and hemorrhage were the most common causes of morbidity and mortality and the routine administration of platelet transfusions had reduced substantially the fatality rate from hemorrhage.

"Few physicians at that time were interested in the infectious problems of cancer patients, since a negative attitude prevailed regarding the treatment of patients with extensive malignant disease. The fact that neutropenic patients were especially susceptible to infection was universally recognized, but many infectious disease experts were of the opinion that therapy was ineffective in these patients.

"A previous study relating platelet count to hemorrhagic complications served as the model for this study of 54 consecutive leukemic patients.[2] All blood counts determined in these patients from diagnosis until death (in some patients this represented more than one year) were included. Since absolute neutrophil and lymphocyte counts were not available, they had to be calculated from the total white blood count and differential percentages. Calculators were not nearly as sophisticated in those days and we had to share ours with other investigators! Most of the work was tedious and repetitious and became interesting only when all of the data had been tabulated. Because of the many numbers involved, calculations had to be checked and rechecked, a frustrating venture when errors were discovered. Finally, everything was in order and we consulted Y. Sathe and Marvin Zelen for a statistical analysis. We were somewhat surprised when they told us that statistical analyses were unnecessary because of the large number of observations and the magnitude of the differences—hence, no sacred p values!

"The information derived from this study has served as a reference for many subsequent investigations. The risk of infection was shown to increase only when the neutrophil count fell below 1,000/mm^3. Hence, oncologists designing chemotherapeutic studies with myelosuppressive drugs select doses of such drugs that will not cause the neutrophil count to fall below this level for extended periods of time.

"During the last 15 years, we have studied new antibiotics and antibiotic regimens for the treatment of infection in cancer patients. The knowledge gained from this initial study led us to evaluate therapeutic efficacy related to the patients' initial neutrophil count and to changes in their neutrophil count during infection. We showed that aminoglycoside antibiotics were less effective in neutropenic patients and that response depended upon whether the neutrophil count increased or decreased during the infection.[3] Subsequently, we found that this relationship between response and neutrophil count did not apply to all antibiotics—the antipseudomonal penicillins were effective even in persistently neutropenic patients.[4] These observations have been confirmed by other investigators and cooperative groups."

1. **Hersh E M, Bodey G P, Nies B A & Freireich E J.** Causes of death in acute leukemia: a ten-year study of 414 patients from 1954-1963. *J. Amer. Med. Assn.* **193**:105-9, 1965. [Citation Classic. *Current Contents/Clinical Practice* **8**(1):10, 7 January 1980.]
2. **Gaydos L A, Freireich E J & Mantel N.** The quantitative relation between platelet count and hemorrhage in patients with acute leukemia. *N. Engl. J. Med.* **266**:905-9, 1962.
3. **Bodey G P, Middleman E, Umsawasdi T & Rodriguez V.** Infections in cancer patients—results with gentamicin sulfate therapy. *Cancer* **29**:1697-701, 1972.
4. **Bodey G P, Whitecar J P, Jr., Middleman E & Rodriguez V.** Carbenicillin therapy of *Pseudomonas* infections. *J. Amer. Med. Assn.* **218**:62-6, 1971.

This Week's Citation Classic

Park B H, Fikrig S M & Smithwick E M. Infection and nitroblue-tetrazolium reduction by neutrophils: a diagnostic aid. *Lancet* **2**:532-4, 1968. [Dept. Pediatrics, State Univ. New York, NY]

This paper described a supravital staining of phagocytes in fresh unstimulated whole blood using nitroblue tetrazolium (NBT) dye, and classified neutrophils as 'NBT positive' and 'NBT negative.' The proportion and absolute number of the former was increased in patients with certain types of bacterial infections. [The *SCI®* indicates that this paper has been cited over 500 times since 1968.]

Byung Hak Park
Department of Pediatrics
State University of New York
and
Children's Hospital
Buffalo, NY 14222

October 10, 1981

"In April 1967, at the annual meeting of the American Pediatric Society, I heard Baehner and Nathan's report[1] that neutrophils from chronic granulomatous disease failed to reduce NBT dye, which was attributed to the defective oxidative metabolism and phagocytic defect. I thought that one might extend this finding to other conditions associated with phagocytic dysfunction, such as patients receiving steroid therapy.

"With initial help from Fikrig and Smithwick, I could demonstrate the reduction of NBT dye in normal neutrophils. In July 1967, Fikrig sent me with 'the slide' to Nathan in Boston, who kindly identified the 'NBT-positive' cell. Since I was an acting chief resident, as well as an immunology fellow, most of the experiment was done in the evening hours and on weekends. For the next five months my results were entirely negative.

"My project came to a turning point when I was on call on Christmas Eve 1967. While I was browsing through the journals in the library, I came across a report by Gluck,[2] who used whole blood for testing phagocytic function in newborns. It was already 2 am, and I promptly went to the laboratory, which was on the seventh floor of King's County Hospital, one floor up from the library. After many 'feeble' attempts to lance my finger, and with some sweat on my forehead, I finally collected a few drops of blood into a plastic tube. Using 'unstimulated' whole blood this time, I found only one NBT-positive cell in the entire slide, which was in contrast to the usual number of about 20 percent. It was 4 am. Feeling tired, I went back to my room in the dormitory.

"Why were there so few NBT-positive cells? Suddenly it occurred to me: 'It might be due to the way the WBC was handled *in vitro,* i.e., minimal stimulation. The one NBT-positive cell might represent a small proportion of neutrophils in activated conditions in the blood of a healthy person. Therefore, one might find an increased number of these cells during natural infection.' At that moment I was seized by a kind of strange feeling, a sort of excitement, hard to describe for lack of proper words.

"For the next two months I improved and standardized the method. I tried to avoid stimulation of WBCs *in vitro* while making the method so simple that it could be performed with minimum equipment in developing countries.

"The reasons for the paper's receiving so many citations are probably due to: 1) a new idea and simplicity of methodology, 2) description of methodology which left many 'critical' aspects undefined, 3) its potential clinical use, and 4) discordant results and heated controversy due to different methodology and sometimes erroneous interpretations based on insufficient data.

"I believe that my hypothesis of activated neutrophils during natural infection is largely correct, with a few exceptions.[3,4] Since the publication of this paper, I have learned a great deal about the art of scientific investigation while the original idea has grown and matured. In this personal sense, this paper may be affectionately called 'a classic.' "

1. **Baehner R L & Nathan D G.** Chronic granulomatous disease: an X-linked deficiency of leukocyte NADH oxidase. *Pediat. Res.* **1**:306-7, 1967.
2. **Gluck L & Silverman W A.** Phagocytosis in premature infants. *Pediatrics* **20**:951-7, 1957.
3. **Park B H.** The use and limitations of NBT-test as a diagnostic aid. *J. Pediatrics* **78**:376-8, 1971.
4. **Kite P.** *The evaluation and some applications of the nitroblue tetrazolium test.* PhD thesis. Leeds, England: University of Leeds, 1980.

This Week's Citation Classic

Lerner P I & Weinstein L. Infective endocarditis in the antibiotic era.
N. Engl. J. Med. **274**:199-206; 259-66; 323-31; 388-93, 1966.
[Infectious Disease Serv., New England Med. Ctr. Hosps., and Dept. Med.,
Tufts Univ. Sch. Med., Boston, MA]

A review of eight years' experience with endocarditis at a large referral center formed the basis for a comprehensive analysis of this multifaceted infection, at a critical point in the natural evolution of the disease, and on the threshold of a revolution in the surgical management of the disorder. [The *SCI*® indicates that these papers have been cited over 1,025 times in 448 papers since 1966.]

Phillip I. Lerner
Department of Infectious Diseases
Mt. Sinai Medical Center
Department of Medicine
Case Western Reserve University
School of Medicine
Cleveland, OH 44106
and
Louis Weinstein
Department of Medicine
Infectious Disease Division
Brigham and Women's Hospital
Harvard Medical School
Boston, MA 02115

October 15, 1981

"Resurrecting the term 'infective endocarditis,' as distinct from 'bacterial endocarditis,' was most timely, since the natural history of this once uniformly fatal cardiac infection appeared to be undergoing a remarkable evolution for various reasons, some recognized, some unknown. The manuscript was a joint effort by my mentor, Louis Weinstein, and me. Our review of 100 patients at the New England Medical Center in Boston formed the basis for a comprehensive analysis of endocardial infection, as there had been no in-depth examination of this topic since Kerr's monograph in 1955.[1] The opportunity to present this material in an almost open-ended forum (the Medical Progress section of four consecutive issues of the *New England Journal of Medicine*) demanded that this analysis be as comprehensive as possible. The protean manifestations of endocarditis remain a fascination to practitioners, generalists and specialists alike, for this is truly an entity that encompasses the breadth of medicine. Rheumatologists, neurologists, cardiologists, immunologists, nephrologists, infectious disease specialists, and now cardiac surgeons all find endocarditis one of medicine's most fascinating and challenging diseases. This article has been so widely cited because of the prestige of the journal, the topic's widespread appeal to many physicians and particularly specialists, and, I would like to think, for the quality of the analysis.

"Both Weinstein[2,3] and I[4] have continued to reexamine this topic over the years, as we have witnessed some areas of remarkable progress. While we devoted but two brief paragraphs to the surgical aspects of this disease, stating that 'surgical repair of the ravages of healed endocarditis is also being undertaken cautiously,' today a comprehensive review of the aggressive surgical management of endocarditis could easily be as long as our entire paper! The development of a practical experimental animal model represents another major advance toward the understanding and management of this disease since our review was published. The non-invasive technique of cardiac echography also promises to promote a minor revolution in our approach to diagnosis and therapy.

"Disappointingly, however, we still don't know the correct dose, duration, or combination of antibiotics necessary to treat most cases, and, indeed, we probably overtreat the majority of our patients because we lack this knowledge. Even more discouragingly, early diagnosis remains an elusive goal, thereby delaying the initiation of appropriate therapy, which unfortunately still determines the ultimate outcome in most patients with infective endocarditis."

1. **Kerr A, Jr.** *Subacute bacterial endocarditis.* Springfield, IL: Thomas, 1955. 343 p.
2. **Weinstein L & Rubin R H.** Infective endocarditis—1973. *Progr. Cardiovasc. Dis.* **16**:239-74, 1973.
[Citation Classic. *Current Contents/Clinical Practice* **10**(12): 20, 22 March 1982.]
3. **Weinstein L & Schlesinger J.** Treatment of infective endocarditis—1973. *Progr. Cardiovasc. Dis.* **16**:275-302, 1973.
4. **Lerner P I.** Infective endocarditis: a review of selected topics. *Med. Clin. N. Amer.* **58**:605-22, 1974.

This Week's Citation Classic

Weinstein L & Rubin R H. Infective endocarditis—1973.
Progr. Cardiovasc. Dis. **16**:239-74, 1973.
[Infectious Disease Serv., New England Medical Ctr. Hosps., and Dept. Med., Tufts Univ. Sch. Med., Boston, MA]

The definition of the basic microbiological, pathoanatomical, pathophysiological, and immunological factors involved in the pathogenesis and clinical behavior of infective endocarditis has led to a better understanding of the disease and restoration of great interest in it. [The *SCI*® indicates that this paper has been cited over 165 times since 1973.]

Louis Weinstein
Department of Medicine
Infectious Disease Division
Brigham and Women's Hospital
Harvard Medical School
Boston, MA 02115

November 16, 1981

"Infective endocarditis has occupied my attention over almost 40 years during which it has become clear that all the mechanisms involved in the pathogenesis of the disease as well as those operating after infection develops have been defined. It is now possible to understand this disease and to predict with considerable accuracy both its uncomplicated and complicated course as well as to anticipate the need for special therapeutic maneuvers.

"My interest in infective endocarditis was first aroused as an intern in medicine at University Hospital in Boston in 1942-1943. I had the opportunity then to study a large number of patients and to participate in the first trial of treatment with penicillin under the aegis of Chester S. Keefer, the physician-in-chief at the hospital, who controlled the use of penicillin in the US during a study conducted by the National Academy of Sciences. A large number of patients with this infection from all over the country were admitted to the hospital. Treatment consisted of 5,000 units of penicillin given intravenously every three hours for ten days. This dose of the antibiotic proved far too small and was used only because the supply of the drug was very limited. None of the patients survived.

"The opportunity to study a large number of cases that came to autopsy was a very important experience because of the opportunity to correlate the clinical behavior of the disease with important anatomical changes. I have now studied over 900 cases of this disease, concentrating on correlating its microbiological, immunological, pathoanatomical, and pathophysiological abnormalities with its clinical behavior.

"One of the most important experiences to come out of this study has been the observation that remarkable changes have taken place, without any identifiable causes, in the clinical features of subacute infective endocarditis. The classical and sometimes diagnostic findings are all seen much less frequently now than they were years ago. Most remarkable has been a striking change in the age distribution of the disease, so that the bulk of patients are now in their 50s and 60s. It has become clear that if the diagnostic criteria, short of 'positive' blood cultures, employed years ago were used today, the diagnosis would be overlooked in better than 80-90 percent of cases.

"I believe this paper is a *Citation Classic* for two reasons. It was the first publication that stressed the importance of the multiple factors involved in the pathogenesis and clinical manifestations of the disease. Because of its increasing incidence, especially of complicated cases, an understanding of the mechanisms involved, as detailed in this paper, has stimulated growing interest in infective endocarditis and has led to publication of a large number of papers by me[1-6] and many other investigators.

"Honors received for my studies in infective endocarditis include a medal from the American College of Chest Physicians, and the Bristol and the Finland Awards from the Infectious Diseases Society of America."

1. **Lerner P & Weinstein L.** Infective endocarditis in the antibiotic era. *N. Engl. J. Med.* **274**:199-206; 259-66; 323-31; 388-93, 1966.
2. **Weinstein L & Schlesinger J.** Treatment of infective endocarditis—1973. *Progr. Cardiovasc. Dis.* **16**:275-302, 1973.
3. ----------------------------------. Pathoanatomic, pathophysiologic and clinical correlations in endocarditis. I and II. *N. Engl. J. Med.* **291**:832-7; 1122-6, 1974.
4. **Weinstein L.** "Modern" infective endocarditis. *J. Amer. Med. Assn.* **233**:260-3, 1975.
5. **Cohen P S, Maguire J H & Weinstein L.** Infective endocarditis caused by gram-negative bacteria. *Progr. Cardiovasc. Dis.* **22**:205-42, 1980.
6. **Weinstein L.** Infective endocarditis. (Braunwald E, ed.) *Heart disease. A textbook of cardiovascular medicine.* Philadelphia: Saunders, 1980. p. 1166-220.

Ridley D S & Jopling W H. Classification of leprosy according to immunity: a five-group system. *Int. J. Leprosy* **34**:255-73, 1966. [Hospital for Tropical Diseases, London, and Jordan Hospital, Redhill, Surrey, England]

It is proposed that the classification of leprosy should be revised by relating the clinical and histological features used for classification to the resistance of the patient, which is what determines the course of the disease. A five-group spectrum is defined accordingly. [The *SCI*® indicates that this paper has been cited over 275 times since 1966.]

Dennis S. Ridley
Pathology Laboratory
Hospital for Tropical Diseases
London NW1 0PE
England

June 19, 1981

"The origin of this work lay in the assumption (which proved false) that the response of leprosy patients to chemotherapy could be determined by observing the rate of disappearance of bacilli from the lesions, and in the view (probably valid) that this rate could best be determined from skin biopsies. Accordingly, in the middle-1950s, W.H. Jopling started to send me regular serial biopsies of his drug trial patients at the Jordan Hospital in Surrey. The trials were planned by Sir Neil Fairley, a methodical investigator who did not lightly give up. Leprosy being a chronic disease, it was some years before we were satisfied that the outcome was determined not by the drug (except that the infection had to be under control) but by the type of leprosy. The first International Leprosy Congress we attended was at Tokyo in 1958, and I was much impressed by the way the vexed confusion over classification brought so many discussions to an impasse. From this arose the idea that the rate of elimination of dead bacilli from skin lesions, which was evidently an immune response, would provide an objective basis for a prognostic and clinically useful system of classification. An over hasty paper was rejected: 'Everyone is tired of classification; give it a rest.'

"I then set about correlating every possible histological feature of the initial biopsies with subsequent bacteriological response. Jopling, working on the clinical side, used other immunological parameters such as the lepromin test. And in the final analysis we concerted our conclusions to define five groups in the spectrum from tuberculoid, through borderline, to lepromatous, which we designated TT, BT, BB, BL, and LL. To make the new scheme acceptable, we arranged the groups as far as possible in conformity with previous ideas about the spectrum, and the outcome was by no means revolutionary. After the results had been confirmed at the Medical Research Council Unit in Malaysia with the assistance in particular of J.A. McFadzean and M.F.R. Waters, they were published in a preliminary report[1] in 1962 and later amplified in the paper cited. At this time it was still not known that immunity in leprosy was cell mediated, but later it became possible to corroborate the spectrum by reference to the lymphocyte transformation test, and an expanded and slightly modified histological classification was produced.[2,3]

"This work has been widely quoted partly because classification in leprosy is clinically important; partly because the spectrum of leprosy serves as the model for other infectious diseases and so it is useful to immunologists and pathologists. Above all, this classification is comprehensive and comprehensible. There is another reason why it has to be cited as 'Ridley-Jopling': it has never been officially adopted and so has to be distinguished from the official classification of leprosy, which is still that of the Madrid Congress of 1953."

1. **Ridley D S & Jopling W H.** A classification of leprosy for research purposes. *Leprosy Rev.* **33**:119-28, 1962.
2. **Ridley D S.** Histological classification and the immunological spectrum of leprosy. *Bull. WHO* **51**:451-65, 1974.
3. ---------------. *Skin biopsy in leprosy.* Basel, Switzerland: Documenta Geigy, 1977. 57 p.

This Week's Citation Classic™

CC/NUMBER 33
AUGUST 13, 1984

Maki D G, Goldmann D A & Rhame F S. Infection control in intravenous therapy. *Ann. Intern. Med.* **79**:867-87, 1973.

[Hosp. Infections Sect., Bacterial Dis. Br., Epidemiol. Program, Ctr. for Dis. Control, Health Serv. and Mental Health Admin., HEW, Atlanta, GA, and Harvard Med. Serv., Boston City Hosp., MA]

The intravenous infusion has become indispensable in modern medical therapy, but infection, especially infusion-related septicemia, remains a life-threatening hazard. This review pointed up the magnitude, clinical and microbiological profile, and epidemiology of infections complicating intravenous therapy and provided specific recommendations for prevention of these infections. [The *SCI*® indicates that this paper has been cited in over 200 publications since 1973.]

Dennis G. Maki
Section of Infectious Diseases
Department of Medicine
University of Wisconsin Medical School
Madison, WI 53792

June 20, 1984

"Although intravenous therapy had been in wide use in hospitals throughout the world for over 35 years, it was not until the late 1960s that it began to be recognized that intravenous cannulas were a major cause of serious iatrogenic infection, usually with *Staphylococcus aureus*. I became interested in the problem of nosocomial (hospital-acquired) infection and, particularly, bacteremias deriving from intravascular devices during a two-year appointment as an Epidemic Intelligence Service Officer with the US Center for Disease Control (CDC) in Atlanta, Georgia, between 1969 and 1971.

"For nearly six months in 1970-1971, we worked 100 hours per week in wide-ranging investigations of an extraordinary nationwide epidemic caused by the contaminated intravenous products of one US manufacturer.[1-3] This outbreak awakened medicine to the considerable potential of intravenous therapy to produce life-threatening iatrogenic disease. Our investigations demonstrated conclusively that intravenous fluid could become contaminated, during its manufacture or during administration in the hospital, by gram-negative bacilli, particularly *Enterobacter* species, and produce devastating bacteremic illness. The source of the epidemic was ultimately traced to the company's manufacturing plants where, paradoxically, microorganisms in the plant environment were being introduced into intravenous products after the autoclaving stage of production.[4]

"By July, I was back in Boston resuming my postgraduate training in internal medicine and infectious diseases at Harvard Medical School. Most of my free time away from my residency training at the Massachusetts General Hospital that year was spent completing manuscripts dealing with research done at CDC during the preceding two years.

"By 1972, ever-increasing numbers of patients in US hospitals were receiving infusion therapy in some form, no longer simply for administration of fluid and electrolytes and blood products, but increasingly for delivery of parenteral drugs, hemodynamic monitoring, or hyperalimentation (total parenteral nutrition)—which had recently been introduced into clinical practice. Moreover, knowledge of the nature and magnitude of nosocomial infections complicating intravenous therapy and, especially, measures to reduce the risk of these infections was rapidly advancing. It was apparent to me and two of my former CDC coworkers, Frank Rhame and Don Goldmann, yet at CDC in the second year of their appointments as Epidemic Intelligence Service Officers, that a well-written review could greatly enhance awareness of the risk of infusion-related infections and help improve hospital infection control practices aimed at prevention.

"Thus, during a serendipitously quiet weekend in the spring of 1972 while on-call as the hospital senior medical resident, between occasional calls to assist interns or provide consultation on surgical patients, working around the clock, I wrote the first draft of the needed review, including incorporation of the nearly 300 citations. I sent the manuscript to my two CDC colleagues who further added to and revised the paper, after which we submitted it to the *Annals of Internal Medicine*. Edward Huth, editor of the *Annals*, called me several weeks later to say that his editorial board liked the paper and wanted to publish it, but would like us to also submit an accompanying short article summarizing our recommendations for prevention of infection in intravenous therapy, which we did.[5]

"We have been gratified by the reception the paper has received through the years. We believe it achieved our goals and has been frequently cited in great measure because of its timing: the 1970-1971 nationwide outbreak was yet painfully fresh in the minds of American infection control personnel, and there was a clear-cut need for a comprehensive review of this newly recognized iatrogenic health care problem. All of us have remained in academic medicine and are actively involved in research on the epidemiology of nosocomial infection. I have continued to pursue the increasingly complex problem of infection related to intravascular devices and have published several updated reviews."[6,7]

1. **Center for Disease Control.** Nosocomial bacteremias associated with intravenous fluid therapy—USA. *Morbid. Mortal. Weekly Rep.* **20**(Suppl. 9), 1971. 2 p.
2. **Maki D G, Rhame F S, Mackel D C & Bennett J V.** Nationwide epidemic of septicemia caused by contaminated intravenous products. I. Epidemiological and clinical features. *Amer. J. Med.* **60**:471-85, 1976.
3. **Goldmann D A, Fulkerson C C, Dixon R E, Maki D G & Bennett J V.** Nationwide epidemic of septicemia caused by contaminated intravenous products. II. Assessment of the problem by a national nosocomial infection surveillance system. *Amer. J. Epidemiol.* **108**:207-13, 1978.
4. **Mackel D C, Maki D G, Anderson R L & Bennett J V.** Nationwide epidemic of septicemia caused by contaminated intravenous products. III. Mechanisms of contamination during manufacture. *J. Clin. Microbiol.* **2**:486-96, 1975.
5. **Goldmann D A, Maki D G, Rhame F S, Kaiser A B, Tenney J H & Bennett J V.** Guidelines for infection control in intravenous therapy. *Ann. Intern. Med.* **79**:848-50, 1973. (Cited 55 times.)
6. **Maki D G.** Nosocomial bacteremia. An epidemiologic overview. *Amer. J. Med.* **70**:719-32, 1981.
7. **Maki D G.** Infections associated with intravascular lines. (Swartz M & Remington J, eds.) *Current topics in clinical infectious disease.* New York: McGraw-Hill, 1982. p. 309-63.

CC/NUMBER 30
JULY 25, 1983

This Week's Citation Classic

Young R C, Bennett J E, Vogel C L, Carbone P P & DeVita V T. Aspergillosis: the spectrum of the disease in 98 patients. *Medicine* **49**:147-73, 1970.
[Solid Tumor Serv., Med. Branch, Natl. Cancer Inst., and Infectious Disease Sect., Lab. Clin. Investigation, Natl. Inst. Allergy and Infectious Diseases, Natl. Insts. Health, Bethesda, MD]

The clinicopathologic spectrum of aspergillosis in 98 patients from a single institution served to characterize the disease seen in the immunosuppressed host. In such patients, invasive manifestations predominated over the allergic and colonizing forms of the disease seen in other patients. [The *SCI*® indicates that this paper has been cited in over 290 publications since 1970.]

Robert C. Young
Medicine Branch
National Cancer Institute
National Institutes of Health
Bethesda, MD 20205

June 1, 1983

"As a fledgling member of the attending staff of the National Cancer Institute's Medicine Branch, I arrived at a time when the program was alive with enthusiasm about the role of intensive combination chemotherapy in the treatment of disseminated malignancies. The initial successes with such treatment for Hodgkin's disease had already produced a report destined to become another *Citation Classic*.[1] However, it was also apparent that unusual infectious complications, different from those to which we had all been accustomed on general medical services, were being seen with increasing frequency. While the predominant infections were bacterial, fully 20-25 percent of the fatal complications seen in our patients were fungal. Although complications involving *Candida* organisms were most common, we saw at least one fatal case of aspergillosis a month during my first year on the senior staff.

"My chief, Vincent T. DeVita, Jr., pointed out that we were in the unusual position of seeing more of these unique infections than most specialists in infectious disease. Out of these discussions and a growing feeling that the manifestations of the disease were different in the immunocompromised host, we undertook the comprehensive review. I was also fortunate to have the expertise of John E. Bennett, whose in-depth knowledge of the common manifestations of *Aspergillus* infections in other patient populations convinced us that the disease described in the literature was not the disease we were seeing. Invasive disease had replaced fungus balls and allergic bronchopulmonary aspergillosis. I remember with great delight the excitement of being alone in the record room of the National Institutes of Health late at night extracting the data from the clinical and pathology records of patients known and unknown to me which together served to characterize aspergillosis in the immunosuppressed host.

"This paper has been highly cited for the following reasons. Not only was the study the first to describe in detail the clinicopathologic spectrum of this disease in a large number of patients, but it emphasized the importance of the underlying disease, its treatment, and the difficulty of diagnosis. Few of these basic observations have changed in the past 13 years since the paper was published but the importance of infectious complications in immunosuppressed hosts has become increasingly important in immunodeficiency syndromes and with widespread use of immunosuppressive chemotherapy, not only for malignant disorders but for other serious nonmalignant systemic diseases as well as organ transplantation. Aspergillosis continues to be a frequent complication of such illnesses and available treatments have not developed sufficiently to have altered either the frequency or the manifestations of the disease greatly since our publication. The continued importance of this area of infectious disease has been comprehensively discussed recently."[2]

1. **DeVita V T, Jr., Serpick A A & Carbone P P.** Combination chemotherapy in the treatment of advanced Hodgkin's disease. *Ann. Intern. Med.* 73:881-95, 1970.
[Citation Classic. *Current Contents/Clinical Practice* 7(12):10, 19 March 1979.]
2. **Pizzo P A & Young R C.** Management of infections of the cancer patient. (DeVita V T, Hellman S & Rosenberg S A, eds.) *Cancer: principles and practice of oncology*. Philadelphia: Lippincott, 1982. p. 1677-703.

This Week's Citation Classic

CC/NUMBER 34
AUGUST 24, 1981

London W T, DiFiglia M, Sutnick A I & Blumberg B S. An epidemic of hepatitis in a chronic-hemodialysis unit: Australia antigen and differences in host response. *N. Engl. J. Med.* 281:571-8, 1969.
[Inst. for Cancer Res., Fox Chase, and Dept. Nephrology, Jefferson Med. Coll. Hosp., Philadelphia, PA]

This paper made two new points: 1) Australia antigen, a marker of hepatitis B virus, was prevalent in patients treated in a chronic hemodialysis unit; 2) the infected patients had a mild, persistent, anicteric hepatitis whereas staff members exposed to the same virus contracted an acute, icteric, transient illness. This demonstrated the essential role of the host immune response in the clinical manifestations of the hepatitis. [The *SCI*® indicates that this paper has been cited over 230 times since 1969.]

W. Thomas London
Institute for Cancer Research
Fox Chase Cancer Center
7701 Burholme Avenue
Philadelphia, PA 19111

July 10, 1981

"In 1968, Blumberg, Sutnick, and I were in need of human antibodies to what was then called Australia antigen. This antigen, now called hepatitis B surface antigen (abbreviated HBsAg), is the outer coat of the hepatitis B virus. Our best sources of antibody had been patients who had received many blood transfusions. Therefore, in collaboration with P.J. McKenna, we began screening serum from patients at Thomas Jefferson University Hospital who had received five or more blood transfusions. Of the first 39 patients tested, we were surprised to find six whose blood contained Australia antigen, not the antibody to it. On investigation it turned out that five of the six were patients with end-stage renal disease who were being treated in the hospital's chronic hemodialysis unit. Since there were only nine patients receiving hemodialysis, we knew that we had stumbled on to an interesting situation. At that time, Marion DiFiglia was a fellow on the nephrology service. She told us about several cases of viral hepatitis among staff members, but she was unaware of hepatitis problems among the patients. This observation became the major focus of our investigation and the subsequent paper.

"Ultimately, we found that eight of the nine hemodialysis patients were HBsAg(+), and the one HBsAg(-) patient was only tested once before she died. At autopsy she had evidence of mild chronic hepatitis. Six of the 15 staff members developed hepatitis, and the two that we were able to test were HBsAg(+). Laboratory studies confirmed DiFiglia's initial clinical observation. The dialyzed patients had a chronic anicteric illness without symptoms of hepatitis, whereas the staff members had acute hepatitis with high serum bilirubin levels and markedly elevated serum transaminase levels. We hypothesized that the differences in response to the virus infection were due to impairment of the immune systems of the patients with chronic renal disease. From this we concluded that it was the immune response to the infection, rather than replication of the virus, which caused liver damage and the clinical signs and symptoms of hepatitis.

"After our paper was published, many investigators in the United States and Europe reported similar findings. I think it was the great prevalence of silent hepatitis B infections in dialysis units that led to the numerous citations of our paper. Following our initial report, we began a long-term study of patients and staff in chronic hemodialysis units in Philadelphia, which still continues, and has resulted in several interesting findings.[1,2]

"The hepatitis B vaccine, which should be available shortly, will most likely be administered to the patients and staff of hemodialysis units. My guess is that hepatitis B infection will be eliminated from dialysis units within 15 years of the discovery of the problem."

1. **London W T, Drew J S, Lustbader E D, Werner B G & Blumberg B S.** Host responses to hepatitis B infection in patients in a chronic hemodialysis unit. *Kidney Int.* **12**:51-8, 1977.
2. **London W T & Drew J S.** Sex differences in response to hepatitis B infection among patients receiving chronic dialysis treatment. *Proc. Nat. Acad. Sci. US* **74**:2561-3, 1977.

This Week's Citation Classic

Dane D S, Cameron C H & Briggs M. Virus-like particles in serum of patients with Australia-antigen-associated hepatitis. *Lancet* **1**:695-8, 1970.
[Bland-Sutton Inst., Middlesex Hosp., London, England]

Virus-like particles 42 nm in diameter were found in the blood of three patients infected with hepatitis B virus. These particles were thought to be complete virions and the much more numerous 22 nm particles and long forms excess virus-coat material. [The *SCI*® indicates that this paper has been cited over 455 times since 1970.]

D.S. Dane
Department of Microbiology
School of Pathology
Middlesex Hospital Medical School
London W1P 7LD
England

October 17, 1980

"In 1965 at the Queen's University, Northern Ireland, I started a research programme which aimed at identifying human hepatitis viruses by electron microscopy (EM). Conventional methods of isolating and growing viruses in tissue-culture or small laboratory animals had been unsuccessful for hepatitis and I thought that EM and negative staining techniques had developed to the stage where they could be used by virologists in rather the same way as light microscopy was used by bacteriologists. As a first step Moya Briggs and I looked at as many different morphological types of viruses as we could using negative staining and concentrating on the recognition of viruses in unpurified preparations.

"This work was brought to an end by a move to the Middlesex Hospital, London, in 1966. We did not start again until 1969 when a hematologist friend, J.W. Stewart, persuaded me to test some of his patients for the mysterious 'Australia antigen.'[1] This antigen was found in the blood of patients with hepatitis B virus infections in the form of spherical 22 nm diameter particles which were often present in enormous numbers. A few long forms of the antigen which were 22 nm wide might also have been present. The antigen particles did not contain nucleic acid and therefore could not be conventional virions. Some people even doubted whether Australia antigen was specifically related to hepatitis B virus.

"One of the first blood samples we were given was from a hemophiliac patient who complained of feeling 'liverish.' Colin Cameron demonstrated Australia antigen by immunodiffusion and we then looked at it by EM. Among the enormous numbers of the small round and long antigen particles described by others we saw just a few quite different, larger particles with inner cores. They looked like virions and it was a simple matter to show that in other Australia antigen positive blood samples there were small numbers of these larger 42 nm diameter particles which had a core surrounded by an outer coat. Cameron showed that they were denser than the other particles and might therefore contain nucleic acid. In appearance and also immunologically the outer coat of the 42 nm particles seemed to be made of the same material as the much more numerous small round and long particles. We suggested that the 42 nm particle was the infective virus and that the other particles consisted of surplus coat material. This explanation of Australia antigen was later reinforced when our friend June Almeida demonstrated the immunological specificity of core antigen,[2] and DNA and DNA polymerase were found to be associated with cores.

"Hepatitis B research has been something of a growth industry in recent years and many papers have been published. When mention has been made of the virus particle our paper has often been quoted. The 42 nm particle was christened the Dane particle, but I never discovered whether the person who originally referred to it in this way was a well-wisher who thought we were right or someone who hoped we were wrong."

1. **Blumberg B S, Alter H J & Visnich S.** A "new" antigen in leukemia sera. *J. Amer. Med. Ass.* **191**:541-6, 1965.
[Citation Classic. *Current Contents/Life Sciences* (51):14, 17 December 1979.]
2. **Almeida J D, Rubenstein D & Scott E J.** New antigen-antibody system in Australia-antigen-positive hepatitis. *Lancet* **2**:1225-7, 1971.

This Week's Citation Classic

Weller T H & Hanshaw J B. Virologic and clinical observations on cytomegalic inclusion disease. *New Eng. J. Med.* **266**:1233-44, 1962.
[Department of Tropical Public Health, Harvard School of Public Health, Department of Medicine, Children's Hospital Medical Center, Boston, MA]

The authors delineate virologic and clinical features of congenital cytomegalic inclusion disease in 17 infants, diagnosed by isolation of cytomegalovirus from urine or liver biopsy material. Cytomegalovirus is incriminated as a cause of intrauterine brain damage, and persistent viruria established as a characteristic manifestation of infection. [The *SCI*® indicates that this paper has been cited over 260 times since 1962.]

Thomas H. Weller
Department of Tropical Public Health
School of Public Health
Harvard University
Boston, MA 02115

February 21, 1978

"In 1955, we described a virus isolated from the liver of an infant initially thought to have congenital toxoplasmosis, and then from the urine of two infants exhibiting hepatosplenomegaly and evidence of central nervous system damage.[1] We suggested that the new viruses played an etiologic role. (The historical circumstances and the concurrent isolation of similar viruses by two other groups had been published.[2]) Thus, when James B. Hanshaw (now professor and head, Department of Pediatrics, University of Massachusetts Medical School, Worcester) joined us as a post-doctoral fellow in 1958, we desired to establish the etiologic role of the new agents in congenitally acquired disease and to define the consequences.

"We sought infants who exhibited frank disease in the neonatal period. Generous cooperation was offered by pediatricians at hospitals in Boston, New York, and Philadelphia. By 1962, we had accumulated a group of 17 virologically confirmed cases of congenitally acquired cytomegalic inclusion disease, and had observed them for periods of 11 months to four years. In the interim we had proposed the now accepted name 'cytomegaloviruses' for the agents. We also introduced the obvious term 'viruria' for the phenomenon of urinary excretion of virus, and had presented the first evidence that the viruses constituted a related but antigenically non-homogeneous group.[3]

"Our publication in 1962 embodied these virologic concepts, established isolation of cytomegalovirus from urine as a diagnostic procedure, and delineated the blatant insults of congenital infection with cytomegalovirus, one extreme of a now recognized clinical spectrum. Microcephaly was common. Persistent cytomegaloviruria, often for years, was recorded. At the conclusion of the study, 16 were alive, 13 exhibited mental retardation, 12 had motor disability and three had already been institutionalized. Thus the societal impact of cytomegaloviral infection was documented, a social tax now recognized as exceeding that imposed by rubella virus in the pre-vaccination era.

"Since 1962, the cytomegaloviruses have been shown to be ubiquitous in distribution and protean in their clinical manifestations. Transmission may be vertical or longitudinal by a variety of methods, including the venereal route. Exhibiting characteristic herpeslike latency, they reactivate in the immunosuppressed host and complicate the handling of the transplant recipient. The field is active and the literature continues to expand rapidly. This provides an opportunity for frequent citation of our clinico-virologic study."

1. **Weller T H, Macaulay J C, Craig J M & Wirth P.** Isolation of intranuclear inclusion producing agents from illnesses resembling cytomegalic inclusion disease. *Proc. Soc. Exper. Biol. Med.* **94**:4-12, 1957.
2. **Weller T H.** Cytomegaloviruses: the difficult years. *J. Infec. Dis.* **122**:532-9, 1970.
3. **Weller T H, Hanshaw J B & Scott D E.** Serologic differentiation of viruses responsible for cytomegalic inclusion disease. *Virology* **12**:130-2, 1960.

This Week's Citation Classic

CC/NUMBER 17
APRIL 25, 1983

Weller T H. The cytomegaloviruses: ubiquitous agents with protean clinical manifestations. *N. Engl. J. Med.* **285**:203-14; 267-74, 1971.
[Department of Tropical Public Health, Harvard School of Public Health, Boston, MA]

This review provided a comprehensive and integrative summary of the expanding knowledge of the human cytomegaloviruses (CMV) that had occurred in the 15-year period following their discovery.[1-4] Emphasizing the broad clinical implications of infection produced by CMV, the content was of interest to virologists and to clinicians from diverse subspecialties. [The *SCI*® indicates that these papers have been cited over 590 times in 396 publications since 1971.]

Thomas H. Weller
Department of Tropical Public Health
Harvard School of Public Health
Boston, MA 02115

February 22, 1983

"The paper falls in the category of *Citation Classics* that are review articles and thus contrasts with an earlier similarly cited paper[5] on the cytomegaloviruses (CMV) that was experimental in scope. There are obvious reasons for the usefulness of the review. Appearing in a readily available publication, and emphasizing the great breadth of clinical manifestations induced by CMV, the review also attempted a synthesis of the natural history of CMV-host relationships.[5] These concepts, based on fact and augmented with a degree of speculation, have stood the test of time and the summary figure in the paper has been reproduced extensively. We also attempted to assess the social significance of CMV, and indicated that in terms of personal tragedy and economic loss, the toll exacted by CMV far exceeded that produced by congenital rubella infections. The problem posed by the antigenic heterogenicity of strains of human CMV, a concept then contentious, was emphasized. The review promoted relatively new concepts that are now generally accepted and in addition stimulated investigations by other workers. For example, it was suggested that CMV should be sought in the tears and feces of infected individuals; reports of isolations of virus from these materials appeared shortly thereafter.[6,7]

"In all probability, the frequent citation of this review reflects another facet of current scientific writing that is to be deplored. Citation of a review ever more frequently supplants a reasoned, critical historical introduction. This tendency is enhanced by the increasing use of computerized literature searches with a limited time span. One can only speculate as to what proportion of the authors utilizing this review as a starting point are aware that the discovery of CMV stemmed from concurrent studies in St. Louis, Bethesda, and Boston? Probably few have read the original papers, although the review referenced a then current summary of the circumstances of the independent isolation of CMV by three groups of investigators.[8]

"Parenthetically, having been involved in the original isolation of varicella-zoster virus,[9] of rubella virus,[10] and of CMV,[1,4] I am bemused by the fact that none of the papers describing these contributions, except the paper on rubella virus, have achieved the citation rate of a *Citation Classic*. However, it is a source of satisfaction that some ten years after its appearance, this review of CMV is still commonly cited as a basic reference. Whether this usage is a reflection of the content of the review, or a reflection of contemporary customs of preparation of a scientific paper, or a combination thereof, is not clear."

1. **Weller T H.** Problems revealed by the expanding use of tissue culture procedures in studies on infectious agents. *Amer. J. Trop. Med. Hyg.* **5**:422-9, 1956.
2. **Smith M G.** Propagation in tissue cultures of cytopathogenic virus from human salivary gland (SGV) disease. *Proc. Soc. Exp. Biol. Med.* **92**:424-30, 1956.
3. **Rowe W P, Hartley J W, Waterman S, Turner H C & Huebner R J.** Cytopathogenic agent resembling human salivary gland virus recovered from tissue cultures of human adenoids. *Proc. Soc. Exp. Biol. Med.* **92**:418-24, 1956.
4. **Weller T H, Macaulay J C, Craig J M & Wirth P.** Isolation of intranuclear inclusion producing agents from infants with illnesses resembling cytomegalic inclusion disease. *Proc. Soc. Exp. Biol. Med.* **94**:4-12, 1957. [The *SCI* indicates that this paper has been cited in over 190 publications since 1961.]
5. **Weller T H & Hanshaw J B.** Virologic and clinical observations on cytomegalic inclusion disease. *N. Engl. J. Med.* **226**:1233-44, 1962. [Citation Classic. *Current Contents/Clinical Practice* 7(39):12, 24 September 1979.]
6. **Cox F & Hughes W T.** Fecal excretion of cytomegalovirus in disseminated cytomegalic inclusion disease. *J. Infec. Dis.* **129**:732-6, 1974.
7. **Cox F, Meyer D & Hughes W T.** Cytomegalovirus in tears from patients with normal eyes and with acute cytomegalovirus retinitis. *Amer. J. Ophthalmol.* **80**:817-24, 1975.
8. **Weller T H.** Cytomegaloviruses: the difficult years. *J. Infec. Dis.* **122**:532-9, 1970.
9. --------------. Serial propagation *in vitro* of agents producing inclusion bodies derived from varicella and herpes zoster. *Proc. Soc. Exp. Biol. Med.* **83**:340-6, 1953. [The *SCI* indicates that this paper has been cited in over 85 publications since 1961.]
10. **Weller T H & Neva F A.** Propagation in tissue culture of cytopathic agents from patients with rubella-like illness. *Proc. Soc. Exp. Biol. Med.* **111**:215-25, 1962. [The *SCI* indicates that this paper has been cited in over 315 publications since 1962.]

This Week's Citation Classic™

Chany C, Lépine P, Lelong M, Le-Tan-Vinh, Satgé P & Virat J. Severe and fatal pneumonia in infants and young children associated with adenovirus infections. *Amer. J. Hygiene* **67**:367-78, 1958.
[Service des Virus, Institut Pasteur & Hôpital St.-Vincent-de-Paul, Paris, France]

During an epidemic of acute respiratory disease in young children in December 1955 and sporadic cases up to February 1957, we recorded 23 cases of acute pneumonia of which four were fatal. The associated clinical manifestations were given and the pathological lesions described in the necrotic areas found in the bronchi. Specific cellular lesions of adenovirus were detected, identical to those seen in tissue culture. This adenovirus inclusion pneumonia seemed to be comparable to the Goodpasture inclusion pneumonia reported in 1939.[1] [The *SCI*® indicates that this paper has been cited in over 150 publications since 1958.]

Charles Chany
Unité de Recherches sur les Virus
Hôpital Saint-Vincent-de-Paul
Institut National de la Santé
et de la Recherche Médicale, U. 43
75014 Paris
France

November 10, 1983

"I was appointed as an intern to the Saint-Vincent-de-Paul Hospital in 1953 in the pediatric department headed by M. Lelong. Our institution is descended directly from the one founded by Saint Vincent de Paul himself, who created the first foundling home for children in the seventeenth century.

"I first worked directly with Satgé and Viallatte, who were responsible for the care of the abandoned children. As a medical student, I was particularly interested in viral diseases and had just finished a special course in fundamental virology at Pasteur Institute. I was impressed by a number of epidemics of unknown etiology which occurred in this relatively close children's community, especially in the winter months. As a rule, we spoke about virus infections when we were not able to find any other explanation for the diseases we encountered.

"Equipped with my fresh and limited knowledge, I decided to try to label these unknown diseases. My decision was also supported by the observations of Huebner and Rowe[2] and Hilleman *et al.*,**[3] who described, at that time, adenoviruses as possible causes for acute respiratory diseases.**

"For a period of 15 months between December 1955 and February 1957, I collected specimens during my rounds in the morning and worked on them in the afternoon at Pasteur Institute in Lépine's laboratory. The first epidemics in December 1955 led us directly to adenovirus pneumonia, with four fatal cases. In most instances, viral pneumonia was associated with other symptoms that we had listed, especially encephalitis. At that time, Barsky (with whom I worked at Pasteur Institute) and I discovered that adenoviruses were responsible for a specific cytopathic effect in tissue culture. We focused our attention on the detection of these lesions *in vivo*. **In association with our pathologist, Le-Tan-Vinh, the lesions were indeed found in the necrotic areas of bronchi, which therefore enabled us to support more directly the role of adenoviruses.**

"In further studies we explored possible reasons for such an unusual gravity of the disease in this age group. The association with whooping cough or measles probably worsened the disease. In one case, chlorpromazine therapy and hibernation, which effectively decreased the fever, aggravated the infection, as we later learned from Lwoff's work.[4]

"The study of these foundling children and the necessity to survey such a vulnerable population led us later to another interesting discovery, namely, the description of the hemagglutinating and hemolytic properties of measles virus, which enabled us to diagnose rapidly this frequently occurring and dangerous disease.[5,6]

"Presently, abandoned children are no longer kept for long periods in the hospital and are placed in foster families as soon as possible. The studies we reported contributed certainly in part to the decision of the authorities to end long-term internship of orphans in institutions.

"The interest which arose from our publication is perhaps linked to the unexpected nature of our observations since adenovirus infections were considered harmless at that time. Furthermore, it resolved the etiological problem of Goodpasture's inclusion pneumonia."

1. **Goodpasture E W, Auerbach S H, Swanson H S & Cotter E F.** Virus pneumonia of infants secondary to epidemic infections. *Amer. J. Dis. Child.* **57**:997-1011, 1939. (Cited 40 times since 1955.)
2. **Huebner R J & Rowe W P.** Adenoviruses as etiologic agents in conjunctivitis and keratoconjunctivitis. *Amer. J. Ophthalmol.* **43**:20-5, 1957. (Cited 20 times since 1957.)
3. **Hilleman M R, Werner J H, Adair C V & Dreisbach A R.** Outbreak of acute respiratory illness caused by RI-67 and influenza A viruses, Fort Leonard Wood, 1952-1953. *Amer. J. Hygiene* **61**:163-73, 1955. (Cited 70 times since 1955.)
4. **Lwoff A & Lwoff M.** Sur les facteurs du développement viral et leur rôle dans l'évolution de l'infection. *Ann. Inst. Pasteur* **98**:173-203, 1960. (Cited 95 times since 1960.)
5. **Perles J R & Chany C.** Activité hémagglutinanate et hémolytique du virus morbilleux. *C.R. Acad. Sci* **251**:820-1, 1960. (Cited 70 times since 1960.)
6. ---------------------------. Studies on measles virus hemagglutination. *Proc. Soc. Exp. Biol. Med.* **110**:477-82, 1962.

This Week's Citation Classic

CC/NUMBER 10
MARCH 9, 1981

Connolly J H, Allen I V, Hurwitz L J & Millar J H D. Measles-virus antibody and antigen in subacute sclerosing panencephalitis. *Lancet* **1**:542-4, 1967. [Depts. Microbiology and Pathology, Queen's Univ., and Royal Victoria Hospital, Belfast, Northern Ireland]

Measles antibody was found in serum and cerebrospinal fluid of three boys with subacute sclerosing panencephalitis and serum/CSF antibody ratios were low. Serum titres were high in two boys while in one the titre increased 16-fold during the illness. Measles virus antigen was present in the brain. [The *SCI*® indicates that this paper has been cited over 285 times since 1967.]

John H. Connolly
Department of Microbiology
and Immunobiology
Queen's University
Belfast BT12 6BN
Northern Ireland

February 10, 1981

"Subacute sclerosing panencephalitis (SSPE) is a very rare disease yet in 1965 within a three month period, three boys from different areas of Northern Ireland were diagnosed by the Royal Victoria Hospital neurologists, Lewis Hurwitz and Harold Millar. Northern Ireland had a population of only 1.5 million people so this was an unusual event. I was doing diagnostic virology in the Queen's University, department of microbiology, and Hurwitz, whom I knew well, encouraged me to examine the patients. Seeing the boys with this devastating disease was a powerful stimulus to do some investigative work. We asked the parents about the boys' childhood illnesses, animal contacts, and whether they had been in contact with each other. No clues emerged. The success of this project owed much to the enthusiasm of Hurwitz, who ensured that all specimens asked for were delivered and who encouraged us during the whole investigation.

"Serum and cerebrospinal fluid (CSF) specimens taken on the same day were tested against several viral complement fixing antigens including a recently acquired measles antigen. When I saw the first measles antibody titrations I was surprised at the height of the titres, then doubts appeared because we knew the boys had had measles 11 to 13 years previously. The results were confirmed using the haemagglutination-inhibition test. It seemed contradictory that childhood measles, which was then a universal illness, should be associated with this rare disease.

"We were anxious to isolate measles virus from the brain although numerous attempts with CSF were unsuccessful. When the three boys died, the neuropathologist Ingrid Allen from Queen's University, department of pathology, carried out the post-mortems within a few hours of death, so that any virus present would still be viable. Two post-mortems were done in the middle of the night. However, all attempts at virus isolation were unsuccessful. The histological features of SSPE including the virus-like type A inclusions first described by Dawson[1] were seen.

"Shortly after this, Kenneth Fraser came to the department of microbiology. He was experienced in the immunofluorescence technique and we discussed the possibility of using it to detect measles antigen in the brains. Measles antisera were labelled with fluorescein isothiocynate. Brain sections stained with these antisera showed intranuclear and intracytoplasmic measles antigen. Subsequent work[2,3] extended these observations and showed the production of immunoglobulins within the central nervous system. There is still, however, an incomplete understanding of the pathogenic mechanisms involved in SSPE.

"I think this paper is often cited because it was the first to show measles antibody in serum and CSF and measles antigen in the brain in SSPE and there was widespread interest in slow and persistent viral infections of the central nervous system."

1. **Dawson J R.** Cellular inclusions in cerebral lesions of lethargic encephalitis. *Amer. J. Pathol.* **9**:7-15, 1933.
2. **Connolly J H, Allen I V, Hurwitz L J & Millar J H D.** Subacute sclerosing panencephalitis: clinical, pathological, epidemiological and virological findings in three patients. *Quart. J. Med.* **37**:625-44, 1968.
3. **Thomson D, Connolly J H, Underwood B O & Brown F.** A study of immunoglobulin M antibody to measles, canine distemper and rinderpest viruses in sera of patients with subacute sclerosing panencephalitis. *J. Clin. Pathol.* **28**:543-6, 1975.

CC/NUMBER 44
OCTOBER 29, 1984

This Week's Citation Classic™

Evans A S, Niederman J C & McCollum R W. Seroepidemiologic studies of infectious mononucleosis with EB virus. *N. Engl. J. Med.* **279**:1121-7, 1968.
[Dept. Epidemiology and Public Health, Yale Univ. Sch. Med., New Haven, CT]

This seroepidemiological study of infectious mononucleosis (IM) demonstrated antibody to Epstein-Barr virus (EBV) to be absent prior to development of IM, to appear regularly during illness, and to persist for years. This relationship was not found in other infectious diseases. EBV is the probable cause of IM. [The *SCI*® indicates that this paper has been cited in over 265 publications since 1968.]

Alfred S. Evans
Department of Epidemiology and Public Health
Yale University School of Medicine
New Haven, CT 06510

August 1, 1984

"This study examined the possible relationship between antibody to EBV and IM in three serum collections. In one, sera collected by Jim Niederman from 362 Yale University freshmen who had been bled on entry into college from 1958 to 1963 and again at the time when 40 developed IM over the next four years were taken from our freezers and tested for EBV antibody. Of 268 students lacking antibody on entry, 19.4 percent developed IM over the next four years. In contrast, of 94 students entering with antibody, none subsequently developed IM. The second collection obtained and frozen by me was from patients with IM who had been admitted to the University of Wisconsin student infirmary, and the third collection was sera sent to the Wisconsin State Laboratory of Hygiene for heterophile antibody determinations. Of 135 sera from heterophile antibody cases of IM in all three collections, all were found to have EBV virus capsid antigen IgG antibody. Pre-illness sera available from 56 of these patients were uniformly negative for EBV antibody. Of 16 patients who were persistently negative for heterophile antibody but who fulfilled clinical and hematologic criteria for IM, six were EBV antibody positive, indicating that EBV might cause heterophile-negative cases, and nine were EBV antibody negative, suggesting that agents in addition to EBV could produce a mononucleosis-like syndrome.

"This study confirmed and extended the preliminary report by Niederman, Bob McCollum, and the Henles[1] that EBV antibody was absent from the pre-illness sera and developed early in the course of IM in 29 patients, some showing a rising titer of antibody. Our study clearly indicated that EBV was implicated in the causation of IM and not simply a passenger virus. The evidence was based on: 1) EBV antibody was consistently present in 135 cases of IM and invariably present in other infections and healthy controls, 2) the antibody was absent in pre-illness sera from 58 persons and appeared during illness, 3) a rising titer of antibody was observed in some patients, 4) the absence of EBV antibody indicated susceptibility to the subsequent development of IM, whereas its presence indicated immunity, 5) a past history of IM was found only in students whose serum had EBV antibody, 6) EBV antibody persisted for years as expected of a true antibody and in contrast to the transient heterophile antibody, 7) the association of EBV antibody with IM was consistent with available epidemiological data on IM, and 8) the study also implicated EBV as one of the causes of heterophile-negative IM.

"My own interest in IM had begun years before this 1968 study. It started in 1946 when I had returned from service in the Army and was offered a fellowship at Yale by John R. Paul, who had discovered the heterophile antibody of IM in 1932 with W.W. Bunnell[2] (the Paul-Bunnell test) and had maintained an active interest in the disease. We believed that IM was probably due to a filterable agent, but many attempts made by me[3,4] and later by Niederman and Scott[5] to transmit the infection to volunteers were unsuccessful or at best equivocal. Some of the sera from volunteers were frozen and stored and when EBV antibody was discovered, we retested them and learned that almost all possessed antibody at the time we had inoculated them. Thus, working with immune subjects is not the best way to carry out such experiments. In 1950-1952, I re-entered the Army and carried out unsuccessful experiments in the Army Hepatitis Research Center in Munich, to transmit both EBV and viral hepatitis to monkeys.[6] On leaving the service, I went to the University of Wisconsin, where I continued my interest in IM, making vigorous but unsuccessful attempts to isolate the elusive causative agent from throat washings, sera, and buffy coats from cases of IM.[7] I did confirm Hoagland's concept[8] that IM might be transmitted by intimate oral contact and proposed a concept of pathogenesis of the viral etiology of IM that has turned out to be substantially correct.[7] Thus, after over 20 years of working with IM, I was well prepared, as were my associates, to evaluate the observation of Henle *et al.* that EBV might be the cause of IM.[9] For a recent review, see reference 10."

1. **Niederman J C, McCollum R W, Henle G & Henle W.** Infectious mononucleosis. Clinical manifestations in relation to EB virus antibodies. *JAMA—J. Am. Med. Assn.* **203**:205-9, 1968. (Cited 325 times.)
2. **Paul J R & Bunnell W W.** The presence of heterophile antibodies in infectious mononucleosis. *Amer. J. Med. Sci.* **183**:91-104, 1932. (Cited 225 times since 1955.)
3. **Evans A S.** Attempts to transmit infectious mononucleosis to man. *Yale J. Biol. Med.* **20**:19-26, 1948.
4. -------------. Further experimental attempts to transmit infectious mononucleosis to man. *J. Clin. Invest.* **29**:508-12, 1950.
5. **Niederman J C & Scott R B.** Studies on infectious mononucleosis. Attempts to transmit the disease to human volunteers. *Yale J. Biol. Med.* **38**:1-10, 1965.
6. **Evans A S, Evans B K & Sturtz V.** Standards for hepatic and hematologic tests in monkeys: observations during experiments with hepatitis and mononucleosis. *Proc. Soc. Exp. Biol. Med.* **82**:437-40, 1953.
7. **Evans A S.** Infectious mononucleosis in University of Wisconsin students: report of a five year investigation. *Amer. J. Hyg.* **71**:342-62, 1960. (Cited 95 times since 1960.)
8. **Hoagland R J.** The transmission of infectious mononucleosis. *Amer. J. Med. Sci.* **229**:262-72, 1955. (Cited 80 times since 1955.)
9. **Henle G, Henle W & Diehl V.** Relation of Burkitt's tumor-associated herpes-type virus to infectious mononucleosis. *Proc. Nat. Acad. Sci. US* **59**:94-101, 1968. (Cited 740 times.)
10. **Evans A S & Niederman J C.** The Epstein-Barr virus. (Evans A S, ed.) *Viral infections of humans: epidemiology and control.* New York: Plenum Press, 1982. p. 253-81.

Chapter

2

Clinical Pathology

The Citation Classics described in this chapter were grouped on the basis of their common emphasis of laboratory procedures for the detection or determination of medically important molecules. This grouping overlaps with some topics in Chapter 3 on Immunology and Rheumatology and Chapter 7 on Endocrinology and Metabolic Disease, and these chapters should also be consulted.

Citation Classics that have been cited 1,000 or more times are unusual in this volume on Clinical Medicine, yet three such papers are contained in this chapter. These are the article on hydroxycorticoid determination by Mattingly (cited 1,056 times), the article on the serum glutamic oxaloacetic and glutamic pyruvic transaminases by Reitman and Frankel (cited 1,304 times), and the article on enzymatic determination of glucose developed by Huggett and Nixon (cited 1,045 times).

The last owes its popularity to the need for a specific method to quantitate glucose in the clinical evaluation of diabetics. The method that Huggett and Nixon advanced was equally applicable to the measurement of glucose in urine or blood and eliminated the necessity for the dual determination of total reducing sugar and of fructose. The "This Week's Citation Classic" (TWCC) was written by the wives of the scientists involved. The most valuable application of the transaminase paper is in assisting the diagnosis of myocardial infarction. This was also one of the first methods to be available as a reagent kit. Prior to this time enzymatic methods had not been used to evaluate heart disease, and this article became the forerunner of what is now considered a routine clinical determination. Mattingly's steroid classic probably owes its popularity to the combined interest in endocrinology of the adrenal cortex and to the simplicity and sensitivity of the fluorimetric assay which made it superior to numerous procedures that were published earlier. Mattingly experienced considerable difficulty in perfecting his method as a result of impurities in the reagents then available in Britain. The great popularity of these articles is emphasized by the fact that only three other articles among the 21 Citation Classics in this chapter were cited more than 350 times.

Though the remaining 18 articles have not had such a high citation frequency, several of them are remarkable for other qualities. Zak's TWCC on his report that described the quantitation of serum cholesterol is but one of his three articles on cholesterol methodology that became Citation Classics. His other two are in an earlier volume (*Contemporary Classics in the Life Sciences, volume 2, The Molecules of Life*). Nelson is a contributor to two Citation Classics in this chapter. As a young postdoctoral fellow, Nelson developed with Samuels a method for determining the concentration of cortisol in blood, and nearly simultaneously with Glenn used β-glucuronidase to hydrolyze the steroid-glucuronide conjugate so that the free steroid could be measured quantitatively. It is certainly uncommon for two of the first articles of a junior scientist to reach Classic status. Glenn's commentary in the first paragraph of the second TWCC is of interest. The attraction of stray dogs to clothing, briefcases, etc., that had become perfumed during the heating process required to dissociate steroids in urine from their carrier glucuronides must have created a number of embarrassing situations. Glenn's paragraph on their string trio, the barefoot guitarist, and laboratory songfests indicates that a multi-talented group participated in their important biochemical discovery.

The contribution of junior-level scientists to steroid research noticeable in the comments of Nelson and Glenn is again evidenced by Klopper's development of the pregnanediol method for his Ph.D. dissertation. Other commentaries on phosphoribosylpyrophosphate (PRPP) (p. 49) and iron determination (p. 54) also identify a significant role of junior scientists in these studies. Returning to Klopper's TWCC, note that his attempt to incorporate 3 years of bench work in his manuscript's first draft is an experience similar to that shared by many scientists in their first writing effort. Nevertheless, he did not cause his advisor any "rude shocks" from his relatively unsupervised bench work.

As might be expected, several of these TWCCs were written because the original Citation Classic described a medical first. This is the case with the article on PRPP that first demonstrated the medical importance of this enzyme. The report of the role of the enzyme phosphofructokinase (PFK) in glycogenosis and the result of a genetic deficiency of this enzyme is another medical first. PFK is the major regulatory enzyme of the glycolytic pathway that converts glucose to lactic acid. Since lactic acid did not increase in the blood of three patients after exercise, Tarui and his assistants began a search for the defective muscle enzyme in the Embden-Meyerhof pathway. This was identified as PFK; however, erythrocyte PFK was only slightly affected, thus also first indicating the isozymic nature of this enzyme. Layzer's TWCC is also about hereditary PFK deficiency and its isozymes, including an immunological demonstration of the latter.

But turning away from Citation Classics as important "firsts" or highly cited articles, the remainder are clearly important for other reasons.

Odell's assessment of the toxicity of bilirubin as a free molecule rather than when bound to albumin clarified why it is that neonates under certain drug regimens expressed bilirubin toxicity (kernicterus). The answer lay in the ability of sulfa drugs, as an example, to dissociate bilirubin from its non-toxic conjugate with albumin and liberate the free, toxic molecule.

Sequentially following the previously mentioned TWCC on the transaminases are three on phosphatases. The phosphatases, perhaps more often the alkaline than the acid forms, have been of considerable interest to medical scientists. The ability to associate low levels of the enzyme with chronic myelocytic leukemia and elevated levels with other granulocytoses (p. 46) emphasized the importance of a sensitive and rapid cytochemical assay for the enzyme (p. 47). Eventually, through initially crude heat stability studies, serum alkaline phosphatase was determined to derive from several tissues, thus clarifying its isoenzyme nature to all but the editor of the *American Journal of Medicine,* who rejected the manuscript.

The TWCCs on PRPP and glucose oxidase precede that written by Gibson, who noted that mothers of patients with cystic fibrosis were reluctant to enter, nude, into the plastic bags used for sweat collections. This modesty seemed to have a positive correlation with body weight. Because of this and the need to examine the electrolyte content of sweat, Gibson, then a medical resident, advanced the electro-osmotic use of pilocarpine as a sweat inducer.

Bilirubin-derived pigments in amniotic fluid, identified spectrophotometrically, became a useful early indicator of hemolytic disease of the newborn. This surpassed the value of determining maternal anti-Rh antibody titrations since, despite the presence of such antibodies, the fetus could still be Rh negative and thus be unnecessarily taken by premature delivery. At the present time, prevention of the original maternal sensitization to the Rh antigen has limited the use of amniocentesis for these bilirubin determinations and has the prospect to totally eliminate hemolytic disease of the newborn infant due to this cause.

Thyroid disease has been evaluated by the protein-bound iodine test or by T3 (triiodothyronine) quantitation since the early 1950s. Clark and Horn found that the product of these tests expressed as the free thyroxine index was superior to either of these tests alone. Serum iron concentrations have been markedly expedited by the automation of this procedure, still in use 20 years after its initial description. Another method conceived 20 years ago is the microbiological growth assay for folic acid. Finally, a TWCC on a cytochemical method to stain fibrin in its various stages of alteration to pseudocollagen closes this chapter.

Anatomic pathology is an important segment of clinical pathology although it is not represented in this chapter, which has clinical chemistry as its main theme. A search through *Index Medicus* for review articles directly related to the subjects of the Citation Classics in this chapter will prove disappointing. Apparently the steroid and enzyme "quantifiers" have achieved satisfaction with the methods they now use to determine the levels of steroids, glucose, alkaline phosphatase, and transaminases in blood and urine. However, in a search through *Advances in Clinical Chemistry, Clinics in Laboratory Medicine, Annual Review of Medicine, Advances in Internal Medicine, CRC Critical Reviews in Clinical Laboratory Science, Pathology Annual, International Review of Experimental Pathology, Seminars in Diagnostic Pathology,* and several other journals, the following articles pertinent to these Citation Classics were uncovered.

Defreese J D & Wang T S-C. Properties and determination of serum bilirubin. *CRC Crit. Rev. Clin. Lab. Sci.* **19:**267–96, 1984.

Delves H T. Assessment of trace element status. *Clin. Endocrinol. Metab.* **14:**725–60, 1985.

Howanitz P J & Howanitz J H. Hypercortisolism. *Clin. Lab. Med.* **4:**683–702, 1984.

Kapadia C P & Donaldson R M Jr. Disorders of cobalamin (vitamin B_{12}) absorption and transport. *Annu. Rev. Med.* **36:**93–110, 1985.

Lott J A & Landesman P W. The enzymology of skeletal muscle disorders. *CRC Crit. Rev. Clin. Lab. Sci.* **20:**153–90, 1984.

Odell G B & Childs B. Hereditary hyperbilirubinemias. *Prog. Med. Genet.* **4:**103–134, 1980.

Posen S & Doherty E. The measurement of serum alkaline phosphatase in clinical medicine. *Adv. Clin. Chem.* **22:**165–245, 1981.

Schwartz M, Schwartz S, Wenk R E & Cohen M. Amniotic fluid and advances in prenatal diagnosis. *Clin. Lab. Med.* **5:**371–87, 1985.

Trainer T D & Howard P L. Thyroid function tests in thyroid and nonthyroid disease. *CRC Crit. Rev. Clin. Lab. Sci.* **19:**135–71, 1983.

CC/NUMBER 1
JANUARY 5, 1981

This Week's Citation Classic

Nelson D H & Samuels L T. A method for the determination of 17-hydroxycorticosteroids in blood: 17-hydroxycorticosterone in the peripheral circulation. *J. Clin. Endocrinol. Metab.* **12**:519-26, 1952.
[Dept. Biochemistry, Univ. Utah Coll. Med., Salt Lake City, UT]

Cortisol or 17-hydroxycorticosterone is found to be present in the peripheral circulation of man. A method is described for the measurement of this steroid in blood. [The *SCI*® indicates that this paper has been cited over 270 times since 1961.]

Don H. Nelson
Department of Medicine
University of Utah
Endocrine Research Laboratory
Salt Lake City, UT 84103

November 12, 1980

"Early in 1949 I came as a postdoctoral fellow into the laboratory of Leo T. Samuels, head of the department of biochemistry, University of Utah College of Medicine. Samuels' laboratory was heavily involved in studying the synthesis and metabolism of the androgenic steroids. He thought that it would be of interest to also look at the corticosteroids and thus the task assigned to me on arrival in the laboratory was to evaluate methods for the estimation of the corticosteroids. Each of those available proved to be nonspecific and the results obtained were highly variable. I was enough of a novice in the field of endocrinology that it came as a surprise to me that no one had identified the major corticosteroid secreted by the adrenal cortex and thus I took as my first task identification of the major steroids secreted by the gland. After many trials and errors we were able to demonstrate that 17-hydroxycorticosterone was the major corticosteroid in the adrenal-venous blood of dogs.[1] This was accomplished using a lipid extraction followed by chromatographic separation and measurement by ultraviolet absorption of the steroids present in blood coming from a cannulae placed in the adrenal veins of dogs. Application of this technique to peripheral blood failed to demonstrate any steroids due to the much lower levels of the hormone present.

"At about this time Porter and Silber described a new color reaction with some specificity for the dihydroxyacetone structure found in the 17, 21-dihydroxy-20-ketone of cortisol. Their initial applications of this procedure had also failed to demonstrate measurable hormone in peripheral blood.[2] Using much larger quantities of blood and paper chromatography which recently had become available, we then demonstrated cortisol in the peripheral blood of man. As we now knew the hormone that was present and approximate amount we combined our extraction and chromatography procedure, which had been successful in the isolation of cortisol from blood, with a micromodification of the color reaction of Porter and Silber and were able to measure cortisol in the peripheral blood of man. This procedure was then employed by us and others to measure cortisol in blood including normal levels, demonstration of diurnal variation, and response to ACTH and other physiologic stimuli. We introduced the term '17-hydroxycorticosteroid' to indicate that the color reaction was not totally specific for cortisol, although this was by far the major steroid in the circulation measured by the procedure. This method was replaced by a simplified application of the Porter-Silber reaction which did not require chromatography, a protein binding assay, and radioimmunoassays.

"The many citations of the paper are probably due to the fact that this was not only the first reproducible method for the measurement of '17-hydroxycorticosteroids' in peripheral blood or plasma but also the first demonstration that cortisol was the major circulating corticosteroid, and establishment of the amounts present in the circulation. We have always been pleased that although the methodology was somewhat primitive by modern standards, the levels of cortisol in blood measured by this method were essentially the same as those which continue to be measured by other procedures."

1. **Nelson D H, Reich H & Samuels L T.** Isolation of a steroid hormone from the adrenal-vein of dogs. *Science* **111**:578-9, 1950.
2. **Porter C C & Silber R H.** A quantitative color reaction for cortisone and related 17, 21-dihydroxy-20-ketosteroids. *J. Biol. Chem.* **185**:201-7, 1950.

This Week's Citation Classic

Glenn E M & Nelson D H. Chemical method for the determination of 17-hydroxy-corticosteroids and 17-ketosteroids in urine following hydrolysis with β-glucuronidase. *J. Clin. Endocrinol. Metab.* **13**:911-21, 1953.
[Dept. Biological Chemistry, Univ. Utah Coll. Med., Salt Lake City, UT]

17-Hydroxycorticosteroids and 17-ketosteroids were determined and quantitatively separated in urine treated with β-glucuronidase. The procedure gave good separation and high reproducibility along with good recoveries of added steroids. The methods were more specific than other methods previously described. [The *SCI*® indicates that this paper has been cited over 280 times since 1961.]

E. Myles Glenn
Hypersensitivity Diseases
The Upjohn Company
Kalamazoo, MI 49001

May 29, 1980

"During the late 1940s I had been investigating the isolation and determination of various steroids from the urines of experimental animals and man with Roy Hertz, Benton Westfall and, especially, Erich Heftmann, at the National Institutes of Health. At that time, the splitting of the steroid ester conjugates in urine was a tedious, unsatisfactory, and stinking affair requiring acid hydrolysis of urine at elevated temperatures. One knew the essential nature of the work when stray dogs mistook one's briefcase or trouser leg for a mobile fireplug and used them accordingly. The smelly laboratory procedures required differential solvent extractions to extricate the desired steroidal alcohols for final colorimetric analysis—procedures which, at best, were unpredictable because of the lack of air-conditioning and high humidity in Bethesda at the time.

"Max Sweat and Kathryn Knowlton, working in adjacent laboratories, made it possible for me to become associated with Leo Samuels and Don Nelson in the department of biochemistry at the University of Utah School of Medicine. They were investigating steroid levels in human blood, as well as their synthetic pathways in various isolated tissues of experimental animals. My contribution, consequently, occurred from being at the right place, at the appropriate time; in association with interesting scientists; all working on similar biomedical problems.

"Nelson[1] had already devised successful methods for the extraction and separation of 17-hydroxycorticosteroids from human serum, using Florisil columns. My contribution consisted of β-glucuronidase hydrolysis of urine, followed by solvent extractions and separation of the two major steroid components on Florisil columns and their subsequent quantitation by well-established colorimetric procedures. This procedure allowed future studies to be done easily concerning adrenocortical and probable testicular function in man.

"Along with Nelson, Kristen Eik-Nes also worked alongside me on another project involving steroid secretion rates from the adrenal cortex of dogs treated with endotoxin. Eik-Nes was a tall and gifted Norwegian. Working in his bare feet some of the time, he played the guitar and sang, especially while working at midnight and beyond. He was accompanied by Pete and Oley Johnson, two Mormon youngsters playing ukuleles and singing while washing our dirty glassware—young men who were later to become members of the medical fraternity. Then, there were the beautiful and talented Rosie and Carma, capably assisting all of us in the many diversified experiments.

"After the intense labor on the methodologies was completed, Avery Sandberg[2] and I applied them to a study of steroid metabolism and excretion in both healthy patients and those with various endocrine diseases. This voluminous clinical work gained the attention of the great endocrinologist and teacher, George Sayers, with whom I later became associated and from whom, subsequently, I received the PhD degree in physiology at Western Reserve University School of Medicine.

"The frequency of citation of this article—although I was unaware of it until now—resulted, probably, from the simplicity, reproducibility, and applicability of the methodology to the study of steroid excretion rates, steroid metabolism, and various endocrinologic diseases in man."

1. **Nelson D H & Samuels L T.** Method for the determination of 17-hydroxycorticosteroids in blood: 17-hydroxycorticosterone in the peripheral circulation. *J. Clin. Endocrinol. Metab.* **12**:519-26, 1952.
2. **Sandberg A A, Nelson D H, Glenn E M, Tyler F & Samuels L T.** 17-Hydroxycorticosteroids and 17-ketosteroids in urine of human subjects: clinical application of a method employing β-glucuronidase hydrolysis. *J. Clin. Endocrinol. Metab.* **13**:1445-64, 1953.

This Week's Citation Classic

NUMBER 8
FEBRUARY 19, 1979

Mattingly D. A simple fluorimetric method for the estimation of free 11-hydroxycorticoids in human plasma. *J. Clin. Pathol.* **15**: 374-9, 1962.

11-hydroxycorticoids have a structure which is unique to steroids of adrenal origin. Their plasma concentration is a valuable measure of adrenocortical activity, provided that the normal circadian rhythm is taken into account. This paper describes a simple fluorimetric assay which is ideal for routine clinical use. [The *SCI®* indicates that this paper has been cited 1,056 times since 1962.]

D. Mattingly
University of Exeter
Postgraduate Medical Institute
Exeter EX2 5DW, England

February 28, 1978

"The dramatic introduction of the corticosteroids into clinical practice in 1948 provided an enormous impetus to the study of the role of the adrenal glands in health and disease. Despite their beneficial effects it soon became obvious that pharmacological doses of these drugs had many undesirable side-effects, not least being the inhibition of the normal pituitary-adrenal response to stress. Attempts to investigate this phenomenon in individual patients were frustrated by the lack of suitable steroid assays which could be carried out in the routine laboratory.

"Cortisol, or hydrocortisone as it is better known to the clinician, is the main hormone secreted by the human adrenal cortex and accounts for most of the 11-hydroxycorticoids presented in the blood. However, since the plasma levels of this life-maintaining steroid are extremely small, even in normal unstressed individuals, the techniques used to estimate it must be particularly sensitive. The reaction between these steroids and concentrated sulphuric acid produces highly potent fluorophores, but it was not until 1960 that DeMoor and his colleagues published the first practical fluorimetric method for the estimation of plasma 11-hydroxycorticoids in man.[1]

"At the time that their paper appeared I was working with Cuthbert Cope at Hammersmith Hospital and we were attracted by the potential advantages of fluorimetry over the much more laborious and less precise colorimetric methods which were then available. Unfortunately we could not duplicate the results obtained by DeMoor's group and our interest in their method waned until I discovered that this failure was largely due to impurities in the reagents available in Britain. The petroleum ether used in the preliminary de-fatting wash and the methylene chloride employed to extract the steroids from the plasma were particularly fertile sources of spurious fluorescence. Rigorous purification of the methylene chloride and omission of the petroleum ether and alkali washes eliminated most of the non-specific fluorescence, simplified the procedure considerably and, rather to our surprise, did not reduce the accuracy or precision of the method.

"The value of this simple and rapid steroid assay in the investigation of adrenal problems at the bedside soon became apparent, especially in cases of suspected adrenal failure. Since the synthetic corticosteroids did not fluoresce, it was possible to study endogenous adrenal activity during their administration.

"The fact that this paper has been chosen as a 'Citation Classic' shows that many workers have found this method of use in the elucidation of disorders of the adrenal cortex, and also indicates how the simplification of a more elaborate procedure can lead to quicker and more accurate diagnoses in clinical practice."

REFERENCE

1. **DeMoor P, Steeno O, Raskin M & Hendrikx A.** Fluorimetric determination of free plasma 11-hydroxycorticosteroids in man. *Acta Endocrinol.* **33**:297-307, 1960.

CC/NUMBER 25
JUNE 22, 1981

This Week's Citation Classic

Klopper A, Michie E A & Brown J B. A method for the determination of urinary pregnanediol. *J. Endocrinology* **12**:209-19, 1955.
[Clinical Endocrinology Research Unit, Medical Research Council, Univ. Edinburgh, Scotland]

Pregnanediol is the chief metabolite of the sex hormone progesterone. At the time when this work was done, it was not yet possible to measure progesterone itself. We managed to measure pregnanediol by boiling urine with hydrochloric acid to free the steroid from its combination with glucuronic acid. The free pregnanediol was extracted from the urine and the crude extract purified by chromatography on alumina columns. The purified material was acetylated and rechromatographed. The nearly pure pregnanediol acetate gave a yellow colour with sulphuric acid which enabled spectrophotometric measurements to be made. [The *SCI*® indicates that this paper has been cited over 455 times since 1961.]

Arnold Klopper
Department of Obstetrics & Gynaecology
University of Aberdeen
Royal Infirmary
Foresterhill, Aberdeen AB9 2ZB
Scotland

May 27, 1981

"Invent a new mousetrap and the world will beat a path to your door. The pregnanediol method was just that—a gimmick, no more, and it is this which accounts for the article's frequent citation. It was certainly no great trick, although it took me three years to work it out and fed me for a good many more. In one form or another the various parts of the technique had been worked out either for pregnanediol or for other steroids and it was just a case of fitting all the ideas together. Probably the most original idea was to make the derivative of pregnanediol and that was Jim Brown's sole contribution to the work, a notion produced over beer in the pub round the corner from the Medical Research Council laboratory where we worked. He was much too busy with his own classic work on estrogen estimation to do more.[1] Brown's work has dominated the field for more than a quarter of a century. If that computer in Philadelphia does not identify that as a *Citation Classic*, it can't count.

"Although the pregnanediol method was really the centrepiece of my PhD thesis, Guy Marrian brought in Eileen Michie at the last stages to give bench expertise and biochemical respectability to the work. He had suffered some rude shocks by letting young medicals work unsupervised. In the end I got just the right amount of supervision from Marrian himself. He was a towering figure in the world of steroid chemistry, having himself been the first to isolate estriol and pregnanediol.[2] With the perspective of time I can see how difficult it must have been not to simply take over and tell us what to do. Happily he was too busy isolating and identifying half a dozen new estrogens himself. Indeed, if there is any single reason for the creativity of the laboratory at that time it was because everybody had their own thing to do.

"Marrian did do one thing for me. He had a passion for brief and factual writing. My first draft of the pregnanediol method contained everything that I had learned in three years and much besides. Marrian tore it up after a glance and told me to start again. The shock of seeing my brainchild destroyed before my eyes comes back to me every time I put pen to paper. The experience may not have put much into my writing but it certainly took a lot out.

"The pregnanediol method was to be a tool to elucidate the physiology of progesterone. In the end it took us only a little way down the road. We were analysing exhaust fumes and trying to deduce the nature of the internal combustion engine. The estimation of pregnanediol in urine has now largely been superseded by the measurement of the original active hormone, progesterone, in blood."

1. **Brown J B.** A chemical method for the determination of estriol, estrone, and estradiol in human urine. *Biochemical J.* **60**:185-9, 1955. [The *SCI*® indicates that this paper has been cited over 1,010 times since 1961.]
2. **Marrian G F.** The chemistry of oestrone. 1. Preparation from urine and the separation from an unidentified solid alcohol. *Biochemical J.* **23**:1090-2, 1929.

This Week's Citation Classic

CC/NUMBER 48
NOVEMBER 29, 1982

Vlahcevic Z R, Bell C C, Jr., Buhac I, Farrar J T & Swell L. Diminished bile acid pool size in patients with gallstones. *Gastroenterology* **59**:165-73, 1970. [Veterans Admin. Hosp., and Depts. Medicine, Surgery, and Biochemistry, Medical College of Virginia, Richmond, VA]

Patients with gallstones were found to have a significantly smaller total bile acid pool than subjects without evidence of gallstones. The findings suggested that a diminished bile acid pool could be an important factor responsible for the production of the abnormal (lithogenic) bile found in patients with gallstones. [The ***SCI®*** **indicates that this paper has been cited in over 305 publications since 1970.]**

Z.R. Vlahcevic
Gastroenterology Section
McGuire Veterans Administration
Medical Center
Richmond, VA 23249

September 16, 1982

"Cholesterol has been recognized as the major constituent of human gallstones since it was first isolated from that source by Poulletier de la Salle in 1763.[1,2] However, it is only within recent years that we have developed an understanding as to how cholesterol is solubilized in bile as a mixed micelle. Adequate proportions of bile acids and lecithin in bile have been found to be essential for the proper solubilization of biliary cholesterol.

"In 1967, Leon Swell had worked with Cecil Entenman at Berkeley and had made the interesting observation that biliary lecithin secretion by the perfused rat liver is directly linked to the availability of bile acids in the system.[3] This was an exciting finding since it suggested that circulating bile acids might play an important role in regulating biliary lecithin secretion *in vivo*, which could have important implications for the proper solubilization of biliary cholesterol.

"It seemed to us that a logical next step to test this hypothesis would be to ascertain if there was any alteration in the amount of bile acids circulating in the enterohepatic circuit in human subjects with gallstones. Accordingly, we measured the bile acid pool by isotope dilution in subjects with and without gallstones. The data indicated that patients with gallstones had a greatly diminished bile acid pool which was approximately one half that of the subjects without gallstones. Later studies in female and male Caucasians and American Indians confirmed these findings and also showed that the fractional turnover rate of the bile acids was significantly increased.[4,5] The mechanism responsible for the reduction in bile acid pool size was therefore attributed to an increased loss of bile acids coupled with a failure of the liver to synthesize adequate amounts of bile acids to maintain the pool size. We then postulated that gallstone formation in man may be initiated by a decrease in bile acid pool size, which would lead to an inordinate decrease in the secretion of biliary bile acids and lecithin, resulting in bile containing cholesterol microcrystals. More up-to-date information on the present concepts of pathogenesis of cholesterol gallstones has recently been published.[6]

"This paper has been highly cited because it provided a new perspective on the gallstone pathogenesis and served as an impetus for a number of investigations by other workers related to the factors regulating the solubilization of biliary cholesterol. Also, this work formed a basis (at least initially) for the rationale of gallstone dissolution by oral administration of bile salts to expand the bile acid pool. The initial 1970 study was the beginning of a very active scientific collaboration and friendship between myself and Swell, which has continued uninterrupted until the present time."

1. **de Fourcroy M.** Examen chimique de la substance feuilletée et cristalline contenue dans les calculs biliaires, et de la nature des concrétions cystiques cristallisées. *Ann. Chim. Phys. Series 1* **3**:242-52, 1789.
2. **Bills C E.** Physiology of the sterols, including vitamin D. *Physiol. Rev.* **15**:1-97, 1935.
3. **Swell L, Entenman C, Leong G F & Holloway R J.** Bile acids and lipid metabolism. IV. Influence of bile acids on biliary and liver organelle phospholipids and cholesterol. *Amer. J. Physiol.* **215**:1390-6, 1968.
4. **Vlahcevic Z R, Bell C C, Jr., Gregory D H, Buker G, Juttijudata P & Swell L.** Relationship of bile acid pool size to the formation of lithogenic bile in female Indians of the Southwest. *Gastroenterology* **62**:73-83, 1972.
5. **Bell C C, Jr., McCormick W C, III, Gregory D H, Law D H, Vlahcevic Z R & Swell L.** Relationship of bile acid pool size to the formation of lithogenous bile in male Indians of the Southwest. *Surg. Gynecol. Obstet.* **134**:473-8, 1972.
6. **Shaffer S A.** Gallstones: current concepts of pathogenesis and medical dissolution. *Can. J. Surg.* **23**:517-29, 1980.

CC/NUMBER 12
MARCH 21, 1983

This Week's Citation Classic

Zak B. Simple rapid microtechnic for serum total cholesterol. *Amer. J. Clin. Pathol.* **27**:583-8, 1957. [Labs. of the Depts. Pathology, Wayne State Univ. Coll. Med., and Detroit Receiving Hospital, Detroit, MI]

A bifunctional reagent, ferric chloride in acetic acid, was designed for the determination of serum cholesterol. One function was to precipitate the serum proteins while leaching cholesterols from their lipoproteins and solubilizing them in the acetic acid. The other function was to become the color reagent when an aliquot was mixed with sulfuric acid. [The *SCI*® indicates that this paper has been cited in over 445 publications since 1961.]

B. Zak
Department of Pathology
Wayne State University School of Medicine
and
Detroit Receiving Hospital
University Health Center
Detroit, MI 48201

December 22, 1982

"It is devastating when one is criticized in the literature for what appears to be a serious error. It is even worse that such a happening could warrant any credence. As a novice clinical chemist at the time, the potential procedural interference that surfaced in my case was the possibility of a Hopkins-Cole reaction with the tryptophane of the serum proteins. This generated an overlapping spectrum to the one formed by cholesterol, the analyte of interest, when using a ferric chloride reaction in a sulfuric acid-acetic acid medium. The tryptophane reaction requires that glyoxal, a natural impurity of acetic acid, be present. Without it, no such side reaction would take place. In addition, and ideally for the interference, the Hopkins-Cole reaction works well when ferric iron is present. We had inherited 24 one-lb. bottles of glyoxal-free glacial acetic acid from a recently departed professor who had obtained it for some project of his own, a project about which we knew nothing. Using this purified solvent, we optimized a reaction we had developed for the determination of cholesterol in rabbit serum and then applied it to a direct reaction using whole serum rather than an organic extract in the reaction medium. Because of the absence of glyoxal, we obtained results that were similar to those that we arrived at on comparing this direct procedure to an acceptable extraction.

"We described the process as one using 100 percent glacial acetic acid. Had others known this and used a purification process such as a Kuhn-Roth treatment, then the tryptophane interference could have been avoided as it was in our own studies using the manufacturer purified glacial acetic acid. This publication was popular and it became a *Citation Classic*.[1]

"Another naturally occurring interference was bilirubin. It, like tryptophane, has been a critical substance because it generates a side reaction on its easy oxidation to a stable bilirubin. This resulted in an additive error of 0.7 mg of cholesterol per mg of bilirubin. However, the popular Liebermann-Burchard reaction, which is still commonly used in automation, results in an error of at least 5 mg of cholesterol per mg of bilirubin. Because of some criticism on the tryptophane problem, we began work on the development of procedures that would minimize it as an interference and thus evolved two extraction procedures that removed the proteins and their tryptophane as well as much of the bilirubin. The first of these, also a *Citation Classic*,[2] became popular with researchers looking for what they must have considered to be more suitable cholesterol methodology than those available to them at the time.

"I believe that the method that was developed became a *Citation Classic* because it offered a simple way to remove all proteins, at the same time easily leaching the cholesterols from their binding sites on the lipoproteins. In a somewhat novel approach, the precipitating agent was also the color reagent when it was mixed with sulfuric acid, the final reagent. Another advantage afforded to investigators along with procedural simplicity was the formation of a stable, intensely colored equilibrium form that provided a molar absorptivity about eight times that of the unstable Liebermann-Burchard reaction. This allowed one to apply the procedure and its stable reaction to a large number of small samples, making it eminently suitable for small animal research.

"On surveying the literature for a comparison to other procedures for the determination of cholesterol in biological fluids early on, a review of the available methodologies resulted. Since that time, requests have been received to write four subsequent reviews where the latest contributions[3,4] include a description of the more modern use of enzymes as reagents in spectrophotometric procedures allowing a more selective approach to the assay of serum and cerebrospinal fluid cholesterol[(81)]."

1. **Zlatkis A, Zak B & Boyle A J.** A new method for the direct determination of serum cholesterol. *J. Lab. Clin. Med.* **41**:486-92, 1953. [Citation Classic. *Current Contents/Life Sciences* **24**(12):20, 23 March 1981.]
2. **Zak B, Dickenman R C, White E G, Burnett H & Cherney P J.** Rapid estimation of free and total cholesterol. *Amer. J. Clin. Pathol.* **24**:1307-15, 1954. [Citation Classic. *Current Contents/Life Sciences* **24**(18):16, 4 May 1981.]
3. **Zak B.** Cholesterol methodologies: a review. *Clin. Chem.* **23**:1201-14, 1977.
4. --------. Cholesterol methodology for human studies. *Lipids* **15**:698-704, 1980.

CC/NUMBER 47
NOVEMBER 19, 1984

This Week's Citation Classic™

Tarui S, Okuno G, Ikura Y, Tanaka T, Suda M & Nishikawa M.
Phosphofructokinase deficiency in skeletal muscle. A new type of glycogenosis.
Biochem. Biophys. Res. Commun. **19**:517-23, 1965.
[Second Dept. Internal Medicine, Osaka Univ. Med. Sch., Japan]

This paper describes a novel entity of glycogenosis due to muscle-type phosphofructokinase deficiency. It also indicates that erythrocyte phosphofructokinase is partially affected, resulting in increased hemolysis in this disease, and suggests the possible existence of isozymes of phosphofructokinase. [The *SCI*® indicates that this paper has been cited in over 190 publications since 1965.]

Seiichiro Tarui
Second Department of Internal Medicine
Osaka University Medical School
Fukushima-ku, Osaka 553
Japan

August 22, 1984

"In 1964, I was doing clinical research at the Second Department of Internal Medicine, Osaka University Medical School. My emphasis was on analysis of disorders of carbohydrate metabolism. We were visited by five siblings from a single family, three of whom complained unanimously of quickly induced fatigue and inability to keep pace with their classmates. Since ischemic forearm exercise failed to cause any rise in venous lactate in the three subjects, and their parents were first cousins, we at first thought they were suffering from muscle glycogenosis due to phosphorylase deficiency.

"As I had expected, a significant increase in the glycogen concentration in their muscles was clearly demonstrated. However, completely normal activity of muscle phosphorylase greatly surprised me. Therefore, we had to analyze all the steps below glucose-1-phosphate in the Embden-Meyerhof glycolytic pathway.

"The approximately 60-year history of studies of glycogenosis had taught us that the cooperation of investigators in clinical and basic science fields occasionally bears rich fruit: Wagner-Parnas, von Gierke-Schönheimer, and van Creveld-Huijing are just a few examples. Fortunately, at that time I received much good advice from Tanaka, my classmate in Osaka University Medical School, who was famous for his studies on pyruvate kinase.[1] Consequently, the identification of the defective enzyme was not so difficult. Marked increases in hexose monophosphates and an extreme decrease in fructose-1,6-bisphosphate in muscles indicated the distinct crossover in the phosphofructokinase step.

"Of interest was the fact that erythrocyte phosphofructokinase was only partially affected in contrast to the almost complete lack of muscle phosphofructokinase activity. It provided a challenge for further intensive study of the isozymes of phosphofructokinase.[2,3] These fundamental features of the disease have been confirmed by many case studies reported in the US, France, England, Canada, Spain, and Italy.[4]

"This clinical entity was classified as Type VII glycogenosis by Brown and Brown.[5] No controversy has hitherto occurred concerning the eponym. At present, Type VII glycogenosis (Tarui disease) is not infrequently described in textbooks of metabolism, hematology, neurology, biochemistry, internal medicine, and pediatrics.

"The popularity of this paper seems to rest on the following points. First, it added a novel clinical entity not only to glycogenosis but also to enzymopenic hemolytic anemia. Second, the defective enzyme demonstrated is nothing else but phosphofructokinase, which plays a key regulatory role in glycolysis through its complicated allosteric properties. Third, it provided the indication of the possible existence of the isozymes of phosphofructokinase and also gave an impetus to the study of phosphofructokinase in a number of nonhuman mammalian species.[3] Finally, it represented a unique experiment of nature and could open a new way to the understanding of the cause of alterations in glycolytic intermediates, e.g., the close relationship between phosphofructokinase and 2,3-bisphosphoglycerate in erythrocytes."[6]

1. **Tanaka T, Harano Y, Sue F & Morimura H.** Crystallization, characterization and metabolic regulation of two types of pyruvate kinase isolated from rat tissues. *J. Biochem. Tokyo* **62**:71-91, 1967. (Cited 420 times.)
2. **Tarui S, Kono N, Nasu T & Nishikawa M.** Enzymatic basis for the coexistence of myopathy and hemolytic disease in inherited muscle phosphofructokinase deficiency. *Biochem. Biophys. Res. Commun.* **34**:77-83, 1969. (Cited 75 times.)
3. **Vora S.** Isozymes of phosphofructokinase. *Curr. Top. Biol. Med. Res.* **6**:119-67, 1982.
4. **Tarui S, Mineo I, Shimizu T, Sumi S & Norio K.** Muscle phosphofructokinase deficiency and related disorders. (Serratrice G, Cros D, Desnuelle C, Gastaut J L, Pellissier J F, Pouget J & Schiano A, eds.) *Neuromuscular diseases.* New York: Raven Press, 1984. p. 71-6.
5. **Brown I B & Brown D H.** Glycogen-storage diseases: type I, III, IV, V, VII and unclassified glycogenosis. (Deckens F, Randle P J & Whelan W J, eds.) *Carbohydrate metabolism and its disorders.* London: Academic Press, 1968. Vol. 2. p. 123-50.
6. **Tarui S, Kono N, Kuwajima M & Kitani T.** Hereditary and acquired abnormalities in erythrocyte phosphofructokinase activity. The close association with altered 2,3-diphosphoglycerate levels. *Hemoglobin* **4**:581-92, 1980.

CC/NUMBER 48
NOVEMBER 26, 1984

This Week's Citation Classic™

Layzer R B, Rowland L P & Ranney H M. Muscle phosphofructokinase deficiency. *Arch. Neurol.* **17**:512-23, 1967.

[Dept. Neurol., Coll. Physicians and Surgeons, Columbia Univ.; Neurological Clinical Res. Ctr., Neurological Inst., Columbia-Presbyterian Medical Ctr.; and Heredity Clinic and Dept. Medicine, Albert Einstein Coll. Medicine, Yeshiva Univ., New York, NY]

Clinical and biochemical studies of a patient with muscle phosphofructokinase (PFK) deficiency confirmed the presence of a block in muscle glycolysis at the PFK step. Immunologic studies suggested that the disease was caused by hereditary absence of the muscle-type subunit of PFK, which is normally present in red cells but not in white cells. [The *SCI*® indicates that this paper has been cited in over 160 publications since 1967.]

**Robert B. Layzer
Department of Neurology
School of Medicine
University of California
San Francisco, CA 94143**

February 13, 1984

"This was my second scientific article, and for the most part it was not very original. It reported a second family with muscle phosphofructokinase (PFK) deficiency, a rare hereditary disorder with symptoms resembling those of McArdle's disease (muscle phosphorylase deficiency). The first such family had been reported not long before in an excellent paper by Tarui *et al.*[1] and many of our studies merely confirmed their results.

"We did make some new observations, however. Tarui *et al.* had shown that red-cell PFK was about half of normal in affected persons; we found that PFK activity was normal in white blood cells. At that date (1966), nothing was known about PFK isoenzymes. We realized that the simplest hypothesis to explain the different degrees of PFK deficiency in muscle, red cells, and white cells was that PFK existed in multiple molecular forms composed of at least two nonidentical subunits, only one of which (the muscle type) was affected by the genetic defect. By this theory, muscle PFK should contain only muscle-type subunits; red-cell PFK should contain both the muscle-type subunit and another type; and white-cell PFK should contain no muscle-type subunits.

"To test this hypothesis, we prepared antiserum to purified human muscle PFK and checked its ability to inhibit the PFK activity of muscle and red-cell extracts. Sure enough, the antiserum inhibited the PFK activity of normal muscle and red cells but did not inhibit the patient's red-cell PFK. We also found no immunologically cross-reactive material in the patient's muscle extracts. These results came through just in time to be included as 'unpublished data' in the last paragraph of the article. We were nervous about not having repeated the experiment, but we wanted to scoop Tarui's group, who, we suspected, might be working along similar lines. Fortunately, the results turned out to be repeatable and were later confirmed by the Japanese workers.[2]

"This research helped me to obtain a National Institutes of Health Career Development Award in 1968. I worked on PFK isoenzymes for several years after that and succeeded in separating the two subunits of red-cell PFK, though others eventually did a better job of elucidating the subunit composition of PFK isoenzymes.[3] Meanwhile, many new metabolic myopathies were discovered, and medical interest in PFK deficiency dwindled, while the rise of nucleic acid chemistry made isoenzyme biochemistry seem quaintly out of date. Why, then, has this paper been cited so often? I really have no idea, unless it is because the paper was very well written."

1. **Tarui S, Okuno G, Ikura Y, Tanaka T, Suda M & Nishikawa M.** Phosphofructokinase deficiency in skeletal muscle. A new type of glycogenosis. *Biochem. Biophys. Res. Commun.* **19**:517-23, 1965. [See also: **Tarui S.** Citation Classic. *Current Contents/Clinical Practice* **12**(47):20, 19 November 1984.]
2. **Tarui S, Kono N, Nasu T & Nishikawa M.** Enzymatic basis for the coexistence of myopathy and hemolytic disease in inherited muscle phosphofructokinase deficiency. *Biochem. Biophys. Res. Commun.* **34**:77-83, 1969. (Cited 75 times.)
3. **Vora S, Corash L, Engel W K, Durham S, Seaman C & Piomelli S.** The molecular mechanism of the inherited phosphofructokinase deficiency associated with hemolysis and myopathy. *Blood* **55**:629-35, 1980.

This Week's Citation Classic

NUMBER 15
APRIL 9, 1979

Odell G B. The dissociation of bilirubin from albumin and its clinical implications. *J. Pediat.* **55:** 268-79, 1959.

The cytoxicity of bilirubin cannot be accurately assessed from its total concentration in plasma, because bilirubin is bound to albumin. The current studies demonstrate the ability of albumin to bind bilirubin is significantly reduced when other organic anions (e.g. sulfisoxazole, benzoate, and hematin, which also bind to albumin) coexist in the plasma of neonatal infants with hyperbilirubinemia. The results indicate that the pathogenesis of bilirubin toxicity is more closely related to that fraction of the circulating bilirubin which is dissociated from albumin or indirectly to the relative saturation of the albumin with bilirubin. [The *SCI*® indicates that this paper has been cited over 205 times since 1961.]

Gerard B. Odell
Department of Pediatrics
University of Wisconsin School of Medicine
Madison, WI 53706

February 4, 1976

"The genesis of these studies can be appropriately ascribed to 'undisciplined' thinking about the chemo-physiology of bilirubin. I use the term 'undisciplined,' for most investigators in clinical medicine who study bilirubin metabolism have been trained in either gastroenterology or hematology. My research interests and training were in electrolyte physiology and maturation of renal function. This was interrupted by two years of military service and a year as Chief Resident. The research for this paper took place at the Harriet Lane Home at the Johns Hopkins School of Medicine. When I got back to the laboratory bench, I found the major aspects of salt and water homeostasis had been well described. The forbearance of my mentors, R. E. Cooke and H. H. Gordon, allowed me to switch directions, and I decided to study organic anion secretion by the kidney.

"I selected bilirubin as a clinically important anion, particularly during the period of neonatal jaundice. The molecule has two propionic acid side-chains, and I reasoned that by non-ionic diffusion, one should be able to promote its renal excretion during neonatal jaundice. On an alkaline-ash diet the unconjugated anion of bilirubin was not excreted in significant amounts in the urine! In-vitro ultrafiltration experiments demonstrated it would not be filtered at the glomerulus; but why was it not subject, like other protein-bound anions to tubular secretory processes, such as those for para-aminohippuric acid or salicylate?

"It was at that juncture that I was motivated to study the albumin-binding of bilirubin. While working for the chemistry department during college, I was allowed to take a certain number of courses tuition-free and for fun I took colloidal chemistry. When thinking about the protein-binding of bilirubin, a highly apolar molecule, to the macromolecule of albumin with apolar binding sites, I realized my undergraduate education might prove useful. Thus I read with renewed interest about Freundlich and Langmuir adsorption isotherms, Scatchard plots and Klotz's classic analysis of the binding of small molecular anions to albumin.

"I was also taught and believed that even a lead pipe has a vapor pressure of lead around it. It was in the latter context that I viewed the equilibrium of bilirubin between albumin and its aqueous environment, and thus described it in terms of the chemical laws of mass action, even though the concentration of bilirubin in plasma water had at the time never been measured.

"I suspect this paper has been frequently quoted because it appealed to the scientific training of its readers. The application of the principles of colloidal and physical chemistry to a clinical problem provided an explanation whereby some infants with the same extravascular concentrations of bilirubin could in one instance suffer no injury, while others either died of bilirubin toxicity or exhibited chronic morbidity. The reported observations in this paper demonstrated how the administration of drugs to prevent infection in jaundiced neonates could result in higher mortality and morbidity from bilirubin toxicity because the drugs reduced the albumin binding capacity for bilirubin."

This Week's Citation Classic

Reitman S & Frankel S. A colorimetric method for the determination of serum glutamic oxalacetic and glutamic pyruvic transaminases. *Amer. J. Clin. Pathol.* **28**: 56-63, 1957.

A simple method for the estimation of transaminase activity in serum takes advantage of the differences in the extinction coefficients of alkaline solutions of the 2,4-dinitrophenylhydrazones of alpha-ketoglutarate, oxalacetate, and pyruvate, permitting the reaction rate to be measured by determining the timed change in absorbancy. [The *SCI*® indicates that this paper has been cited 1304 times since 1961.]

Sam Frankel
Midwest Medical Laboratory
4141 Forest Park Blvd.
St. Louis, MO 63108

February 4, 1978

"Both Dr. Reitman and I are extremely pleased to be asked to submit a brief summary of the events leading to the development of our transaminase procedures.

"The key factor responsible for the decision to devise a method sufficiently simple to be used in any laboratory was a patient incorrectly diagnosed as having had an acute myocardial infarction. The diagnosis had been made solely on clinical grounds, since the services of an electrocardiogram and of cardiac enzyme assays were not available in his home town. The patient was instructed to drastically curtail his activity, and felt compelled to sell his business. When subsequently he was seen at the Jewish Hospital of St. Louis, however, the diagnosis was not confirmed.

"Shortly after the appearance of an article by Karmen[1] describing a method for measuring transaminase activity in serum, Chinsky and Shmagranoff,[2] residents in medicine at Jewish Hospital, initiated an extensive project which supported the importance of this test in the diagnosis of acute myocardial infarction. Reitman, also a resident in medicine at that time, remarked that the patient might have been spared serious consequences if a simple test had been available to the physician in that small town. The Chief of Medicine, hearing of this comment, suggested that he begin work on such a procedure. I was then Director of Clinical Chemistry at the hospital, and was contacted for assistance in developing a method that would be simple enough to be run in any medical laboratory without the need of special equipment.

"In making the procedure simple, a few rules of 'good' chemistry were either broken or severely bent. It developed that the reagents required were very critical and there was fear that some laboratories would have difficulty in their preparation. Therefore, it was decided to request the assistance of the Sigma Chemical Company.

"A survey indicated that at one time 95% of all laboratories performing the tests were using the Reitman-Frankel procedures, and current information shows that they are still in use today, more than twenty years later. In our opinion, this remarkable popularity can be attributed to the Sigma Chemical Company, which was the first to manufacture the reagents and standards necessary for good performance.

"Perhaps the most pleasing reward from this entire experience has been seeing the methods in use throughout the world. Although it was originally intended that they would fill a need of the smaller laboratories until such time as better equipment and techniques became available, it is gratifying that not only was the original purpose accomplished, but that they still find considerable use in many areas of this country and abroad."

1. **Karmen A.** A note on the spectrophotometric assay of glutamic oxalacetic transaminase in human blood serum. *J. Clin. Invest.* **34**:131-3, 1955.
2. **Chinsky M., Shmagranoff G L & Sherry S.** Serum transaminase activity. *J. Lab. Clin. Med.* **47**: 108-18, 1956.

CC/NUMBER 38
SEPTEMBER 20, 1982

This Week's Citation Classic

Valentine W N & Beck W S. Biochemical studies on leucocytes. I. Phosphatase activity in health, leucocytosis, and myelocytic leucemia.
J. Lab. Clin. Med. **38**:39-55, 1951.
[School of Medicine, University of California, Los Angeles, CA]

This paper reported quantitative data on the alkaline and acid phosphatase content of separated human leukocytes. Markedly different alkaline phosphatase activity patterns were demonstrable. In chronic myelocytic leukemia (CML) activity was very low; in most nonleukemic granulocytosis it was strikingly elevated. [The *SCI*® indicates that this paper has been cited in over 215 publications since 1961.]

William N. Valentine
Department of Medicine
School of Medicine
Center for the Health Sciences
University of California
Los Angeles, CA 90024

August 6, 1982

"In 1948, I came to the newly founded UCLA medical school with J.S. Lawrence, the first chairman of its department of medicine. Earlier research work at the University of Rochester had centered on thalassemia and hematologic aspects of radiation biology. However, I had become convinced that studies of blood cell metabolism at the molecular level should widen the vistas of classical morphology. My coauthor, Bill Beck, now professor of medicine at Harvard and director of the Hematology Research Laboratory at Massachusetts General Hospital, joined our laboratory after his residency at Wadsworth Veterans Administration Hospital. We determined to investigate the phosphatase activity of human leukocytes (isolation techniques were now available), and correlate this quantitatively with hematologic parameters and disease entities.

"This fortunate choice was motivated largely by the fact that certain leukocytes were known to possess alkaline phosphatase activity, and the techniques involved were within the capabilities of our modest laboratory. We soon became excited by the uniformly low activity in chronic myelocytic leukemia (CML) and the contrastingly striking elevations in most nonleukemic granulocytosis. Perhaps more exciting was the observation that in polycythemia vera (PRV) and certain myeloproliferative syndromes, granulocyte populations morphologically similar to those of CML possessed very high alkaline phosphatase activity (reported in a companion paper[1]). At one point, with the help of John H. Lawrence, director of the Donnor Laboratory, Beck and I packed up our instrumentation and traveled to Berkeley. There, in 48 hours, we studied 15 subjects with CML, PRV, and other myeloproliferative syndromes. These were patients in the large clinic supervised by Lawrence. The companion report[1] also documented the characteristically low alkaline phosphatase activity in the leukocytes in paroxysmal nocturnal hemoglobinuria. Although it had received essentially no attention by clinicians and we initially had missed it, Beck and I soon realized that what we believed to be a 'first' was not. Wachstein had observed similar metabolic patterns in CML and PRV utilizing histochemical techniques.[2]

"Beck later left Los Angeles to work with Severo Ochoa and to be recruited by the late Walter Bauer to the Harvard faculty. During the next several years, my laboratory made additional observations on the high and low activity patterns in different morbid states, the effect of corticosteroids on leukocyte alkaline phosphatase, and on the role of Zn^{++} and the substrate specificities of the enzyme. The widely variant patterns in morphologically similar cells in myeloproliferative syndromes strongly suggested heterogeneous etiologies. The observation that a few (but by no means most) therapeutically induced remissions in CML were accompanied by apparent reversion of leukocyte alkaline phosphatase to normal with restoration of normal responsiveness to corticosteroids prompted us to raise the possibility that in CML a suppressed normal clone would still exist in conjunction with a dominant leukemic clone.[3,4]

"This paper has been highly cited largely because of the interest in the correlations of enzyme activity with certain disease states such as those observed in various myeloproliferative disorders. Recently, Hayhoe and Quaglino[5] have extensively reviewed the literature on leukocyte alkaline phosphatase in health and disease."

1. **Beck W S & Valentine W N.** Biochemical studies on leucocytes. II. Phosphatase activity in chronic lymphatic leucemia, acute leucemia, and miscellaneous hematologic conditions. *J. Lab. Clin. Med.* **38**:245-53, 1951.
2. **Wachstein M.** Alkaline phosphatase activity in normal and abnormal blood and bone marrow cells. *J. Lab. Clin. Med.* **31**:1-17, 1946.
3. **Valentine W N, Follette J H, Solomon D H & Reynolds J.** Biochemical and enzymatic characteristics of normal and leukemic leukocytes (with particular reference to leukocyte alkaline phosphatase). (Rebuck J W, Bethell F H & Monto R W, eds.) *The leukemias: etiology, pathophysiology, and treatment.* New York: Academic Press, 1957. p. 457-65.
4. **Valentine W N.** The metabolism of the leukemic leucocyte. *Amer. J. Med.* **28**:699-710, 1960.
5. **Hayhoe F G J & Quaglino D.** *Haematological cytochemistry*. London: Churchill Livingston, 1980. p. 105-45.

CC/NUMBER 5
FEBRUARY 1, 1982

This Week's Citation Classic

Hayhoe F G J & Quaglino D. Cytochemical demonstration and measurement of leucocyte alkaline phosphatase activity in normal and pathological states by a modified azo-dye coupling technique. *Brit. J. Haematol.* **4**:375-89, 1958.
[Department of Medicine, University of Cambridge, Cambridge, England]

This paper describes a cytochemical technique for demonstrating alkaline phosphatase in haemic cells and gives the results of applying a semiquantitative scoring method to assess positivity in neutrophil leucocytes in health and in leukaemias, leukaemoid reactions, lymphomas, metastasising malignancies, and miscellaneous blood diseases. [The *SCI*® indicates that this paper has been cited over 160 times since 1961.]

F.G.J. Hayhoe
Department of Haematological Medicine
University of Cambridge
Clinical School
Cambridge CB2 2QL
England

November 23, 1981

"I had used the Gomori methods for acid and alkaline phosphatase in blood and marrow cells between 1950 and 1955 with the somewhat erratic results many other investigators had found. When Kaplow published an azo-dye coupling procedure in 1955[1] that gave consistent and satisfactory results for alkaline phosphatase in his hands, I attempted to apply it in collaboration with Dennis Quaglino, then starting a PhD research project on haematological cytochemistry in my laboratory. The variability in constitution of commercial azo-dyes was such that we couldn't actually make Kaplow's method work very well in our laboratory using the available fast blue RR salt, but from a range of other diazonium salts tried, fast garnet G.B.C. gave excellent results. Using this simple modification we explored the leucocyte alkaline phosphatase (LAP) score in 50 healthy subjects and in 102 patients with various diseases attending my haematology and lymphoma clinics. Patterns of LAP score in major disease groups were delineated—very low in CML, normal in non-Hodgkin's lymphoma, high in Hodgkin's disease, in infectious leucocytosis, in polycythaemia vera and myelofibrosis, and in disseminated carcinoma.

"The report seems likely to have been frequently cited because the modified technique described was found easy to use by others and perhaps because it contains data on many if not most of the disorders associated with abnormal LAP scores. It was the first of a series of about 20 papers and communications on cytochemistry of haemic cells which Dennis, Roger Flemans, and I were to produce in the period between 1958 and 1964 before Dennis returned to Italy. Among these works was a monograph on the cytology and cytochemistry of acute leukaemia[2] which probably played some part in encouraging the development of cytochemistry as a regular procedure in haematological diagnosis.

"Although the distance between Modena, in northern Italy, and Cambridge (even in East Anglia rather than Massachusetts) prevented regular subsequent collaboration in research, Dennis and I recently put together our experiences of 25 years in cytochemical practice in a monograph entitled *Haematological Cytochemistry.*[3] We were encouraged and a little relieved to find that neither our own subsequent experience nor an exhaustive review of the literature led us to contradict or withdraw the findings of that original 1958 paper which forms the subject of this commentary."

1. **Kaplow L S.** A histochemical procedure for localizing and evaluating leukocyte alkaline phosphatase activity in smears of blood and marrow. *Blood* **10**:1023-9, 1955.
2. **Hayhoe F G J, Quaglino D & Doll R.** *The cytology and cytochemistry of acute leukaemia: a study of 140 cases.* London: HMSO, 1964. 105 p.
3. **Hayhoe F G J & Quaglino D.** *Haematological cytochemistry.* Edinburgh: Churchill Livingstone, 1980. 336 p.

CC/NUMBER 17
APRIL 23, 1984

This Week's Citation Classic™

Posen S, Neale F C & Clubb J S. Heat inactivation in the study of human alkaline phosphatases. *Ann. Intern. Med.* **62**:1234-43, 1965.
[Dept. Medicine, Univ. Sydney, and Dept. Biochemistry, Sydney Hosp., New South Wales, Australia]

This paper describes differences in the heat inactivation rates of alkaline phosphatase in sera from different groups of patients. Alkaline phosphatase in serum from patients with skeletal disorders was inactivated at a more rapid rate than serum alkaline phosphatase from patients with hepatobiliary disorders. [The *SCI*® indicates that this paper has been cited explicitly in over 180 publications since 1965.]

Solomon Posen
Royal North Shore Hospital
St. Leonards, New South Wales 2065
Australia

January 17, 1984

"During 1963, a number of patients at Sydney Hospital were found to have unexpected, transient, and spectacular elevations of their serum alkaline phosphatase values. John Clubb, who was then a resident, found that all these patients had received infusions of albumin prepared from human placentas,[1] and we discussed ways and means to distinguish this contaminant alkaline phosphatase (presumably of placental origin), from the endogenously occurring material.

"At Frank Neale's suggestion we tried heat denaturation. We chose 56°C in the first instance because the thermostat of a water bath in the microbiology department (used for complement work) was set at that temperature. It soon became clear that human placental alkaline phosphatase, whether obtained from fresh placentas, from maternal pregnancy serum, from placental albumin preparations, or from the serum of recipients, was uniquely heat stable and differed from other human alkaline phosphatases in a variety of other parameters.[2]

"Differences between serum alkaline phosphatase from patients with skeletal disorders and patients with hepatobiliary disorders were less spectacular but, nevertheless, highly significant.

"Skeletal material (whether derived from bone or from blood) was more readily denatured by physical and chemical agents than biliary alkaline phosphatase ('bone breaks'). We concluded, 'Serum alkaline phosphatase in subjects with skeletal disorders is of bony origin while in hepatic disorders the enzyme is derived from the contents of the biliary tree.'

"When this paper was submitted to the *American Journal of Medicine*, the then editor (Alexander B. Gutman—a great believer in the 'unitary' nature of alkaline phosphatase) returned it with a curt note saying that it needed more than such a crude method to convince him that there were multiple tissue origins of this enzyme.

"After its publication in the *Annals of Internal Medicine*, this method generated a good deal of interest for a variety of reasons. Serum alkaline phosphatase assays constitute one of the most commonly performed tests in clinical medicine.[3] The heat denaturation technique is universally available so that our results were rapidly confirmed in other laboratories.

"In spite of its inherent inaccuracies (no worse than those of electrophoretic methods), the test is still widely employed in the study of tissue sources of circulating alkaline phosphatases. Most importantly, this paper changed clinical thinking about the mechanism of serum alkaline phosphatase elevation in hepatic disease.

"More work needs to be done to clarify the nature of the differences between skeletal and biliary alkaline phosphatases which are probably due to posttranslational factors."[4]

1. **Neale F C, Clubb J S & Posen S.** Artificial elevation of the serum alkaline phosphatase concentration. (Letter to the editor.) *Med. J. Australia* **2**:684, 1963.
2. **Posen S, Cornish C J, Horne M & Saini P K.** Placental alkaline phosphatase and pregnancy. *Ann. NY Acad. Sci.* **166**:733-44, 1969.
3. **McComb R B, Bowers G N & Posen S.** *Alkaline phosphatase.* New York: Plenum Press, 1979. 1004 p.
4. **Goldstein D J, Rogers C & Harris H.** Evolution of alkaline phosphatase in primates. *Proc. Nat. Acad. Sci. US* **79**:879-83, 1982.

This Week's Citation Classic™

CC/NUMBER 15
APRIL 9, 1984

Fox I H & Kelley W N. Phosphoribosylpyrophosphate in man: biochemical and clinical significance. *Ann. Intern. Med.* **74**:424-33, 1971.
[Div. Rheumatic and Genetic Diseases, Depts. Medicine and Biochemistry, Duke Univ. Medical Center, Durham, NC]

The intracellular concentration of phosphoribosylpyrophosphate (PRPP), a high energy, 1,5-substituted ribose sugar, has been demonstrated to have a critical role in the regulation of purine metabolism in man. Increased intracellular levels of PRPP may be important in the pathogenesis of excessive uric acid production in patients with primary gout and the Lesch-Nyhan syndrome. In addition, intracellular PRPP levels are altered by several compounds and certain trophic hormones. [The *SCI*® indicates that this paper has been cited in over 150 publications since 1971.]

Irving H. Fox
Clinical Research Center
University Hospital
University of Michigan
Ann Arbor, MI 48109

January 31, 1984

"In July 1969, my assignment at the start of my postdoctoral fellowship work was to develop an assay for phosphoribosylpyrophosphate (PRPP). William N. Kelley, who was my supervisor, believed that this compound might be important in human purine metabolism and that it would be worthwhile studying. Despite my lack of previous training in the methods of biochemical research, I enthusiastically undertook this project. In my initial attempts to develop an assay for PRPP, I followed the methods of Henderson and Khoo.[1] After a few months of intensive effort, the assay was established.

"In one series of studies, we attempted to understand the role of PRPP in the regulation of purine biosynthesis *de novo*. In these experiments in cultured fibroblasts, we made correlations between the rate of purine biosynthesis *de novo* and changes in the intracellular levels of PRPP. The other line of research involved studies in humans to test the hypothesis that alterations in PRPP concentrations might be important in the pathogenesis of hyperuricemia and gout. Previous work had suggested that this was possible.[2-4] With these studies, we examined a large number of patients with gout. The results of these studies indicated to us that PRPP was indeed a rate-limiting substrate in *de novo* purine synthesis and that it was involved in the pathogenesis of hyperuricemia, at least in hypoxanthine-guanine phosphoribosyltransferase deficiency. We also initiated studies to observe whether the administration of various drugs or other compounds might modulate PRPP levels *in vivo*. One of our first studies with allopurinol was published in the *New England Journal of Medicine* in November 1970[5] and this study and others demonstrated, indeed, that specific purine and pyrimidine compounds could modulate PRPP levels *in vivo*.

"After one year's work in this area, we realized that PRPP was a critical compound in the regulation of purine synthesis in humans, was altered in some human disease states, and could be modulated by administration of drugs. To crystallize these concepts, in 1970, we began writing a review article for a medical journal which would describe the biochemistry of the compound and its alterations in different clinical states. Although it was a review article, we had performed a number of studies of PRPP metabolism in humans which had not been published. These included the evaluation of patients with gout and the administration of some purine and pyrimidine compounds which did show alterations in PRPP levels. In the course of writing this review, we added this new data to the article.

"I believe that this article has been frequently quoted because it provided clinicians and scientists, for the first time, with a description of PRPP and its relevance to human disease. The appeal of this article was reflected in the acceptance of it, virtually unchanged, within five days of our submission of the manuscript to the *Annals of Internal Medicine*. It is interesting that one or two years after the publication of this article, the discovery of a PRPP synthetase mutation with enzyme overactivity as a cause of gout was reported by Odette Sperling[6] in Israel and Michael Becker[7] in the US. The majority of the information in the article remains as correct today as it was in 1971."

1. **Henderson J F & Khoo K Y.** Synthesis of 5-phosphoribosyl-1-pyrophosphate from glucose in Ehrlich ascites tumor cells *in vitro*. *J. Biol. Chem.* **240**:2349-57, 1965. (Cited 160 times.)
2. **Greene M L & Seegmiller J E.** Erythrocyte 5-phosphoribosyl-1-pyrophosphate (PRPP) in gout: importance of PRPP in the regulation of human purine synthesis. (Abstract.) *Arthritis Rheum.* **12**:666-7, 1969.
3. **Jones O W, Ashton D M & Wyngaarden J B.** Accelerated turnover of phosphoribosylpyrophosphate, a purine nucleotide precursor, in certain gouty subjects. *J. Clin. Invest.* **41**:1805-15, 1962.
4. **Hershko A, Hershko C & Mager J.** Increased formation of 5-phosphoribosyl-1-pyrophosphate in red blood cells of some gouty patients. *Isr. Med. J.* **4**:939-44, 1968.
5. **Fox I H, Wyngaarden J B & Kelley W N.** Depletion of erythrocyte phosphoribosylpyrophosphate (PRPP) in man: a newly observed effect of allopurinol. *N. Engl. J. Med.* **283**:1177-82, 1970. (Cited 80 times.)
6. **Sperling O, Boer P, Persky-Brosh S, Kanarek E & deVries A.** Altered kinetic property of erythrocyte phosphoribosylpyrophosphate synthetase in excessive purine production. *Rev. Eur. Etud. Clin. Biol.* **17**:703-6, 1972. (Cited 70 times.)
7. **Becker M A, Meyer L J, Wood A W & Seegmiller J E.** Purine overproduction in man associated with increased phosphoribosylpyrophosphate synthetase activity. *Science* **179**:1123-6, 1973. (Cited 80 times.)

This Week's Citation Classic

Huggett A St. G & Nixon D A. Use of glucose oxidase, peroxidase, and o-dianisidine in determination of blood and urinary glucose. *Lancet* **2**:368-70, 1957. [Dept. Physiol., Univ. London, and Dept. Physiol., St. Mary's Hosp. Med. Sch., London, England]

A method for estimating glucose specifically by the use of a fungal oxidase preparation and a chromogenic oxygen acceptor was described. It has proved of considerable value for the measurement of blood glucose in clinical medicine, as well as in other fields. [The *SCI®* indicates that this paper has been cited over 1,045 times since 1961.]

Marion Nixon
Wellcome Institute for the
History of Medicine
183 Euston Road
London NW1 2BP
and
Helen Huggett
49E Beaumont Street
London W1N IRE
England

April 13, 1981

"It is very sad that neither Professor Huggett, FRS, nor Dr. D.A. Nixon is alive to learn of the request for this *Citation Classic*. By the mid-1960s, both men realised that the paper was often referred to, and a number of scientists also visited the laboratory to discuss the method with them. The frequent citation of this paper is not difficult to understand for it provided a method for measuring glucose specifically and this has had widespread daily use in clinical medicine. It can perhaps best be regarded as a 'classical' method since it has now been in use for 20 years.

"Huggett's main interest was foetal and placental physiology, and his development of Caesarian section during late pregnancy of sheep and goats enabled him and his colleagues to study functions of the living foetus while still attached to the mother.

"In these investigations, Huggett and Nixon made many estimates of blood glucose in both foetal and maternal circulations. Since the blood of the sheep foetus contains fructose as well as glucose, the glucose was determined as the difference between total reducing power, measured by reduction of copper, and a direct estimate of fructose. Clearly a direct estimate of glucose was desirable. In 1956, a method based on the enzymic oxidation of glucose to gluconic acid with simultaneous production of hydrogen peroxide, which in turn, in the presence of peroxidase, acted on a chromophore whose oxidation product could be determined colourimetrically was discovered by A.S. Keston and J.D. Teller.[1,2] Keston applied his reagent to filter paper for testing urinary glucose. Teller modified the reagent and used it to test for glucose in blood plasma or serum. Huggett and Nixon modified Teller's method and worked out details suitable for estimating glucose in deproteinised blood and in decolourised urine using glucose oxidase prepared from *Penicillin notatum*. Their procedure requires a reagent simple to prepare, a constant temperature bath at 37°C, and a colourimeter or spectrophotometer. Colour develops in an hour and is stable for several hours."

1. **Keston A S.** Specific colorimetric enzymatic analytical reagents for glucose. *Abstracts of papers of the 129th meeting of the American Chemical Society, 8-13 April 1956, Dallas, Texas.* Washington, DC: American Chemical Society, 1956. p. 31-2C.
2. **Teller J D.** Direct, quantitative, colorimetric determination of serum or plasma glucose. *Abstracts of papers of the 130th meeting of the American Chemical Society, 16-21 September 1956, Atlantic City, New Jersey.* Washington, DC: American Chemical Society, 1956. p. 69C.

This Week's Citation Classic

CC/NUMBER 21
MAY 21, 1979

Gibson L E & Cooke R E. A test for concentration of electrolytes in sweat in cystic fibrosis of the pancreas utilizing pilocarpine by iontophoresis. *Pediatrics* **23**:545-49, 1959.

A method of inducing localized sweating by the iontophoretic induction of pilocarpine into the skin is described. It is shown that when this sweat is collected appropriately and analyzed for its sodium or chloride content the method is a simple and rapid means of diagnosing cystic fibrosis. [The *SCI*® indicates that this paper has been cited over 205 times since 1961.]

Lewis E. Gibson
Loyola University
Stritch School of Medicine
2160 South First Avenue
Maywood, IL 60253

March 17, 1978

"It is a pleasure to write this commentary since I enjoy recalling the stimulating, somewhat unstructured, environment in which the work was done and where my abiding fascination with the pathophysiology of cystic fibrosis originated.

"In 1953 Paul di Sant'Agnese discovered the strikingly elevated concentration of salt in the sweat of patients with cystic fibrosis.[1] My interest in these patients was stimulated by Harry Schwachman in 1953-55 when I was a house-officer in Boston. Therefore, when I became a clinical associate at the NIH in 1955, I welcomed the opportunity to study a group of CF patients. The fact that I worked in the Institute of Allergy and Infectious Diseases and that I was investigating the physiology of a genetic disease did not seem to bother anybody.

"I became interested in the effects of autonomically active drugs upon human sweat. Side effects made systemic administration unsatisfactory so I looked for a method of local stimulation. Iontophoresis was found to be ideal. Soon a number of drugs could be iontophoresed. Pilocarpine, also iontophoresed, was found to be a convenient cholinergic stimulator of the sweat I was attempting to modify.

"At that time the usual way of performing a sweat test for the diagnosis of CF was to place the subject's, usually nude, body in a plastic bag which fitted tightly around the neck. The procedure was time consuming, uncomfortable, and sometimes even dangerous. Iontophoresis obviously needed to move from the research to the diagnostic laboratory.

"The greatest impetus to make this move, however, came during a study of the sweat of obligate CF heterozygotes. Frequently the subjects were the mothers of CF patients. Their modesty seemed to have a positive correlation with their body weight. The task of persuading ladies with sweat soaked girdles to remain in hot plastic bags proved too difficult and iontophoresis became diagnostic.

"As a senior pediatric resident at Johns Hopkins, I found that the departmental chairman, Robert E. Cooke, shared my interest in CF sweat. He believed that the iontophoretic method of performing the sweat test was of sufficient importance to deserve publication and encouraged me to gather the data necessary to prove its efficacy.

"A method of stimulating localized sweating more convenient than pilocarpine iontophoresis has not been found, so our original paper continues to be cited. Sometimes, however, the manufacturers of $100.00 plus, current sources forget us for a fairly good reason: We stated that our current source cost $7.00. This included a zero labor cost which, though almost accurate for a resident physician at that time, could not apply to an electrician. We also forgot to price the EKG electrodes which were 'permanently borrowed' from Helen Tausig."

1. **di Sant'Agnese P A, Darling R C, Perera G A & Shea E.** Abnormal electrolyte composition of sweat in cystic fibrosis of the pancreas. *Pediatrics* **12**:549, 1953.

NUMBER 36
SEPTEMBER 3, 1979

This Week's Citation Classic

Liley A W. Liquor amnii analysis in the management of the pregnancy complicated by rhesus sensitization. *Amer. J. Obstet. Gynecol.* **82:**1359-70, 1961. [Postgraduate School of Obstetrics and Gynaecology, National Women's Hospital, Auckland, New Zealand]

A correlation was shown between the spectrophotometrically estimated bilirubinoid pigment concentration in amniotic fluid and the severity of fetal anemia in Rh hemolytic disease. The paper presents a method by which this correlation could be used with precision in selecting the optimal time for delivery of each baby. [The *SCI*® indicates that this paper has been cited over 285 times since 1961.]

A.W. Liley
University of Auckland
National Women's Hospital
Auckland 3, New Zealand

May 24, 1979

"Experience with newborn Rh babies in the mid 1950s persuaded me that, 15 years after the elucidation of the concept of hemolytic disease, the pediatric achievement had outstripped the obstetricians' ability.[1] The pediatricians, like the parents, were helplessly dependent on what time, luck, intrauterine life, and the obstetrician presented them with at birth. A carefully controlled study under the auspices of the British Medical Research Council had shown that routine premature delivery had nothing to offer. But logically some babies needed premature delivery to avoid stillbirth and some needed leaving alone.[2] At that time the only guides to likely severity were antibody titres and past history of affliction. While these were valid enough as statistical generalizations they were frequently very wide of the mark in individual babies.

"The most tragic blunder was the premature delivery of a baby on the strength of previous stillbirths only to find the baby was Rh negative and unaffected—and then to have the baby die from some complication of unnecessary prematurity. A concentration of several such episodes was the spur to introduce amniocentesis as British researchers had already shown the amniotic fluid was pigmented yellow with affected babies. The decision of whether to intervene and when had already been made from antibody titres and history and the only information sought from amniotic fluid was a written guarantee that the fetus was affected at all. This information was easy to supply but made little difference in the outcome. If the baby was unaffected no interference was necessary and if it was affected the severity was often such that intervention was unavailing. By this time, however, confidence had been gained in the technique of amniocentesis and the ability to recognize gradations of severity of anemia if allowance was made for maturity. Therefore policy was altered to extend amniocentesis to all women with antibodies of titre capable of harming a fetus irrespective of history. This permitted precise management by leaving to term those babies with no or insignificant affliction and progressively more premature delivery for more severely affected babies.

"The Rh baby was no longer treated in terms of statistical risk but for each individual baby the best compromise between anemia and prematurity could be achieved. This work has led not only to many other analyses of amniotic fluid to achieve precise fetal diagnosis in a variety of disorders but also directly, three years later, to intrauterine blood transfusion of the severely anemic Rh fetus unable to reach a deliverable maturity unaided.[3] Now for the first time an unborn baby could be ill, could be specifically diagnosed, and could receive and respond to treatment just like a patient in any other age group."

1. **Levine P, Katzin E M & Burnham L.** Isoimmunisation in pregnancy: its possible bearing on the etiology of erythroblastosis fetalis. *J. Amer. Med. Ass.* **116:**825-7, 1941.
2. **Mollison P L & Walker W.** Controlled trials of the treamtent of haemolytic disease of the newborn. *Lancet* **1:** 429-33, 1952.
3. **Liley A W.** Intrauterine transfusion of the foetus in haemolytic disease. *Brit. Med. J.* **2:**1107-9, 1963.

CC/NUMBER 49
DECEMBER 8, 1980

This Week's Citation Classic

Clark F & Horn D B. Assessment of thyroid function by the combined use of the serum protein-bound iodine and resin uptake of ^{131}I-triiodothyronine.
J. Clin. Endocrinol. Metab. **25**:39-45, 1965.
[Depts. Med. and Clin. Chem., Med. Sch., Univ. Newcastle upon Tyne and Royal Victoria Infirmary, Newcastle upon Tyne, UK]

A comparison was made of the diagnostic accuracy of the PBI, the resin uptake of ^{131}I-T3 and their mathematical product: the free thyroxine index. The latter was shown to give the better diagnostic discrimination in patients with thyroid disease and corrected for variations in protein binding of thyroid hormones seen in certain conditions, e.g., pregnancy. [The *SCI*® indicates that this paper has been cited over 250 times since 1965.]

Frederick Clark
Department of Medicine and Geriatrics
Freeman Hospital
Newcastle upon Tyne NE7 7DN
England

October 30, 1980

"This work evolved out of the investigation of the use of the red cell and resin uptake test of labelled thyroid hormones as a test of thyroid function following upon the earlier studies by Hamolsky, *et al.*,[1] Mitchell, *et al.*,[2] and Tabachnick.[3] Following the observations of Osorio, *et al.*,[4] in 1961 that the red cell uptake of I^{131} triiodothyronine was inversely related to the unsaturated or free binding sites on thyroxine binding proteins in plasma (FTBP), and their subsequent demonstration that an assessment of free thyroxine (FT4) in plasma (the generally accepted determinant of the thyroid status of an individual) could be obtained from the relationship between plasma protein-bound iodine (PBI) and the red cell uptake (Osorio, *et al.*[5]), we decided to examine the diagnostic reliability of the PBI, of the resin uptake of I^{131} triiodothyronine (resin uptake ratio RUR), and of their mathematical product the 'free thyroxine' index (FTI) which is an arbitrary figure assumed to be proportional to the concentrations of free thyroxine in the blood: FT 4 + FTBP = TBP.T4.

At equilibrium: $\frac{(FTBP)\ (FT4)}{(TBP.T4)} = K$ or

$1/K\ FT4 = \frac{TBPT4}{FTBP}$ assuming that

$FTBP = K'\ \frac{1}{RUR}$ and $TBPT4 = PBI$

$1/K'\ FT4(FTI) = PBI \times RUR.$

"The derived free thyroxine index so obtained correlated well with the clinical thyroid status of the patient (confirmed when necessary by supplementary tests) and in addition offered for better diagnostic discrimination than the PBI or resin uptake test alone. Furthermore in those subjects whose total thyroid hormones concentration was altered because of a change in the concentration of thyroid hormone binding protein (pregnancy, nephrotic syndrome) and was therefore misleading, the free thyroxine index largely corrected for the disparity.

"The original premise appears to have been borne out and we presume that this is the reason for the frequency of quotation. In addition the concept has been used to evaluate the binding of ligands to plasma proteins in other fields, e.g., clinical pharmacology.

"The work was carried out in the department of medicine and department of clinical biochemistry, University of Newcastle upon Tyne, by myself (as senior Luccock research fellow) and D.B. Horn largely during 1963 and owes much to the encouragement of Sir George A. Smart, professor of medicine, and A.L. Latner, professor of biochemistry at that time. Our particular thanks are due to the constant help and advice of S.G. Owen, former reader in medicine, University of Newcastle upon Tyne (presently at the Medical Research Council, London). The paper was submitted solely to the *Journal of Clinical Endocrinology and Metabolism* in May 1964 and was accepted by the editor after minor amendments and published in January of the following year. Horn is currently at the department of clinical chemistry, Western General Hospital, Edinburgh, Scotland."

1. **Hamolsky M W, Stein M & Freedberg A S.** The thyroid hormone-plasma protein complex in man. II. A new *in vitro* method for study of "uptake" of labelled hormonal components by human erythrocytes. *J. Clin. Endocrinol. Metab.* **17**:33-44, 1957. [Citation Classic. *Current Contents/Clinical Practice* (46):18, 17 November 1980.]
2. **Mitchell M L, Harden A B & O'Rourke M E.** The *in vitro* resin sponge uptake of triiodothyronine I^{131} from serum in thyroid disease and in pregnancy. *J. Clin. Endocrinol. Metab.* **20**:1474-83, 1960.
3. **Sterling K & Tabachnick M.** Resin uptake of I^{131} triiodothyronine as a test of thyroid function. *J. Clin. Endocrinol. Metab.* **21**:456-64, 1961.
4. **Osorio C, Jackson D J, Gartside J M & Goolden A W G.** The uptake of ^{131}I triiodothyronine by red cells in relation to the binding of thyroid hormones by plasma proteins. *Clin. Sci.* **21**:355-65, 1961.
5. --. The assessment of free thyroxine in plasma. *Clin. Sci.* **23**:525-30, 1962.

CC/NUMBER 26
JUNE 29, 1981

This Week's Citation Classic

Young D S & Hicks J M. Method for the automatic determination of serum iron. *J. Clin. Pathol.* **18**:98-102, 1965.
[Dept. Chemical Pathology, Postgraduate Medical School, London, England]

The existing time-consuming and cumbersome procedures for the determination of serum iron and iron-binding capacity prompted the adaptation of the method to the Technicon AutoAnalyzer. This greatly simplified the performance of the test in routine clinical laboratories. [The *SCI*® indicates that this paper has been cited over 220 times since 1965.]

Donald S. Young
Section of Clinical Chemistry
Department of Laboratory Medicine
Mayo Clinic
Rochester, MN 55901

May 28, 1981

"I started this work after I had completed my PhD and shortly after I had begun a residency in the department of chemical pathology at the Royal Postgraduate Medical School in London. Jocelyn Hicks, now director of clinical laboratories at Children's Hospital National Medical Center in Washington, DC, was at that time a biochemist in the same department and responsible for several of the tests in the routine laboratory.

"As part of their training in clinical chemistry, residents were expected to become familiar with all the routine tests. For me to learn the intricacies of AutoAnalyzer operation, it seemed logical to attempt to set up a new method on the instrument that might improve the efficiency of the laboratory. We decided to adapt the serum iron method to the AutoAnalyzer because the then manual procedure[1] for measuring iron was time-consuming and required great care in the preparation of glassware and reagents to ensure that they were iron-free. The need for absolutely iron-free reagents and equipment could be avoided with the AutoAnalyzer as a low iron background could be tolerated. To adapt the procedure to the AutoAnalyzer meant experimenting with one of the two AutoAnalyzer systems available in the laboratory, but not until after the daily workload of other tests had been completed and neither instrument was required for routine tests.

"The major problems encountered in setting up the procedure were identifying the most effective reducing agent, avoidance of turbidity caused by the use of acid to disrupt the iron-protein complex, and obtaining adequate sensitivity so that low concentrations of iron could be accurately determined. To minimize the latter problem, a large volume of serum had to be aspirated into the analytical system. This actually caused some differences in the rate of dialysis of iron from the serum and standard solutions, which we did not recognize at the time, which led to some inaccuracy in results. This was pointed out by Babson and Kleinman,[2] who overcame the problem by a simple modification of the original procedure. With the second generation of AutoAnalyzers inadequate sensitivity has been much less of a problem.

"Even though AutoAnalyzers are now used much less in clinical laboratories for single tests on a specimen, they are still widely used for iron measurements because totally iron-free reagents and equipment are not necessary as each specimen is read against a continuous reagent blank. There are several other widely used serum iron methods on AutoAnalyzers including procedures by Zak and Epstein[3] and Giovanniello *et al.*,[4] and because of this I am surprised that our paper has been cited so often."

1. **Ramsay W N M.** The determination of iron in blood plasma or serum. *Biochemical J.* **53**:227-31, 1953.
2. **Babson A L & Kleinman N M.** A source of error in an AutoAnalyzer determination of serum iron. *Clin. Chem.* **13**:163-6, 1967.
3. **Zak B & Epstein E.** Automated determination of serum iron. *Clin. Chem.* **11**:641-4, 1965.
4. **Giovanniello T J, Di Benedetto G, Palmer D W & Peters T, Jr.** Fully and semi-automated methods for the determination of serum iron and total iron-binding capacity. *J. Lab. Clin. Med.* **71**:874-83, 1968.

CC/NUMBER 45
NOVEMBER 8, 1982

This Week's Citation Classic

Hoffbrand A V, Newcombe B F A & Mollin D L. Method of assay of red cell folate activity and the value of the assay as a test for folate deficiency. *J. Clin. Pathol.* **19**:17-28, 1966.
[MRC Group for the Investigation of Megaloblastic and Sideroblastic Anaemias and Dept. Haematol., Postgraduate Med. Sch., London, England]

A method of assay of red cell folate was established using a microbiological assay. Red cell folate was then shown to be an excellent guide to tissue folate stores except in certain well-defined circumstances. [The *SCI*® indicates that this paper has been cited in over 265 publications since 1966.]

A. Victor Hoffbrand
Department of Haematology
Royal Free Hospital
London NW3 2QG
England

September 6, 1982

"When I joined David Mollin's laboratory at the Royal Postgraduate Medical School, London, in 1963, the assay of serum folate microbiologically using *Lactobacillus casei* had recently been established. Studies by Victor Herbert[1] in the US and Alan Waters[2] in Mollin's laboratory had shown that folate in serum was not always an accurate measure of the degree of folate deficiency since very low results could be obtained in many patients without any haematological evidence of the deficiency.

"A number of groups in Israel, Sweden, Canada, Holland, and Britain had already reported assays of whole blood folate using *L. casei* or *Streptococcus faecalis* but the results were not consistent or reproducible. It was clear, however, that most of the folate in blood was in the red cells, but, unlike folate in serum, red cell folate was largely in a conjugated (polyglutamated) form and had to be deconjugated before assay. Some workers added a deconjugating enzyme (folate conjugase), e.g., from chick pancreas; others relied on the conjugase present in plasma.

"I joined Beverley Newcombe, who had worked with Waters to determine the conditions necessary to achieve a maximum folate concentration in whole blood. Early experiments showed that distilled water was preferable to buffers for release of folate from red cells. As with the serum folate assay, it was necessary to add ascorbic acid to protect the folate from oxidative destruction in subsequent autoclaving. We showed that one in ten dilution of whole blood in distilled water containing one gram ascorbic acid per 100 ml gave a haemolysate with optimal release and stabilisation of folate. By happy coincidence, this ascorbate concentration lowered the pH of the haemolysate to approximately 4.6 which is optimum for the conjugase in plasma to deconjugate folate polyglutamates in red cells to microbiologically active monoglutamates.

"The presence of Barbara Anderson in the same laboratory, who had determined the optimum conditions for the serum vitamin B_{12} assay using *Euglena gracilis*,[3] ensured that the new assay would be fully tested by reproducibility and recovery experiments. It was then shown that the red cell folate was an excellent guide to tissue folate stores except in patients who had recently been transfused or had raised reticulocyte counts, or had vitamin B_{12} deficiency. In both vitamin B_{12} and folate deficiencies, the most anaemic patients had the lowest red cell folate levels, implying that the degree of depletion of tissue folate stores determined the severity of anaemia in both deficiencies.

"The assay became standard in studies of folate deficiency and metabolism. Moreover, the results in the paper indicated that the red cell folate assay was in general the best test for folate deficiency. It formed a cornerstone for subsequent studies[4] on folate deficiency in a wide variety of diseases. The fact that the paper has been so widely quoted is largely due to the determination of Mollin to leave no loose ends before publication, either in studies of the method or studies of the significance of the results obtained. The assay remains a standard diagnostic test for tissue folate status."

1. **Herbert V.** The assay and nature of folic acid activity in human serum. *J. Clin. Invest.* **40**:81-91, 1961.
2. **Waters A H & Mollin D L.** Studies on the folic acid activity of human serum. *J. Clin. Pathol.* **14**:335-44, 1961.
3. **Anderson B B.** Investigation into the Euglena method for the assay of vitamin B_{12} in serum. *J. Clin. Pathol.* **17**:14-26, 1964.
4. **Chanarin I.** Folate in blood, CSF and tissues. *The megaloblastic anaemias.* Oxford: Blackwell Scientific, 1979. p. 187-97.

CC/NUMBER 41
OCTOBER 11, 1982

This Week's Citation Classic

Lendrum A C, Fraser D S, Slidders W & Henderson R. Studies on the character and staining of fibrin. *J. Clin. Pathol.* **15**:401-13, 1962.
[University of St. Andrews Department of Pathology, Royal Infirmary, Dundee, Scotland]

The technical aim was methods sensitive for fibrin with coincident portrayal of local tissues; the pathological aim was to elucidate different fibrinous vasculoses. Fibrinous vasculosis is deposition of fibrin within, and possibly beyond, the wall of blood vessels without visible fibrin in the lumen. This interstitial fibrin undergoes change with time, showing affinity for larger molecule dyes. The last stage is a pseudo-collagen. [The *SCI*® indicates that this paper has been cited in over 290 publications since 1962.]

A.C. Lendrum
Department of Pathology
Royal Infirmary
Dundee DD1 9ND
Scotland

August 23, 1982

"An almost explosive interest in the structural character of renal disease followed the conjunction in medical practice of needle-biopsy and EM techniques. The time was therefore ripe for a simple trichromic staining method able to show, at the variable magnifications of the light microscope, not only the presence but also the actual situation of fibrinous deposits. Our attempt to explain the underlying principle of trichromic methods and to illustrate the results in colour may well have enticed histopathologists, other than nephrologists, to adopt the methods and to apply them in the study of the group of diseases characterized by zonal hyperpermeability of blood vessels. These diseases cover a wide range: from urticaria to polyarteritis nodosa; from the kidney of diabetes mellitus to that of malignant hypertension; from the fibrin-soaked vessel walls of a torsed tissue to the hyaline broadening of the intima in senile arteries.

"Subsequent studies on the methods and their applications particularly to the diabetic kidney showed that the fibrinous deposits within the vessel walls and beyond (what we called 'fibrinous vasculosis'), eliciting no xenophobic reaction, undergo intrinsic alteration with time. As it ages, the fibrin loses its affinity for the small anionic dyes and takes the larger anionic dyes that characteristically in trichromic methods stain collagen. Thus, the old fibrin becomes a pseudo-collagen and we have to question the canonical views on hyalin.[1,2] The fact that the sites and shapes of amyloid deposits in the kidney so remarkably resemble the fibrinous deposits in the diabetic kidney[2] is surely of significance to those interested in amyloidosis. Finally, considering the growing interest in dysoria,[3] definable as an upset of the normal balance between the selective permeability of the vessel's wall and the pressure within the vessel, and the fact that fibrinous vasculosis is the visible result of the less sudden and less destructive degrees of dysoria, it is perhaps not surprising that there is increasing interest in staining methods for fibrin.

"Another possible explanation of the interest in our article could be enticement by the excellent colour reproduction of the photomicrographs, and I now submit that the printers did even better in two related subsequent publications.[1,2] To this I would add the wise caution[3] of the same H. Edward MacMahon who was at the birth of dysoria,[4] 'Most of us are inclined to regard an investigator's first paper as his final opinion on a particular subject.' As far as I am concerned the paper of 1962 is neither the first nor the last on this particular matter.

"It has been my good fortune in Glasgow and then Dundee to have as fellow workers senior technicians who have collaborated wholeheartedly and played their part in contributing their skill and their ideas. It was, therefore, a great thrill and surprise to receive, as had my onetime encouraging teacher and later colleague, the late D.F. Cappell, the rare honour of the Sims Woodhead Medal for Services to Medical Laboratory Technology, presented by the Institute of Medical Laboratory Sciences."

1. **Lendrum A C.** The validation of fibrin and its significance in the story of hyalin. (Association of Clinical Pathologists) *Trends in clinical pathology: essays in honour of Gordon Signy.* London: British Medical Association, 1969. p. 160-87.
2. **Lendrum A C, Slidders W & Fraser D S.** Renal hyalin, a study of amyloidosis and diabetic fibrinous vasculosis with new staining methods. *J. Clin. Pathol.* **25**:373-96, 1972.
3. **MacMahon H E.** Malignant nephrosclerosis. (Sommers S C, ed.) *Pathology annual.* New York: Meredith, 1958. p. 297-334.
4. **Schürmann P & MacMahon H E.** Die maligne Nephrosklerose zugleich ein Beitrage zur Frage der Bedeutung der Blutgewebsschranke. *Virchows Arch. Path. Anat.* **291**:47-218, 1933.

Chapter

3

Immunology and Rheumatology

Traditionalists will surely not quarrel with the division of this chapter into those two historic sectors (the word domains probably should have been used) of cellular and humoral immunology. The only weakness here that the traditionalists might seize upon is the placement of the Citation Classics on cellular aspects of immunology before those on the humoral topics.

Cellular Immunology

The emphasis on cellular immunology noted in volume 1 of *Contemporary Classics in the Life Sciences* is evidenced here also by the grouping of 29 of the 46 Classics on immunologic topics in this section of the chapter. Other Classics in Chapter 4 on Oncology and Chapter 5 on Hematology are related to some of those grouped here.

The journal article derived from Bain's Ph.D. dissertation on the topic of mixed leukocyte culturing (MLC) introduces this chapter. T cells are stimulated into a reproductive cycle when lymphocytes from genetically unrelated individuals are mixed. These cells are effector cells in graft rejection and in the elimination of virus-infected cells and tumor cells. The MLC reaction is still performed today for the selection of suitable tissue donors for transplantation surgery. Moore's Classic is somewhat related in that he and his colleagues, with the aid of tissue culture medium RPMI 1640, were able to establish long-term cultures of normal—nonmalignant—lymphocytes for the first time. Whether the injection of billions of these cells into an individual is absolute proof of nonmalignancy of the total population could be questioned by hard-line skeptics, but certainly the population contained an insufficient number of such cells to establish a malignant growth (leukemia) *in vivo.*

Moore seems disappointed (see his last paragraph) that their method was so successful that it is now considered only as a "service function" to provide large quantities of cells for other purposes. Markers on lymphocyte surfaces have been valuable in the separation and identification of T-cell subsets because these cells are not easily distinguished by differences in morphology. Though at first rejecting Seligmann's advice to study surface-bound immunoglobulins on human lymphocytes, Preud'homme returned to this topic successfully with the discovery that lymphoproliferative disorders could be classified according to the presence or absence of this surface marker. Some of the B-cell leukemias would fall into the first category. Aisenberg and Bloch published a similar study in the same year on chronic lymphocytic leukemia. They also determined that the surface immunoglobulin was of a single structural class, thus supporting the clonal concept of oncogenesis. The statement in the next to last paragraph of their "This Week's Citation Classic" (TWCC) that this "was to be the last manuscript on a subject as outlandish as lymphocyte surface markers to be published by the journal," which the authors attribute to the editors of the *New England Journal of Medicine,* is an historic example of overstatement.

In the 1960s, following earlier studies in chickens, mammalian lymphocytes were learned to exist as a separate subset of B and T cells. In 1964, Nezelof and his colleagues identified the rare condition of hereditary thymic aplasia in which the T-cell population is absent or markedly diminished. The penalty of this genetic condition was a severe immunodeficiency. The reward was a recognition that thymocytes and plasmocytes were of independent cellular lineage. The next year, Di George reported basically the same form of immunodeficiency from a non-inheritable defect in thymic embryogenesis. During this period, many investigators sought to identify the exact role of T cells in host immunity. Claman and Chaperon, in pursuit of this goal, uncovered the role of helper T cells as necessary partners of the B cells in the production of antibodies (at least to one set of antigens, the T-cell-dependent antigens). Their use of the "test tube mouse," a lethally irradiated animal that could be reconstituted with lymphocytes mixtures chosen by the experimenter was a key to their success. This innovation was soon adopted by many immunologists.

Loss of thymic function as a result of protein-calorie nutrition (p. 70), or in neoplastic transformations such as Hodgkin's disease, renders the individual more susceptible to infectious disease and alters the response to BCG vaccination (p. 71). At the cellular level this is reflected by a failure of the T lymphocyte to demonstrate positive responses to certain antigens or mitogens (p. 72). The balance of the helper and suppressor subpopulations of T cells is important in many immunologic phenomena, including autoimmunity. This is discussed by Allison, who rightly states that a loss of T suppressors or a dominance by T helpers may result in the unwanted, self-directed activity of the immune system that results in autoimmune disease.

Malignantly transformed T cells were shown by Edelson et al. to be the basis for cutaneous lymphocytic lymphoma, often referred to as Sezary syndrome. Lymphomas or leukemias that did not significantly involve the skin were predominantly B cell in origin. An understanding of T- and B-cell markers and an application of the proper reagents permitted this conclusion to be achieved and to be supported by later investigators.

The normal behavior of T cells can often be analyzed by their influence on other cells since T cells excrete numerous cytokines. Clausen forwarded an agarose plate technique for quantitating the excretion by T cells of a substance that would inhibit the motility of macrophages, the macrophage migration inhibitor. This method is inexpensive and facile, and allows for numerous determinations on a single plate. Weissmann's article described in a more general vein how enzymes released from phagocytic cells, particularly their lysosomes, could provoke an acute inflammatory response.

Although surface markers are now in extensive use for identifying white blood cells, cytochemical procedures were used earlier for this purpose and remain useful, as described in the TWCC by Yam and Li.

The uncommon genetic failure to synthesize the α_2 neuraminoglycoprotein, a molecule that controls the activated form of the first component of the complement system, causes the condition known as hereditary angioneurotic edema (p. 78). This illness, partially misnamed since it has no relationship to neurosis, was the first described as due to the loss of a complement-regulating molecule.

The TWCCs on autoimmune diseases are introduced by Doniach's commentary and the observation that patients with primary biliary cirrhosis, but not most other liver diseases, contained autoantibodies in their sera that reacted with mitochondria. The two autoimmune dermatologic conditions, pemphigus and bullous pemphigoid, were among the first of the autoimmune states to be described, yet until recently have been hidden in the shadows of better known autoimmune conditions such as Hashimoto's thyroiditis and systemic lupus erythematosus. In the first paragraph of Beutner's TWCC on these two dermodestructive diseases, he includes some personal data about his family's past in medical science. His second and third paragraphs beg for a more quantitative approach to immunocytochemistry.

The next three TWCCs on systemic lupus erythematosus (SLE) amply support the role of DNA-anti-DNA complexes in the pathophysiology of this disease. The deposition of these complexes in the kidney is responsible for SLE nephritis. The presence of circulating antibodies to double-stranded DNA in patient sera is useful in the diagnosis of this disease, though numerous other antigen-antibody systems under current study may prove superior. Pincus attributes the success of his contribution to the role of DNA-binding globulins in SLE to the enlightened leadership of his mentors and the unstructured working environment that permitted a successful conclusion from a poorly articulated research plan. The third TWCC on SLE is the result of a committee study to classify this disease entity. Among the criteria suggested, one of the most important was autoantibodies.

The relative risk relationship of the autoimmune disease ankylosing spondylitis to the presence of antigen HLA-27 (now HLA-B27) exceeds 90 percent. The proximity of the genes for the transplantation antigens with those that control immune responses on human chromosome 6 is the basis for this phenomenal association. The study that reached this conclusion (p. 84) was criticized for failing to demonstrate a statistical proof that 96 percent (72 of 75 patients) and 4 percent (3 of 75 controls) were statistically different. Years earlier (p. 85), it had been learned that the lymphocytes of patients with ankylosing spondylitis were fragile to X-rays.

Sarcoidosis and amyloidosis are two diseases with immunologic components that have not yet been assigned specific causes. The startling events that preceded the publication of the Citation Classic by Kissmeyer-Nielsen et al. would be humorous in a different setting. First there was the denial of a lecture opportunity at an international conference. This was followed by a limitation of 3 minutes for a lecture in which "only one slide" was allowed at a second international conference. Then the rejection of their manuscript by *Lancet* became the final blow. Ultimately, *Lancet* accepted the article. In the 5 years following the publication, Kissmeyer-Nielsen received four prizes for showing that preexisting antibodies were the cause of hyperacute graft rejection. Truly a trial by fire with a happy ending.

The two-part review by Thomas et al. on bone marrow transplantation has been cited more than 800 times. The transplant team at the University of Washington is world renowned for their development and improvement of this procedure. Most readers will surely be unaware that 1,179 marrow transplants had been conducted by early 1982.

The next three Citation Classics turn to immunodeficiency. The first is on malignancy in immunodeficiency states, the second is on the absence of the enzyme adenosine deaminase (ADA) in one class of patients with a T-cell deficiency, and the third is on a phagocytic deficiency. Lack of the ADA enzyme or the closely related purine nucleotide phosphorylase (PNP) allows the suicidal accumulation of deoxyribonucleotides within T lymphocytes. Erythrocyte infusions provide the needed enzymes and temporary relief from this deficiency. The last paper identifies the hereditary disease chronic granulomatous disease as a defect in oxidative metabolism by granulocytes. This genetic fault is detected by the failure of these cells to reduce nitroblue tetrazolium (NBT) to its insoluble formazan state. When reduced, the dye is visually detectable in the cells, from which it can then be extracted for spectrophotometric determination. This article is related to the NBT-based article in Chapter 1, Microbiology and Infectious Disease.

Immunoglobulins and Serologic Reactions

Bruton's discovery of human agammaglobulinemia is an oft-told tale, frequently presented to medical students as an introduction to a lecture series on immunodeficiency diseases. It is a pleasure to read his own account of how this condition was diagnosed in a young boy (it is a sex-linked character) who was treated for pneumococcal infections with penicillin on 10 separate occasions prior to diagnosis and successful treatment. Although it is easy to detect a total loss of immunoglobulins, it was not until 1966 (p. 94) that standard serum values of these antibodies were established for infants, children, and adults. From these data partial losses could then be identified, or conversely, excessive quantities could be recognized. This second possibility is useful in establishing the existence of in utero infections or aberrations in globulin synthesis. Axelsson et al. found that 64 of the 6,995 adults examined had an increased quantity of an immunoglobulin in their circulation. This excess is the result of immunoglobulin synthesis by myeloma cells, hence the term M-component. This conclusion would not have been possible in the absence of a table of normal values unless the M-component was so excessive as to be detectable by ordinary electrophoresis as a spike in the serum globulin profile. Overproduction of only the heavy-chain portion of IgG is described in Franklin's TWCC, which also includes the prediction, later met, that aberrant heavy chains of the other immunoglobulins would eventually be found.

A "series" of three hepatitis patients fortuitously falling into the categories of carrier, fatal outcome, and chronic liver disease enabled Almeida and Waterson to recognize immune complexes of hepatitis B virus in blood and to determine that the virus was most virulent when complexed with antibody. The concept of disease due to an immune response had encountered serious opposition after the suggestion of this possibility by von Pirquet, but contemporary immunologists recognize that molecules of the immunoglobulin and complement series are instrumental agents in many inflammatory reactions. The most powerful support of this idea is found in IgE, recognized by the Ishizakas and Hornbrook to be identical to the allergic reagin found in the blood of persons with atopic illness. Their study was contemporary with that of the Swedish scientists who had identified an IgE myeloma protein and then learned that IgE levels were unusually high in persons with atopic dermatitis (p. 99) or in Ethiopian children where the incidence of intestinal worm infestations is high (p. 100). Ovary's review on immediate-type skin reactions in experimental animals measures the lower animal homolog of human IgE and is thus related to the two immediately preceding Citation Classics.

The only other Classic based on the development of a serologic reaction other than a radioimmunoassay is that described by Vyas. The ease by which erythrocytes bind extraneous proteins and polysaccharides makes them useful carriers for antigens and a sensitive indicator via hemagglutination of any reaction of that antigen with antibody. This type of passive hemagglutination was advanced in the 1950s by Boyden. The popularity of the article by Vyas and Shulman was dependent upon the need for a rapid and simple assay for hepatitis B virus. It is remarkable, even given the simplicity of the hemagglutination assay, that a patentable project and respected publication could be accomplished in only 6 days of bench time. In a different context the statements by Vyas' chairman are also remarkable.

The next seven Citation Classics all describe articles on radioimmunoassays (RIAs)—for insulin, digoxin, angiotensin, testosterone, chorionic gonadotropin, and prolactin. Despite the proven need for procedures to quantitate these molecules and the obvious value that these RIAs have had in clinical laboratory medicine, one can't escape that jaded feeling of "Oh, another RIA" when reading the titles of the original articles. It is shameful how history has skewed our perspective. In the 1960s when these procedures were being developed, RIA methodology was one of the most exciting advances in immunology. By the late 1970s, RIAs were legion and available to measure virtually any molecule with the faintest semblance of importance. Consequently, in looking at these seven Classics from this point in time, they appear as seven among scores, or even hundreds, of similar articles. This is not at all intended as a disparaging remark. What must *not* be overlooked is the importance that these articles had in their own time. This is indicated in Soeldner's TWCC in which he states that over 100 visitors learned the RIA procedure for insulin in their laboratory, and in Nieschlag's statement that samples of the critical antiserum were distributed to more than 140 laboratories. Sinha states that his group shared reagents with clinicians and investigators throughout the world. The RIA procedures were obviously important advances at their time and, though modified many times (see Nieschlag's TWCC), have had an important role in human medicine, even though largely supplanted by enzyme-linked immunosorbent assay (ELISA) methods by the 1980s.

The large number of Citation Classics in this chapter prevent a uniform reflection of their content through the selection of a few recent reviews. Nevertheless, newly published articles on T and B cells, complement, IgE, autoimmune disease, immunodeficiency, and transplantation are provided. These references to some extent reflect the wide assortment of review journals available in immunology. In addition to those listed here, review articles can be found in such journals as *Monographs in Allergy, Contemporary Topics in Molecular Immunology, Current Topics in Microbiology and Immunology,* and *Seminars in Arthritis and Rheumatology.* Because of the topical interest in immunology in all parts of medicine, significant publications in this field can be found in a wide array of journals.

Bach M A. Immunoregulatory T cells in multiple sclerosis: markers and functions. *Springer Semin. Immunopathol.* **8:**45–56, 1986.

Chirigos M A & Talmadge J E. Immunotherapeutic agents: their role in cellular immunity and their therapeutic potential. *Springer Semin. Immunopathol.* **8:**327–46, 1985.

Giles R C & Capra J D. Structure, function, and genetics of human class II molecules. *Adv. Immunol.* **37:**1–71, 1985.

Howard M. Soluble-factor induction of B cell growth. *Contemp. Top. Mol. Immunol.* **10:**181–93, 1985.

Ishizaka T & Ishizaka K. Activation of mast cells for mediator release through IgE receptors. *Prog. Allergy* **34:**188–235, 1984.

Jordan B R & 15 co-authors. HLA class I genes: from structure to expression, serology and function. *Immunol. Rev.* **84:**73–92, 1985.

Kay A B. Eosinophils as effector cells in immunity and hypersensitivity disorders. *Clin. Exp. Immunol.* **62:**1–12, 1985.

Lane H C & Fauci A S. Immunologic abnormalities in the acquired immune deficiency syndrome. *Annu. Rev. Immunol.* **3:**477–500, 1985.

Leung D T M & Geha R S. Regulation of IgE synthesis in man. *Clin. Immunol. Rev.* **3:**1–24, 1984.

Nusinow S R, Zuraw B L & Curd J G. The hereditary and acquired deficiencies of complement. *Med. Clin. North Am.* **69:**487–504, 1985.

Rogers J & Wall R. Immunoglobulin RNA rearrangements in B lymphocyte differentiation. *Adv. Immunol.* **35:**39–59, 1984.

Salinas F A, Wee K H & Silver H K. Clinical relevance of immune complexes, associated antigen, and antibody in cancer. *Contemp. Top. Immunobiol.* **15:**55–109, 1985.

Schrader J W. Bone marrow differentiation *in vitro. CRC Crit. Rev. Immunol.* **4:**197–277, 1983.

Towbin H & Gordon J. Immunoblotting and dot immunobinding—current status and outlook. *J. Immunol. Methods* **72:**313–40, 1984.

Tsokos G C & Balow J E. Cellular immune responses in systemic lupus erythematosus. *Prog. Allergy* **35:**93–161, 1984.

Vitetta E S & Uhr J W. Immunotoxins. *Annu. Rev. Immunol.* **3:**197–212, 1985.

Warr G W, Vasta G R, Marchalo J J, Allen R C & Anderson D P. Molecular analysis of the lymphocyte membrane. *Dev. Comp. Immunol.* **8:**757–72, 1984.

NUMBER 11
MARCH 12, 1979

Bain B, Vas M R & Lowenstein L. The development of large immature mononuclear cells in mixed leukocyte cultures. *Blood* **23**: 108-16, 1964.

In mixed leukocyte cultures prepared from pairs of normal unrelated donors, some of the lymphocytes became transformed to large cells capable of mitosis. Subsequent experiments indicated that transformation was stimulated by genetically determined factors in leukocytes. A relationship to transplantation immunity was suggested. [The *SCI*® indicates that this paper has been cited over 505 times since 1964.]

Barbara Bain
Zoology Department
University of Western Ontario
London, Ontario, Canada N6A 5B7

March 4, 1978

"My observation of the mixed leukocyte reaction is a classical example of a discovery that was bound to happen. It happened to me because I was in the right place at the right time.

"In the early 1960s, Magdalene Vas came to the Royal Victoria Hospital in Montreal to do research on leukocyte cultures. I was employed as her technician, and I soon became so interested in these studies that I wanted to continue them as a Ph.D. student. Our chief, the late Louis Lowenstein, was enthusiastic about the idea and had me enrolled at McGill University before I had a chance to change my mind.

"Just around this time, Peter Nowell published a paper showing that the bean extract phytohemagglutinin (PHA) could induce normal leukocytes to undergo mitosis.[1] Vas and I (undoubtedly along with many others) tried the technique and found that it worked. Very soon thereafter, it was demonstrated that tuberculin caused mitosis in leukocyte cultures from sensitive individuals, and evidence accumulated that small lymphocytes were the responding cells. It was suggested that PHA and tuberculin stimulated lymphocytes in a manner analogous to immune responses *in vivo.*

"These notions were roaming around inside my head when I read a paper by Schrek and Donnelly, in which they reported large, primitive mitotic cells in a culture containing mixed leukocytes from two donors.[2] Their main objectives in the study were along other lines, so they made no further comment on this phenomenon. Because of the way my mind was tuned at the time, I suspected that the changes observed in the mixed culture were the result of antigenic differences between the two donors. I immediately recruited two of my colleagues to donate blood for cultures, and five days later I found primitive cells, mitoses, and a topic for my Ph.D. thesis.

"My initial assumption, based on no logic whatsoever, was that ABO blood group differences were causing the stimulation. Therefore my first pairs of donors were A and B combinations. I then decided to run a 'negative' control using Vas and myself, both group O. The result was by no means negative, which disproved my poorly conceived hypothesis and cleared the way for a more rational approach to the mixed leukocyte reaction.

"I believe that the interest in my work was due to the novelty of the observation, set against a background of progress and excitement in the areas of lymphocyte function and transplantation immunity. As I indicated at the beginning of this article, I was very fortunate to have a head start in the discovery of the mixed leukocyte reaction: Chapman and Dutton,[3] and their rabbits, were close behind!"

REFERENCES

1. **Nowell P C.** Phytohemagglutinin: an initiator of mitosis in cultures of normal human leukocytes. *Cancer Res.* **20**: 462-6, 1960.
2. **Schrek R & Donnelly W J.** Differences between lymphocytes of leukemic and non-leukemic patients with respect to morphologic features, motility, and sensitivity to guinea pig serum. *Blood* **18**: 561-71, 1961.
3. **Chapman N D & Dutton R W.** The simulation of DNA synthesis in cultures of rabbit lymph node and spleen cell suspensions by homologous cells. *J. Exp. Med.* **121**: 85-100, 1965.

This Week's Citation Classic

Moore G E, Gerner R E & Franklin H A. Culture of normal human leukocytes.
J. Amer. Med. Ass. **199**:519-24, 1967.
[Dept. Surgery, Roswell Park Memorial Institute, Buffalo, NY]

This paper describes establishment of continuous permanent normal lymphocyte cell lines derived from the peripheral blood which many 'basic' scientists said couldn't be done and was actually a malignant transformation. Culture medium RPMI 1640 was an evolution of over 1000 media designed for human cells. [The *SCI*® indicates that this paper has been cited over 390 times since 1967.]

George E. Moore
Division of Surgical Oncology
Denver General Hospital
Denver, CO 80204

May 30, 1980

"I began cell culture in an attempt to grow cancer cells circulating in the blood in order to prove that such cells were viable even though only a few of them ever established metastases. It's the sort of research a surgeon can do between cases.

"The epic paper by Epstein and Barr[1] on the successful culture of Burkitt's lymphoma cells provoked a heated argument as to why normal lymphocytes and other bone marrow cells couldn't be established as cell lines. Other scientists had undoubtedly derived normal B-lymphocyte cell lines from bone marrow and leukemia blood but could not accept the theses: 1) that normal cells could be 'immortalized,' and 2) that cell lines from patients with leukemias and lymphomas could be other than malignant.

"The presence of an innocuous and perhaps useful passenger EB-virus in normal B-lymphocytes was and is a difficult concept for most scientists to accept despite the acceptance that sterility of the gut is detrimental.

"Once we established these B-lymphoid cell lines, we immediately attempted to grow cells from patients with genetic disorders, and unique malignant cells, and to design a cell plant for the growth of kilogram amounts of normal lymphoid cells for virus research and in the hope that they could be used for cancer therapy. We did grow about 90 kilograms of cells one year in a cell plant, and infused large amounts of cells in several volunteer patients with advanced malignant disease. This early attempt at cellular therapy for malignant disease was inhibited by our failure to increase the ratio of killer B-cells. The normalcy of the billions of infused cells was confirmed by subsequent freedom of any evidence of leukemia.

"I foresee a future in which we will culture and establish many normal functional human cells as cell lines. The dogma of the finite life of some cells may not be true of many other cells.

"The era of genetic and biochemical studies of bacteria is gradually being superseded by studies of mammalian (and human) cells. The lymphoid cell lines derived from a few drops of peripheral blood provide convenient means for screening and for comparative studies of those amazing sausages of information—the chromosomes. Intermediate methodology such as hybridomas and the growth of malignant cells will be replaced by the culture of functional normal cells as growth factors are identified. The production of interferon is a crude example of the future ability to produce in the laboratory specific hormones, proteins, enzymes, antigens, and antibodies from cultured cells. Special media without foreign protein will be used to grow large amounts of cells for cellular therapy—the replacement of erythroid and megakaryocyte precursors, islet cells for diabetics, autochthonous leukocytes to combat infection, skin cells to cover burns, and the culture of lymphoid cells to search out and destroy malignant cells.

"Our comments in this article are rarely quoted despite or because they proved to be quite accurate and now just 13 years later these studies are described in a grant critique as 'service functions!' "

1. **Epstein M A & Barr Y M.** Cultivation in vitro of human lymphoblasts from Burkitt's malignant lymphoma. *Lancet* **1**:252-3, 1964.

CC/NUMBER 47
NOVEMBER 22, 1982

This Week's Citation Classic

Preud'homme J L & Seligmann M. Surface bound immunoglobulins as a cell marker in human lymphoproliferative diseases. *Blood* **40**:777-94, 1972. [Lab. Immunochemistry and Immunopathology, Research Inst. on Blood Diseases, Hôpital Saint-Louis, Paris, France]

The paper provides evidence for the monoclonality of human B cell proliferations and introduces several concepts such as those of blocked or persistent maturation of proliferating cells, biclonal proliferation, and changes in the nature of proliferating clones. It shows the frequent exogenous origin of surface immunoglobulins, especially IgG. [The *SCI*® indicates that this paper has been cited in over 465 publications since 1972.]

Jean Louis Preud'homme
Laboratory of Immunology
and Immunopathology
C.H.U.R. La Milétrie
86021 Poitiers
France

September 20, 1982

"By the end of the 1960s, data on surface immunoglobulins (SIg) of mouse and rabbit lymphocytes were reported at several meetings. I worked in Paris in INSERM Research Unit No. 108 with Maxime Seligmann. He was immediately convinced that SIg were potentially a fantastic tool for studying human lymphocytes and advised me very strongly to work in this area. I refused. Indeed, I was not ready to admit from available data that SIg were not merely cytophilic immunoglobulins. Some months later, a long conversation with Ben Pernis during a meeting made me believe enough of the story to spend some time in his laboratory in Milan, where Luciana Forni showed me her methods for SIg staining and eventually convinced me that it was worth doing some preliminary experiments.

"Back in Paris, it soon became apparent that the microscope and reagents which we had long used for cytoplasmic staining were inadequate. Getting a microscope equipped with Ploem's illuminator was easy. Preparing conjugated antisera suitable for surface immunofluorescence turned out to require hard work. In fact, this is still a major problem today (only a few laboratories have clean reagents) and it is not surprising that it took us a long time to obtain strong monospecific conjugates devoid of nonspecific staining. Developing a reproducible method to prove SIg synthesis (based upon *in vitro* regrowth after stripping by proteolytic enzymes) was not easy either.

"Due to my initial skepticism, I began studying SIg on human lymphocytes much later than certain other investigators. However, I believe it to be the major reason why our work was sound and subsequently confirmed by other—sometimes very recent and elegant—studies.[1,2] Indeed, being already late to begin with, I was not in a hurry and took all the time needed to work out a reliable methodology. Then, with the exceptional clinical material from the Hôpital Saint-Louis's hematology department, cells from a number (116) of selected patients could be studied relatively quickly. We could therefore draw firm conclusions on the B cell nature and monoclonality (based upon SIg isotype and antibody activity restriction) of most lymphoproliferative diseases and describe maturation blocks or persistent differentiation of proliferating clones, biclonal proliferations, non-IgM Waldenstroem-like syndrome, and B cell acute leukemia. We also suggested the T cell nature of Sezary cells and first reported results on cold agglutinin disease and heavy chain diseases, mentioned the difficulties in the study of hairy cells, and pointed out that immunoglobulins found on fresh cells are not necessarily actual cell products.

"The paper therefore deals with many aspects of immunoproliferative diseases and B cell physiology. In view of the incredible inflation of the literature in clinical immunology, it is not very surprising that it is cited quite often. However, reasons for its citation are not always the ones discussed earlier. The paper was indeed often misquoted (to support opposite conclusions or contradictorily to introduce reports of similar findings) and also sometimes carefully omitted from reference lists.

"For a report of recent work in the field, see *Leukemia Markers*."[3]

1. **Fu S M, Winchester R J, Feizi T, Walzer P D & Kunkel H G.** Idiotypic specificity of surface immunoglobulin and the maturation of leukemic bone marrow derived lymphocytes. *Proc. Nat. Acad. Sci. US* **71**:4487-91, 1974.
2. **Stevenson F K, Hamblin T J, Stevenson G T & Tutt A L.** Extra-cellular idiotypic immunoglobulin arising from human leukemic B lymphocytes. *J. Exp. Med.* **152**:1484-96, 1980.
3. **Knapp W**, ed. *Leukemia markers*. London: Academic Press, 1981. 574 p.

CC/NUMBER 24
JUNE 14, 1982

This Week's Citation Classic

Aisenberg A C & Bloch K J. Immunoglobulins on the surface of neoplastic lymphocytes. *N. Engl. J. Med.* **287**:272-6, 1972.
[John Collins Warren Labs., Huntington Memorial Hosp., Harvard Univ., and Robt. W. Lovett Memorial Group for the Study of Diseases Causing Deformities, Massachusetts General Hosp., Boston, MA]

The neoplastic lymphocytes of nearly all of 25 patients with chronic lymphocytic leukemia (CLL) were shown to bear surface immunoglobulin (Ig) molecules of a single heavy (mu) and light chain (either kappa or lambda) type. B lymphocytes show a similar restriction of their surface Ig to a single heavy and light chain type. Thus, the observations in CLL provided evidence for the clonal origin of the neoplastic cells and established their B-cell lineage. [The *SCI*® indicates that this paper has been cited over 350 times since 1972.]

Alan C. Aisenberg
and
Kurt J. Bloch
Department of Medicine
Massachusetts General Hospital
Boston, MA 02114

April 9, 1982

"In 1970, Martin Raff[1] presented a seminar at Massachusetts General Hospital describing the identification of murine B lymphocytes by the presence of immunoglobulin (Ig) in their surface membrane. It was apparent that this simple method could be directly applied to human cells. Lymphocytes from patients with chronic lymphocytic leukemia (CLL) seemed to be an especially appropriate cell type to be studied by Raff's technique, because there already existed suggestive, but not conclusive, evidence that CLL represented a B-cell proliferative disorder.

"In the work described, we took a number of shortcuts because of the limited funds available and the realization that there was need for some urgency since other investigators would also be stimulated by Raff's observation. Thus, instead of producing our own fluoresceinated anti-immunoglobulin antisera, we bought commercial products, albeit those of highest quality. We examined cells stained with these reagents by fluorescence microscopy rather than using quantitative assays. The presence of contaminating antibodies in some commercial products posed difficulties which were overcome by appropriate absorptions. With that detail attended to, 25 patients with CLL and a small number of individuals with other lymphomas were studied with gratifying results: the neoplastic cells from nearly all cases of CLL and most of the other lymphomas were unequivocally of B-cell lineage. The surface Ig of the neoplastic cells had mu heavy chains and *either* kappa *or* lambda light chains, reducing the possibility of nonspecific staining, a constant worry with fluorescence microscopy. In addition, several patients presented with circulating M-components of the same heavy and light chain type as the surface Ig. This observation permitted us to verify the specificity of the novel surface marker technique by conventional immunochemical methods applied to the secreted product of the neoplastic cell. In four, a second heavy chain, that of IgD (delta), was detected in the plasma membrane of the neoplastic cells. Although we commented on this finding, we did not follow through on this observation and thus missed the opportunity to discover that most normal B lymphocytes bear immunoglobulin molecules of the IgM *and* IgD classes.

"After minor revision the manuscript was accepted by the *New England Journal of Medicine*, the first journal to which it was submitted. Word leaked back from the editors that this report was to be the last manuscript on a subject as outlandish as lymphocyte surface markers to be published by the journal. But the editors must be given their due; the manuscript was accepted.

"We believe that the paper is cited frequently because it is an easily understood and novel application of modern immunological theory (the T and B cell concept) and technique to clinical medicine. The experimental findings were particularly uniform. For the present, the detection of surface-incorporated immunoglobulin remains the most reliable technique for identifying B lymphocytes.[2] The entire field of lymphocyte surface markers has proliferated at a hectic pace in the past decade.[3] The identification of lymphocyte surface markers has been especially useful in advancing our understanding of the lymphoproliferative diseases."

1. **Raff M C.** Two distinct populations of peripheral lymphocytes in mice distinguishable by immunofluorescence. *Immunology* **19**:637-50, 1970.
2. **Aisenberg A C.** Cell-surface markers in lymphoproliferative disease. *N. Engl. J. Med.* **304**:331-6, 1981.
3. **Knapp W.** *Leukemia markers.* New York: Academic Press, 1981. 574 p.

CC/NUMBER 15
APRIL 12, 1982

This Week's Citation Classic

Nezelof C, Jammet M L, Lortholary P, Labrune B & Lamy M. L'hypoplasie héréditaire du thymus: sa place et sa responsabilité dans une observation d'aplasie lymphocytaire, normoplasmocytaire et normoglobulinenique du nourrisson. *Arch. Fr. Pédiat.* **21**:897-920, 1964.

This paper reports a new form of hereditary immunodeficiency, characterized by peripheral alymphocytosis, thymic hypoplasia, and the presence of plasma cells and normal or subnormal serum immunoglobulins. This form demonstrates in man the functional, morphologic, and genetic delineation in lymphoid tissue development. [The ***SCI®*** **indicates that this paper has been cited over 155 times since 1964. This is the most-cited paper from this journal 1961-1980.]**

C. Nezelof
Groupe de Recherche
Pathologie Pédiatrique
Institut National de la Santé
et de la Recherche Médicale
Hôpital Necker Enfants Malades
75730 Paris
France

February 17, 1982

"In 1961, I was a pediatrician and was just finishing my training as a pathologist. Clinical immunology was still in its infancy and, at the time, to most pediatricians, could be summed up as the findings of immunoelectrophoresis and antibody evaluation. The thymus was then considered to be an organ for storing lymphocytes which somehow aided growth.

"By chance, in the department of the esteemed Maurice Lamy at Hôpital des Enfants Malades in Paris, we encountered a 14-month-old boy who, from the age of three months, had suffered from repeated digestive and respiratory infections.

"This history and a persistent blood lymphopenia suggested a primary immune deficiency, of course, but this diagnosis was finally and resolutely eliminated on the basis of normal electrophoreses and the presence of a small amount of anti-APC antibodies. The child died at 16 months and his autopsy revealed two disturbing facts: first, a thymic tissue lacking both thymocytes and corpuscles, so unusual that I had some difficulty in identifying it as such; and secondly, a peripheral alymphocytosis affecting essentially the small lymphocytes but, strangely and unexpectedly, sparing the plasma cells.

"Perplexed by the contradictory findings published in the 1960 *Ciba Foundation Symposium on Cellular Aspects of Immunity*,[1] I did not immediately grasp the significance of the case. Fortunately, through reading the excellent general review published by G. Fabiani and A. Delaunay[2] and attending a symposium organized by R.A. Good in the Netherlands, I became acquainted with the experimental work done by J.F.A.P. Miller[3] and Good and his co-workers[4] on the role of the thymus in the development of cellular immunity and on the probable dichotomy of lymphoid tissue.

"From then on, the almost experimental character of the case history became clear, for it demonstrated for the first time that the lymphocytic and plasmocytic lineages were independent. These lineages were soon to be dubbed 'thymo-dependent' and 'burso-dependent.' It also revealed the crucial nature of thymic lesions.

"This paper has been highly cited for the following reason: like the cases of congenitally absent thymus, reported by Di George in 1966,[5] this publication was well received and drew a large audience because it appeared *at the right moment*, that is to say, at a time when immunologists needed to document in humans the experimental findings of T and B dichotomy of lymphoid tissue, already well established in chickens, and to demonstrate in man the vital role of thymic epithelial tissue in the maturation of peripheral lymphoid tissue, as well as to establish a coherent classification of primary immunodeficiency diseases. Furthermore, it kindled hopes of discovering, in man, the equivalent of the bursa of Fabricius. The golden age of thymology had begun.

"Fifteen years later, we are still surprised by the success which this single case history has had, because, in fact, it reported only clinical pathological findings and did not contain any real immunological investigation. At any rate, this case report opened up the gates of immunopathology for me, which at the time were narrow, and allowed me to deal with T cell immunodeficiencies."[6]

1. **Wolstenholme G E W & O'Connor M,** eds. *Ciba Foundation Symposium on Cellular Aspects of Immunity.* Boston: Little, Brown, 1960. 495 p.
2. **Fabiani G & Delaunay A.** Un problème d'actualité: la place du thymus en immunologie. *Biol. Méd.* **52**:446-91, 1963.
3. **Miller J F A P.** Immunity and the thymus. *Lancet* **1**:43-5, 1963.
4. **Good R A, Martinez C, Archer O K & Papermaster B W.** Role of the thymus in development of immunity. *J. Clin. Invest.* **41**:1361, 1962.
5. **Di George A M, Dacou C, Lischner H W & Arey J B.** Congenital absence of the thymus and its immunologic consequences concurrent with congenital hypoparathyroidism. *Program and abstracts: Seventy-Sixth Annual Meeting of the American Pediatric Society, 27-28 April 1966, Atlantic City.* St. Louis: American Pediatric Society, 1966. p. 29.
6. **Gosseye S & Nezelof C.** T system immunodeficiencies in infancy and childhood. *Pathol. Res. Pract.* **171**:142-58, 1981.

This Week's Citation Classic

Claman H N & Chaperon E A. Immunologic complementation between thymus and marrow cells—a model for the two-cell theory of immunocompetence. *Transplant. Rev.* **1**:92-113, 1969.
[Div. Clinical Immunol., Univ. Colorado Med. Ctr., Denver, CO and Dept. Microbiol., Creighton Univ. Sch. Med., Omaha, NE]

This paper reviews and expands the idea that antibody production requires both thymus-derived cells (now called T cells) and bone marrow-derived (B) cells. [The *SCI*® indicates that this paper has been cited in over 480 publications since 1969.]

Henry N. Claman
Department of Medicine and
Microbiology/Immunology
University of Colorado Medical School
Denver, CO 80262

July 1, 1982

"In the early-1960s, there was great excitement in immunology. The role of the thymus (one of the last 'mystery' organs in the body) was being unraveled. The work of J.F.A.P. Miller,[1] R.A. Good,[2] and A.J.S. Davies[3] and their colleagues showed that the presence of the thymus was needed for the proper development of the immune system. Nevertheless, it was quite clear that thymus cells themselves did not make antibody *in vivo*. Why not? At the same time, there were data to indicate a 'blood-thymus barrier' so that the failure to make antibody in the thymus might be due to the fact that antigen never got to the thymic lymphocytes. The critical experiments were done in 1965.[4]

"Using the then recently developed methods of cell transfer, we wondered if thymus cells could respond to antigen if they were removed from the thymus and injected (with antigen) into lethally irradiated syngeneic recipients (which had been irradiated to render them nonresponsive). This would bypass the blood-thymus barrier. The results were unequivocal. Normal spleen cells plus sheep rbc antigen given to irradiated mice produced antibody (showing that the spleen has all the necessary immunologic machinery), but transferred thymus cells plus antigen were inert.

"The important experiment involved pure serendipity. We felt that the transferred thymus cells might be either too immature or too 'sluggish' to respond, so we gave the recipients thymus cells and *two* injections of antigen. By the time there might possibly have been a response to the second dose of antigen, the recipients had died (from the radiation). We knew that bone marrow infusions would protect the recipients from irradiation death. When we added syngeneic bone marrow to thymus cells plus antigen, much antibody was made! By adjusting the cell and radiation doses, we showed that neither thymus cells nor bone marrow cells alone would respond to antigen by making antibody, but a *mixture* of both cell types would do so. We hypothesized that bone marrow cells made the antibody while thymus cells acted in some auxiliary fashion. We were unable to prove this, but, as G.F. Mitchell and Miller showed, this was correct.[5]

"I believe that this article has been highly cited for three reasons: (a) It reviews the first experiments showing cell-cell interactions in immunology. This concept has since become crucial in understanding immune responses. (b) It was clearly written and posed a number of simple questions for further research. (c) It appeared in the first volume of a series of publications together with three other articles on similar topics (by Miller and Mitchell,[6] by Davies,[7] and by R.B. Taylor[8]). Each of these papers explored (in different ways) the results of the interaction between antigen and thymus-derived cells.

"The precise nature of T-B cell interaction is still not quite clear. There have been hundreds of experiments, some of which are reviewed in the paper by R.N. Germain and B. Benacerraf."[9]

1. **Miller J F A P.** Immunological function of the thymus. *Lancet* **2**:748-9, 1961.
[Citation Classic. *Current Contents* (24):11, 12 June 1978.]
2. **Good R A, Dalmasso A P, Martinez C, Archer O K, Pierce J C & Papermaster B W.** The role of the thymus in development of immunological capacity in rabbits and mice. *J. Exp. Med.* **116**:773-96, 1962.
3. **Davies A J S, Leuchars E, Wallis V & Koller P C.** The mitotic response of thymus-derived cells to antigenic stimulus. *Transplantation* **4**:438-51, 1966.
4. **Claman H N, Chaperon E A & Triplett R F.** Thymus-marrow cell combinations. Synergism in antibody production. *Proc. Soc. Exp. Biol. Med.* **122**:1167-71, 1966.
5. **Mitchell G F & Miller J F A P.** Cell to cell interaction in the immune response. II. The source of hemolysin-forming cells in irradiated mice given bone marrow and thymus or thoracic duct lymphocytes. *J. Exp. Med.* **128**:821-37, 1968.
6. **Miller J F A P & Mitchell G F.** Thymus and antigen-reactive cells. *Transplant. Rev.* **1**:3-42, 1969.
7. **Davies A J S.** The thymus and the cellular basis of immunity. *Transplant. Rev.* **1**:43-91, 1969.
8. **Taylor R B.** Cellular cooperation in the antibody response of mice to two serum albumins: specific function of thymus cells. *Transplant. Rev.* **1**:114-49, 1969.
9. **Germain R N & Benacerraf B.** Helper and suppressor T cell factors. *Springer Semin. Immunopathol.* **3**:93-127, 1980.

CC/NUMBER 52
DECEMBER 29, 1980

This Week's Citation Classic

Smythe P M, Schonland M, Brereton-Stiles G G, Coovadia H M, Grace H J, Loening W E K, Mafoyane A, Parent M A & Vos G H. Thymolymphatic deficiency and depression of cell-mediated immunity in protein-calorie malnutrition. *Lancet* **2**:939-44, 1971. [Depts. Paediat. and Pathol. and Natal Inst. Immunol., Univ. Natal, and King Edward VIII Hosp., Durban, South Africa]

Investigation of the thymolymphatic system and cell mediated immunity in children with protein-calorie–malnutrition (PCM) showed a decrease in: tonsil size, chemical sensitisation of the skin, rate of lymphocyte transformation, the haemolytic serum complement, and thymic and peripheral lymphoid tissue. Lymphopenia below 2,500 prognosed death. In measles less than half had a rash and a giant-celled pneumonia was common. [The *SCI*® indicates that this paper has been cited over 330 times since 1971.]

P. M. Smythe
Department of Paediatrics
and Child Health
University of Natal
Congella 4013, Durban
South Africa

November 11, 1980

"In the early days most research on PCM was centred on supplementary foods and biochemical and electrolyte disturbances. My concern was that despite correction of diet and electrolytes so many children still died. Attendances at autopsies drew attention to the possibility that infection unrecognised clinically could be an important cause of death. Blood cultures identified a high frequency of gram-negative septicaemia as a frequent cause of death, and it was noted that these children were usually afebrile and had little leucocyte response.[1] Taken together with the tendency for Herpes simplex infections to disseminate, the severity of monilial infections, the frequency of a negative tuberculin test in the presence of active tuberculosis, the fulminating course taken by measles, the pattern was that of depressed immunological response, especially of cell-mediated immunity. The final stimulus had a touch of serendipity in that the chance observation that the mitotic figures seen in smears from bone-marrow of children with PCM often showed bizarre configurations and what appeared to be non-dysjunction. When chromosome studies became available an approach was made to one of the coauthors (H.J.G.) to try to ascertain the significance of this observation. Samples were submitted for phytohaemagglutinin stimulation. What was found was the marked inability of lymphocytes to transform.

"One can only surmise as to why this article has been highly cited. Perhaps because it was multifactorial, drawing together clinical, immunological, and pathological observations, including a number of observations made by earlier workers into a coherent picture of significant immunological depression. Perhaps it was opportune, coming at a time when there was widespread interest both in immunology and nutrition. Perhaps it was a product of clinical observations, coupled with advances in laboratory investigations. Of interest is how pure clinical observations can precede scientific explanation. For years one had taught that children suspected of active tuberculosis with a negative tuberculin test should have active anti-tuberculosis treatment. If after three weeks' treatment the tuberculin test remained negative treatment could be stopped, as by that time tuberculin sensitivity would have been reestablished. This is the precise period found for delayed hypersensitivity to be reestablished in PCM.

"The research was carried out in the departments of paediatrics and pathology and the Natal Institute of Immunology of the University of Natal and King Edward VIII Hospital, Durban, South Africa. All the coauthors made significant contributions. Particularly helpful was the work done on lymphocyte transformation (H.J.G.), the serology (G.H.V.), and the detailed pathological studies (M.S.)."

1. **Smythe P M & Campbell J A H.** The significance of the bacteraemia of kwashiorkor. *S. Afr. Med. J.* **33**:777, 1959.

Sokal J E & Primikirios N. The delayed skin test response in Hodgkin's disease and lymphosarcoma. Effect of disease activity. *Cancer* **14**:597-607, 1961.
[Division of Medicine, Roswell Park Memorial Institute, Buffalo, NY]

Impairment of delayed skin test responses correlated with disease activity. However, in Hodgkin's disease, anergy to recall antigens was common even during remission. Serial patient studies confirmed the relationship of skin test responses to disease activity and showed a trend toward progressive loss of reactivity. Patients with quiescent Hodgkin's disease responded normally to bacillus Calmette-Guérin (BCG) vaccination, while a small group with active disease and systemic manifestations exhibited neither local reactions to vaccination nor conversion of tuberculin responses. [The *SCI*® indicates that this paper has been cited in over 180 publications since 1961.]

Joseph E. Sokal
Department of Medicine
Hematology-Oncology Division
Duke University Medical Center
Durham, NC 27710

October 13, 1983

"My interests in tumor immunology and in Hodgkin's disease dated back to my fellowship years at Yale University, but Roswell Park Memorial Institute afforded me an ideal opportunity for long-term studies in a sizable and cooperative patient population, as well as providing funding for research associates such as N. Primikirios. At the time, several groups were studying the immunology of Hodgkin's disease, and some of the work reported in this paper only confirmed more elegant studies by others. Our major contributions consisted of a critical review of the literature (including reanalysis of the data in one publication by a more powerful statistical technique, resulting in a different conclusion) and application of bacillus Calmette-Guérin (BCG) vaccination as a test of cellular immune reactivity. Perhaps the latter is the reason this paper has been cited frequently. This may have represented the first systematic use of BCG to test immunologic function in neoplastic disease (at least, in the US). Others had already used skin sensitization to chemicals, and one group had applied the ultimate test of immunologic competence—transplantation of skin from unrelated donors.[1]

"We needed a method to test primary sensitization, which could form the basis for repeated subsequent recall testing. I considered skin sensitization with dinitrochlorobenzene (DNCB), used by several investigators, but rejected it because: a) serial testing of reactivity would require repeat applications of DNCB, which would constitute booster sensitization and complicate interpretation of the results; b) it was difficult to see what argument, other than serving science, could be used to persuade subjects (particularly, healthy controls) to accept DNCB sensitization; on the other hand, stimulation of resistance against tuberculosis, then still a common disease, could be offered as a personal benefit from BCG vaccination; and c) frequent use of DNCB posed some hazard of sensitization and morbidity for those handling the chemical. (As it turned out, working with BCG wasn't entirely free of risk either; eventually, both I and one of my colleagues accidentally inoculated ourselves with vaccine. We escaped without any lesions, after brief courses of isoniazid.)

"In the concluding paragraph of the paper, we speculated that there might be a correlation between delayed hypersensitivity responses and prognosis in Hodgkin's disease. I undertook a formal study of this question subsequently, using both a battery of recall skin tests and BCG vaccination to measure immunologic reactivity. Since I wasn't sure what effects BCG might have in addition to converting the tuberculin response, I included appropriate controls. Thus started the first stratified, prospectively controlled study of BCG vaccination in malignant lymphoma. Response to BCG proved to be a rather good prognostic indicator for patients with disseminated Hodgkin's disease.[2] We also found that BCG was a general stimulant of delayed hypersensitivity responses in man[3] and that it might exert a favorable effect in malignant lymphoma of limited extent."[4]

1. **Kelly W D, Good R A & Varco R L.** Anergy and skin homograft survival in Hodgkin's disease. *Surg. Gynecol. Obstet.* **107**:565-70, 1958. (Cited 115 times.)
2. **Sokal J E & Aungst C W.** Response to BCG vaccination and survival in advanced Hodgkin's disease. *Cancer* **24**:128-34, 1969.
3. **Sokal J E, Aungst C W & Han T.** Effect of BCG on delayed hypersensitivity responses of patients with neoplastic disease. *Int. J. Cancer* **12**:242-9, 1973.
4. **Sokal J E, Aungst C W & Snyderman M.** Delay in progression of malignant lymphoma after BCG vaccination. *N. Engl. J. Med.* **291**:1226-34, 1974.

CC/NUMBER 13
MARCH 28, 1983

This Week's Citation Classic

Hersh E M & Oppenheim J J. Impaired *in vitro* lymphocyte transformation in Hodgkin's disease. *N. Engl. J. Med.* **273**:1006-12, 1965.
[Medicine Branch, National Cancer Institute, Natl. Insts. Health, Bethesda, MD]

Lymphocyte blastogenic responses to phytohemagglutinin and vaccinia were measured in 23 patients with Hodgkin's disease and 35 controls. Diminished blastogenic responses were seen in 87 percent and correlated with skin test anergy, stage of disease, and presence of symptoms. Serum factors were not responsible for the impairment. [The *SCI*® indicates that this paper has been cited in over 400 publications since 1965.]

Evan M. Hersh
Department of Clinical Immunology
and Biological Therapy
University of Texas System Cancer Center
M.D. Anderson Hospital and
Tumor Institute
Houston, TX 77030
and
Joost J. Oppenheim
Laboratory of Microbiology and Immunology
National Institute of Dental Research
National Institutes of Health
Bethesda, MD 20205

January 4, 1983

"In 1956, a young woman was accepted to the 1960 class of Columbia University College of Physicians and Surgeons. Prior to the start of the first year, René Dede was discovered to have Hodgkin's disease. The dean, Aura E. Severinghaus, encouraged her to pursue her studies in spite of her disease, and she completed radiotherapy just prior to the start of the first semester. Two of her classmates, who became her close friends, are the authors of the above cited paper. In 1959, René relapsed and, for the first time, revealed that she was a victim of Hodgkin's disease. In spite of additional radiotherapy, nitrogen mustard, and corticosteroids, René died after repeated episodes of viral infection, prior to the start of the fourth year of medical school.

"In 1962, the authors of the paper became clinical associates of the National Cancer Institute (NCI), working under the supervision of Emil Frei III, and Emil J. Freireich. Clinical investigation of Hodgkin's disease was an active Medicine Branch program at that time and resulted in the development of curative chemotherapy.[1] During our clinical year we were impressed with the manifestations of host defense failure in Hodgkin's and other cancer patients.

"Interaction with immunologists and hematologists at NCI made us aware that phytohemagglutinin, recall antigens, and allogeneic cells could stimulate lymphoblastoid proliferation of peripheral blood leukocytes and that lymphocyte blastogenesis was an *in vitro* analogue of the immune response. Therefore, coupling the findings of skin test anergy and impaired resistance to infection in Hodgkin's disease with this concept of blastogenesis, we investigated whether the impaired *in vivo* immunocompetence was related to an intrinsic lymphocyte defect expressed by impaired *in vitro* blastogenic response. At that time, blastogenesis was measured, not by tritiated thymidine incorporation, but by counting the number of enlarged cells with prominent nuclei and basophilic cytoplasm and the number of mitoses in mitogen and antigen stimulated cultures. We did indeed find impaired blastogenesis and mitoses in patients' lymphocytes compared to controls. It correlated with skin test anergy and the stage of disease and the prognosis.

"We dedicated the paper to the memory of our valiant and beloved classmate. The paper is frequently cited because it was one of the first to relate impaired lymphocyte competence to stage of disease and prognosis in malignancy. With curative therapy as immunity recovers, the *in vitro* lymphocyte reactivity returns to normal. The fundamental etiology of the anergy and impaired immune reactivity in Hodgkin's disease is still not fully understood. There is evidence that macrophage suppressor cell activity is prominent in patients with impaired immune competence and that this relates to excessive production of prostaglandins and superoxides by macrophages. There is other evidence, however, that an intrinsic lymphocyte defect may also be present which is manifested by impaired E-rosette formation, T cell chemotaxis, T cell colony formation, and cap formation by lymphocytes. Serum factors binding to lymphocytes and blocking of surface receptors may also play a role in the immunodeficiency.[2,3]

"Finally, it is interesting to note that both of us have continued our careers in immunology. One of us (E.M.H.) is in clinical immunological research as the chairman of the department of clinical immunology and biological therapy at M.D. Anderson Hospital and Tumor Institute of the University of Texas, and one of us (J.J.O.) is in basic immunology research as the head of the section of immunology of the National Institute of Dental Research. This is illustrative of the fact that early career experiences may provide the driving force for an entire scientific career."

1. **De Vita V T, Jr., Serpick A & Carbone P P.** Combination chemotherapy in the treatment of advanced Hodgkin's disease. *Ann. Intern. Med.* **73**:881-95, 1970.
2. **Kaplan H S.** Hodgkin's disease: unfolding concepts concerning its nature, management and prognosis. *Cancer* **45**:2439-74, 1980.
3. **Schulof R S, Bockman R S, Garofalo J A, Cirrincione C, Cunningham-Rundles S, Fernandes G, Day N K, Pinsky C M, Incefy G S, Thaler H T, Good R A & Gupta S.** Multivariate analysis of T cell functional defects and circulating serum factors in Hodgkin's disease. *Cancer* **48**:964-73, 1981.

This Week's Citation Classic

Allison A C, Denman A M & Barnes R D. Cooperating and controlling functions of thymus-derived lymphocytes in relation to autoimmunity. *Lancet* **2**:135-40, 1971. [Clinical Research Centre, Harrow, Middlesex, England]

It is suggested that thymus-derived lymphocytes play two roles in preventing autoimmunity. T-lymphocytes, but not B-lymphocytes, are unresponsive to autoantigens. Ways in which the requirement for autoreactive T-lymphocytes can be bypassed are discussed. These result in stimulation of B-lymphocytes to secrete autoantibodies. Suppressor T-lymphocytes can also inhibit autoimmune reactions. [The *SCI*® indicates that this paper has been cited over 410 times since 1971.]

Anthony C. Allison
International Laboratory for Research on Animal Diseases
P.O. Box 30709
Nairobi
Kenya

November 22, 1979

"This article was an attempt to resolve a long-standing difficulty in immunology. Since animals do not as a rule make antibodies against their own body constituents, it had been thought that lymphocytes with capacity to produce such autoantibodies are eliminated or inactivated in embryonic or early postnatal life. Yet certain manipulations (e.g., injection of autologous tissues in adjuvants or of heterologous cross-reactive proteins) lead to autoantibody formation. We offered two explanations for this apparent paradox, one reinforcing the other. The first proposal was that tolerance to self-antigens is selective, involving only T-lymphocytes, and leaving B-lymphocytes with the capacity to make autoantibodies when suitably stimulated. The requirements for autoantigen-specific helper T-lymphocytes could be bypassed in different ways, for example by adjuvants, graft-versus-host reactions, virus infections, or immunization with heterologous cross-reactive proteins. In the article several predictions were made on the basis of this hypothesis, and during the years that followed publication these were confirmed experimentally in our laboratory and others.

"The second proposal was that suppressor T-lymphocytes normally prevent autoimmune reactions. Before the article was published, I attended a meeting on immune regulation at Brook Lodge, Michigan. I suggested that T-lymphocytes must have suppressor as well as helper functions, quoting observations on autoimmunity that had been made by my colleagues Denman and Barnes. Remarkably, three other participants at the meeting (Gershon, Herzenberg, and Tada) had independently reached the same conclusion from different experimental observations. Thus the concept of suppressor T-lymphocytes was launched. It is now known that these represent a distinct subpopulation of cells, investigation of which has led to major advances in cellular immunology in the last eight years.

"What is so gratifying about our paper is not only that it is widely cited, but that the predictions in the article generated a great deal of experimental work. Traveling in Britain, Europe, North and South America, and Australia, I have met many young investigators who tell me how they were stimulated by the article and began their experiments to test the hypotheses presented. Several of these research workers have already made well known contributions to the field, some as visiting scientists in my laboratory. Thus the article was timely and had a substantial impact. Much experimental evidence in support of both hypotheses in this paper has accumulated, as subsequently reviewed.[1]

"My own researches on immunological tolerance have continued with several colleagues, leading to the use of the drug Cyclosporin A to elicit specific tolerance to allografts.[2,3] Selective inhibition by the drug of helper and cytotoxic-T-lymphocytes, while allowing the generation of specific suppressor cells, is evidently involved. Since this is what transplantation immunologists have been attempting to do for decades, we believe these articles should also become *Citation Classics,* and it will be interesting to see what happens."

1. **Allison A C.** Autoimmune diseases: concepts of pathogenesis and control. (Talal N, ed.) *Autoimmunity: genetic, immunologic, virologic, and clinical aspects.* New York: Academic Press, 1977. p. 91-139.
2. **Green C J, Allison A C & Precious S.** Induction of specific tolerance in rabbits by kidney allografting and short periods of Cyclosporin A treatment. *Lancet* **2**:123-5, 1979.
3. **Tutschka P, Beschorner W E, Allison A C, Burns W H & Santos G W.** Use of Cyclosporin A in allogeneic bone marrow transplantation in the rat. *Nature* **280**:148-51, 1979.

CC/NUMBER 14
APRIL 2, 1984

This Week's Citation Classic™

Edelson R L, Kirkpatrick C H, Shevach E M, Schein P S, Smith R W, Green I & Lutzner M. Preferential cutaneous infiltration by neoplastic thymus-derived lymphocytes: morphologic and functional studies.
Ann. Intern. Med. **80**:685-92, 1974.

[Dermatol., Med., and Immunol. Branches, Natl. Cancer Inst., and Labs. Clin. Invest. and Immunol., Natl. Inst. Allergy and Infectious Dis., NIH, Bethesda, MD]

Malignant lymphocytes from each of seven patients with widespread involvement of skin were shown to be of T- (thymus-derived) cell lineage. These cells had a characteristic tissue distribution: preferential infiltration of skin and T-cell zones of lymph nodes and sparing of bone marrow. These findings suggested that lymphomas and leukemias with widespread cutaneous infiltration are frequently T-cell malignancies with several distinguishing features. [The *SCI*® indicates that this paper has been cited in over 225 publications since 1974.]

Richard L. Edelson
Department of Dermatology
Columbia-Presbyterian Medical Center
New York, NY 10032

January 27, 1984

"At the time of my arrival as a clinical associate at the National Institutes of Health (NIH) in 1972, the discipline of human cellular immunology was in its early infancy. Techniques for identification of human B (bone marrow-derived) and T (thymus-derived) lymphocytes had recently been established. I was fortunate to receive substantial guidance from four senior investigators who had already made major contributions to this new science (Ira Green, Michael Frank, Ethan Shevach, and Charles Kirkpatrick).

"The above mentioned paper was actually only the second one which I published. We were quite surprised to discover that malignancies of lymphocytes with a tendency to invade broad expanses of skin were almost invariably T-cell lymphomas or leukemias. In marked contrast, lymphomas and leukemias in which the skin was not significantly infiltrated were almost always malignancies of B lymphocytes. One particularly unusual finding in the patients with T-cell leukemias was the sparing of the bone marrow, a finding explained by the circulatory patterns of T cells.

"This paper was the point of departure for much of my research over the next ten years, which is summarized in two recent editorials.[1,2] It permitted unification, under the classification 'cutaneous T-cell lymphoma' (CTCL),[3] of an artificially splintered group of lymphocytic malignancies that previously went by such noncontributory names as 'mycosis fungoides,' 'Sézary syndrome,' or 'leukemia cutis.' CTCL is now being studied in many laboratories around the world and is widely recognized to be a malignancy of phenotypic helper T cells with an extraordinary affinity for epidermis. It may, in fact, be the most common form of adult lymphoma with an incidence greater than that of Hodgkin's disease. It is noteworthy that CTCL was identified as a single disease with diverse clinical manifestations only through T-cell marker studies.

"On the basis of this work at the NIH, I received an Irma T. Hirschl Career Investigator Award (1976-1981), which is given to promising junior faculty members at research institutes in New York City. This early support, along with subsequently obtained NIH grants, has permitted me to continue to study the basic biology of CTCL. In collaboration with my close colleague, Carole Berger, at Columbia University, monoclonal antibodies with specificity for CTCL cells have been produced and are useful as diagnostic and investigational tools. The affinity of the malignant T cells for epidermis led to the initial suggestion of a role for this tissue in normal T-cell maturation,[3] which is now being supported by the finding that this tissue produces thymic-like factors.

"The number of citations which this paper received is almost certainly a reflection of the clinical significance of CTCL. It is far more common than we anticipated and remains a devastating disease for those afflicted with it. Hopefully, exciting new observations, such as Robert Gallo's that CTCL is associated with an RNA retrovirus (human T lymphoma virus), will contribute to elucidation of its pathogenesis. The subject is one of ever-increasing excitement, and I am privileged to have been there at the beginning."

1. **Patterson J A K & Edelson R L.** Interaction of T cells with the epidermis. (Comment.) *Brit. J. Dermatol.* **107**:117-22, 1982.
2. **Edelson R L.** Pathogenesis of T cell lymphoma of skin. (Editorial.) *J. Amer. Acad. Dermatol.* **9**:957-60, 1983.
3. ----------------. Cutaneous T cell lymphomas: clues of a skin-thymus interaction. *J. Invest. Dermatol.* **67**:419-24, 1976.

CC/NUMBER 11
MARCH 12, 1984

This Week's Citation Classic™

Clausen J E. Tuberculin-induced migration inhibition of human peripheral leucocytes in agarose medium. *Acta Allergol.* **26**:56-80, 1971.
[Medical Department A, Rigshospitalet, University Hospital, Copenhagen, Denmark]

An agarose technique able to demonstrate tuberculin-induced migration inhibition of human peripheral leucocytes is described. The inhibition was well correlated to the sensitivity of the cell donor as expressed by the delayed intracutaneous reaction to tuberculin. [The *SCI*® indicates that this paper has been cited in over 250 publications since 1971, making it the most-cited paper published in this journal to date.]

Jens Erik Clausen
Department of Medicine
Ringsted County Hospital
DK-4100 Ringsted
Denmark

January 6, 1984

"My interest in cell-mediated immunity was initiated in 1967 when I was an intern in medicine at Rigshospitalet, University Hospital of Copenhagen. There, I was stimulated by close contact with Gunnar Bendixen and Mogens Søborg, who had adapted the capillary tube technique for the study of cell-mediated immunity in man.[1] Even though the capillary tube technique was valuable in the study of cell-mediated immunity in laboratory animals as well as in man, techniques more sensitive were needed.

"In guinea pig experiments, Carpenter *et al.*[2] observed that splenic and peritoneal exudate cells placed in wells cut into agar medium migrated out beneath the gel. Therefore, I started to develop an agarose migration inhibition technique for *in vitro* demonstration of cell-mediated immunity in man.

"My studies showed that the agarose technique was suited to demonstrate antigen-induced leucocyte migration inhibition and was more sensitive than the capillary tube technique. Furthermore, results obtained by the agarose technique were easier to reproduce. But the test will be useless if all the steps are not thoroughly standardized. It is, for example, very important to use a physiological pH and temperature and to make sure that the cell cultures are incubated in air saturated with water during the culture period. Nevertheless, difficulties may arise because of variations from batch to batch of agarose or culture medium.

"The agarose migration technique has also been used to demonstrate migration inhibitory factor in cell-free supernatants from stimulated leucocyte cultures and to examine the role of the various leucocyte types in the migration reaction.

"A review[3] and my previously published papers were accepted as a doctoral thesis by the University of Copenhagen in 1975. Since 1976, I have been chief physician of a medical department in a small county hospital and therefore unable to continue the immunological studies. In my last study,[4] I demonstrated that the agarose technique was suitable also in investigations of phytohemagglutinin (PHA)-stimulated leucocytes.

"I believe that my paper is frequently cited because techniques to demonstrate the leucocyte migration inhibition reaction as an *in vitro* parameter of cell-mediated immunity had been urgently needed. Even if I am no longer working with the test myself, I am glad to know that the agarose migration technique is still used in the Laboratory of Clinical Immunology at Rigshospitalet, where most of my studies were carried out."

1. **Søborg M & Bendixen G.** Human lymphocyte migration as a parameter of hypersensitivity. *Acta Med. Scand.* **181**:247-56, 1967. (Cited 575 times.)
2. **Carpenter R R, Barsales P B & Ganchan R P.** Antigen-induced inhibition of cell migration in agar gel, plasma clot, and liquid media. *J. Reticuloendothel. Soc.* **5**:472-83, 1968.
3. **Clausen J E.** The agarose migration inhibition technique for in vitro demonstration of cell-mediated immunity in man. A review. *Dan. Med. Bull.* **22**:181-94, 1975.
4. ---------------, Migration inhibition of human leucocytes mixed with phytohemagglutinin-preincubated leucocytes. *Acta Allergol.* **30**:239-49, 1975.

CC/NUMBER 15
APRIL 13, 1981

This Week's Citation Classic

Weissmann G. Lysosomes and joint disease. *Arthritis Rheum.* **9**:834-40, 1966. [Department of Medicine, New York University, School of Medicine, New York, NY]

The hypothesis is presented that lysosomal constituents are released from phagocytic cells following direct injury or endocytosis of immune complexes. Lysosomal enzymes, chiefly proteases, provoke acute inflammation and degrade extracellular structures, including the proteoglycans of cartilage. This view implies that tissues such as the joint destroy themselves by a 'final common pathway' under stimuli that vary from disease to disease. [The *SCI*® indicates that this paper has been cited over 165 times since 1966.]

Gerald Weissmann
Department of Medicine
School of Medicine
New York University Medical Center
New York, NY 10016

March 18, 1981

"This article was a summary of work carried out at New York University (with Lewis Thomas), and the Strangeways Research Laboratory in Cambridge (with John Dingle and Honor B. Fell). By 1966, we had concluded that lysosomes could play a role in tissue injury, although we were ignorant of the exact means whereby their corrosive intracellular ferments were extruded from cells. In this review, the hypothesis was first articulated that cells such as granulocytes, macrophages, or synovial lining cells might release lysosomal enzymes consequent to their encounter with immune complexes or urate crystals.

"It has required another decade of experimental work to validate this youthful restatement of Metchnikoff's contention, that 'the organism digests materials which it encounters outside the gastrointestinal tract by means of an inflammatory reaction.'[1] But, I presume that the heuristic value of this 1966 article was due to the encapsulation, for the clinician, of the previous decade's analysis of the lysosomal apparatus, by Christian de Duve, Alex Novikoff, Zanvil Cohn, and James G. Hirsch.[2] It carried, as a long footnote, definitions of such lysosomal neologisms as 'endocytosis,' 'autophagy,' 'heterophagy,' 'phagolysosome,' and 'residual body.' It was also suggested that anti-inflammatory steroids, by interacting with biomembranes, would diminish extrusion of lysosomal contents.

"The major hypothesis elaborated in this review has since been appropriately tested in our own, and other, laboratories. Indeed, phagocytic cells exposed to particulate invaders or immune complexes secrete lysosomal enzymes by a process now termed 'regurgitation during feeding,' whereas their encounter with crystals such as monosodium urate leads to 'perforation from within' the intracellular gastrointestinal tract. The interaction of *neutral* proteases from lysosomes (elastase, cathepsin G) with circulating, inflammatory materials (complement, kinin, and clotting cascades) has become partially elucidated. Finally, the role of these proteases in degrading extracellular matrices has been carefully documented.

"It is surprising that this speculative review, in a journal devoted to my clinical subspecialty, has proved useful to so many. Especially, I might add, for younger investigators, since Dingle and I had submitted a similar hypothesis to the same journal five years earlier. It was rejected with the (proper) advice that we do more experiments, and the (improper) suggestion that the lysosome was an artifact of the biochemical literature. Claude Bernard once compared the process of science to a progression from a warren of dark and busy kitchens to an occasional, brilliantly-lit hall. Busy in the kitchen of the 1970s, it is reassuring to have once passed fairly close to a bright salon.

"Although I have been informed that the most highly cited paper from my laboratory is 'Studies on lysosomes,'[3] it was not until 1966 that it became possible to extend this experimental work in rabbits to an analysis of human disease. A recent summary of these developments has been published by J.E. Smolen, H.M. Korchak, and myself."[4]

1. **Metchnikoff E.** *Immunity in infective diseases.* London: Johnson Reprint Co. (reprinted from Cambridge Univ. Press, 1905 edition), 1968. p. 210.
2. **de Duve C.** The lysosome in retrospect. (Dingle J T & Fell H B, eds.) *Lysosomes in biology and pathology.* Amsterdam: North Holland, 1969. Vol. I. p. 3-42.
3. **Weissmann G & Thomas L.** Studies on lysosomes. I. The effect of endotoxin, endotoxin tolerance, and cortisone on the release of acid hydrolases from a granular fraction on rabbit liver. *J. Exp. Med.* **116**:433-50, 1962. [The *SCI*® indicates that this paper has been cited over 385 times since 1962.]
4. **Weissmann G, Smolen J E & Korchak H M.** Release of inflammatory mediators from stimulated neutrophils. *N. Engl. J. Med.* **303**:27-34, 1980.

CC/NUMBER 50
DECEMBER 15, 1980

This Week's Citation Classic

Yam L T, Li C Y & Crosby W H. Cytochemical identification of monocytes and granulocytes. *Amer. J. Clin. Pathol.* **55**:283-90, 1971.
[Blood Res. Lab., New England Med. Ctr. Hosps., and Dept. Med., Tufts Univ. Sch. Med., Boston, MA]

Several cytochemical methods were developed to identify the monocytes and the granulocytes. These methods are simple, sensitive, easily reproducible, and can be used either singly or in combination. They may be used as objective means for accurate identification of the human blood cells. [The *SCI*® indicates that this paper has been cited over 615 times since 1971.]

Lung T. Yam
Section of Hematology
Veterans Administration Medical Center
Louisville, KY 40202
&
Chin Yang Li
Mayo Clinic
Rochester, MN 55901

November 11, 1980

"Accurate identification of blood cells is important for diagnosis and management of patients with blood diseases. It is essential for the studies involving functions, interactions, and immunity of various types of cells. Cell identification is usually based on morphologic observation. This method is not objective, but rather an 'art' and not a 'science.'

"In 1967, while working as staff members in the cytology laboratory of the hematology service under the direction of William H. Crosby, we were detailed the responsibility of cytodiagnosis for all patients with blood diseases. We were also charged with assisting researchers in identifying various types of cells in human subjects and experimental animals. These assignments proved to be difficult due to frequent encounters with unusual and exotic clinical cases. In addition, the variety of animals and experimental conditions used by our colleagues also complicated our job. We told Crosby our problems and with his blessings began searching for a more objective and specific method of cell identification. Our research approach was often met with cynicism. It wasn't uncommon to hear comments doubting our competency in cytodiagnosis. We soon found useful cytochemical markers for blood cell identification and established techniques for our procedures, yet we were reluctant to publish our observations. The mounting skepticism expressed by others undermined our own confidence.

"In the fall of 1969, we attended a meeting on lymphocyte cultures in New Hampshire. We also took our families along to enjoy the area. The meeting consisted of two grueling days and left little time for our loved ones. At the close of the meeting, as the exhausted participants were preparing to leave, one member of the group shocked us awake with a final question: 'Are you guys sure you're studying the lymphocytes? What is a lymphocyte anyway?' We shyly mentioned our work on the cytochemical markers but again met with little enthusiasm or interest.

"While returning to our motel, we began discussing our experience in cell identification and our moods changed from despair and frustration to that of anger and rage. We decided to report our observation and begin this paper before our emotions cooled. At the motel, using paper towels, we sat on the front lawn amid happy shouts of our playing children and protests from our wives, and laid down the essential groundwork of our paper in less than one hour. We insisted on inviting Crosby to be a coauthor because of his indispensable support and encouragement to us on this work and he should not go unrecognized.

"Our paper is cited often because the several methods for objective cell identification described are simple, practical, and indispensable both in patient care and cell research. We are, however, rather amused that this 'quickie' has withstood the test of time and has been useful to many, including those working in automation of the leukocyte differential count, and that it has helped to curtail comments regarding our competency in cytodiagnosis."

CC/NUMBER 30
JULY 28, 1980

This Week's Citation Classic

Donaldson V H & Evans R R. A biochemical abnormality in hereditary angioneurotic edema. Absence of serum inhibitor of C'1-esterase. *Amer. J. Med.* **35**:37-44, 1963.
[Res. Div. and Dept. Allergy, Cleveland Clinic Foundation, and Dept. Med., Western Reserve Univ. Sch. Med., Cleveland, OH]

Affected members of kindred with hereditary angioneurotic edema were markedly deficient in the serum inhibitor of the activated first component of complement (C'1-esterase inhibitor, C$\bar{1}$-Inhibitor, or C$\bar{1}$-INH). The deficiency and susceptibility to attacks of edema were transmitted as autosomal dominant traits. [The *SCI*® indicates that this paper has been cited over 330 times since 1963.]

Virginia H. Donaldson
Children's Hospital Research
Foundation and Department of Pediatrics
College of Medicine
University of Cincinnati
Cincinnati, OH 45229

June 10, 1980

"The serum complement system consists of a group of proteins, some of which are enzymes, which participate in immune reactions. When the first component of complement (C$\bar{1}$) is activated it acquires esterase activity.[1] Normally, an α-2 glycoprotein called serum inhibitor of C$\bar{1}$ (C$\bar{1}$-INH) regulates the action of activated C$\bar{1}$ or C'1-esterase.[2] The deficiency of this serum inhibitor in hereditary angioneurotic edema was inadvertently observed during laboratory studies examining the effect of the fibrinolytic enzyme, plasmin, upon serum complement. The goal of these experiments was to determine if C$\bar{1}$ became activated by plasmin through a two-step mechanism in which plasmin first destroyed C$\bar{1}$-Inhibitor, thus permitting autocatalytic activation of C$\bar{1}$.

"While at lunch with a colleague during these studies, my attention was drawn to a patient with hereditary angioneurotic edema whose symptoms had been treated with a large amount of adrenalin, albeit to no avail. Adrenalin is known to activate fibrinolytic mechanisms *in vivo*, but does not accomplish this *in vitro*, and it was possible that it might have an effect on complement *in vivo* not demonstrable in the test tube. I therefore pursued the possibility that this means of plasminogen activation might affect C$\bar{1}$-Inhibitor and C$\bar{1}$. When the patient's serum was found to lack C$\bar{1}$-Inhibitor activity it was thought that this might have occurred through this hypothetical mechanism. The same observation, however, was made on serum collected after swellings had subsided, and when other members of the family who were subjected to these swellings were tested, all affected adults were found to have this deficiency even when their symptoms were in remission. Moreover, some of the children in this and other kindred who had not yet had attacks of hereditary angioneurotic edema were deficient in serum C$\bar{1}$-Inhibitor; these children have since developed the classical symptoms of the disease. Therefore, the detection of this deficiency is a diagnostic feature of hereditary angioneurotic edema, and this inherited defect demonstrates the participation of the complement system in a human disease. In the face of this deficiency there is ready activation of the first component of complement with consequent destruction of the hemolytic activity of the fourth component, because it is easily destroyed by active C$\bar{1}$.

"This disorder represents a unique disease due to an inherited deficiency of an inhibitor protein of blood plasma. This study is probably frequently cited because it was the first published description of a disease process associated with a deficiency of a clearly defined regulatory protein of serum, and because it was the first description of a disease picture associated with perturbed serum complement reflecting an inherited abnormality of the system."

1. **Ratnoff O D & Lepow I H.** Some properties of an esterase derived from preparations of the first component of complement. *J. Exp. Med.* **106**:327-43, 1957.
2. **Levy L R & Lepow I H.** Assay and properties of serum inhibitor C'1-esterase. *Proc. Soc. Exp. Biol. Med.* **101**:608-11, 1959.

NUMBER 6
FEBRUARY 5, 1979

This Week's Citation Classic

Doniach D, Roitt I M, Walker J G & Sherlock S. Tissue antibodies in primary biliary cirrhosis, active chronic (lupoid) hepatitis, cryptogenic cirrhosis and other liver diseases and their clinical implications. *Clin. Exp. Immunol.* **1**: 237-62, 1966.

The finding of mitochondrial antibodies in the serum of almost all cases of primary biliary cirrhosis and in very few patients having other clinically similar disorders, made it possible to avoid unnecessary and harmful laparotomies by a correct preoperative diagnosis of the 'autoimmune' cases. [The *SCI*® indicates that this paper has been cited 235 times since 1966.]

Deborah Doniach
Department of Immunology
The Middlesex Hospital Medical School
London W1 England

January 31, 1978

"This paper contained the fullest account of the serological studies which led to the identification of mitochondrial antibodies, and the realization of their importance in the differential diagnosis of chronic liver diseases. The work was a direct extension of the initial discovery by Ivan Roitt and myself in 1956 that human lymphoid thyroiditis was an 'autoimmune' disorder, when we found precipitins to normal thyroglobulin in the sea of patients with Hashimoto goitres.[1] This was soon followed by the detection of adrenal antibodies in Addison's disease with 'idiopathic' adrenal atrophy, and of gastric autoimmunity in pernicious anaemia. These two conditions were known to occur in clinical association with chronic thyroiditis.

"Autoimmune mechanisms had been suspected in hepatic cirrhosis since the beginning of the century when the complement fixation reaction (CFT) was first discovered. This was found to be positive to high titres in certain cases of cirrhosis when liver extracts were used as antigens.

"In the early 1960s we had acquired our first ultraviolet microscope and had mastered the art of immunofluorescence, the method developed by Albert Coons, which has contributed more than any other to unravelling the mysteries of organ and tissue antibodies. We then felt that we ought to look for evidence of autoimmunity in liver diseases. We approached the distinguished hepatologist, Prof. Sheila Sherlock, and asked her to send us the sera of cases likely to belong to the autoimmune group. Her young resident at the time was Geoffrey Walker, who is now a consultant and much loved teacher in clinical gastroenterology. He was the go-between for us autoimmunologists. We worked together for several years and spent many hours puzzling over the data described in the cited paper. It proved impossible to demonstrate liver-specific antibodies at that time but instead, when the results on over 200 cases were decoded, we found that a defined immunofluorescence pattern, which we identified as mitochondrial, was seen mostly in middle-aged women with a disease in which there is a progressive destruction of the small bile ductules inside the liver, giving rise to an obstructive jaundice difficult to distinguish from that produced by lesions affecting the larger extrahepatic ducts, for which surgery is mandatory. The anti-mitochondrial-antibody (AMA) test has now been adopted world-wide as one of the essential diagnostic parameters for this and related diseases. Later Peter Berg, now Professor of Clinical Immunology in Tubingen, joined our research team and contributed important studies relating to the location and nature of the mitochondrial antigens. He is now expanding this work in many fruitful directions.

"I was always an endocrinologist at heart and in the past four years I have had the good fortune to train another gifted autoimmunologist, Dr. Franco Bottazzo, whose work led to the discovery of pancreatic islet-cell antibodies in 'insulin-dependent' diabetes mellitus,[2] a disease more common and causing even more suffering than hepatic cirrhosis. If this 'autoimmune' marker allows us to predict the onset of the disease in predisposed families this will be ample reward for my 30 years spent in trying to fathom the causes of human ailments."

1. **Doniach D & Roitt I M.** 'Autoimmune thyroid disease' in *Textbook of immunopathology.* (Miescher P A & Muller-Eberhard H J. ed.) Vol. II, 2nd edition, Grune & Stratton N.Y., 1976, p. 715-735.

2. **Doniach D & Bottazzo G F.** Autoimmunity and the endocrine pancreas in *Pathobiology Annual* Vol. 7 (Iochim H L. ed.) Appleton-Century-Crofts N.Y., 1977, p. 327-346.

This Week's Citation Classic

Beutner E H, Jordon R E & Chorzelski T P. The immunopathology of pemphigus and bullous pemphigoid. *J. Invest. Dermatol.* **51**:63-80, 1968.
[State Univ. New York Sch. Med., Dept. Microbiology, Buffalo. NY]

Pemphigus and pemphigoid are rare blistering diseases with mortality rates in untreated cases of 95% and 25% respectively. Both are associated with circulating IgG class autoantibodies to stratified epithelia. In pemphigus these antibodies react with a surface protein on epithelial cells, and in bullous pemphigoid they fix to the basement membrane, as seen by indirect immunofluorescence (IF) tests of sera on normal epithelia. Direct IF tests of patients' biopsies show that these antibodies react in vivo with normal skin and oral mucosa. [The *SCI*® indicates that this paper has been cited over 145 times since 1968.]

Ernst H. Beutner
Department of Microbiology
State University of New York
Buffalo, NY 14214

February 7, 1978

"As a third generation researcher in the health sciences, it is clear to me that many well-based efforts fail. One of my grandparents worked with Robert Koch when he tried to treat tuberculous patients with old tuberculin. In fact, I think Koch was right, but all he succeeded in doing was to kill some people, mislead some devoted followers, and cast doubt on his reputation; all because he failed to quantitate. Also my father devoted his entire life to work on the physical chemistry of the biogenesis of electric currents in the heart, brain, and other tissue. Though I think he was right about much of what he wrote, he was unable to convince physiologists of his time that the ambient theories on the sodium pump were in error.

"Added to this background is the contrast between the excitement of my first chief, Stuart Mudd, at the time he made me a charter member of the Society of Histochemistry and Cytochemistry almost 30 years ago, and the pathetic yield of useful information from this discipline to date, largely because of a lack of quantitation. To be successful, I think that we must either pick or help to create fields that are soundly based with a minimum of theories and a maximum of quantitation methods.

"Fortunately, Ernest Witebsky, my chief from 1956 to 1969, persuaded us of the folly of the use of IF methods as mere 'immunohistochemical' tools and the need for a quantitative serologic approach. When Bob Jordon and I first found the antibodies of pemphigus and pemphigoid in a summer project his father had suggested, we knew they were important but that the IF methods could not hold up under criticism. Accordingly, I spent most of 1965 to 1970 developing 'defined IF staining' methods. It paid off well. Defined IF staining is now used widely. With this technique, it has been possible to show, that pemphigus antibodies cause pemphigus, that IF tests are of value in diagnosis, and that psoriasis also involves autoimmunity.

"All three of us are now full professors and are carrying on fruitful studies in the field to this day. We offer summer courses, put out a second edition of *Immunopathology of the Skin*,[1] and run a small non-profit foundation (the ISIL) devoted to helping others to use defined IF methods."

1. **Beutner E, Chorzelski T P & Bean S F,** eds. *Immunopathology of the skin.* New York: Wiley, 1979. 496 p.

This Week's Citation Classic

Koffler D, Schur P H & Kunkel H G. Immunological studies concerning the nephritis of systemic lupus erythematosus. *J. Exp. Med.* **126**:607-24, 1967. [Rockefeller Univ., and Dept. Pathol., Mt. Sinai Sch. Med., New York, NY]

Anti-DNA and several other antinuclear antibodies were eluted from glomeruli of kidneys showing SLE nephritis. Deposits of DNA antigen associated with immunoglobulin and complement were observed using immunofluorescence. These results suggest a pathogenetic role for DNA-anti-DNA immune complexes. [The *SCI*® indicates that this paper has been cited over 465 times since 1967.]

David Koffler
Department of Laboratory Medicine
Hahnemann Medical College &
Hospital of Philadelphia
Philadelphia, PA 19102

August 12, 1980

"These studies were performed in my first year as a postdoctoral fellow studying immunology in the laboratory of Henry Kunkel at Rockefeller University. I had come to this laboratory for training in immunology having had some experience in immunopathology acquired during a pathology residency. A strong interest in SLE had developed as a result of my own immunopathology studies of this disease and conversations with Paul Klemperer, retired chairman of pathology at the Mount Sinai Hospital, who had devoted many years to the study of this disease. I was most impressed by the insights into potential pathogenetic mechanisms that he had obtained by simple light microscopic studies, which were thoughtfully and critically analyzed.

"When I moved to the laboratory at the Rockefeller University, I became associated with investigators who had a major interest in the immunology of SLE. The serological studies of Kunkel and his colleagues had provided compelling evidence that anti-DNA antibodies were closely related to the pathogenesis of the disease. It appeared reasonable, therefore, that complexes containing both antibody and antigen were present in the kidneys of patients affected by glomerulonephritis. Prior attempts to demonstrate the antigen in tissue had not been successful probably because the antigen was concealed in a complex with antibody. Acid buffer elution of tissue sections removed sufficient antibody to permit demonstration of the antigen. Deoxyribonuclease enzyme treatments of the isolated glomeruli facilitated the preferential release of anti-DNA antibody from tissue providing further support for the immune complex hypothesis involving DNA.

"The evidence obtained from these studies was one of the early demonstrations that a specific antigen (DNA) and antibody were associated with renal glomerular injury. The techniques utilized were of potential importance for the identification of antigens and antibodies in other forms of immune complex type glomerulonephritis. Subsequently, similar techniques were utilized to demonstrate DNA antigen and antibodies in a murine model of human SLE. Although the precise mechanism of immune injury in this disease remains to be established, a large number of investigators have continued to evaluate, characterize and demonstrate the importance of the DNA system for the pathogenesis of SLE. The disease is of considerable interest, not only as an entity more common than originally believed, but because it serves as a prototype of immune manifestations of several other human diseases. These factors have probably contributed to the frequent citation of this study."

CC/NUMBER 2
JANUARY 10, 1983

This Week's Citation Classic

Pincus T, Schur P H, Rose J A, Decker J L & Talal N. Measurement of serum DNA-binding activity in systemic lupus erythematosus. *N. Engl. J. Med.* **281**:701-5, 1969. [Labs. Viral Dis. and Biol. Viruses, Natl. Inst. Allergy and Infect. Dis., Arthritis and Rheumatism Br., Natl. Inst. Arthritis and Metabolic Dis., NIH, Bethesda, MD and Robert Breck Brigham Hosp., Boston, MA]

The Farr ammonium sulfate technique was applied to measurement of antibodies to double-stranded DNA found in patients with systemic lupus erythematosus (SLE). The method provides an easily performed specific clinical test for diagnosis and management of SLE. [The *SCI*® indicates that this paper has been cited in over 335 publications since 1969.]

Theodore Pincus
Division of Rheumatology & Immunology
Department of Medicine
Vanderbilt University
Nashville, TN 37232

December 15, 1982

"DNA antibodies were recognized in active systemic lupus erythematosus (SLE) in 1957, but measurement of these antibodies was largely confined to research laboratories in 1967. The possibility of using the Farr ammonium sulfate precipitation technique to provide a simple clinical measure of DNA antibodies was raised initially in a discussion with Norman Talal at a social gathering in the home of Ron Lamont-Havers. I had learned this technique as a medical student in the laboratory of Charles Christian, and was invited by Talal to work on the assay as a spare-time project, despite my background as a surgical intern and affiliation with a tumor virus laboratory. There were many other sources of help, including Jim Rose, who taught me how to prepare radiolabeled DNA, and Peter Schur, who provided well-characterized SLE sera. After about three months of informal experimentation, it became apparent that the research might lead to a useful clinical test. My supervisor, Wallace Rowe, generously allowed me to spend nine months away from tumor virus studies, while John Decker kindly provided space in the Arthritis Branch to complete the work. I then returned to more basic research on endogenous murine retroviruses with Rowe, which has continued over the years, and have not pursued further research on DNA antibodies. I did enjoy introducing the technique to colleagues, including Alfred Steinberg,[1] and Graham Hughes and Rob Lightfoot,[2] whose studies were responsible for its wide use.

"In retrospect, the resources and unstructured environment at NIH provided an optimal environment for problem solving, under the enlightened leadership of Rowe, Talal, and Decker. I had no formal affiliation with the Arthritis Branch nor identity as a rheumatology trainee during this entire period, though eight studies with six members of the Branch were completed during the year of informal collaboration. These studies did not result from well-articulated planning, but rather from empirical 'hands on' intuitive probing, as has been the case in most of my interesting research as well as in many advances from other laboratories far more important than my work. Yet it remains curious that scientific progress is frequently described as resulting primarily from orderly predictable planning rather than unstructured high-risk intuition, prior expertise rather than a will to solve a problem, the number of workers or dollars involved rather than the enthusiasm of the workers, and formal administrative organization rather than ideas and a positive environment.

"I believe the relatively trivial observation in this study has been highly cited because it was published in a most respected and well-read journal, and contains clinically significant diagnostic, management, and pathogenetic observations in a single source—it is unfortunate that consolidation of data into potentially important papers may be discouraged by a tendency to assess scientific accomplishment in terms of the quantity rather than quality of publications. My experiences at NIH led to reorientation of my career from surgery to rheumatology, with continued study of host variables in disease in a milieu of inquiry at Vanderbilt University under Grant Liddle, involving the two themes which provided so much satisfaction during that period, i.e., basic research on regulatory mechanisms involving endogenous retroviruses,[3] and clinical research toward better assessment in diagnosis and therapy of inflammatory rheumatic diseases. My recent clinical research has been outside the laboratory, toward assessment of patient function, demographic variables, and attitudes in the course of chronic rheumatic diseases, as limitations to the use of laboratory data in optimally defining patient status which were apparent in 1969 are even more appreciated today. Basic laboratory research, including recent elegant studies of nucleic acid antibodies,[4] will provide ultimate solutions, but improved clinical measurements are needed to advance ongoing patient care in chronic rheumatic diseases."

1. **Steinberg A D, Raveche E S, Laskin C A, Miller M L & Steinberg R T.** Genetic, environmental, and cellular factors in the pathogenesis of systemic lupus erythematosus. *Arthritis Rheum.* **25**:734-43, 1982.
2. **Lightfoot R W, Jr. & Hughes G R V.** Significance of persisting serologic abnormalities in SLE. *Arthritis Rheum.* **19**:837-43, 1976.
3. **Pincus T.** Studies regarding a possible function for viruses in the pathogenesis of systemic lupus erythematosus. *Arthritis Rheum.* **25**:847-56, 1982.
4. **Koffler D,** ed. Current perspectives on the immunology of systemic lupus erythematosus. (Whole issue.) *Arthritis Rheum.* **25**(7), 1982. p. 721-910.

CC/NUMBER 11
MARCH 15, 1982

This Week's Citation Classic

Cohen A S, Reynolds W E, Franklin E C, Kulka J P, Ropes M W, Shulman L E & Wallace S L. Preliminary criteria for the classification of systemic lupus erythematosus. *Bull. Rheum. Dis.* **21**:643-8, 1971.
[Diagnostic and Therapeutic Criteria Committee of the American Rheumatism Assn. Sect. of the Arthritis Foundation, New York, NY]

A system to classify a patient's disease as systemic lupus erythematosus (SLE) was devised from data obtained from 900 patients. Fourteen manifestations were selected by sensitivity-specificity testing. If four or more of these manifestations were present, there was a 90 percent sensitivity and 99 percent specificity for SLE against rheumatoid arthritis and 98 percent specificity against 'other diseases.' [The *SCI*® indicates that this paper has been cited over 790 times since 1971.]

Alan S. Cohen
Thorndike Memorial Laboratory
Department of Medicine
Boston City Hospital
Boston University School of Medicine
Boston, MA 02118

November 4, 1981

"This study had its origin in 1962, when the American Rheumatism Association (ARA) had the foresight to realize the difficulties ahead in our understanding of SLE, a disease of unknown etiology and multisystem manifestations. The criteria were created to achieve uniform classification of defined groups of patients in order to compare data from different sources concerning the natural history, evaluation of therapy, and epidemiologic description of SLE. There was considerable debate as to whether such a classification scheme should be undertaken, but there was the precedent of the Jones criteria for rheumatic fever and the ARA criteria for rheumatoid arthritis.[1] Acknowledgement should go to the 59 hospitals and clinics which contributed to the data base, and to the full membership of the ARA Criteria Committee, especially Bill Reynolds, who worked so effectively with the mathematics and statistical handling of the data.

"The several years of study, the multiple meetings, and the generation of 900 completed data sheets on patients with SLE, possible SLE, rheumatoid arthritis, and other diseases were a huge undertaking. We on the committee learned an enormous amount about the disease itself, about how it was viewed and followed by experts in various parts of the country, and how difficult an undertaking a study of this type is. We felt very strongly that these were criteria for the classification, not for the diagnosis, of SLE. It is interesting that our review in 1979 of how the criteria were being utilized demonstrated that they were more appropriately used with the passage of time, and that most large series of cases utilized them, while small series and single case reports tended to use explicit case descriptions.[2] The sensitivity of 90 percent was found to hold up while the specificity studies have yielded more conflicting data.

"When the data were first evaluated, a cluster analysis was developed and subsets of patients defined. Those efforts anticipated the current trend which increasingly identifies SLE subsets with different serologic findings, different clinical patterns and prognoses, and presumably different treatments. Although the cluster analysis yielded such data, the more cumbersome determination of sensitivity and specificity of each item (of 74) alone and in combination was ultimately used to select the individual criteria.

"It seems that the criteria have been widely quoted as they did indeed fill a need, since studies of SLE occupy such a large part of the current rheumatologic literature, and because the criteria themselves have been a focus of discussion. The SLE criteria have led to a series of further committee studies to classify rheumatologic diseases. Criteria for the classification of juvenile rheumatoid arthritis, gout, and scleroderma have been completed while a study on the classification of vasculitis is in progress. The criteria have also proven useful in allowing the delineation of subsets with negative antinuclear antibody tests in a reproducible fashion.

"It was apparent when the SLE criteria were published that newer laboratory data such as antinuclear antibodies and complement would have to be considered for inclusion. This update is currently in progress and it is anticipated that revised criteria will be made available in the not too distant future."

1. **Ropes M W, Bennett G A, Cobb S, Jacox R & Jessar R A.** 1958 revision of diagnostic criteria for rheumatoid arthritis. *Bull. Rheum. Dis.* **9**:175, 1958.
2. **Canoso J J & Cohen A S.** A review of the use, evaluations and criticisms of the preliminary criteria for the classification of systemic lupus erythematosus. *Arthritis Rheum.* **22**:917-21, 1981.

CC/NUMBER 29
JULY 21, 1980

This Week's Citation Classic

Brewerton D A, Caffrey M, Hart F D, James D C O, Nicholls A & Sturrock R D. Ankylosing spondylitis and HL-A 27. *Lancet* 1:904-7, 1973. [Westminster Hospital, London, England]

The inherited antigen now known as HLA B27 was found in 72 of 75 patients with the rheumatic disease ankylosing spondylitis and in three of 75 matched controls. The same antigen was also present in 31 of 60 first-degree relatives. [The *SCI®* indicates that this paper has been cited over 385 times since 1973.]

Derrick Brewerton
Westminster Hospital
Horseferry Road
London SW1P 2AP
England

June 12, 1980

"It was lunch in the common room at Westminster Hospital on a hot summer day in 1971. As a rheumatologist I had been fascinated for many years by the enigma of ankylosing spondylitis, which is primarily a chronic inflammation of the spine. Its aetiology was unknown except that family studies had indicated a hereditary component. My colleague, David James (head of our tissue-typing laboratory), had recently returned from an international conference at which there were reports of associations between histocompatibility antigens and inherited immune responses in mice and a paper indicating a possible link between HLA antigens and Hodgkin's disease. Over the salad we decided to investigate the frequency of HLA antigens in ankylosing spondylitis.

"There were delays while grant-giving bodies declined to support the project. Caffrey joined James to do the tissue-typing. Nicholls helped me in clinical assessments. Hart and Sturrock were planning a drug trial of patients with spondylitis. Once we had started, the association between HLA B27 and spondylitis was obvious. Although it now seems strange, we made a joint decision in 1972 that James and Caffrey would write a brief (laboratory oriented) report for *Nature,*[1] while I wrote a longer (more clinical) paper for the *Lancet.* At first the research results appeared too good to be true. We worried that they might be false results produced by an unrecognized component of the disease or by treatment, so we turned to the first-degree relatives, most of whom would not have spondylitis or received treatment. The *Lancet* article was delayed until we learned—to our relief—that 31 of 60 relatives had B27.

"Unknown to us, the association between B27 and spondylitis had been discovered independently by a team in Los Angeles led by Bluestone and Terasaki. Their article in the *New England Journal of Medicine*[2] was published between our *Nature* and *Lancet* reports, all three appearing within a few weeks. Subsequently, James, Bluestone, and I shared the Robecchi (European) and Geigy (International) prizes for arthritis research. I won the Bose prize of the Royal College of Physicians.

"Before writing the *Lancet* article, we had already established that HLA B27 was also strongly associated with acute anterior uveitis (iritis), seronegative limb arthritis, Reiter's disease, and the spondylitis in patients with psoriasis, ulcerative colitis, and Crohn's disease. In the article we hinted that this might be so but held back the material for three subsequent articles in the *Lancet.* A review was published in 1978.[3] From the outset we hoped that B27 would help in the identification of infective agents. The hunt for such agents is now our main endeavour. We received one criticism of our article: it contained no statistical proof that 96 percent and 4 percent were significantly different."

1. **Caffrey M F P & James D C O.** Human lymphocyte antigen association in ankylosing spondylitis. *Nature* **242**:121, 1973.
2. **Schlosstein L, Terasaki P I, Bluestone R & Pearson C M.** High association of an HL-A antigen, W27, with ankylosing spondylitis. *N. Engl. J. Med.* **288**:704-6, 1973.
3. **Brewerton D A.** Inherited susceptibility to rheumatic disease. *J. Roy. Soc. Med.* **71**:331-8, 1978.

CC/NUMBER 46
NOVEMBER 15, 1982

This Week's Citation Classic

Buckton K E, Jacobs P A, Court Brown W M & Doll R. A study of the chromosome damage persisting after X-ray therapy for ankylosing spondylitis. *Lancet* **2**:676-82, 1962. [MRC Clinical Effects of Radiation Res. Unit, Western Gen. Hosp., Edinburgh, Scotland and MRC Statistical Res. Unit, Univ. Coll. Hosp. Med. Sch., London, England]

Immediately after radiotherapy for ankylosing spondylitis (total dose 1,500 r), 32 percent of lymphocytes carried unstable chromosome abnormalities, which gradually disappeared at a rate of 3.5 percent per month. The frequency of cells with stable chromosome abnormalities did not change with time posttreatment. [The *SCI*® indicates that this paper has been cited in over 275 publications since 1962.]

K.E. Buckton
Clinical and Population Cytogenetics Unit
Medical Research Council
Western General Hospital
Edinburgh EH4 2XU
Scotland

September 6, 1982

"This study was initiated by the late Court Brown, who, with his colleague (now Sir) Richard Doll, had made a detailed study of the incidence of leukaemia and other cancers in irradiated ankylosing spondylitis (AS) patients. He felt that 'a knowledge of the effects of radiations at the cellular and subcellular levels might provide clues to the mechanism of leukaemogenesis'; one such subcellular level was the human chromosome. The technique for obtaining chromosome preparations from human peripheral blood, which became available in 1960,[1] was a further stimulus to investigate *in vivo* radiation-induced chromosome damage in man. The AS patients were chosen because of the wealth of knowledge of the long-term effects of irradiation and because the disease, which primarily affects men usually as young adults, is not itself malignant. As our group had its premises in a small part of the department of radiotherapy, the patients were receiving their treatment and attending the follow-up clinics nearby, and therefore were readily available.

"The publication was criticised by one radiation cytogeneticist because it introduced a new classification of different types of chromosome aberrations of which he did not approve. Although we no longer use the nomenclature, the terms 'unstable' and 'stable' aberrations, which were also introduced in this paper, have now been widely accepted.

"This publication was followed by more extensive studies of the radiation-induced chromosome aberrations in AS patients, but it laid the grounding for the direction of future studies and was the first indication that this damage remained in the body for many years posttreatment. As the blood culture technique was fairly new at the time this study was done, we were not aware of a number of pitfalls surrounding the system, and particularly the timing of the first divisions in culture, which led us to suggest that 'many of the cells with unstable abnormalities have divided *in vivo*.' Later studies[2] showed that the majority of cells had divided *in vitro* by three days in culture and this was the reason for dicentrics being present without their accompanying fragments or with two similar fragments.

"As a result of this study, it was realised (1) that there was a population of lymphocytes with a much longer life cycle than had previously been estimated;[3] (2) that chromosome aberrations could be used as a 'biological dosimeter' of both partial and whole body irradiation, even if the irradiation had taken place some years previously;[4] and (3) that the age of the individual at irradiation might be an important factor to be taken into consideration.

"I believe that this paper has been highly cited because it was of interest not only to cytogeneticists, but also to radiation biologists, epidemiologists, and immunologists."

1. **Moorhead P S, Nowell P C, Mellman W J, Battips D M & Hungerford D A.** Chromosome preparations of leucocytes cultured from human peripheral blood. *Exp. Cell Res.* **20**:613-16, 1960.
2. **Buckton K E & Pike M C.** Time in culture. An important variable in studying *in vivo* radiation induced chromosome damage in man. *Int. J. Radiat. Biol.* **8**:439-52, 1964.
3. **Buckton K E, Smith P G & Court Brown W M.** The estimation of lymphocyte lifespan from studies on males treated with X-rays for ankylosing spondylitis. (Evans H J, Court Brown W M & McLean A S, eds.) *Human radiation cytogenetics*. Amsterdam: North Holland, 1967. p. 106-14.
4. **United Nations. Scientific Committee on the Effects of Atomic Radiation.** *Report of the United Nations Scientific Committee on the Effects of Atomic Radiation*. New York: UN, September 1969. 165 p. Document A/7613.

CC/NUMBER 48
NOVEMBER 28, 1983

This Week's Citation Classic

Mayock R L, Bertrand P, Morrison C E & Scott J H. Manifestations of sarcoidosis: analysis of 145 patients, with a review of nine series selected from the literature. *Amer. J. Med.* **35**:67-89, 1963.
[Pulmonary Disease Sect., Dept. Med., Hosp. Univ. Pennsylvania and Univ. Pennsylvania Sch. Med., Philadelphia, PA]

The manifestations of sarcoidosis in 145 patients with generalized proved sarcoidosis were described and compared with other series making a combined group of 1,254 patients. The groups were analyzed with respect to background data, symptoms, frequency and type of organ involvement, laboratory findings, and mortality. Although marked differences were noted among the groups, when combined, a reasonably representative picture of the manifestations of sarcoidosis was presented. [The *SCI*® indicates that this paper has been cited in over 270 publications since 1963.]

Robert L. Mayock
Ravdin Building
Hospital of the University of Pennsylvania
Philadelphia, PA 19104

September 7, 1983

"After completing my medical training in internal medicine at the University of Pennsylvania, I became interested in pulmonary disease and took over a group of patients with sarcoidosis who had been diagnosed throughout the various parts of the medical complex. Although patients with sarcoidosis were reported since the days of Hutchinson,[1] the cases were not recognized as being of a common pathology until the work of Caesar Boeck,[2] as well as others, brought all the different entities together as a combined disease—sarcoidosis. Since the disease is uncommon and is so protean in its manifestations, it was apparent that most of the literature was devoted to case presentations or isolated organ system studies with little emphasis on the whole disease picture.

"As our own cases accumulated, we felt that a summary of the disease was overdue and that it should also include the previously reported larger series in the literature for comparison.

"The selection of series to be reviewed presented a major problem. Diagnostic confusion existed and still exists with diseases such as lymphoma, tuberculosis, and the systemic fungi; therefore series were chosen that consisted of only proved cases that were large enough for analysis. The smallest series was 28 cases.

"In reviewing the authors' descriptions of the source of their case material, a tremendous diversity was noted. Patients available to them ranged all the way from relatively asymptomatic young individuals found during X-ray surveys to clinically ill individuals referred for therapy (Massachusetts General Hospital, Johns Hopkins Hospital). Our own series was of the latter group. Since sarcoidosis is ten to 15 times more common in blacks, racial ratios added to the diversities found in the analyses. It was our hope that combining the disparate series would give a composite picture of the disease and that individual variations due to the above factors could be analyzed or eliminated.

"I believe that our study achieved these goals and over the years has served many specialties and subspecialties as a basis of reference for the frequency of manifestations in their particular area. The frequencies of occurrence have held up well on the whole except for the tracheobronchial tree where newer diagnostic measures, i.e., fiberoptic bronchoscopy and multiple biopsies via this route, have revealed a 15-20 percent incidence of involvement compared to no bronchial involvement found in the collected series. This probably reflects the lack of extensive changes and also the hurried examination required during straight bronchoscopy which resulted in the missing of very small lesions.

"Our major production problems consisted of interpreting the descriptions in the nine reported series and reducing them to numbers that could be tabulated. We spent many hours at this task as well as the cross-checking of tabulations to be sure that the series were correct on the multiple tables.

"I believe our study has been extensively quoted because we achieved our goal of a composite picture of the disease. Thus, our data serve as a starting point for many of the specialty areas of medicine when researchers begin describing and analyzing their own patients with sarcoidosis.

"I am not aware of an equivalent effort since our original report, probably due to the difficulties noted by us here. Perhaps our review was sufficiently well done so as to not warrant repetition.

"Recent studies of the disease have centered around disturbances in the immune system and their relationships to sarcoidosis.[3] At the moment, this approach appears to be the most fruitful in the development of a better understanding of this disease of unknown etiology."

1. **Hutchinson J.** Anomalous disease of skin of the fingers, etc. (papillary psoriasis?). *Illustrations of clinical surgery*. London: Churchill, 1875. p. 42-3.
2. **Boeck C.** Nachmals sur Klinic und zur Stellung des "Benignen Miliarlupoids." *Arch. Derm. Syph. Wein* **121**:707-41, 1916.
3. **Daniele R P, Dauber J H & Rossman M D.** Immunologic abnormalities in sarcoidosis. *Ann. Intern. Med.* **92**:404-16, 1980.

CC/NUMBER 21
MAY 23, 1983

This Week's Citation Classic

Cohen A S. Amyloidosis. *N. Engl. J. Med.* **277**:522-30; 574-83; 628-38, 1967.
[Robert Dawson Evans Dept. Clinical Res., University Hosp., and Dept. Medicine, Boston Univ. Sch. Med., Boston Univ. Med. Ctr., MA]

The delineation of the basic pathobiologic, immunologic, and biochemical factors involved in the genesis of amyloidosis as well as the clinical behavior of the disease has led to a clearer understanding of its manifestations. The description of the various clinical types including an analysis of the increasing numbers of heredofamilial amyloidoses has led to a greater awareness of their presence and greater interest in its diagnosis. [The *SCI*® indicates that these papers have been cited over 855 times in 423 publications since 1967.]

Alan S. Cohen
Thorndike Memorial Laboratory
Boston City Hospital
Boston University School of Medicine
Boston, MA 02118

March 24, 1983

"The study of amyloidosis has been of interest to me for over 25 years, starting with my fellowship in rheumatology at Massachusetts General Hospital in 1956. After our startling observations made in 1957-1958[1] that amyloid has a precise fibrous ultrastructure, we embarked on long-term basic and clinical studies that grew in scope when I moved to Boston University School of Medicine in 1960-1961. It became apparent that this substance, which previously had been regarded as a collection of debris, had a unique fine structure (and subsequently it was shown to have an interesting cross beta conformation on X-ray diffraction) and was a highly ordered molecule or molecules. These studies led to a series of observations by my laboratory and others on the isolation, biochemistry, and immunologic properties of amyloid. It is now known that while the fibrous structure is common to all amyloids, several major biochemical subclasses exist (i.e., AL, that related to immunoglobulin light chain; AA, that related to a new protein SAA also found in the serum; A prealb, that related to circulating prealbumin; and others).

"My review, however, followed a detailed analysis of the pathogenesis of amyloidosis[2] and was meant to bring together in one article the heterogeneous collection of information about types of amyloid, its classification, course, and organ involvement. As I warmed to the subject, the outgoing editor of the *New England Journal of Medicine* viewed with alarm the space requirements of the growing bibliography and tried to persuade me to pare it down to a few general references. When I pointed out that the complete bibliography was more likely to have long-lasting usefulness than the article itself, the editor agreed and the 329 references (about five printed pages) were allowed. The editor, however, did divide the article for publication in three consecutive issues.

"It became apparent to me in the course of writing this article how little opportunity any one clinical investigator had to study more than a handful of patients with any one form of the disease and that an analysis of the natural history of amyloid and its effect on a variety of organ systems was needed. As the opportunity developed for us to embark on such studies, we did so in the course of our basic investigations, and in recent years, a series of discrete clinical studies has appeared.

"I suspect that the article has become a *Citation Classic* since it put together in one place the enormous and confusing literature on etiology and pathogenesis, and suggested the ubiquity of the disease. The multisystem nature of the disorder and its importance to internists, ophthalmologists, dermatologists, hematologists, urologists, etc., led to a fuller understanding of its prevalence and to a broader range of basic investigations. The development led to an expansion from the one or two laboratories studying amyloidosis in the 1950s to the many investigations taking place in the US and abroad at the present time. Indeed, since that time, major international meetings on amyloid have taken place in Holland, Finland, and Spain."[3-5]

1. **Cohen A S & Calkins E.** Electron microscopic observations on a fibrous component in amyloid of diverse origins. *Nature* **183**:1202-3, 1959.
2. **Cohen A S.** Constitution and genesis of amyloid. *Int. Rev. Exp. Pathol.* **4**:159-244, 1965.
3. **Mandema E, Ruinen L, Scholten J H & Cohen A S,** eds. *Amyloidosis: proceedings of the Symposium on Amyloidosis, University of Groningen, the Netherlands, 24-28 September 1967.* Amsterdam: Excerpta Medica, 1968. 465 p.
4. **Wegelius O & Pasternack A,** eds. *Amyloidosis: proceedings of the Fifth Sigrid Juselius Foundation Symposium.* London: Academic Press, 1976. 605 p.
5. **Glenner G G, Costa P P & Freitas F,** eds. *Amyloid and amyloidosis: proceedings of the Third International Symposium on Amyloidosis, Povoa de Varzim, Portugal, 23-28 September 1979.* Amsterdam: Excerpta Medica, 1980. 629 p.

CC/NUMBER 23
JUNE 8, 1981

This Week's Citation Classic

Kissmeyer-Nielsen F, Olsen S, Posborg Petersen V & Fjeldborg O. Hyperacute rejection of kidney allografts, associated with pre-existing humoral antibodies against donor cells. *Lancet* **2**:662-5, 1966.
[Blood Bank and Blood Grouping Lab. and Dept. Surg., Aarhus Kommunehospital, and Depts. Pathol. and Intern. Med., Univ. Aarhus, Aarhus, Denmark]

The paper presents very clearly the association between presence of circulating antibodies active against leucocytes, platelets, and kidney extract, and resulting in hyperacute rejection of two cadaver kidney grafts. When the grafts were removed total cortical necrosis was found caused by micro-thrombi in the glomeruli. Both recipients were females, and the presensitization obviously caused by previous pregnancies and blood transfusions. The antibodies were active against donor specific antigen. [The *SCI*® indicates that this paper has been cited over 280 times since 1966.]

F. Kissmeyer-Nielsen
Tissue Typing Laboratory
Department of Clinical Immunology
University Hospital of Aarhus
DK-8000 Aarhus C
Denmark

April 30, 1981

"Kidney transplantation was started early in 1964 in our centre, and we have by now performed ~600 transplants—mostly from cadavers. The two classical cases were seen in relation to our kidney transplants, Numbers 14 and 17, performed November 4, 1965, and January 1, 1966, respectively. They were remarkably similar in their cause, and we felt absolutely certain that the circulating antibodies were of crucial importance for the 'disaster.'

"It should here be mentioned that allograft rejection at that time was thought mainly to be caused by an attack of immunocompetent cells (i.e., lymphocytes). In mice it had been impossible to transfer the rejection phenomenon by injection of serum from presensitized animals from inbred strains. (Retrospectively, it can be stated that this most probably is caused by too small doses of antibody being transferred by this passive immunization.)

"We were convinced about the importance of our observations—later resulting in the compulsory use of a direct crossmatch between recipient serum and lymphocytes from the donor. However, being untraditional, we experienced great difficulties in getting our data published. First, a lecture at the International Congress for Nephrology in Washington, DC (1966) was rejected. During the first International Congress of Transplantation in Paris (1967), I was allowed to speak for three minutes, and to show one slide and I am quoting now: 'One slide only!'

"We feel that we submitted a very well-documented article to *Lancet* in 1966, but to our surprise it was rejected without any explanation. This was obviously caused by a referee who did not believe in 'serology,' but only a cellular (lymphocyte-mediated) cause for rejection.

"I became slightly desperate, and returned the article to the very nice editor for *Lancet*, and stated shortly that we really felt that our observations were indeed important—and we asked for a second thought by a different reviewer—without changing a comma in the article. Then the article was finally accepted.

"It should here be added that our article resulted in a letter to the editor in *Lancet* from one of the transplant pioneers, W.J. Dempster.[1] He stated that what we described could be 'the same complications (as seen) when newcomers start work in this laboratory'—and he ended his letter with the following sentence: 'To ascribe these two early anurias to pre-existing antibodies (as have Hamburger *et al.* in their first two cases) is to be fashionable at the expense of accuracy. A more humble but less impressive diagnosis would be "unknown." '

"After the publication we became aware that Hamburger[2] had seen similar pathological findings (very similar to the Schwartzmann phenomenon), but they did not correlate with serological findings. Almost simultaneously, Terasaki *et al.*,[3] during a congress in the US, made very similar observations.

"This publication has been highly cited for the following reason. Our findings were controversial, but, as gradually accepted, they were found to be of great practical importance in relation to kidney transplantation—the direct crossmatch problem in particular. For a recent survey the reader can refer to P.J. Morris.[4]

"I do believe that the publication cited here is one of the major reasons for my receiving the following honourable presentations and awards: (1) the Emily Cooly lecture, 1970 (American Association of Blood Banks); (2) Holst Knudsen honorary prize, 1968, from the University of Aarhus; and (3) very recently (February 14, 1981) the Danish Novo prize."

1. **Dempster W J.** Rejection of kidney allografts. (Letter to the editor.) *Lancet* **2**:972-3, 1966.
2. **Hamburger J, Vaysse J, Crosnier J, Auvert J, LaLanne C M & Dormont J.** Six attempted renal homotransplantations in humans after irradiation of the recipient. *Rev. Fr. Étud. Clin. Biol.* 7:20-39, 1962.
3. **Terasaki P I, Thrasher D L & Hauber T H.** Serotyping for homotransplantation. XIII. Immediate kidney transplant rejection and associated preformed antibodies. (Dausset J, Hamburger J & Mathe G, eds.) *Advances in transplantation.* Baltimore: Williams and Wilkins, 1967. p. 225-9.
4. **Morris P J,** ed. *Kidney transplantation: principles and practice.* London: Academic Press, 1979. 408 p.

CC/NUMBER 21
MAY 24, 1982

This Week's Citation Classic

Thomas E D, Storb R, Clift R A, Fefer A, Johnson F L, Neiman P E, Lerner K G, Glucksberg H & Buckner C D. Bone-marrow transplantation. *N. Engl. J. Med.* **292**:832-43; 895-902, 1975.
[Dept. Medicine, Div. Oncology, Univ. Washington Sch. Med., Providence Med. Ctr., and Fred Hutchinson Cancer Res. Ctr., Seattle, WA]

This paper reviewed studies of marrow transplantation in rodents, dogs, and primates. The experiences in man regarding histocompatibility typing, preparation of the recipient, the technique of marrow transplantation, and supportive care of the patient without marrow function were described. Clinical data were presented and problems associated with marrow engraftment, graft-versus-host disease, opportunistic infections, and recurrence of malignancy were summarized. [The *SCI*® indicates that these papers have been cited over 800 times in 539 papers since 1975.]

E. Donnall Thomas
Division of Oncology
Department of Medicine
Fred Hutchinson Cancer Research Center
University of Washington
Seattle, WA 98104

March 4, 1982

"By the mid-1950s, it had become apparent that mice exposed to lethal irradiation could survive if given a marrow transplant. Initial clinical enthusiasm was soon tempered by an appreciation of the numerous major problems involved.[1] My colleagues and I spent the next decade working with the dog as an outbred model for studies of marrow transplantation biology. Initial encouragement came from the fact that some of our beagles given allogeneic marrow grafts survived to become excellent rabbit hounds. Progress on many fronts made it possible for several marrow transplant teams to attempt clinical application again by the end of the 1960s.

"In 1972, I wrote to my old friend Franz Inglefinger, editor of the *New England Journal of Medicine*, to criticize the quality of some articles that had been published in the journal. Franz responded with an eloquent dissertation about the variability of manuscript reviews presented to an editor by presumed experts in the field. Also, he invited me to submit an article on bone marrow transplantation for the Medical Progress section of the journal. I replied that I thought the time was not quite right. After some further correspondence we agreed on a submission date at the end of 1974 and in due time my colleagues and I submitted the article.

"In retrospect, the manuscript was a potpourri of topics including a brief history of the field, a review of the more significant advances based on work in animals, particularly the canine model, and a review of the developments that set the stage for marrow transplantation in man. Unlike most reviews, the article contained a great deal of clinical data and interpretation that had not been published previously.

"Because of all of these factors the article has provided a convenient reference for those who have subsequently written on the subject of marrow transplantation. Of even greater importance, perhaps, is the fact that this article appeared at that junction in time marking the emergence of marrow transplantation from an experimental laboratory procedure and/or a desperate clinical undertaking to an accepted form of therapy for selected patients with severe aplastic anemia or patients with acute leukemia who had failed combination chemotherapy. Indeed, many of the patients described in the article continue to be living and well and apparently cured of the disease.[2]

"At the time the article appeared, the Seattle Marrow Transplant Team had carried out 149 transplants. We have now done 1,179. There has been an impressive increase in the number of centers doing marrow transplants. Many problems still require solution, but investigations in many centers on the use of monoclonal antibodies, interferon, cyclosporin A, fractionated irradiation, and unrelated donors will undoubtedly provide insight into the basic principles of transplantation biology and will extend the success rate and the kinds of diseases that may benefit from marrow transplantation."

1. **Thomas E D, Lochte H L, Jr., Lu W C & Ferrebee J W.** Intravenous infusion of bone marrow in patients receiving radiation and chemotherapy. *N. Engl. J. Med.* **257**:491-6, 1957.
2. **Thomas E D.** Bone marrow transplantation. (Burchenal J H & Oettgen H F, eds.) *Cancer: achievements, challenges, and prospects for the 1980s.* New York: Grune & Stratton, 1981. Vol. 2. p. 625-38.

CC/NUMBER 40
OCTOBER 5, 1981

This Week's Citation Classic

Gatti R A & Good R A. Occurrence of malignancy in immunodeficiency diseases: a literature review. *Cancer* **28**:89-98, 1971.
[Depts. Pediatrics and Pathology, Univ. Minnesota, Minneapolis, MN]

This report reviews the frequency and types of cancer which are seen among patients, mainly children, with various forms of immunodeficiencies. While the frequency we originally reported was probably overestimated, it is still a dramatic fact that such patients develop cancer between 100-1,000 times more commonly than the general population of similar age. Lymphoid cancer far predominates other kinds, although this spectrum alters slightly from one primary immunodeficiency to another. [The *SCI*® indicates that this paper has been cited over 285 times since 1971.]

Richard A. Gatti
Department of Pathology
School of Medicine
University of California
Los Angeles, CA 90024

August 1, 1981

"This report added great credibility to the then-incubating hypothesis that defective immunosurveillance mechanisms might underlie the pathogenesis of cancer. When I arrived for my fellowship in immunology with R. A. Good, there was a consensus that the cancer incidence was higher than normal among patients with immunodeficiencies and those receiving long-term immunosuppression following renal transplants. In the literature, I found mainly anecdotes and hypotheses about immunosurveillance, so Good and I felt it important to document the frequency and types of malignancy in patients with immunodeficiencies.

"With time, tumor-*specific* antigens were shown to be tumor-*associated*. Law's neonatally thymectomized mice with abundant tumors were overshadowed by the observation that nude mice, born without thymuses, develop little or no cancer.[1] The idea that blocking antibodies protect neuroblastoma cells from destruction by circulating killer lymphocytes bogged down in technological controversy. The latest fashionable hypothesis is that interferon turns on natural killer cells and that these cells *may* be important in immunosurveillance, if that exists. What remains the single most convincing observation to support a role for immunosurveillance is our review showing that patients with primary immunodeficiencies do develop cancer with a consistently high frequency. No doubt this accounts for the frequent citing of the reference.

"Good suggested that we establish an international Immunodeficiency-Cancer Registry so as to learn more about this provocative relationship. In late 1971, shortly before I left Minneapolis to join George Klein's department of tumor biology at the Karolinska Institute, I handed over my bulging files to Kersey and Spector, who then initiated such a registry. The registry now contains over 350 case reports.[2] The expanded data base has confirmed the dominance of lymphoid cancer among immunodeficiency patients. It has also made us recognize that if immunodeficiency were the primary defect responsible for oncogenesis, the spectrum of cancers seen in these patients would not differ substantially from those seen among the general population.

"That 'a *major* role for immunity in oncogenesis seems almost certain,' now seems uncertain. A *minor* role now seems more certain! Immunologic responses are a secondary or, possibly even, tertiary event in tumor development: the initial transformation occurs at a genetic level. Our recent focus on immunogenetics is now yielding more basic information as we try to map cancer susceptibility genes in high-cancer risk families.[3] Perhaps we jumped too quickly away from biochemistry and virology, then too quickly again from serological immunology into the vagaries of cellular immunology. Perhaps after the basic mechanisms of malignant transformation have been elucidated, the principles of tumor immunology will take on new significance, for example, in immunotherapy.

"Anecdote: The degree of 'DABP' (as appears after MD in the original publication) was my way of rebelling against pediatricians who often cite in their papers the title 'FAAP' (i.e., Fellow of the American Academy of Pediatrics). The difference: if you pass your pediatrics board exams, you become a Diplomat of the American Board of Pediatrics (DABP). If you then contribute $180.00 a year, you are an FAAP. DABP seems the more relevant of the two."

1. **Law L W.** Studies of thymic function with emphasis on the role of the thymus in oncogenesis. *Cancer Res.* **26**:551-74,1966.
2. **Spector B, Perry G & Kersey J.** Genetically-determined immunodeficiency diseases (GDID) and malignancy. Report from the Immunodeficiency-Cancer Registry. *Clin. Immunol. Immunopathol.* **11**:12-29, 1978.
3. **Gatti R A, Spence A, Sparkes R, Harris N & Freidin M.** Association of cancer susceptibility with the major histocompatibility complex (MHC). *Proc. Amer. Assn. Cancer Res.* **22**:67a, 1981.

CC/NUMBER 22
MAY 31, 1982

This Week's Citation Classic

Giblett E R, Anderson J E, Cohen F, Pollara B & Meuwissen H J. Adenosine-deaminase deficiency in two patients with severely impaired cellular immunity. *Lancet* **2**:1067-9, 1972. [King County Central Blood Bank, Inc., Seattle, WA; Children's Hosp. Michigan, Dept. Pediat., Wayne State Univ., Detroit, MI; and Dept. Pediat., Albany Med. Coll., Kidney Dis. and Birth Defects Insts., State of NY Dept. Health, Albany, NY]

This paper describes two unrelated children with severe immunodeficiency whose blood cells contain no adenosine deaminase activity. It suggests that the parents in each case are heterozygous and the children homozygous for a 'silent' allele and that adenosine deaminase may be necessary for normal immune function. [The ***SCI***® **indicates that this paper has been cited over 555 times since 1972.]**

Eloise R. Giblett
Puget Sound Blood Center
Terry at Madison
Seattle, WA 98104

March 9, 1982

"Working in a blood bank provides an excellent opportunity to investigate human genetic systems involving blood cell antigens, electrophoretic polymorphisms, and plasma protein variants. Studies of such genetic markers formed the basis of a book I wrote in 1969,[1] and I often receive blood specimens sent for tests to evaluate, for example, the fate of transplanted bone marrow. In 1972, Albany pediatricians Hilaire Meuwissen and Bernard Pollara asked me to determine the red cell antigens and isozymes of a child with combined immunodeficiency and her mother, the potential bone marrow donor. In Seattle, Jeanne Anderson (my assistant) and I were astonished to find that adenosine deaminase (ADA, a polymorphic enzyme) was missing from the child's blood cells, and her (consanguineous) parents had very low ADA levels. These findings suggested that the parents were heterozygous and the child homozygous for a 'silent' allele at the structural gene locus for ADA. Several weeks later, I received a telephone call from my old friend Flossie Cohen—a pediatric immunologist visiting Seattle from Detroit. I asked her if she had any patient with severe immunodeficiency disease whose blood we might test for ADA and she said yes. To our amazement, we found the same ADA anomalies in that patient and family. We reported this remarkable coincidence of two cases of ADA deficiency with immunodeficiency in the *Lancet* paper. Subsequently, over 30 more cases have been described.

"Because of our serendipitous finding, we set up assays for several additional enzymes in the purine, pyrimidine, and nucleic acid pathways. In 1975, Arthur Ammann, Diane Wara, and Louis K. Diamond at the University of California sent us blood from a child with normal B cells but a numerical and functional T-cell deficiency. We found that her blood cells had normal ADA but no measurable purine nucleoside phosphorylase (PNP) activity, and her (consanguineous) parents had low PNP levels.[2] Ten more children with this inherited anomaly and selective T-cell dysfunction were later described.

"The paper on ADA deficiency is frequently cited because it demonstrated the unique importance of purine metabolism in lymphoid cells and showed that some cases of immune deficiency have a biochemical basis. Many laboratory investigators were stimulated into action by that paper; I wish there were sufficient space to mention all their names, especially my colleagues at the University of Washington. Most participated in two 1978 symposia that brought together the genetic, immunologic, biochemical, clinical, and therapeutic findings in ADA and PNP deficiency.[3,4] The impaired immunity in these patients is now ascribed to the unique kinases in lymphoid cells that (in the absence of ADA or PNP) cause accumulation of deoxyribonucleotides. The latter inhibit the action of ribonucleotide reductase and thereby the synthesis of DNA. Inhibition of S-adenosylhomocysteine hydrolase may also play a role. Differences between the kinases, and perhaps the nucleotidases, in B and T cells account for the selective susceptibility of T cells to PNP deficiency.[5] I am confident that further research will uncover additional biochemical defects that cause immunodeficiency."

1. **Giblett E R.** *Genetic markers in human blood.* Oxford: Blackwell Scientific Publishers, 1969. 629 p.
2. **Giblett E R, Ammann A A, Wara D W, Sandman R & Diamond L K.** Nucleoside phosphorylase deficiency in a child with severely defective T-cell immunity and normal B-cell immunity. *Lancet* **1**:1010-13, 1975.
3. **Pollara B, Pickering R J, Meuwissen H J & Porter I H,** eds. *Inborn errors of specific immunity: proceedings of a Symposium on Inborn Errors of Specific Immunity, held in Albany, New York, 16-18 October 1978.* New York: Academic Press, 1979. 469 p.
4. **Elliott K & Whelan J,** eds. *Symposium on Enzyme Defects and Immune Dysfunction, London, 1978.* Amsterdam: Excerpta Medica, 1979. 289 p.
5. **Carson D A, Lakow E, Wasson D B & Kamatani N.** Lymphocyte dysfunction caused by deficiencies in purine metabolism. *Immunol. Today* **2**:234-8, 1981.

CC/NUMBER 44
NOVEMBER 1, 1982

This Week's Citation Classic

Baehner R L & Nathan D G. Quantitative nitroblue tetrazolium test in chronic granulomatous disease. *N. Engl. J. Med.* **278**:971-6, 1968.
[Hematology Res. Lab., Dept. Medicine, Children's Hosp. Medical Ctr., and Dept. Pediatrics, Harvard Medical Sch., Boston, MA]

Chronic granulomatous disease is a hereditary defect in the killing of certain bacteria by peripheral blood granulocytes and can be detected with the nitroblue tetrazolium (NBT) test. The rate and reduction of NBT by normal leukocytes is stimulated by phagocytosis. It also depends on cell number, pH, and temperature. Granulocytes of affected patients failed to reduce NBT to blue formazan during phagocytosis whereas leukocytes of carrier females, of the X-linked form, demonstrated intermediate dye reduction. Parents' leukocytes of the autosomal recessive form had normal dye reduction rather than intermediate values. [The *SCI*® indicates that this paper has been cited in over 570 publications since 1968.]

Robert L. Baehner
Section of Pediatric Hematology-Oncology
Department of Pediatrics
James Whitcomb Riley Hospital for Children
Indiana University
School of Medicine
Indianapolis, IN 46223

September 7, 1982

"Almost 15 years have elapsed since David Nathan and I stumbled on the idea that nitroblue tetrazolium (NBT) might be employed to monitor the activation of normal blood neutrophil oxidase. The initial manuscript was published after a series of controversial reviews because some doubted the biological significance and clinical relevance of the test. Nathan had used redox dyes for studies of red cells deficient in glucose-6-phosphate dehydrogenase. Manfred Karnovsky and his group at Harvard Medical School had previously shown that the respiratory burst of phagocytizing PMN was catalyzed by an FAD-enzyme complex which required reduced pyridine nucleotide (NADPH) as substrate.[1] Thus, the stage was set by these scientists to enable me as an inexperienced hematology fellow at the Children's Hospital Medical Center in Boston to walk on. Two samples of blood neutrophils, one from myself and the other from my three-year-old patient, a former patient of Louis K. Diamond, were studied. The child had lifelong anemia and suppurative infections resulting in liver and lung granulomas and abscesses. Nathan and I observed that my patient's PMNs could not reduce NBT whereas my PMNs became coated with and internalized the purple formazan. In a short time, I found a way to extract the dye and quantify spectrophotometrically the extent of NBT reduction. We identified several other patients with the same PMN response. Not only was the test completely accurate in identifying all subsequent patients with chronic granulomatous disease, but we and Dorothy Windhorst and Robert Good at Minnesota also found it to be useful to identify the female carriers for the X-linked form of the disease.[2]

"Subsequent studies in our laboratory at Indiana University's James Whitcomb Riley Hospital for Children have shown that the biochemical basis for NBT reduction in PMN is the release of superoxide anion, a univalent reduced product of oxygen.[3] Morphometric studies indicated that NBT reduction was in phagolysosomes.[4] Klebanoff reported, about the same time, that the dismutated form of superoxide anion, hydrogen peroxide, was responsible for effective bactericidal activity in PMN.[5] Quie and his group in Minnesota as well as our own studies confirmed the inability of PMNs deficient in both superoxide anion and hydrogen peroxide to effectively kill bacteria employing *in vitro* tests.[6,7]

"Because the NBT test is so simple in design and is easy to perform, its clinical appeal and popularity increased rapidly during the 1970s. Clinicians employed it to evaluate the oxidation capacities of blood PMNs from children and adults in a wide assortment of disease states. Several slide tests were adapted to assess NBT reduction by individual cells and to establish the diagnosis of chronic granulomatous disease prenatally.[8] The test is now standard in many clinical and research laboratories throughout the world. Perhaps our comments on the NBT test will stimulate young investigators who initially receive rejections of their work to continue to refine it and persist in their attempts to have it published especially when they are convinced of its scientific merit."

1. **Karnovsky M L.** Metabolic basis of phagocytic activity. *Physiol. Rev.* **42**:143-68, 1962.
2. **Windhorst D B, Holmes B & Good R A.** A newly defined X-linked trait in man with demonstration of the Lyon effect in carrier females. *Lancet* **1**:737-9, 1967.
3. **Baehner R L, Boxer L A & Davis J.** The biochemical basis of nitroblue tetrazolium reduction in normal human and chronic granulomatous disease polymorphonuclear leukocytes. *Blood* **48**:309-13, 1976.
4. **Nathan D G, Baehner R L & Weaver D K.** Failure of nitro blue tetrazolium reduction in the phagocytic vacuoles of leukocytes in chronic granulomatous disease. *J. Clin. Invest.* **48**:1895-904, 1969.
5. **Klebanoff S J.** Myeloperoxidase-halide-hydrogen peroxide antibacterial system. *J. Bacteriology* **95**:2131-8, 1968.
6. **Quie P G, White J G, Holmes B & Good R A.** *In vitro* bactericidal capacity of human polymorphonuclear leukocytes: diminished activity in chronic granulomatous disease of childhood. *J. Clin. Invest.* **46**:668-79, 1967.
7. **Baehner R L & Nathan D G.** Leukocyte oxidase: defective activity in chronic granulomatous disease. *Science* **155**:835-6, 1967.
8. **Newburger P E, Cohen H J, Rothchild S B, Hobbins J C, Malawista S E & Mahoney M J.** Prenatal diagnosis of chronic granulomatous disease. *N. Engl. J. Med.* **300**:178-81, 1979.

CC/NUMBER 49
DECEMBER 6, 1982

This Week's Citation Classic

Bruton O C. Agammaglobulinemia. *Pediatrics* 9:722-8, 1952.
[Pediatric Sect., Medical Service, Walter Reed Army Hospital, Washington, DC]

This paper presents observations over a four-year period on a four- to eight-year-old boy who had numerous serious infections and pneumococcal septicemia ten times. He was found to have no gamma globulin and when treated with gamma globulin his severe infections ceased. [The *SCI®* indicates that this paper has been cited in over 335 publications since 1961.]

Ogden C. Bruton
13227 Betty Lane
Silver Spring, MD 20904

October 15, 1982

"After World War II, I was assigned to the Walter Reed Army Hospital to initiate a pediatric training program. It was there that I observed a four-year-old boy who had numerous infections and pneumococcal septicemia ten times. As chief of the service, with frequent rotation of interns and residents, it was necessary to assume personal responsibility for this very serious and most difficult medical problem. Essentially, I was on call to the boy around the clock. The onset of his attacks appeared quite suddenly; he often left home for school apparently well, only to have his teacher call to say that he was very ill with chills and fever. Fortunately, he always responded to penicillin and his blood culture was positive for pneumococci ten times. One can only speculate on the significance that penicillin was discovered the year he was born, and thus explain why someone had not discovered this condition previously. These patients probably just did not live long enough for their true deficiency to be recognized.

"It was obvious early on his second admission to the hospital in 1946 that he had a very unique disease, which many consultants and the literature were not helpful in solving. In the meantime, I could keep him alive with penicillin and give him pneumococcal vaccines in hopes of boosting these antibodies. There was no antibody increase with the pneumococcal vaccines used, and no response to several other bacterial vaccines given him.

"With repeated, very severe infections it was expected that his blood gamma globulin would be abnormally high; however, when this laboratory test became available, we found that just the opposite was true. He had no measurable gamma globulin in his blood serum according to the electrophoretic method used to determine it; thus, he had agammaglobulinemia.

"No gamma globulin—give him some. This I did and with very gratifying results. He no longer had the severe infections and/or septicemia with the administration of gamma globulin at monthly intervals. Treatment was continued for 14 months before I felt confident enough to publish these unique findings and was completely unprepared for the interest engendered by the report. It suggested many avenues for investigation, resulting in a flood of papers pertaining to the immune mechanism,[1] as well as an enlarging of the nomenclature of immunodeficiency diseases in man.

"Honors have been few as a result of this paper; however, a quote from Robert A. Good's introduction to the third workshop, 1967, on immunodeficiency diseases in man, is highly prized: 'Bruton's discovery of agammaglobulinemia in 1952 not only introduced a new concept of human disease, but opened a veritable Pandora's box for immunobiology.' This has proved to be true as any current general textbook of medicine or pediatrics will reveal.

"I believe my paper has become a *Citation Classic* because it opened for study a most important system in the human body, one which had been neglected for a long time."

1. **Norman P S & Lichtenstein L M.** Immune responses in man. (Harvey A M, Johns R J, McKusick V A, Owens A H & Ross R S, eds.) *The principles and practice of medicine.* New York: Appleton-Century-Crofts, 1980. p. 1073-9.

CC/NUMBER 51
DECEMBER 17, 1979

Stiehm E R & Fudenberg H H. Serum levels of immune globulins in health and disease: a survey. Pediatrics **37**:715-27, 1966.
[Dept. Pediatrics and Hematology Unit, Dept. Med., Univ. California Sch. Med., San Francisco, CA]

Serum levels of IgG, IgM, and IgA immunoglobulins were determined on 296 normal infants and children at various ages and in 30 adults. The technique employed radial immunodiffusion in agar, using monospecific antisera. The marked alterations of immunoglobulins with age, particularly in the first year of life, necessitate comparison of the immunoglobulins obtained on any pediatric patient with appropriate age-matched controls. [The *SCI*® indicates that this paper has been cited over 425 times since 1966.]

E. Richard Stiehm
Department of Pediatrics
School of Medicine
University of California
Los Angeles, CA 90024

April 10, 1978

"This paper, prepared during a pediatric immunology fellowship in Hugh Fudenberg's laboratory at the University of California-San Francisco Medical Center, was conceived because of three factors. The need throughout pediatrics for standard values of immunoglobulins at different ages; the availability of a then unpublished new method, radial immunodiffusion, for quantitating immunoglobulin levels with a minimum of antiserum and effort; and the availability of 300 sera from infants and young children at various ages as a result of an ongoing trial of killed measles vaccine.

"In 1963, when this work was started, the only study of IgG, IgM, and IgA immunoglobulin levels in infants and children was by C.D. West, R. Hong, and N.H. Holland, in which the levels for IgA and IgM were reported in units, and the method was a cumbersome and inaccurate quantitative immunoelectrophoresis.[1] J.P. Vaerman of Belgium, a postdoctoral scholar in Fudenberg's laboratory, had worked with radial immunodiffusion in the laboratory of the late J.F. Heremans, and taught it to me prior to publication. We prepared rabbit antisera against human IgG (Cohn Fraction II), IgA myeloma, and IgM macroglobulinemia proteins, and absorbed them repeatedly with agammaglobulinemic serum, and other immunoglobulins until they were monospecific. The antisera available commercially at that time was of limited availability and of poor strength and specificity.

"The method was an important advance, permitting 20 or more analyses with .1-.2 ml of antisera and with reproducibility of ±10%. Subsequently, it was (and is) used, with minor modifications, by numerous hospital laboratories and in commercial kits. The paper usually quoted for the radial immunodiffusion method is J.L. Fahey and E.M. McKelvey[2] or G. Mancini *et al.*[3]

"The marked alterations in immunoglobulin levels with age and the expanding recognition of primary antibody immunodeficiencies in young infants necessitated this detailed study to correctly interpret immunoglobulin levels at any age. The tables and graphs of IgG, IgM, and IgA changes with age have been reproduced in innumerable textbooks of pediatrics, immunology, and laboratory methods; they are still the standard reference in most studies of immunoglobulin levels in children.

"Two other aspects of this study have been frequently quoted. One is the immunoglobulin abnormality of mongolism (high levels of IgG and IgA, and low IgM) which has contributed to an extensive literature on the immunologic defect in this genetic disorder. Second, and considerably more important, is the IgM levels in cord blood from normal infants. Elevated levels of cord blood IgM (>20 mg/dl) were noted in a subsequent study of newborns with congenital infection (i.e., rubella, cytomegalovirus, etc.).[4] This led to the IgM screening test used in nurseries to identify infants with suspected congenital infection. Without the normal values established by the 1966 paper, we would not have been able to recognize the subtle but definite IgM elevations present in congenitally infected infants."

1. **West C D, Hong R & Holland N H.** Immunoglobulin levels from the newborn period to adulthood and in immunoglobulin deficiency states. *J. Clin. Invest.* **41**:2054-64, 1962.
2. **Fahey J L & McKelvey E M.** Quantitative determination of serum immunoglobulins in antibody-agar plates. *J. Immunology* **94**:84-90, 1965.
3. **Mancini G, Carbonara A O & Heremans J F.** Immunochemical quantitation of antigens by single radial immunodiffusion. *Immunochemistry* **2**:235-54, 1965.
4. **Stiehm E R, Ammann A J & Cherry J D.** Elevated cord macroglobulins in the diagnosis of intrauterine infections. *N. Engl. J. Med.* **275**:971-5, 1966.

This Week's Citation Classic™

Axelsson U, Bachmann R & Hällén J. Frequency of pathological proteins (M-components) in 6,995 sera from an adult population. *Acta Med. Scand.* **179**:235-47, 1966.
[Depts. Internal Medicine and Clinical Chemistry, Univ. Lund, Malmö General Hosp., Sweden]

This paper presented a large-scale study of the occurrence of M-components in 6,995 people representing 79 percent of an unselected population above 25 years of age. The frequency and the Ig classes in different age groups were analysed. Sixty-four cases were given a full clinical examination. [The *SCI*® indicates that this paper has been cited in over 215 publications since 1966.]

Uno Axelsson
Department of Medicine
Central Hospital
S-651 85 Karlstad
Sweden

January 10, 1984

"In the early 1960s, many people at the General Hospital of Malmö were busy studying plasma proteins. Hällén and I worked in Jan Waldenström's department and Bachmann was in C.-B. Laurell's lab. It was known that elderly people often had M-components without associated disease. But how about the frequency outside institutions? I was at that time invited by the State Board of Mental Health to supervise the clinical part of a mass health screening project where every day blood was drawn from 300 'healthy' people. After some rather hard negotiations, we were allowed to draw an extra sample for plasma protein studies. The blood and I were 600 kilometres north of Malmö so we had to arrange cool night train transports to Hällén in Malmö, who built a small 'factory' for paper electrophoresis outside the routine lab.

"Hällén notified me that he had identified 64 strips which had M-components, and I asked all 64 persons to come back for a clinical examination. All were very cooperative but sometimes embarrassed. The area of the study was scientifically virginal from a medical point of view and hitherto not used for population studies. So when I started to draw marrow from the sternal bone and ask for X rays of the skull, a certain excitement could be observed in the neighbourhood. When telling this, I like to point out that the area chosen for the study is not in the backwoods but in the heartland of the Swedish steel industry which has attracted for centuries working people of all kinds, thereby eliminating the risk of genetic isolation.

"One of the important results of the study was that we got knowledge of what was going on in the immune system of the total population and what a lot of apparently benign M-components are found when looking for one indicating malignant disease.

"I believe that the paper is frequently cited because it was the first sufficiently large study in its field that was thoroughly performed combining detailed chemical and clinical work. The latest follow-up was published in 1977."[1]

1. **Axelsson U.** An eleven-year follow-up on 64 subjects with M-components. *Acta Med. Scand.* **201**:173-5, 1977.

CC/NUMBER 14
APRIL 6, 1981

This Week's Citation Classic

Franklin E C, Lowenstein J, Bigelow B & Meltzer M. Heavy chain disease—a new disorder of serum γ-globulins: *report of the first case.* *Amer. J. Med.* **37**:332-50, 1964.
[Depts. Med. and Pathol. and Rheumatic Diseases Study Group, New York Univ. Sch. Med., New York, NY]

This paper described a patient with γ heavy chain disease, the first example of a plasma cell neoplasm associated with the production of an abnormal, internally deleted heavy chain. It was predicted that similar disorders involving the other immunoglobulin polypeptide chains would be found. [The *SCI*® indicates that this paper has been cited over 260 times since 1964.]

Edward C. Franklin
Department of Medicine
New York University Medical Center
School of Medicine
New York, NY 10016

February 11, 1981

"This report clearly illustrates how sudden and often unexpected discoveries made in a clinical setting can contribute to our understanding of biologic problems. A major reason for its frequent citation is the impact it has had on clinical medicine as well as on basic molecular science.

"Patient CRA had been studied for about a year for an unexplained disease, possibly a lymphoma. As is often the case with diagnostic problems of this type, repeated laboratory examinations are ordered by the house staff, in this case Lowenstein and Guggenheim, in the hope of uncovering a clue. One of these tests, the electrophoretic analysis of serum and urine, done on December 24, 1962, showed unexpectedly an enormous β globulin spike which had the same configuration in both fluids. Since this had not been present two months previously and was unlike anything we had seen before, we set out to characterize the proteins. Within three days we had identified proteins which resembled the Fc fragment of the heavy chain of IgG and shortly demonstrated them to be synthetic products. With the deadline for the submission of abstracts to the FASEB meeting almost upon us, we decided to submit our findings on December 30, 1962, despite some fear that we might be wrong. Fortunately, our conclusion held up and led to the description of the heavy chain diseases (HCD), a term coined by Elliot Osserman who, after seeing our patient, identified four additional examples of γ HCD by analysis of stored samples.[1] Since then, the entity has expanded to include α HCD which is the most frequent, a few patients with μ HCD, and only one reported instance of δ HCD. ε HCD has not yet been identified.

"The report aroused the interest of clinicians because it delineated a new clinically recognizable variant of the plasmacytic-lymphocytic neoplasms, associated with a new type of biochemical abnormality characterized by the synthesis of abnormal molecules (immunoglobulin variants) rather than intact immunoglobulins and immunoglobulin light chains. For immunologists and molecular biologists, these proteins have provided profound insights into the genetic control of Igs. Based on the nonrandom and by now rather predictable nature of the internal deletions characteristic of these proteins, we were able to predict that multiple genes might code for the heavy chain[2] several years before the demonstration of discontinuous genes by DNA cloning. The suggestion that the domains and the hinge of the heavy chain are each under the control of a separate genetic element was based on the finding that the internal deletions in these and related variants usually begin or end at the interdomain regions which are now known to correspond to the sites of excision of intervening sequences and the joining of exons.[3] Many questions remain. These deal with the reason for the almost invariably associated failure of light chain synthesis and the query whether the defect lies in the DNA, transcription, or processing. Answers to these questions should be forthcoming shortly as they are likely to emerge from DNA cloning and sequencing techniques applied to cells from such individuals."

1. **Osserman E F & Takatsuki K.** Clinical and immunochemical studies of four cases of Hγ^2 chain disease. *Amer. J. Med.* **37**:351-73, 1964.
2. **Franklin E C.** Structural studies of human 7S γ-Globulin (G Immunoglobulin). *J. Exp. Med.* **120**:691-709, 1964.
3. **Frangione B & Franklin E C.** Correlation between fragmented immunoglobulin genes and heavy chain deletion mutants. *Nature* **281**:600-2, 1979.

This Week's Citation Classic

CC/NUMBER 27
JULY 7, 1980

Almeida J D & Waterson A P. Immune complexes in hepatitis. *Lancet* **2**:983-6, 1969.
[Dept. Virology, Royal Postgraduate Medical School, London, England]

Serum from three cases positive for hepatitis B antigen were examined in the electron microscope (E/M). The subjects were: a silent carrier, a chronic hepatitic, and a fatal case of fulminant hepatitis. In each instance the distribution of the antigen differed in the E/M. These appearances were related to the presence or absence of antibody and a theory was proposed that the effect of HBAg was immune mediated. [The *SCI®* indicates that this paper has been cited over 310 times since 1969.]

June D. Almeida
Wellcome Research Laboratories
Wellcome Foundation Ltd.
Langley Court
Beckenham, Kent BR3 3BS
England

June 4, 1980

"This paper is a prime example of being in the right place at the right time. The place was the Royal Postgraduate Medical School, London, and the time was just a year after the Australian antigen, later to become the hepatitis B antigen (HBAg), was first visualised in the electron microscope. A.P. Waterson was, and still is, the head of the virology department there and we had managed to enter the virological side of the hepatitis B story at an early stage mainly through the even earlier interest of A.J. Zuckerman. At that time there were none of the present-day sophisticated methods for the detection of HBsAg. The antigen was recognised serologically by immuno-diffusion or counter immunoelectrophoresis, or visually by negative staining in the E/M. As might be imagined we looked in the E/M at anything that might potentially be hepatitis B, and in so doing recognised that the antigen was usually randomly distributed but on occasion it was clumped. My own long-term interest and study throughout the years has been the use of negative staining to visualise the interaction of virus-antigen and antibody. It was therefore natural to consider that the change in distribution seen in different specimens was due to the presence or absence of immune complexes. At this point serendipity entered and, looking back, it seems almost unbelievable that the three cases described occurred almost simultaneously. They were: a silent carrier known to have been positive for HBAg for 20 years; a tragic fatal case of hepatitis in a young nurse; and a long standing chronic hepatitic. The antigen had obviously been harmless in the carrier, fatal in the nurse, and had produced chronic disease in the last subject. The micrographs from the three cases turned up in one batch and, to use a hackneyed English expression, the penny dropped!

"It seemed that the antigen itself did not do the damage without an immune response being mounted against it. This was so exciting that what happened next can only be described as reprehensible. We published on a series of three! However, it appears that this was the right thing to do; more data would almost certainly have muddied the picture, and made the theory less attractive. If there is a moral to this story it is that journals should occasionally take a chance by publishing papers that, although based on observations, also contain a certain amount of surmise, which is exactly what *Lancet* did for us.

"Why has this paper been cited? It came at a time when hepatitis B antigen was very new; in the paper it is still referred to as Australia-serum hepatitis antigen (Au-SH). It is therefore one of the earliest papers to suggest that hepatitis B antigen was God's gift not just to virologists, but to immunologists as well."

CC/NUMBER 8
FEBRUARY 25, 1980

This Week's Citation Classic

Ishizaka K, Ishizaka T & Hornbrook M M. Physicochemical properties of reaginic antibody. V. Correlation of reaginic activity with γE-globulin antibody.
J. Immunology **97**:840-53, 1966.
[Children's Asthma Res. Inst. and Hosp., Denver, CO]

This paper provided convincing evidence that reaginic antibodies in the serum of ragweed sensitive patients are associated with a new immunoglobulin, which we called γE. The physicochemical properties and antigenic structure of γE corresponded to those of reaginic antibodies. [The ***SCI***® **indicates that this paper has been cited over 210 times since 1966.]**

Kimishige Ishizaka
Department of Medicine
and Microbiology
School of Medicine
Johns Hopkins University
Baltimore, MD 21218

December 13, 1979

"When my wife, Teruko Ishizaka, and I were at the California Institute of Technology and Johns Hopkins University from 1957 to 1959, we studied the mechanisms of anaphylaxis in the guinea pig. We reached a hypothesis that bridging of antibody molecules by antigen would induce new biologic activities which trigger allergic reactions. Naturally, we wished to test this hypothesis in humans, and began to study human reaginic antibodies in 1962 after we joined Children's Asthma Research Institute and Hospital in Denver, Colorado.

"The nature of reaginic antibodies in the serum of allergic patients had remained unknown for 40 years since Prausnitz detected skin-sensitizing activity in Küstner's serum.[1] At one time, many immunochemists and allergists reached the conclusion that reaginic antibodies belong to IgA. Indeed, the antibodies were enriched in the IgA fraction of the serum of hay fever patients. We realized, however, that IgA antibodies against conventional antigens, such as blood group substance, did not have the ability to sensitize human skin for allergic reactions. This finding suggested to us the possibility that reaginic antibodies against allergens may belong to impurities present in the IgA fraction. By 1965, we accumulated evidence that the antibodies do not belong to any of the known immunoglobulin classes such as IgG, IgA, IgM, and IgD. In order to detect 'unknown' immunoglobulin with which reaginic antibody is associated, we tried to prepare rabbit antibodies specific for human reaginic antibodies. At that time, the only way to select an antiserum was to assess the skin sensitizing activity of a mixture of a patient's serum and a rabbit antiserum on our skin. Fortunately, we obtained an appropriate rabbit antiserum and detected a new immunoglobulin in a reagin-rich fraction of patient's sera. As we believed that the protein had skin-sensitizing activity, and caused erythema-wheal reactions, we tentatively called this protein γE.[2]

"The paper cited followed studies in which we studied the correlation between γE and reaginic antibodies. Data showed that the distribution of reaginic activity paralleled γE antibody detected *in vitro* when a serum of ragweed sensitive patients was fractionated by various methods and that γE is an immunoglobulin.

"Probable reasons for more frequent citation of this paper than the previous one is that more compelling evidence was provided in the second paper. This work led to purification of γE and confirmed our conclusion. After an atypical myeloma protein with the same antigenic structure as γE was found, γE was approved to represent the fifth immunoglobulin class which is now called IgE. Discovery of IgE enabled us to study immunological mechanisms of reaginic hypersensitivity and led to radioimmunoassay of reaginic antibodies in hay fever patients."

1. **Prausnitz C & Küstner H.** Studien über die überempfindlichkeit.
Zbl. Bakt. Parasitenk. **86**:160-9, 1921.
2. **Ishizaka K, Ishizaka T & Hornbrook M M.** Physicochemical properties of human reaginic antibody. IV. Presence of a unique immunoglobulin as a carrier of reaginic activity.
J. Immunology **97**:75-85, 1966.

CC/NUMBER 28
JULY 9, 1984

This Week's Citation Classic™

Juhlin L, Johansson S G O, Bennich H, Högman C & Thyresson N.
Immunoglobulin E in dermatoses: levels in atopic dermatitis and urticaria.
Arch. Dermatol. **100**:12-16, 1969.
[Dept. Dermatology and Blood Center, University Hospital, Uppsala, Sweden]

The serum level of immunoglobulin E was found to be greater than normal in patients with atopic dermatitis. The level was within normal limits in patients with various urticarias and nonatopic skin disorders. [The *SCI*® indicates that this paper has been cited in over 185 publications since 1969.]

Lennart Juhlin
Department of Dermatology
University Hospital
S-75185 Uppsala
Sweden

May 7, 1984

"A new class of immunoglobulins in human serum was described by Gunnar Johansson and Hans Bennich in Uppsala in 1967.[1] It was in the beginning called IgND after the initials of a patient with a myeloma having an earlier unidentified immunoglobulin. It was also found in healthy subjects although in very low levels (-250 ng/ml). At the same time, the Ishizakas[2] in Denver had detected γE-antibodies as carriers of reaginic activity. At a World Health Organization meeting, it was decided that the E globulins and IgND belonged to a new class of immunoglobulins called IgE.

"Gunnar was at that time working at the Blood Center of the University Hospital where Claes Högman was chief. Hans was the chemist who, together with Gunnar, did the determinations of IgE. Gunnar had found that IgE was increased in patients with asthma. I was at that time working in the department of dermatology, University Hospital, headed by Nils Thyresson. I was especially interested in patients with atopic dermatitis and urticaria. We often met for lunch in the hospital and it was natural that we should have a look at patients with other atopic disorders such as urticaria and atopic dermatitis. I therefore did a screening of various dermatological disorders and sent the blood samples to Gunnar. The IgE levels were significantly greater than normal in 23 out of 28 patients with atopic dermatitis. Normal levels were obtained from patients with contact dermatitis, various eczema, acute and chronic urticaria, as well as various other dermatoses.

"At the same time, Leif Wide, Hans, and Gunnar also developed a radioallergosorbent test (RAST) with which one could determine specific antibodies belonging to the IgE class. This test is now commercialized by Pharmacia in Uppsala together with kits for determination of IgE. The relation between clinical findings in atopic dermatitis, asthma, and hay fever with number of esosinophils, RAST, intracutaneous test, and IgE levels resulted in a series of papers from Uppsala especially by S. Öhman,[3] T. Foucard,[4] T. Berg,[5] A. Dannaeus,[6] and E. Fagerberg. The reason why our work has been cited frequently is that it was the first on this specific subject.

"For a review of recent findings see 'The clinical significance of IgE' by S.G.O. Johansson."[7]

1. **Johansson S G O.** Raised levels of a new immunoglobulin class (IgND) in asthma. *Lancet* **2**:951-3, 1967. (Cited 320 times.)
2. **Ishizaka K & Ishizaka T.** Identification of γE-antibodies as a carrier of reaginic activity. *J. Immunology* **99**:1187-98, 1967. (Cited 315 times.)
3. **Öhman S & Johansson S G O.** Immunoglobulins in atopic dermatitis. *Acta Dermato-Venereol.* **54**:193-202, 1974.
4. **Foucard T.** *Studies on reaginic allergy* in vitro *and* in vivo. Uppsala: University of Uppsala, 1973. 39 p.
5. **Berg T & Johansson S G O.** Immunoglobulin levels during childhood, with special regard to IgE. *Acta Paediat. Scand.* **58**:513-24, 1969. (Cited 105 times.)
6. **Dannaeus A & Inganas M.** A follow-up study of children with food allergy. Clinical course in relation to serum IgE- and IgG-antibody levels to milk, egg and fish. *Clin. Allergy* **11**:533-9, 1981.
7. **Johansson S G O.** The clinical significance of IgE. (Franklin E C, ed.) *Clinical immunology update: reviews for physicians.* New York: Elsevier, 1981. p. 123-45.

This Week's Citation Classic

Johansson S G O, Mellbin T & Vahlquist B. Immunoglobulin levels in Ethiopian preschool children with special reference to high concentrations of immunoglobulin E (IgND). *Lancet* **1**:1118-21, 1968.
[Dept. Paediatrics and Blood Ctr., Univ. Hosp., Uppsala, Sweden and Children's Nutrition Unit, Addis Ababa, Ethiopia]

Immunoglobulin levels were determined in serum from Ethiopian children. The IgE concentrations were 16 to 20 times higher than in Swedish children and in a group with *Ascaris lumbricoides* infection the level was 28 times higher. Clinical investigations did not reveal a high incidence of atopic allergy. These findings favour the hypothesis that parasitic infestations are important factors in stimulating IgE production. [The *SCI*® indicates that this paper has been cited over 275 times since 1968.]

S.G.O. Johansson
Department of Clinical Immunology
Karolinska Sjukhuset
S-104 01 Stockholm
Sweden

October 13, 1981

"The allergy immunoglobulin, IgE, was discovered in the late-1960s[1] through the independent work of an American and a Swedish research group. I was, as a medical student, a young and inexperienced member of the latter team.

"From late-1966 to early-1967 we developed a radioimmunoassay for IgE, or IgND as our protein was tentatively named after the initials of a unique myeloma patient I had found.[2] After considerable initial problems we succeeded in the spring of 1967 in determining IgND (IgE) in human serum. The level was extremely low for an immunoglobulin. The first study of normal individuals, a group of 50 blood donors, showed that 49 of them had levels around a few hundred nanograms per ml while one girl had an IgND (IgE) concentration of 6,000 nanograms per ml. She was found to suffer from atopic allergy with asthma due to dog dander sensitivity.

"This finding initiated a study of IgND (IgE) concentrations in serum from patients with asthma.[3] It was shown that patients with atopic, extrinsic asthma had on average six to seven times higher IgND (IgE) concentrations than patients with intrinsic, endogenous asthma or healthy individuals. These data indicated that an IgND (IgE) determination would be useful for differentiation of atopic and non-atopic diseases. I guess one could say that the concept of IgE determination as 'an allergy specific sedimentation rate' was born and today many millions of IgE determinations are performed annually for that routine diagnostic purpose.

"The study on Ethiopian children appointed as a *Citation Classic* started in 1966 and the idea was to determine IgG, IgA, IgM, and IgD. I have to admit that I was not particularly crazy about the study. There were already a couple of papers on immunoglobulin levels in African communities. However, after the discovery of the high IgND (IgE) levels in atopic diseases the interest increased. The idea of looking for atopic diseases among Ethiopian children was of interest. The results that we obtained were surprising and not clearly explained. Despite clinical impressions that allergy is rare among these children, we found extremely high IgE values. Although it was not too obvious at that time it was not too farfetched to think about helminth infestations and we were quite impressed by the relationship we found between the degree of *Ascaris* infestation and the IgND (IgE) level. Attempts to detect specific IgND (IgE) antibodies to *Ascaris* antigens turned out to be more difficult than expected and had to be left with the usual phrase, 'further studies are in progress.'

"I really do not know why this publication has been so highly cited. It is true that many reports have confirmed and extended our findings about IgE in parasitic infestations. Parasites are also commonly used in experimental situations to study the mechanisms behind the production of IgE. However, the above mentioned article on IgE in asthma[3] would in my mind better deserve to be a *Citation Classic*. IgE in parasitic infestations has been covered by several recent review articles, some stressing the clinical applications and others the experimental ones."[4]

1. **Bennich H H, Ishizaka K, Johansson S G O, Rowe D S, Stanworth D R & Terry W D.** Immunoglobulin E, a new class of human immunoglobulin. *Bull. WHO* **38**:151-2, 1968.
2. **Johansson S G O & Bennich H.** Immunological studies of an atypical (myeloma) immunoglobulin. *Immunology* **13**:381-94, 1967.
3. **Johansson S G O.** Raised levels of a new immunoglobulin class (IgND) in asthma. *Lancet* **2**:951-3, 1967.
4. **Johansson S G O & Foucard T.** IgE in immunity and disease. (Middleton E, Jr., Reed C E & Ellis E F, eds.) *Allergy. Principles and practice.* St. Louis, MO: Mosby, 1978. p. 551-62.

CC/NUMBER 16
APRIL 19, 1982

This Week's Citation Classic

Ovary Z. Immediate reactions in the skin of experimental animals provoked by antibody-antigen interaction. *Progr. Allergy* 5:459-508, 1958.
[Department of Microbiology, Johns Hopkins University, Baltimore, MD]

This article described immediate type skin reactions in experimental animals emphasizing passive cutaneous anaphylaxis (PCA), which is a widely used, simple, very sensitive, and reliable method for detecting and quantifying sensitizing antibodies. It is especially useful for detecting antibodies of the IgE class. [The *SCI*® indicates that this paper has been cited over 520 times since 1961.]

Z. Ovary
Department of Pathology
New York University Medical Center
New York, NY 10016

February 19, 1982

"In 1942, I learned from the great Hungarian pharmacologist, M. Jancsó, a technique used to visualize histamine action in the skin. In the late-1940s, while working at the University of Rome, Italy, I proposed to G. Biozzi to do experiments using this technique. Then Biozzi received a one-year fellowship to work in the prestigious laboratory of B. Halpern in Paris. He was so brilliant that the French never let him go back and he is still working in Paris. I remained in Rome and applied what we learned from our work to study histamine release during allergic reactions (my interest stemmed from my allergy to cats). That is how I discovered passive cutaneous anaphylaxis for which I coined the term PCA (a bad term, by the way, as it combines Latin and Greek words). To my amazement, I could detect 0.2 micrograms of rabbit antibody/ml. This was 200 times less than was detectable using other methods then available. I wrote, therefore, to P. Grabar, a professor at the Pasteur Institute in Paris (I worked there in the 1930s), to ask his advice and to see if I could be wrong. He invited me to the Pasteur Institute and gave me several sera to test, of which only he knew the antibody content. Each time I could detect about 200 times less than detectable by other methods known at that time. So, after all, I was right! M. Heidelberger, the dean of immunochemists, happened to be present and on his recommendation, M. Mayer invited me to Johns Hopkins University. It was there that I studied PCA more thoroughly. I made the observation in collaboration with F. Karush that the Fc fragment of the immunoglobulin molecule is necessary for 'skin fixation' (sensitization).[1] This observation led to the study of Ig receptors on cells.

"Monovalent haptens are generally ineffective for challenge of PCA.[2] This observation was at the basis of the bridging hypothesis for immunological triggering.

"In other investigations, concerning complement, the methods described in the *Citation Classic* paper were used, and it was shown for the first time that anaphylatoxin is derived from the last acting component of complement (C3 at that time).[3]

"At New York University with B. Benacerraf and other collaborators, we described that contrary to the unitarian theory, different classes of antibodies carry different biological activities.[4] These biological activities are therefore carried by the Fc fragment. Indirectly, this observation led A.G. Osler to show that two pathways of complement fixation are possible by antibodies[5] (today called classical and alternative) and thus rehabilitated the early work of L. Pillemer on properdin.[6] An unexpected use was later found in the enhancing and suppressing effect of anti-idiotypic antibodies of the IgG1 and IgG2 classes.[7]

"The article was written because P. Kallós, who read my publications, thought that it was time to write a review about the subject and that it would be of general interest to immunologists. It turned out that this happened to be the case, as judged by the frequent citations.

"I think that the article is highly cited because PCA is a very sensitive and reliable method for detection of certain classes of antibodies which sensitize for allergic reactions, especially IgE, and its use permitted the study of some fundamental aspects of many *in vivo* immunological reactions."

1. **Ovary Z & Karush F.** Studies on the immunologic mechanism of anaphylaxis. II. Sensitizing and combining capacity *in vivo* of fractions separated from papain digests of antihapten antibody. *J. Immunology* **86**:146-50, 1961.
2. **Ovary Z.** Activité des substances à faible poids moléculaire dans les réactions antigène-anticorps *in vivo* et *in vitro*. *C.R. Acad. Sci.* **253**:582-3, 1961.
3. **Osler A G, Randall H C, Hill B M & Ovary Z.** The participation of complement in the formation of anaphylatoxin. *J. Exp. Med.* **110**:311-39, 1959.
4. **Ovary Z, Benacerraf B & Bloch K J.** Properties of guinea pig 7 S antibodies. II. Identification of antibodies involved in passive cutaneous and systemic anaphylaxis. *J. Exp. Med.* **117**:951-64, 1963.
5. **Osler A G & Sandberg A L.** Alternate complement pathways. *Progr. Allergy* **17**:51-92, 1973.
6. **Pillemer L, Blum L, Lepow I H, Ross O A, Todd E W & Wardlaw A C.** The properdin system and immunity: I. Demonstration and isolation of a new serum protein, properdin, and its role in immune phenomena. *Science* **120**:279-85, 1954.
7. **Eichmann K & Rajewsky K.** Induction of T and B cell immunity by anti-idiotypic antibody. *Eur. J. Immunol.* **5**:661-6, 1975.

CC/NUMBER 6
FEBRUARY 6, 1984

This Week's Citation Classic™

Vyas G N & Shulman N R. Hemagglutination assay for antigen and antibody associated with viral hepatitis. *Science* **170**:332-3, 1970.
[Dept. Clin. Pathol. and Lab. Med., Univ. California Sch. Med., San Francisco, CA and Clin. Hematol. Branch, Natl. Inst. Arthritis and Metabolic Diseases, Bethesda, MD]

Hemagglutination assays are described for measuring hepatitis-associated Australia antigen and antibody. Red cells coated with isolated antigen, with chromic chloride as a coupling agent, are used for detection of antibodies. Detection of the antigen in serum depends on inhibition of hemagglutination. The test has the sensitivity and rapidity of the best tests available, is simpler to perform, and lends itself to large-scale screening. [The *SCI*® indicates that this paper has been cited in over 535 publications since 1970.]

Girish N. Vyas
Department of Laboratory Medicine
School of Medicine
University of California
San Francisco, CA 94143

December 27, 1983

"The single most important problem in blood transfusion and worldwide public health is the infection with hepatitis B virus (HBV), which causes chronic liver disease and hepatocellular carcinoma (the commonest cancer in Africa and Asia). The discovery of the Australia antigen[1,2] (now termed hepatitis B surface antigen, HBsAg), and the observation of its association with posttransfusion hepatitis, stimulated our studies of the immunochemical properties of HBsAg. Several immunoassays could be employed for the more sensitive and rapid detection of HBsAg and anti-HBs than the gel diffusion analysis then in vogue. I proposed a simple detection of HBsAg and anti-HBs by using a passive hemagglutination assay. I discussed the experiments with George Brecher (then chairman of my department), who suggested that I collaborate with N. Raphael Shulman because a complement fixation assay for the HBsAg and anti-HBs was established in his laboratory at the National Institutes of Health (NIH).[3] The experimental work was accomplished in six days at the NIH. The final draft of the manuscript was written in three days. On the tenth day I was back in San Francisco and gave the manuscript to Brecher for his review and comments. Besides rewriting certain paragraphs to make the text more readable, he removed his name as coauthor and forwarded the manuscript to *Science*. In astonishment I asked him why he removed his name. His answer was, 'I have graduated from this game and all I did was my job as chairman of your department.' This response typified his standards. About two weeks later, I received an acceptance from *Science*. For me this was an unprecedented 'bio-quickie,' an exciting success and the subject of my first US patent (#3,887,697) assigned by us to the government of the US.

"The assay has enabled others to carry out worldwide sero-epidemiologic surveys of viral hepatitis and permitted us to decipher the immunochemical structure of HBsAg. In developing the strategies for the use of the newly licensed HBsAg vaccine against hepatitis B,[4] the late Wolf Szmuness often recalled the usefulness of the hemagglutination test. Through the years since the hemagglutination assay took my own research endeavors beyond its practical usefulness in epidemiologic research, Saul Krugman of New York University has inspired us to study the natural history of the infection and immunity to HBV using new laboratory technology.

"The concept of developing a synthetic peptide vaccine against the hepatitis B infection followed the application of hemagglutination assay to study immune response to HBsAg in man. It took more than ten years of work by Rao, Peterson, Milich, Bhatnagar, Blum, and myself to bring to fruition the first step of this goal.[5] Once again, in 1979, the critical experiment of a synthetic peptide inhibiting human anti-HBs was performed by me using the hemagglutination assay. The fact that the immune response to a synthetic peptide analogue can mimic the natural immune response to HBsAg in humans has recently culminated in my second US patent.[6] Thus, immunochemistry of HBsAg has been an exciting and productive pursuit for several investigators."

1. **Blumberg B S, Alter H J & Visnich S.** A "new" antigen in leukemia sera. *J. Amer. Med. Assn.* **191**:541-6, 1965.
2. **Blumberg B S.** Citation Classic. Commentary on *J. Amer. Med. Assn.* **191**:541-6, 1965. *Current Contents/Life Sciences* **22**(51):14, 17 December 1979.
3. **Shulman N R & Barker L F.** Virus-like antigen, antibody, and antigen-antibody complexes in hepatitis measured by complement fixation. *Science* **165**:304-6, 1969. (Cited 360 times.)
4. **Szmuness W, Stevens C E, Harley E J, Zang E A, Oleszko W R, William D C, Sadovsky R, Morrison J M & Kellner A.** Hepatitis B vaccine: demonstration of efficacy in a controlled clinical trial in a high-risk population in the United States. *N. Engl. J. Med.* **303**:833-41, 1980.
5. **Vyas G N.** Molecular immunology of the hepatitis B surface antigen. (Maupas P & Guesry P, eds.) *Hepatitis B vaccine: proceedings of the International Symposium on Hepatitis B Vaccine held in Paris, 8-9 December 1980.* Amsterdam: Elsevier/North-Holland Biomedical Press, 1981. p. 227-37.
6. ------------. *Synthetic peptide vaccine epitomes of hepatitis B surface antigen.* US Patent 4,415,491. 15 November 1983.

CC/NUMBER 39
SEPTEMBER 29, 1980

This Week's Citation Classic

Soeldner J S & Slone D. Critical variables in the radioimmunoassay of serum insulin using the double antibody technic. *Diabetes* **14**:771-9, 1965.
[E. P. Joslin Res. Lab., Dept. Med., Harvard Med. Sch.; Diabetes Fdn.; and Dept. Med., Peter Bent Brigham Hosp., Boston, MA]

Although a double antibody radioimmunoassay method for serum insulin had been previously proposed, the design of an accurate and reliable method had been elusive. This was achieved by paying careful attention to the duration of time after adding the second antibody to the system to insure adequate precipitation and partitioning of the bound from the free insulin. [The *SCI*® indicates that this paper has been cited over 380 times since 1965.]

J. Stuart Soeldner
Elliott P. Joslin Research Laboratory
Department of Medicine
Harvard Medical School
Boston, MA 02215

July 1, 1980

"Although the original radioimmunoassay for insulin had been described in the late 1950s, and a double antibody technique described in the early 1960s by Morgan and Lazarow,[1] the assay simply wasn't accurate or reliable enough for routine use in the laboratory. My colleague, Dennis Slone, and I spent many months working with M. Grinbergs, our technician, to try to identify the critical variables so that this conceptually excellent assay would have sufficient reliability and accuracy for multiple uses in the laboratory.

"After setting up what could have been the 100th in a series of variations, the final incubation period was both started and completed (as usual) within one morning. It happened to be in this particular instance on a Friday. The centrifugation step to separate the putative bound from the putative free insulin was accomplished, the supernatant was separated from the precipitate and the tubes were placed into an automatic changing gamma counter. This trial assay was rapidly counted and calculated and Slone, Grinbergs, and I saw once again that the assay had failed. By this time it was late in the afternoon of that Friday so rather dejectedly we left the assay tubes in the tube holder of the gamma counter and went our unhappy ways for the weekend.

"On Monday morning, we commenced preparations for another trial radioimmunoassay. As we were removing the tubes from the unsuccessful assay of the previous Friday, to our amazement we noticed that a spontaneous precipitate had formed in the tubes containing the supernatant which we had never previously detected because after each previous trial assay, we inevitably removed and discarded the tubes from the gamma counter. We immediately re-centrifuged the supernatant tubes and counted this 'second' precipitate. When the radioactive counts of the second precipitate were added to the first precipitate and the counts of the supernatant appropriately adjusted, our calculations quickly revealed that the assay had performed exceptionally well. All of the serum samples assayed at multiple dilutions and all of the recoveries now fell into line. We now realized that the most critical variable for the double antibody radioimmunoassay had been identified and within the next few months we did an extended series of studies with both serum and plasma using a wide range of the second incubation times and were able to develop the data that led to the manuscript.

"Prior to publication, I was able to present this at the Fifth Congress of the International Diabetes Federation, held in Toronto, Ontario, Canada on July 1, 1964.

"I suspect that since the study showed in detail how to perform accurate radioimmunoassays using the double antibody technique, many investigators around the world in diabetes and endocrinology rapidly adopted the assay for their particular studies.

"I estimate that over 100 individuals from other laboratories visited us to learn the technique from Grinbergs."

1. **Morgan C R & Lazarow A.** Immunoassay of insulin: two antibody system. Plasma insulin levels of normal, sub-diabetic and diabetic rats. *Diabetes* **12**:115-22, 1963.

CC/NUMBER 43
OCTOBER 27, 1980

This Week's Citation Classic

Odell W D, Wilber J F & Paul W E. Radioimmunoassay of thyrotropin in human serum. *J. Clin. Endocrinol. Metab.* **25**:1179-88, 1965.
[Endocrinol. Branch, National Cancer Institute, Bethesda, MD]

A radioimmunoassay capable of quantifying human thyrotropin (hTSH) in serum was developed. Very scarce, highly purified hTSH was used to immunize two rabbits; each developed high titer antisera. Separation of bound from free hormone was by differential alcohol-saline solubility—antibody bound hTSH was precipitated; free hTSH remained in solution. Data on 101 patients with varied thyroid function were reported (euthyroid, pregnant, hypopituitary, hyperthyroid, and myxedematous). Several patients had repeated measurements of serum TSH during treatment with antithyroid drugs or thyroxine. [The *SCI*® indicates that this paper has been cited over 340 times since 1965.]

William D. Odell
College of Medicine
Department of Internal Medicine
University of Utah Medical Center
Salt Lake City, UT 84112

July 8, 1980

"This was the first description of a radioimmunoassay for TSH which was applicable to human serum or plasma. An earlier publication had described immunological studies of human and bovine BH.[1] Although it was possible then to quantify hTSH in buffer, serum or plasma interfered with the assay. This earlier work was performed at the National Cancer Institute (NCI). Peter Condliffe purified the hTSH and made it available to us (Robert Utiger and myself) for our studies. Following this, Utiger left the NCI to join the faculty at Washington University. I was then senior investigator at NCI, and was joined by my first postdoctoral fellow (Jack Wilber) and W. Paul to develop the hTSH assay for clinical use, as reported in this paper and "Radioimmunoassay of human thyrotropin in serum."[2] We investigated many methods for separating bound and free, finally selecting a simple chemical method based on the unusual solubility of hTSH in 5% NaCl, 55% ETOH. This solubility characteristic was made known to us by personal comment of Robert Bates at NIAMD. We then undertook extensive clinical studies at the NCI using this assay system. Independently, at Washington University, Utiger also developed an assay capable of quantifying hTSH in serum and reported that also at a later date.[3] All these studies used antisera originally obtained from two animals immunized by myself and Utiger in 1962-63. We used this assay method in additional studies related to physiology and pathophysiology of thyrotropin secretion in man.[4,5]

"In addition to frequent citation because it is the first report of an assay applicable to serum, the alcohol-saline separation method is cheap and simple and has been extensively used in many countries where expense of subsequently described methods (e.g., double antibody) was a limiting factor. The alcohol-saline method works for several glycoprotein hormones."

1. **Utiger R D, Odell W D & Condliffe P G.** Immunologic studies of purified human and bovine thyrotropin. *Endocrinology* **73**:359-65, 1963.
2. **Odell W D, Wilber J F & Paul W E.** Radioimmunoassay of human thyrotropin in serum. *Metabolism* **14**:465-7, 1965.
3. **Utiger R D.** Immunoassay of human plasma TSH. (Cassano C & Andreoli M, eds.) *Current topics in thyroid research.* New York: Academic Press, 1965. p. 513-26.
4. **Odell W D, Utiger R D, Wilber J F & Condliffe P G.** Estimation of the secretion rate of thyrotropin in man. *J. Clin. Invest.* **46**:953-9, 1967.
5. **Odell W D, Wilber J F & Utiger R D.** Studies of thyrotropin physiology by means of radioimmunoassay. *Recent Progr. Hormone Res.* **23**:47-78, 1967.

This Week's Citation Classic

CC/NUMBER 47
NOVEMBER 19, 1979

Smith T W, Butler V P, Jr. & Haber E. Determination of therapeutic and toxic serum digoxin concentrations by radioimmunoassay. *New Eng. J. Med.* **281**:1212-6, 1969. [Dept. Med., Harvard Med. School; Cardiac Unit, Med. Service, Massachusetts General Hosp., Boston, MA; Dept. Med., Columbia Univ. Coll. Physicians and Surgeons, New York, NY]

A rapid, sensitive, and specific radioimmunoassay for the cardiac glycoside digoxin is described. The assay was used to show that the mean serum digoxin concentration in a group of patients with cardiac arrhythmias due to digoxin toxicity was significantly greater than for patients without signs of toxicity. [The *SCI*® indicates that this paper has been cited over 390 times since 1969.]

Thomas W. Smith
Department of Medicine
Cardiovascular Division
Peter Bent Brigham Hospital
Boston, MA 02115

August 3, 1979

"Like many previous 'Citation Classics,' this paper is frequently cited because it described a convenient method that has come into common laboratory use. The groundwork for this contribution was laid by the studies of Vincent Butler,[1] who applied approaches developed by Erlanger and Beiser[2] to the problem of eliciting digoxin-specific antibodies, and by further work in our laboratory characterizing these high-affinity antibody populations.[3] Because of a wealth of immunologic expertise and experience with angiotensin radioimmunoassays, the laboratory of Edgar Haber was an ideal environment in which to combine the several concepts and techniques used in the development of the digoxin radioimmunoassay. The close and continuing collaboration in these and related studies among the laboratories of Haber, Butler, and myself remains a source of stimulation and satisfaction.

"An unusual feature of the project was the fact that it was undertaken in my spare time while in training as a clinical fellow in the cardiac catheterization laboratory, with the encouragement of Charles A. Sanders, then director of the laboratory. One hopes that clinical training programs of the future will continue to provide this sort of flexibility.

"The general conclusions of the paper, that serum digoxin concentrations could be measured accurately and conveniently and that mean concentrations are higher in digoxin-toxic patients than in those without toxicity, have been confirmed in at least 30 subsequent published studies. It has also been confirmed that overlap in levels is seen among patients with and without evidence of toxicity. We cautioned then as now that serum digoxin concentrations must be interpreted in the clinical context and weighed together with other factors that influence the response of the individual patient. As might have been expected, the widespread availability of a convenient assay procedure not requiring administration of radioactively labeled substances to patients facilitated clinical studies of digoxin pharmacokinetics.

"In retrospect, one of the most important concepts arising from this work was the recognition that antibody populations of sufficient specificity and affinity allow the measurement of minute concentrations of drugs and endogenous substances in biological fluids without prior separation procedures. Also of importance has been the recognition that antibody populations directed against a non-antigenic drug molecule coupled as a hapten to a carrier macromolecule frequently achieve affinity constants of 10^{10} M^{-1} or greater. Purified Fab fragments of these antibodies have now been used clinically to reverse otherwise fatal, advanced digoxin intoxication."[4]

1. **Butler V P, Jr. & Chen J P.** Digoxin-specific antibodies. *Proc. Nat. Acad. Sci. US* **57**:71-8, 1967.
2. **Erlanger B F & Beiser S M.** Antibodies specific for ribonucleosides and ribonucleotides and their reaction with DNA. *Proc. Nat. Acad. Sci. US* **52**:68-74, 1964.
3. **Smith T W, Butler V P, Jr. & Haber E.** Characterization of antibodies of high affinity and specificity for the digitalis glycoside digoxin. *Biochemistry* **9**:331-7, 1970.
4. **Smith T W, Haber E, Yeatman L & Butler V P, Jr.** Reversal of advanced digoxin intoxication with Fab fragments of digoxin-specific antibodies. *New Eng. J. Med.* **294**:797-800, 1976.

CC/NUMBER 12
MARCH 24, 1980

This Week's Citation Classic

Haber E, Koerner T, Page L B, Kliman B & Purnode A. Application of a radioimmunoassay for angiotensin I to the physiologic measurements of plasma renin activity in normal human subjects. *J. Clin. Endocrinol. Metab.* **29**:1349-55, 1969. [Harvard Med. Sch., and Cardiac Unit, Med. Serv., Mass. Gen Hosp.; Tufts Univ. Sch. Med., and Med. Serv., Newton-Wellesley Hosp., MA]

A radioimmunoassay employing a highly specific antiserum to angiotensin I and its application to the determination of the plasma enzyme renin is described. Plasma renin activity was shown to vary in normal individuals with sodium intake, posture, and the administration of diuretics. The values of renin activity obtained by immunoassay of angiotensin I correspond closely to those observed by bioassay in similar metabolic studies but provide an advantage of relative simplicity, specificity, and reproducibility. [The *SCI*® indicates that this paper has been cited over 1,165 times since 1969.]

Edgar Haber
Cardiac Unit
Massachusetts General Hospital
Harvard Medical School
Boston, MA 02114

January 14, 1980

"Renin, a plasma enzyme synthesized largely in the kidneys, is important in the regulation of blood pressure both in normal and diseased states. Clinical and physiologic investigations of the role of renin in vasomotor control had been impeded by the complexity and lack of general applicability of the bioassays then available. The genesis of my interest in renin was largely fortuitous. I was working on copolymers of several physiologic peptides and polyamino acids as model antigens. I was exploring the question of whether or not a simple antigenic stimulus would result in a less heterogeneous antibody response. Indeed, a far more restricted antibody response occurred with some of these peptides.[1] In a casual conversation in the dining room of the Massachusetts General Hospital with Lot B. Page, then head of the Hypertension Unit, I described some of the antigens I was studying. My luncheon companion immediately recognized the importance of angiotensin antibodies in physiologic and clinical studies and we decided to work on the problem of applying these antibodies to the assay of angiotensin peptides. The first fruit of this collaboration, a report of an immunoassay of angiotensin II, appeared in 1965.[2] Our interests then turned to measurement of the enzymatic activity of renin by determining the rate of generation of angiotensin I in plasma incubated *in vitro*. An angiotensin I antibody was developed by immunizing rabbits with this decapeptide coupled to poly-L-lysine. The assay itself was conventional and proved to be a remarkably straightforward and simple test. The method was reported together with a series of studies in normal human subjects, showing that plasma renin varied as expected with posture, sodium intake, and the administration of diuretics.

"Bernard Kliman and Andre Purnode were endocrinologists who helped us with the human studies on a metabolic ward. Theresa Koerner was a very skillful technical assistant.

"I believe the success of this publication relates to the fact that it represents the first report of a relatively simple method for assessing renin activity. It allowed the widespread application of renin measurement not only in research laboratories but also in hospital clinical laboratories. This method, with slight modification, is still widely used today. This work also illustrates how seemingly irrelevant basic science investigations may lead directly to valuable clinical insights, particularly when pursued in the appropriate environment.

"These early experiments with angiotensin peptides and their antibodies kindled my interest in the renin angiotensin system; investigation in this area has continued actively in my laboratory. I shall receive the Volhard Award of the International Society of Hypertension in May of 1980 for 'important contributions to the biochemistry and physiology of renin and the pathophysiology of hypertension.' "

1. **Haber E, Richards F F, Spragg J, Austen K F, Vallotton M & Page L B.** Modifications in the heterogeneity of the antibody response. *Cold Spring Harbor Symp.* **32**:299-310, 1967.
2. **Haber E, Page L B & Jacoby G A.** Synthesis of antigenic branch-chain copolymers of angiotensin and poly-L-lysine. *Biochemistry* **4**:693-8, 1965.

CC/NUMBER 17
APRIL 26, 1982

This Week's Citation Classic

Nieschlag E & Loriaux D L. Radioimmunoassay for plasma testosterone. *Z. Klin. Chem. Klin. Biochem.* **10**:164-8, 1972. [Reproduction Research Branch, National Institute of Child Health and Human Development, NIH, Bethesda, MD]

The paper describes one of the first radioimmunoassays for testosterone, including the generation of the antiserum with a novel immunization technique. The method is based on the isolation of testosterone by thin-layer chromatography and is applied to plasma samples. [The *SCI*® indicates that this paper has been cited over 185 times since 1972.]

Eberhard Nieschlag
Max Planck Clinical Research Unit
for Reproductive Medicine
D-4400 Münster
Federal Republic of Germany

March 3, 1982

"When I joined M.B. Lipsett at the Reproduction Research Branch of the National Institutes of Health in early-1971, we needed assays for steroids that would allow serial analysis in small volumes of serum. At that time, the first radioimmunoassay for a steroid had just been 'invented' and D.L. Loriaux and I set out to apply this principle to the determination of estrogens and androgens, respectively. When immunizing rabbits with the testosterone conjugate we applied a new immunization technique which was simultaneously applied by J.L. Vaitukaitis to raise antibodies against the hCG subunits. This extremely useful method became another *Citation Classic* in 1980.[1]

"When the radioimmunoassay for testosterone was established, I wanted to publish it. Since, however, one radioimmunoassay for testosterone had already been published[2] (to date there are over 50 published modifications!), it was decided that the manuscript should be submitted 'only' to a German journal and not, as I had hoped, to one of the larger American journals. The paper received some unfriendly comments from one of the reviewers. This reviewer, however, did not hesitate to be one of the first to ask for an antiserum sample, as I learned several years later.

"Soon after publication many people requested the testosterone antiserum and to date my records show that 140 laboratories from all over the world have received samples, several of them repeatedly. A sample of testosterone antiserum has become a well-appreciated gift when visiting other laboratories. While others tried to reap financial reward from their steroid antisera, we gave the samples away free of charge. The antiserum was used, and in many instances also our method, obviously with success. The successful application of this method to many physiological studies explains the frequent citation of the paper.

"After my return to the Federal Republic of Germany in 1972, the method remained a standard method for some time at the Reproduction Research Branch. In the Federal Republic of Germany I applied it to several investigations on the physiology and pathophysiology of testicular function.[3] The method enabled us to investigate, among other topics, the declining testicular function in senescence and to find a correlation between circulating testosterone levels and the male vocal register. Having immunized a number of animals for the production of antisera for assay purposes, we became interested in the biological effects of the testosterone antibodies in the immunized animals. In my opinion, studies in this area arising as a spin-off from the testosterone radioimmunoassay became more important than the assay itself."[4]

1. **Vaitukaitis J L, Robbins J B, Nieschlag E & Ross G T.** A method for producing specific antisera with small doses of immunogen. *J. Clin. Endocrinol. Metab.* **33**:988-91, 1971. [Citation Classic. *Current Contents/Life Sciences* **23**(33):12, 18 August 1980.]
2. **Furuyama S, Mayes D M & Nugent C A.** A radioimmunoassay for plasma testosterone. *Steroids* **16**:415-22, 1970.
3. **Nieschlag E & Wickings E J.** The role of testosterone in the evaluation of testicular functions. (Abraham G E, ed.) *Application of radioassay systems in clinical endocrinology.* New York: Dekker, 1981. p. 169-96.
4. ----------------------------------. Biological effects of antibodies to gonadal steroids. (Munson P L, Glover J, Diczfalusy E & Olson R E, eds.) *Vitamins and hormones: advances in research and applications.* New York: Academic Press, 1978. Vol. 36. p. 165-202.

CC/NUMBER 10
MARCH 7, 1983

This Week's Citation Classic

Vaitukaitis J L, Braunstein G D & Ross G T. A radioimmunoassay which specifically measures human chorionic gonadotropin in the presence of human luteinizing hormone. *Amer. J. Obstet. Gynecol.* **113**:751-8, 1972. [Reproduction Research Branch, Natl. Inst. Child Health and Human Development, Natl. Insts. Health, Bethesda, MD]

This paper presents the first radioimmunoassay capable of selectively measuring low levels of human chorionic gonadotropin (hCG) in blood samples containing luteinizing hormone (LH), hCG, or both hormones. [The *SCI*® indicates that this paper has been cited in over 555 publications since 1972.]

Judith L. Vaitukaitis
Departments of Medicine
and Physiology
Boston University School of Medicine
Thorndike Memorial Laboratory
Boston City Hospital
Boston, MA 02118

December 22, 1982

"Luteinizing hormone (LH) and human chorionic gonadotropin (hCG) share extensive sequence homology which had precluded generating relatively specific antibody to selectively measure low levels of hCG in blood samples containing physiologic concentrations of LH. In the early-1970s, in the course of carrying out studies designed to define the immunologic differences and similarities between the two subunits, alpha and beta, of hCG and the other glycoprotein hormones, we observed that some hCGβ antisera recognized relatively marked immunologic differences between highly purified pituitary LH and hCG, suggesting structural differences between their beta subunits.[1] Human CG and LH share indistinguishable biologic activities and only with insensitive, cumbersome chromatographic techniques could one distinguish between those two glycoprotein hormones.

"Since the amount of highly purified hCG subunits available was limited, we used an intradermal immunization technique we devised to overcome limitations of immunogen availability.[2] Interestingly, the description of that technique has also become a *Citation Classic.* The first animal (SB6) immunized with 50 μg hCGβ produced the best antisera for clinical measurement of hCG in blood. Unfortunately, this assay has been labeled the 'beta subunit assay,' misleading clinicians into thinking that only hCGβ and not the entire hCG molecule is detected. The initial assay technique has been modified to further enhance its specificity and sensitivity for measuring hCG.[3]

"To validate the specific hCG assay, serum samples from several different patients with high physiologic LH concentrations were assayed. Several samples from one of those patients repeatedly yielded high hCG concentrations which we initially thought reflected LH cross-reactivity. At that point, we almost gave up developing the assay. Fortunately, on reviewing the patient's chart, we found that the patient had received hCG injections for the several days his blood samples contained significant hCG levels.

"We realized the hCG was far more sensitive than any other technique. Since the specific hCG assay was sufficiently sensitive to detect hCG in the blood of women several days before onset of expected menses in a menstrual cycle in which they conceived, we chose to publish the technique in an obstetrical journal. Although we initially knew that the assay was an invaluable adjunct to monitor women with gestational trophoblastic neoplasms, we had not anticipated how important the assay would become in monitoring men with germinal cell testicular tumors. This paper became a *Citation Classic* because of its wide clinical applicability to monitoring patients with some hCG-secreting tumors and for the early detection of normal and abnormal pregnancies."

1. **Vaitukaitis J L & Ross G T.** Antigenic similarities among the human glycoprotein hormones and their subunits. (Saxena B, Gandy H & Beling C, eds.) *Gonadotropins.* New York: Wiley, 1972. p. 435-47.
2. **Vaitukaitis J L, Robbins J B, Nieschlag E & Ross G T.** A method for producing specific antisera with small doses of immunogen. *J. Clin. Endocrinol. Metab.* **33**:988-91, 1971. [Citation Classic. *Current Contents/Life Sciences* **23**(33):12, 18 August 1980.]
3. **Vaitukaitis J L.** Specific human chorionic gonadotropin assay. (Jaffee B M & Behrman H R, eds.) *Methods of hormone radioimmunoassay.* New York: Academic Press, 1979. p. 817-29.

CC/NUMBER 23
JUNE 7, 1982

This Week's Citation Classic

Sinha Y N, Selby F W, Lewis U J & VanderLaan W P. A homologous radioimmunoassay for human prolactin. *J. Clin. Endocrinol. Metab.* **36**:509-16, 1973. [Division of Endocrinology, Scripps Clinic and Research Foundation, La Jolla, CA]

This paper described a radioimmunoassay for prolactin that was specific and sensitive enough to measure the hormone in human blood. The reagents for this assay were produced in quantities sufficient to meet the demand for distribution to investigators worldwide. The work contributed to the explosion of scientific publication on the physiology of human prolactin that followed in the 1970s. [The *SCI*® indicates that this paper has been cited over 505 times since 1973.]

Y.N. Sinha
Whittier Institute for Diabetes
and Endocrinology
Scripps Memorial Hospital
La Jolla, CA 92037

April 16, 1982

"I had joined the laboratory of Willard P. VanderLaan as a postdoctoral fellow in the fall of 1969 to work on the problem of prolactin and breast cancer. Just a year before this, U.J. Lewis in the same laboratory had devised an electrophoretic technique for the purification of mouse prolactin.[1] In view of the variety of genetically distinct models of mammary tumors available in mice, this development presented an excellent opportunity to confirm or refute the theory held by many experimental endocrinologists of the time that hypersecretion of prolactin was somehow involved in the induction of breast cancer. My goal was to develop a radioimmunoassay for mouse prolactin sensitive enough to detect it in mouse blood and then to seek a correlation between plasma levels of this hormone and the incidence of the disease. It took almost two years to develop a radioimmunoassay for mouse prolactin, but the experience gained made it possible to devise rapidly a radioimmunoassay for human prolactin once a small quantity of the human hormone was isolated.

"Our isolation of human prolactin was made possible by an extremely rare happening. Prolactin was originally discovered in animals over 50 years ago[2] and since then has been found to exist in a variety of species but, strangely enough, not in primates. The prevailing dogma was that in human beings growth hormone substituted for the lactogenic actions of prolactin. Not satisfied with this explanation, we and others had been examining human pituitary glands electrophoretically for some time with the objective of identifying the component that represented prolactin. Electrophoresis had proved successful in identifying mouse prolactin, but the process did not seem to work for human prolactin. Even fresh pituitary tissue obtained at surgery failed to show a distinct prolactin band. Only when we obtained a gland from a pregnant woman who had died accidentally did we find a new, previously unseen band that we identified as prolactin.[3] That was the first and only time we had the opportunity to examine such a gland. However, once we learned about the electrophoretic characteristics of the protein from this experiment, we looked for the hormone in normal glands and found small amounts of it in a specific fraction.

"We injected bits of this material into two rabbits; one rabbit did not respond, but the other produced antiprolactin serum of a high titer. With this, we were able to develop a radioimmunoassay sensitive enough to detect prolactin in human plasma within a matter of a few weeks. This was a beautiful example of a quick and fruitful application to clinical medicine of experience gained in animal models.

"We shared the reagents developed by us with clinicians and investigators all over the world under the aegis of the Hormone Distribution Program of the National Institutes of Health. I believe this fact plus the fact that this paper described the details of the methodology may have contributed toward it becoming a *Citation Classic*. A review of work in this field has recently been published."[4]

1. **Cheever E F, Seavey B K & Lewis U J.** Prolactin of normal and dwarf mice. *Endocrinology* **85**:698-703, 1969.
2. **Stricker P & Grueter R.** Action du lobe antérieur de l'hypophyse sur la montée laiteuse. *C. R. Soc. Biol.* **99**:1978-80, 1928.
3. **Lewis U J, Singh R N P, Sinha Y N & VanderLaan W P.** Electrophoretic evidence for human prolactin. *J. Clin. Endocrinol. Metab.* **33**:153-6, 1971.
4. **Jaffe R B,** ed. *Prolactin.* New York: Elsevier/North-Holland, 1981. 288 p.

Chapter

4

Oncology

A broad brush of case reports, committee reports, epidemiological surveys, and single observations provide the substance of this chapter. As is the case with other chapters, most of the articles are not heavily cited, ranging between 100 and 400 citations each.

Several of the case reports involved large numbers of patients or tissue samples. The first "This Week's Citation Classic" (TWCC) by Friedman is significant in that two new terms, teratocarcinoma and germinoma, were introduced in his 1946 publication with Moore. Capitalizing on the abundant source material at the Armed Forces Institute of Pathology, they studied 922 testicular tumors. In their study of 202 patients diagnosed to have coeliac disease or steatorrhea, Harris et al. found that both patient groups later developed malignant complications, either lymphoma or esophageal carcinoma. The cause for this was not determined. The largest patient series, 1,414 cases, provided the subject material for a classification of salivary gland tumors (p. 117). The most prevalent of these is pleomorphic adenoma; the least common, adenocarcinoma. The observation that infection was the major cause of death in acute leukemia was determined by a 10-year study of 414 patients (p. 118), and infections following cytotoxic drug therapy remain as a significant obstacle to successful treatment of most malignancies. The article identifying this problem was twice rejected before being published.

The number of tissues or patients examined by other oncologists is not always stated, but it is obvious that Prichard must have examined hundreds of heart tumors before writing his review for the *Archives of Pathology.* Prichard's TWCC is useful on several accounts—first he indirectly states that case studies are not the most intellectually taxing studies to perform, though he next presents a justification for doing them and then, at a personal level, indicates their benefit.

The next nine TWCCs are taken from publications on only two types of cancer—those of the intestinal tract and the leukemia-Hodgkin's grouping. The first three describe studies of intestinal cancer. Spratt made good use of his interest in mathematics to show that colonic polyps were not premalignant.

This was his first paper, and he continued to investigate the nature of colonic tumors which he suggests "may yet be, one day, a preventable disease." The higher incidence of colonic cancer in the United States than in less developed countries has been attributed to differences in diet—high meat, high fat versus low fat, high fiber diets. Burkitt's report was the first to point out this dietary relationship, a discovery which he states should be attributed to Alec Walker at the South African Institute for Medical Research. Colonic cancer is still one of the most frequent manifestations of malignant cell growth in males. The chance occurrence of two patients with gastric acidity enabled Zollinger and Ellison to identify a new malignancy, gastrinoma, in which gastrin-synthesizing cells coexisted with peptic ulcers.

The TWCC by Stewart is the first of six on leukemia and Hodgkin's disease. The British study (p. 123) related 40 percent of childhood leukemias to previous exposure to X-rays. Since 1958, the exposure of children to X-rays has been sharply curtailed. The malignant state of lymphocytic cells in childhood leukemia was demonstrated by the successful long-term cultivation of these cells *in vitro,* a technique that is only successful when large inocula are used. This work was accomplished at the Jimmy Fund Laboratories in Boston by what is essentially a feeder cell culture technique. Several TWCCs on feeder cell methods are contained in *Contemporary Classics in the Life Sciences.*

Treatment of acute lymphoblastic leukemia with large doses of methotrexate may cause a lethal encephalopathy (p. 125). Kay, in his TWCC on this discovery, defends clinical trials as a source of new ideas or discoveries. In this instance, the importance of pre-trial toxicity studies was emphasized. Skipper et al. could have published their paper if some of the detailed data had been deleted, most of the charts eliminated, speculative comments withdrawn, and the page total reduced by 90 percent. In other words, the authors were requested to reduce the 110-page review to 10 pages and render it useless as a review. Combination therapy is a common approach to the problem of resistance mutation, and the MOPP combination achieved a fourfold increase in the number of survivors to Hodgkin's disease (p. 127). The classification of Hodgkin's disease into its several stages by an expert committee has been cited 980 times because of its usefulness in evaluating therapy at the different stages.

Four TWCCs on tumor-specific oncofetal antigens provide information about the use of these antigens in cancer diagnosis. The first of these antigens to be well characterized was CEA (carcinoembryonic antigen), described by Gold and Freedman in 1965 as unique to gastrointestinal tumors and the embryonic digestive system. Routine clinical use of immunoassays for this antigen has been applied to both diagnosis and prognostic evaluations. Caution about the first application is the basis for the Citation Classic described by Laurence. He and his co-authors believe the continuance of elevated CEA plasma levels after therapy or an initial decrease followed by a resurgence of CEA is useful in recognizing regrowth from tumor residues. This is reemphasized by Reynoso et al., who also recovered CEA from the blood of patients with cancer of different organs, not solely the gastrointestinal tract and associated tissue. A second oncofetal antigen, alpha-fetoprotein or AFP, has a parallel relationship in hepatocarcinoma with CEA in gastrointestinal cancers plus a second more unique aspect. In amniotic fluid, AFP is dominantly of fetal origin; most other proteins are of maternal origin. Unexpectedly high AFP levels in amniotic fluid suggest a leakage of AFP from some fetal abnormality. This was confirmed by Brock and Sutcliffe. Spina bifida and anencephaly can now be diagnosed via AFP titering of amniotic fluid.

Although less commonly used as diagnostic or prognostic indicators of cancer, the production of tissue-specific proteins, such as chorionic gonadotropin or prolactin, can be used for such purposes when malignant growth of the hormone-producing tissues develops (p. 134). Braunstein, Vaitukaitis, and Ross, who co-authored the paper on human chorionic gonadotropin, are also authors of another Citation Classic in Chapter 3 on Immunology and Rheumatology.

The appearance of cancers in patients with a damaged immune surveillance system has been observed on several occasions in patients with ataxia telangiectasia or SCID (severe combined immunodeficiency). The immune deficit in Sjögren's syndrome is still incompletely defined, but the development of a malignant lymphoma of B-cell lineage could have several causes, loss of NK cells or loss of cytotoxic T cells being two possibilities. Other causes of cancer include the use of conjugated estrogens, a fact that was established by the study of Ziel and Finkle, whose TWCC describes the casual origin of their study. Their jointly authored commentary contains a final paragraph to which all genuine scientists ascribe. Kellermann's association of a form of lung cancer with the presence of the enzyme marker aryl hydrocarbon hydroxylase was a completely unexpected result of his work.

Three TWCCs address the problem of cancer treatment—the use of the BCG vaccine for melanoma, the creation of an embolism to block the vital circulation to renal adenocarcinomas, and the challenging of tumor cell cultures with drugs that might have an *in vivo* therapeutic potential. The BCG treatment for melanomas has had an on again–off again popularity since its inception, possibly due to differences in the technique used for the vaccinations, as Bluming suggests, or it may be that nonspecific adjuvant therapy is applicable only to a subset of melanoma patients. Soft agar culturing of tumor cells *in vitro* with cytotoxic drugs is one avenue toward selection of cogent therapeutics. In general, drugs that are effective *in vitro* may be effective *in vivo,* but those ineffective *in vitro* are rarely effective *in vivo.* Factors that influence cytotoxic therapy include the basic growth rate of the tumor cell

(p. 140) and, in the case of irradiation, the presence of sufficient oxygen in the tissue to generate the toxic radicals of oxygen that are cytocidal.

No scarcity of review literature exists for those wishing to keep abreast of the current status of cancer. Important review journals in this area include *Advances in Cancer Research, Cancer Treatment Reviews, Clinics in Oncology, CRC Critical Reviews of Oncology and Hematology, Current Problems in Cancer,* and *Seminars in Oncology.* The last of these has been an important forum for discussion of antineoplastic therapy, particularly the newer chemotherapeutic agents. A new series, *Seminars in Oncology Nursing,* was begun in 1985. Periodically, other publications such as the *British Medical Bulletin* devote all or a major portion of an issue to the status of cancer with articles that are summary in tone.

Readers wishing to re-inform themselves about the influence that the Citation Classics in this chapter have had on contemporary studies will have little difficulty in doing so. Although the emphasis in oncology has shifted away from descriptions of tumor pathology and classification, topics of other Citation Classics in this chapter have continued as incompletely resolved problems or as subjects of expanding interest and are thus represented in contemporary writings. The relationship of diet to cancer and adjuvant therapy, described in the following four articles, belong in the first category.

Berstock D A & Baum M. Adjuvant chemotherapy for common solid tumors. *Adv. Cancer Res.* **39:**315–27, 1983.

Byers T & Graham S. The epidemiology of cancer and diet. *Adv. Cancer Res.* **41:**1–71, 1984.

Donaldson S S. The value of adjuvant chemotherapy in the management of sarcomas in children. *Cancer* **55:**2184–97, 1985.

Nair P P. Diet, nutrition intake, and metabolism in populations at high and low risk for colon cancer. Introduction: correlates of diet, nutrition intake, and metabolism in relation to colon cancer. *Am. J. Clin. Nutr.* **40**(Suppl.)**:**880–86, 1984.

Subjects that continue to capture the interest of oncologists include the diagnosis and therapy of cancer. A few recent reviews on these subjects include:

Begent R H J. The value of carcinoembryonic antigen measurement in clinical practice. *Ann. Clin. Biochem.* **21:**231–8, 1984.

Bernstein I, Kersey J, Seeger R & Andrews R. Immunodiagnosis and immunotherapy of childhood malignancies. *Pediatr. Clin. North Am.* **32:**575–99, 1985.

Bleyer W A & Poplack D G. Prophylaxis and treatment of leukemia in the central nervous system and other sanctuaries. *Semin. Oncol.* **12:**131–48, 1985.

Haanen C, Muus P, Raymakers R, Drenthe-Schonk A, Salden M & Wessels J. Studies on the cytotoxicity of cytosine arabinoside. *Semin. Oncol.* **12**(Suppl. 3):120–9, 1985.

Klavins J V. Advances in biological markers for cancer. *Ann. Clin. Lab. Sci.* **13**:275–80, 1983.

Shively J E & Beatty J D. CEA-related antigens: molecular and clinical significance. *CRC Crit. Rev. Oncol. Hematol.* **2**:355–99, 1985.

Zalcberg J R & McKenzie I F C. Tumor-associated antigens—an overview. *J. Clin. Oncol.* **3**:876–82, 1985.

Oncogenes, the role of retroviruses in cancer etiology, and AIDS are among the newer topics of interest in oncology. The entire March 1984 issue of *Seminars in Oncology* was devoted to the human T-cell leukemia viruses and AIDS, and this relationship is under constant re-analysis and review. Much the same can be said for oncogene studies. Five useful reviews on the genetic basis of cancer are listed.

Barbacid M. Oncogenes in human cancers and in chemically induced animal tumors. *Prog. Med. Virol.* **32**:86–100, 1985.

Hunter T. Oncogenes and proto-oncogenes: how do they differ? *J. Natl. Cancer Inst.* **73**:773–86, 1984.

Klein G & Klein E. Oncogene activation and tumor progression. *Carcinogenesis* **5**:429–35, 1984.

Pearson M & Rowley J D. The relation of oncogenesis and cytogenetics in leukemia and lymphoma. *Annu. Rev. Med.* **36**:471–83, 1985.

Varmus H E. The molecular genetics of cellular oncogenes. *Annu. Rev. Genet.* **18**:553–612, 1984.

CC/NUMBER 8
FEBRUARY 21, 1983

This Week's Citation Classic

Friedman N B & Moore R A. Tumors of the testis: a report on 922 cases. *Milit. Surgeon* **99**:573-93, 1946.
[Army Inst. Pathology, Washington, DC and Dept. Pathology, Washington Univ. School of Medicine, St. Louis, MO]

This study brought a simple and clarifying biologic concept to the understanding of testicular germ cell and teratoid tumors. As a general theory it has survived, with modifications, and has been extended to extragenital growths with further ramifications including possibilities of therapeutic differentiation and germ cell programming of immunologic systems. [The *SCI®* indicates that this paper has been cited in over 140 publications since 1961.]

Nathan B. Friedman
Department of Pathology
Cedars-Sinai Medical Center
Los Angeles, CA 90048

December 27, 1982

"This study was carried out during World War II while I was stationed at the old Army Medical Museum in Washington, DC, now the Armed Forces Institute of Pathology. It was prepared as part of a tribute (*festschrift*) to our well-loved commander, Colonel J.E. Ash. It was suggested by my friend, the late Ruell Sloan, then Colonel Ash's executive officer, and written from my notes by my first wife, the late Helen Mc Francis Friedman. The collection of medical materials from our military and civilian sources had been going on since the Civil War. The combination of the enlarged 1942 Army and Colonel Ash's vision led not only to the accumulation of large case groups but to intensive study of diseases of young men.

"Much as a mass of dots in a puzzle can become a figure, so the nearly 1,000 cases of testicular cancer told their own story by the evolution of patterns in primary tumors and their metastases. The basic idea was that most testicular tumors were growths of germ cells expressing the totipotentiality of elements which could give rise to all components of the conceptus, trophoblast, somatoplasm, and germ plasm, and that these tissues could differentiate in various directions at differing times and places. It was this concept which was the basis for the subsequent important work of Pierce[1] which confirmed in animals what had been observed in man, despite the obstinacy of the Willis followers.[2] A parallel development was the identification of germinoma in the pineal by Russell[3] as well as in the thymus by me,[4] the inclusion of extragonadal tumors in the basic concept, and the significance of germ plasm in these loci.[5] Finally, the possibility of induced differentiation as a therapeutic modality in neoplastic disease was given strong impetus.

"The concepts were not entirely brand new. Some of the nineteenth-century German pathologists had anticipated them and Gunnar Teilum published similar interpretations in the 1940s in Scandinavian journals.[6] Peyron[7] had already described embryoid bodies in germ cell tumors in the 1930s.

"The frequency of citation is attributed to this being the first modern paper presenting a simple histogenetic classification of this model cancer. The terms 'teratocarcinoma' and 'germinoma' were first used here and have become standard. The entire subject was brought up to date in a presentation in January 1983, at the opening of the University of Southern California Cancer Center, the proceedings to be published by Grune and Stratton."

1. **Pierce G B, Jr., Dixon F J, Jr. & Verney E L.** Teratocarcinogenic and tissue-forming potentials of the cell types comprising neoplastic embryoid bodies. *Lab. Invest.* **9**:583-602, 1960.
2. **Pugh R C B,** ed. *Pathology of the testis.* Oxford: Blackwell Scientific, 1976. 487 p.
3. **Russell D S.** The pinealoma: its relationship to the teratoma. *J. Pathol. Bact.* **56**:145-50, 1944.
4. **Friedman N B.** The comparative morphogenesis of extragenital and gonadal teratoid tumors. *Cancer* **4**:265-76, 1951.
5. **Friedman N B & Van de Velde R L.** Germ cell tumors in man, pleiotropic mice, and continuity of germplasm and somatoplasm. *Hum. Pathol.* **12**:772-6, 1981.
6. **Teilum G.** Gonocytoma, homologous ovarian and testicular tumors. I. *Acta Pathol. Microbiol. Scand.* **27**:249-61, 1946.
7. **Peyron A.** Faits nouveaux relatifs à l'origine et à l'histogénèse des embryomes. *Bull. Assoc. Fr. Étud. Cancer* **28**:658-81, 1939.

CC/NUMBER 37
SEPTEMBER 12, 1983

This Week's Citation Classic

Harris O D, Cooke W T, Thompson H & Waterhouse J A H. Malignancy in adult coeliac disease and idiopathic steatorrhoea. *Amer. J. Med.* **42**:899-912, 1967.
[Nutrit. and Intestinal Unit, General Hosp., Birmingham, and Depts. Pathol. and Social Med., Birmingham Univ., England]

From a review of 202 patients with adult coeliac disease (ACD) or idiopathic steatorrhoea (IS), evidence is given that both can be complicated by malignancy, either lymphoma or carcinoma (especially oesophageal). It is more significant for men, and a gluten-free diet appeared to decrease the risk of malignancy. [The *SCI*® indicates that this paper has been cited in over 280 publications since 1967.]

Owen D. Harris
Department of Gastroenterology
Princess Alexandra Hospital
Woolloongabba 4102 Brisbane
Queensland
Australia

May 31, 1983

"This study was begun in early 1965 soon after my arrival from Australia. W.T. Cooke had a major interest in small and large bowel disease since 1941, and hence had a huge group of such patients attending his clinic. His nutritional and intestinal unit was a major referral centre from the Midlands of England.

"My research projects were to be centred around coeliac disease (CD). The major project was to review all of the coeliac patients and determine the occurrence of malignancy. Already, the literature contained anecdotal case reports of adenocarcinoma of the small bowel possibly complicating CD, and in 1962, Gough, Read, and Naish[1] had put forward the hypothesis that small bowel reticulosis may develop as a complication of idiopathic steatorrhoea (IS). In 1960, Cooke and his colleagues[2] reported their experience with jejunal biopsy in adult CD (ACD); this produced similar results to the earlier English study by Shiner in 1957.[3] Thus, in my study, these two patient groups were studied—(1) the possibly heterogeneous group without jejunal biopsy (1941-1957) and identified as IS, and (2) the homogeneous group with jejunal biopsy criteria for CD.

"Early in the study a substantial group with lymphoma was found, along with an apparently significant excess of gastrointestinal carcinomas. It was then important to involve the Cancer Registry of the department of social medicine, Birmingham University. They could provide the expected incidence figures for all malignancies, and determine the observed incidence in our patients. Also, Henry Thompson (surgical pathologist) reviewed all jejunal biopsies and the lymphomas.

"The final paper thus represented a critical review of 202 patients with careful clinical and pathological documentation of 31 malignancies that developed in them over a mean follow-up period at this unit for 8.2 years. Of the malignancies, 14 were lymphoma in type, and 13 gastrointestinal. The mean follow-up period had been 7.8 years from the time of diagnosis of the CD (or IS) until the lymphoma was diagnosed. In 11 of these patients, there was asymptomatic follow-up of 8.4 years on a gluten-free diet before the lymphoma developed. This evidence permitted the only conclusion that ACD could be complicated by lymphoma. The remaining three patients were inconclusive in their relationship.

"This study documented that some gastrointestinal cancers (especially oesophageal) can also complicate CD. Lastly, there was some support (not statistically valid) for the beneficial effect of a gluten-free diet on reducing the incidence of malignant complications.

"This paper has become a *Citation Classic* because of the careful documentation of a big group of carefully diagnosed and followed coeliacs; and there were comparative data in the same district for malignancies. The lymphoma is now classified as a histiocytic lymphoma, and the most recent review is 'Coeliac disease and malignancy,' published in *Lancet*."[4]

1. **Gough K R, Read A E & Naish J M.** Intestinal reticulosis as a complication of idiopathic steatorrhoea. *Gut* **3**:232-9, 1962.
2. **Fone D J, Meynell M J, Harris E L, Cooke W T, Brewer D B & Cox E V.** Jejunal biopsy in adult coeliac disease and allied disorders. *Lancet* **1**:933-8, 1960.
3. **Shiner M.** Small intestinal biopsies by the oral route—histopathologic changes in the malabsorption syndrome. *J. Mt. Sinai Hosp.* **24**:273-85, 1957.
4. **Swinson C M, Slavin G, Coles E C & Booth C C.** Coeliac disease and malignancy. *Lancet* **1**:111-15, 1983.

This Week's Citation Classic

Chaudhry A P, Vickers R A & Gorlin R J. Intraoral minor salivary gland tumors: an analysis of 1,414 cases. *Oral Surg. Oral Med. Oral Patho.* **14**:1194-226, 1961. [School of Dentistry, University of Minnesota, Minneapolis, MN]

This study was based on the clinical features, microscopic characteristics, treatment, and prognosis of a large series of 1,414 cases of intraoral minor salivary gland tumors. The most prevalent tumor was pleomorphic adenoma followed by cylindromatous adenocarcinoma, mucoepidermoid, and adenocarcinoma (conventional type). The palate was the site of predilection for all these lesions. Intraoral low-grade mucoepidermoid tumors far exceeded high-grade tumors and responded favorably to adequate local excision. [The *SCI*® indicates that this paper has been cited in over 125 publications since 1961, making it the second most-cited paper published in this journal.]

Anand P. Chaudhry
Department of Pathobiology
and Oral Pathology
New York University Dental Center
New York, NY 10010

March 18, 1983

"In the early-1950s, the histopathologic classification of the major salivary gland tumors and their correlation with biological behavior, treatment modalities, and prognosis were in disarray and undergoing dramatic revisions in the US. Buxton, Maxwell, and French[1] had published their classical work on epithelial tumors of the parotid glands at the University of Michigan Hospital, Ann Arbor, Michigan. At the Memorial Sloan-Kettering Cancer Center, New York, Foote and Frazell[2] had reviewed the largest series of cases of major salivary gland tumors. Their work emerged as the most authoritative on the subject and formed the basis for the Armed Forces Institute of Pathology fascicle.[3]

"It was during 1951-1953, as a resident in oral surgery at the University Hospital at Michigan, that I had the good fortune of attending numerous seminars, discussions, and clinical pathologic conferences on salivary gland tumors. This was the beginning of my interest in the subject which continued while I was a doctoral candidate in experimental pathology at the University of Minnesota Medical Center. In 1958, Robert J. Gorlin provided the necessary incentive, encouragement, and intellectual stimulus to undertake this project. However, it was the late dean, William J. Crawford, who was the inspiring force behind this project. He expected the most and the best of academic excellence in his younger faculty. In 1960, Robert A. Vickers joined the division of oral pathology. He added a new impetus, enthusiasm, and a sense of purpose to the project.

"At that time, knowledge on the subject of intraoral minor salivary gland tumors was still fragmentary and lagged behind what was known about major salivary gland tumors. This was largely due to the much lower incidence of minor salivary gland tumors, roughly 1:10 as compared to major salivary gland tumors. In addition, much of the literature was based on single case reports or small series of cases. This resulted in disparate or contradictory information. This paper has been highly cited for several reasons. As Gorlin has stated, 'This paper was so comprehensive and one of the first to deal with an area of investigation that had heretofore been neglected.' Vickers has added, 'This paper evaluated a large number of intraoral salivary gland tumors from which emerged several findings of biological significance that are even relevant today.'

"The findings of this work were first presented at the Annual Meeting of the Academy of Oral Pathology in 1961 at the University of Michigan. A.J. French, professor and chairman of the department of pathology, University of Michigan School of Medicine, was in attendance at this meeting. His favorable and generous comments provided an incentive to submit this material for publication.

"I have maintained an active research interest in the embryogenesis, regeneration, and neoplasia of the major and minor salivary glands at the cellular and subcellular levels. My most recent work is related to the pathogenesis of various salivary gland diseases and the role myoepithelium plays."[4]

1. **Buxton R W, Maxwell J H & French A J.** Surgical treatment of epithelial tumors of the parotid gland. *Surg. Gynecol. Obstet.* **97**:401-16, 1953.
2. **Foote F W, Jr. & Frazell E L.** Tumors of the major salivary glands. *Cancer* **6**:1065-133, 1953.
3. --. *Tumors of the major salivary glands.* Washington, DC: Armed Forces Institute of Pathology, 1954. 149 p.
4. **Chaudhry A P, Satchidanand S, Peer R & Cutler L S.** Myoepithelial cell adenoma of the parotid gland: a light and ultrastructural study. *Cancer* **49**:288-93, 1982.

CC/NUMBER 1
JANUARY 7, 1980

This Week's Citation Classic

Hersh E M, Bodey G P, Nies B A & Freireich E J. Causes of death in acute leukemia: a ten-year study of 414 patients from 1954-1963. *J. Amer. Med. Ass.* **193**:105-9, 1965. [National Cancer Institute, Acute Leukemia Service, Medicine Branch, Bethesda, MD]

Major causes of death in acute leukemia were infection in 70% of patients and hemorrhage in 52%. In 38% of the patients there was more than one cause of death. Striking changes took place during the ten-year study period. Fatal hemorrhage declined to nearly half the early rate, and fatal staphylococcal infection from 23.5% to 3.1%. At the same time, fatal infections due to fungi increased from 8.2% to 23.2%. [The *SCI*® indicates that this paper has been cited over 235 times since 1965.]

Evan M. Hersh
Department of
Developmental Therapeutics
University of Texas System Cancer Center
M.D. Anderson Hospital and
Tumor Institute
Texas Medical Center
Houston, TX 77030

October 22, 1979

"When we joined the leukemia program at the NCI as clinical associates in 1962, we became aware of the grim prognosis of acute leukemia patients. At that time the remission rate for adults was 10%, and their survival was one year. For children the remission rate was barely 50%, and their survival was less than one year.

"Rather than being discouraged, Emil J. Freireich, chief of the leukemia program, pointed out that this situation was a challenge for clinical research. Data gathering, data analysis, and the use of conclusions from analyzed data to formulate testable hypotheses could result in improved therapy for this disease.

"In 1963, after completing a difficult year caring for patients receiving experimental therapy for acute leukemia (we lost 70 children that year), Gerald P. Bodey, Boyd A. Nies, and I began to review the 414 patients seen at the NCI over the preceding ten years. The data were tabulated and analyzed completely by hand, this preceding the era when biostatistical and computer support were readily available to the clinical investigator.

"The important conclusions of the study were as follows: The most common cause of death was host defense failure and the resultant infection; hemorrhage as a cause of death had declined drastically concurrent with the development of platelet transfusion therapy; few patients died of leukemia (i.e., infiltration of vital organs with malignant cells) but rather from the complications of the disease and/or its treatment.

"This was one of the first clinical studies specifically to evaluate the causes of death in malignant disease and served as a prototype for subsequent similar studies. It proved that supportive care can have a major effect on the course of malignant disease. Most important was the observation that leukemia patients often do not die of the direct effects of the disease. These implications have influenced developments in supportive care, antibiotic therapy, chemotherapy, and immunotherapy. Today the majority of patients with leukemia enter complete remission and 50% of children and 20% of adults are apparently cured.

"Publication of the paper was not easy. It was submitted to and rejected by the *Journal of Clinical Investigation* and the *Annals of Internal Medicine* before its acceptance by the *Journal of the American Medical Association*.

"The study also had a profound effect on my own career. It prompted an interest in host defense mechanisms in cancer, clinical cancer immunology, and immunotherapy which remain my main research interests and have become major components of cancer research.

"Finally, the professional relationships which resulted in this paper have remained remarkably intact during the last 17 years. Freireich, Bodey, and I still work together at the University of Texas M.D. Anderson Hospital: Freireich as chairman of the department of developmental therapeutics, Bodey as chief of chemotherapy and the Clinical Research Center, and myself as deputy department chairman and chief of immunology. Nies is in the private practice of oncology in California. For all of us it continues to be an exciting journey."

This Week's Citation Classic

Prichard R W. Tumors of the heart. *Arch. Pathol.* **51**:98-128, 1951.
[Laboratory of Pathology of the New England Deaconess Hospital and the Harvard Cancer Commission, Boston, MA]

An analytic review of heart tumors, primary and secondary, is supplemented by a description of 150 newly reported tumors. One hypothesis concerning the origin of cardiac myxomas, tested by study of a series of human hearts, could not be confirmed; an alternate suggestion is made. [The *SCI*® indicates that this paper has been cited over 220 times since 1961.]

Robert W. Prichard
Department of Pathology
Wake Forest University
Bowman Gray School of Medicine
Winston-Salem, NC 27013

May 31, 1979

"Finding my 1951 paper on a computer printout with classical examples of basic research is sobering evidence of the machine's impartiality. My first reaction to the invitation to write this piece was to decline; no one should think me unaware of the qualitative difference between my paper and the earlier ones in the series.[1,2] But if my largely analytic and descriptive effort has been useful over more than a quarter century, perhaps there is merit in saying a word for a type of scientific writing often disparaged by people who should know better. Careful description of the natural experiments we call 'cases' have played a major role in the development of scientific medicine and are often a starting point for basic insights into disease and its treatment. I hope young people in medicine will accept case studies as part of their scholarly obligation.

"In spite of their present unpopularity, there was even less money available for case studies in 1949. As a second-year pathology resident, I was dependent on the kindness of my chiefs—Drs. Shields Warren and William Meissner—for the services of their laboratory in preparing sections and taking pictures. I had never heard of a primary heart tumor when the first patient with one came through our autopsy service. The last review in English had appeared in 1931.[3] Convinced that waiting in the wings were developments in diagnosis and surgical treatment that would make at least some of these tumors curable, I took to the literature. Within a few months three more primary tumors came through the autopsy laboratory. The most common primary heart tumor, the myxoma, was not considered a true neoplasm by some authorities. Thinking this might have led to underdiagnosis, I concentrated my efforts on this tumor type, particularly to demonstrate that it is a true tumor.

"Soon after the publication of the paper, I got some inkling that it had been useful. A pioneer cardiac surgeon told me that as he blindly put a finger in a patient's atrium in the old mitral valvulotomy technique he felt something soft and immediately realized he was feeling a myxoma, having recently read about them in my paper. He changed his operative strategy and later removed the tumor. There were other similar experiences. Now there have been major advances in the understanding of cardiac tumors, all of them gratifying because of the curability of some of the tumors. That the humble case study helped is personally satisfying. That the paper was turned down by the first journal to which it was submitted suggests to all authors that persistence is worthwhile!"

1. **Mahaim I.** *Les tumeurs et les polypes du coeur; etude anatomo-clinique.* (The tumors and polyps of the heart: an anatomical study.) Paris: Masson & Cie, 1945, 568 p.
2. **Whorton C M.** Primary malignant tumors of the heart. *Cancer* **2**:245-60, 1949.
3. **Yater W M.** Tumors of the heart and pericardium: pathology, symptomatology, and report of nine cases. *Arch. Int. Med.* **48**:627-66, 1931.

CC/NUMBER 40
OCTOBER 3, 1983

This Week's Citation Classic

Spratt J S, Jr., Ackerman L V & Moyer C A. Relationship of polyps of the colon to colonic cancer. *Ann. Surg.* **148**:682-98, 1958.
[Dept. Surgery and Div. Surgical Pathology, Washington Univ. Sch. Medicine, and Barnes Hosp., St. Louis, MO]

This paper challenged the dogma that all colonic cancers evolved from preexisting benign polyps and initiated a sustained period of restudy of many issues related to the control of colon cancer in man. [The *SCI*® indicates that this paper has been cited in over 185 publications since 1961.]

John S. Spratt, Jr.
Department of Surgery and
Community Health
J. Graham Brown Cancer Center
University of Louisville
Louisville, KY 40202

June 20, 1983

"On my return to Barnes Hospital as a first-year assistant resident in 1955, after being away for two years of post-internship Naval duty, one of my first rotations was in surgical pathology under L.V. Ackerman. As was Ackerman's custom, he gave almost everyone on his service a project. He said, 'Spratt, you go look up polyps.' What he did not know was that my premedical interests had been in mathematics and that I suffered from the unfulfilled ambition to obtain a PhD in mathematics. Southwestern Medical School, near my home and affordable, interposed. At the time I went to 'look up polyps,' I was more of a mathematician than a surgeon, unbeknown to Ackerman. To me the anatomical distributions, sizes, and pathological classifications became mathematical distributions, frequencies, and rates that could be studied and compared. I found, with Carl Moyer's encouragement, many incongruities in the dogma that colon polyps were premalignant lesions or that any public health advantage was being obtained by trying to keep colons free of the ubiquitous benign adenomatous polyp. In fact, the operative mortality rate attending transabdominal colonic polypectomy was found to exceed the age-specific ratio of cancers to polyps. To this day, there is no controlled clinical trial confirming that any particular strategy of benign polyp removal reduces the mortality from colon cancer or adds to human longevity.

"This first paper of mine was presented by Moyer, my now deceased surgical mentor, at the annual meeting of the American Surgical Association and attracted immediate and broad attention because of the documented deviation from past thinking and the economic significance of the study in deflating the justification of high-cost programs for the mass removal of benign polyps. This paper also questioned the credibility with which morphological pathology can be used to predict the rate or frequency of evolution from benign to malignant states.

"Subsequent studies rapidly strengthened these conclusions by defining the properties of small primary cancers,[1] showing that the propensity of colon cancers to metastasize to lymph nodes was independent of the size of the primary cancers,[2] showing the enormous differences in growth rates that exist between cancers and benign polyps,[3] and showing that the same carcinogen could induce both cancers and benign polyps but that the cancers began as cancers and did not go through the polypoid metamorphosis.[4]

"These studies have all stimulated intense arborizations of investigations by many students of colonic cancer. Colonic cancer is still a major health problem that may yet be, one day, a preventable disease."[5]

1. **Spratt J S, Jr. & Ackerman L V.** Small primary adenocarcinomas of the colon and rectum. *J. Amer. Med. Assn.* **179**:337-46, 1962.
2. --. Relationship of the size of colonic tumors to their cellular composition and biological behavior. *Surg. Forum* **10**:56-61, 1960.
3. **Welin S, Youker J & Spratt J S, Jr.** The rates and patterns of growth of 375 tumors of the large intestine and rectum observed serially by double contrast enema study (Malmö technique). *Amer. J. Roentgenol.* **90**:673-87, 1963.
4. **Spjut H J & Spratt J S, Jr.** Endemic and morphologic similarities existing between spontaneous colonic neoplasms in man and 3:2'-dimethyl-4-aminobiphenyl induced colonic neoplasms in rats. *Ann. Surg.* **161**:309-24, 1965.
5. **Spratt J S, Jr. & Greenberg R.** Epidemiology and etiology of cancers of the colon, rectum and anus. *Neoplasms of the large intestine, rectum and anus.* Philadelphia: Saunders. 1984.

CC/NUMBER 12
MARCH 23, 1981

This Week's Citation Classic

Burkitt D P. Epidemiology of cancer of the colon and rectum. *Cancer* **28**:3-13, 1971.

Cancer of the large intestine is the commonest cause of cancer death in North America. It is always uncommon amongst people who still live in a traditional manner in Third World communities. Evidence points to it being primarily the result of environmental factors and consequently it must be considered potentially preventable. [The *SCI*® indicates that this paper has been cited over 345 times since 1971.]

Denis P. Burkitt
Unit of Geographical Pathology
Saint Thomas's Hospital
London SE1 7E7
England

February 24, 1981

"The paper cited was an attempt to show not only that large bowel cancer was more closely associated with the life-style characteristic of modern western culture than is any other form of cancer, but also, that its geographical and socioeconomic distribution is very closely related to that of other characteristically Western diseases.

"These observations indicate that large bowel tumours must be potentially preventable, could causative factors be identified and reduced or eradicated, and in addition that clues to their causation might be provided by studying other diseases that flourish in the same environment and might therefore share common causative factors.

"Bowel cancer and its related diseases are uncommon throughout the Third World and both there and in some Western countries have higher prevalences in urban than in rural communities.

"The pattern of geographical distribution of bowel cancer is closely similar to that of diverticular disease of the colon. In fact, the latter has never been observed to be other than rare until after a rise in incidence of large-bowel cancer had occurred. On the other hand, the low incidence rates for these tumours routinely found in economically poor countries have never been shown to rise until after appendicitis, another disease of Western culture, becomes relatively common.

"It is now generally accepted that the major factor causative of diverticular disease is a deficiency of fibre in the diet, and my colleagues and I[1] have argued that this may also contribute to the causation of appendicitis. Both diseases are related to the consistency and volume of intestinal content, both of which are governed by the fibre content of the diet.

"Bowel behaviour was examined in communities with low, high, and intermediate frequency of colo-rectal cancer, and it was found that where faecal output was 300-500 g/day and mouth to anus transit times around 30 hours, cancer and its associated diseases were rare, but where, as in North America and Western Europe output was only 80-120 g/day, and transit times exceeded three days, these illnesses were common.

"Hypotheses were postulated to endeavour to explain how dietary fibre could be protective against large bowel cancer. It seemed obvious for instance, that any carcinogens concentrated in a small faecal volume and retained a long period in the gut might be more dangerous than those diluted in a large faecal volume, moved along more quickly, and excreted more often.

"At the time this paper appeared nearly all the emphasis was placed on the dangers of fat-rich diets when considering possible causes of large bowel cancer. It is now, however, generally accepted that while fat-rich diets are likely to promote the circumstances responsible for causing bowel tumours, dietary fibre and the fibre of starch staple foods in particular probably exert a protective influence.

"The reason for the frequent citation of this paper is the renewed interest in the role of fibre in human nutrition and its postulated protective role in bowel cancer in particular.

"I was introduced to the enormously important role of refined carbohydrate foods in the causation of some characteristically Western diseases by T.L. Cleave,[2] but it was Alec Walker of the South African Institute for Medical Research in Johannesburg who drew my attention to the possible role of fibre in the causation of colon cancer. The credit which has often been attributed to me for originating the fibre hypothesis for this disease, should by right go to him."

1. **Burkitt D P, Walker A R P & Painter N S.** Dietary fiber and disease. *J. Amer. Med. Assn.* **229**:1068-74, 1974.
2. **Cleave T L.** The neglect of natural principles in current medical practice. *J. Roy. Nav. Med. Serv.* **42**:55-83, 1956.

CC/NUMBER 4
JANUARY 28, 1980

This Week's Citation Classic

Zollinger R M & Ellison E H. Primary peptic ulcerations of the jejunum associated with islet cell tumors of the pancreas. *Ann. Surg.* **142**:709-28, 1955. [Dept. Surg. and Med. Ctr., Ohio State Univ. Coll. Med., Columbus, OH]

Non-insulin producing islet cell tumors of the pancreas were found in two patients with a fulminating ulcer diathesis which eventually required total gastrectomy. It was suggested that a distinct clinical entity resulted from a potent gastric secretagogue produced by these tumors. [The *SCI*® indicates that this paper has been cited over 475 times since 1961.]

Robert M. Zollinger
Department of Surgery
College of Medicine
Ohio State University
Columbus, OH 43210

July 25, 1979

"Edwin Ellison and I simultaneously discovered that each of us was treating a patient who produced excessive gastric juice despite repeated radical surgical procedures culminating in total removal of the stomach. A planned total gastrectomy in one patient, a young girl, prompted a colleague, Hilger Jenkins, to suggest that I evaluate the pancreas, because he had observed ulcer recurrence in a patient who had an insulin-producing islet cell tumor. Peptic ulcer had been associated with insulinoma by R. Strøm and with other endocrine adenomata by P. Wermer.[1,2] This patient, indeed, had two small lymph nodes near the pancreas, containing metastatic islet cell tumor of the non-insulin producing type. She is still living 23 years after total gastrectomy. The other patient died, and autopsy disclosed a non-beta islet cell tumor in the pancreas.

"This chance experience with two rare cases stimulated Ellison and me to postulate a clinical entity comprised of hypersecretion, hyperacidity, and atypical ulceration associated with non-insulin producing islet cell tumors of the pancreas. We reported on the two patients in this 1955 article, and stated: 'If these observations accomplish nothing more than a renewal of interest in the ulcer problem with new avenues of study, we will feel justified in reporting these two cases.'

"Our hypothesis was accepted by many and challenged by many during the next five years. But within ten years, a thousand or more case reports established the clinical ulcerogenic Z-E syndrome (gastrinoma). Proof that these tumors were a rich source of gastrin by R.A. Gregory and H.J. Tracy of Liverpool stimulated great interest in the gastro-intestinal polypeptides, which was implemented by the development of a reliable gastrin immunoassay by J.E. McGuigan.[3,4]

"Ellison and I were amazed to observe the ramifications into many fields which followed our report of a daring concept based on two cases. Recently, the syndrome has been extensively cited because of the introduction of H_2 blockers, which for the first time permit drug control of the excessive gastric hypersecretion.

"Peptic ulcer remains a common and disabling disorder. While the original paper was concerned only with management of patients with the rare islet cell ulcerogenic syndrome, its thrust has been to challenge the research and clinical imaginations of many disciplines to solve the enigma of the gastrointestinal tract."

1. **Strøm R.** A case of peptic ulcer and insuloma. *Acta Chir. Scand.* **104**:252-60, 1952.
2. **Wermer P.** Genetic aspects of adenomatosis of endocrine glands. *Amer. J. Med.* **16**:363-71, 1954.
3. **Gregory R A, Tracy H J, French J M & Sircus W.** Extraction of a gastrin-like substance from a pancreatic tumour in a case of Zollinger-Ellison syndrome. *Lancet* **1**:1045-8, 1960.
4. **McGuigan J E & Trudeau W L.** Immunochemical measurement of elevated levels of gastrin in the serum of patients with pancreatic tumors of the Zollinger-Ellison variety. *N. Eng. J. Med.* **278**:1308-13, 1968.

NUMBER 46
NOVEMBER 12, 1979

This Week's Citation Classic

Stewart A, Webb J & Hewitt D. A survey of childhood malignancies.
Brit. Med. J. **1**:1495-508, 1958.
[Department of Social Medicine, Oxford University, England]

An association between fetal irradiation and cancers exists which is difficult to detect because childhood cancers may have near-conception origins and early (pre-cancer) effects which increase the risk of dying at an early stage of development. The principal effect of preleukemia is loss of immunological incompetence, but there may also be intolerance of the anoxic conditions of parturition. [The ***SCI*®** **indicates that this paper has been cited over 315 times since 1961.]**

Alice M. Stewart
Regional Cancer Registry
Queen Elizabeth Medical Center
Birmingham B15 2TH
England

March 28, 1978

"The fetal irradiation story is a triumph for a small group of epidemiologists who used a retrospective survey to detect the cancer association and the same approach to show why so many prospective surveys had negative findings. We were anxious to discover why the post-war increase in leukemia had produced an early peak of leukemia mortality consisting only of lymphatic cases, but we had difficulty in coming to grips with the problem because, even with the increase, leukemia remained a rare cause of childhood deaths. We drew up a plan which entailed asking a nationwide network of medical officers of health to interview mothers of cases and controls under standardized conditions, but this was rejected by the MRC. However, we had enough money to pay for the necessary train fares, so we went it alone with the results shown in the 1958 paper.

"In this paper there are no answers to our original problem, but it paved the way for a study of any cancer effects of fetal irradiation which eventually showed that 40% of our X-rayed cases (leukemia and solid tumors) were radiation-induced. These cases proved to be a fraction older than a much larger number of idiopathic cases, so we incidentally discovered that all childhood cancers have fetal origins. The paper mentions an association between pneumonia and leukemia which told us that cancers of the immune system might be influencing reactions to other diseases before they were clinically recognizable. With this thought in mind we eventually uncovered a number of facts which led to two conclusions: (1) Infections and injuries are important causes of *pre-cancer* deaths; and (2) These deaths may take the form of abortions, stillbirths, or cot deaths. According to one of our estimates, based on our own data and official statistics, children who develop pneumonia when in an advanced stage of preleukemia are 300 times as likely to have a fatal attack as a normal child!

"For several years, negative findings of prospective surveys were threatening the very existence of our survey. However, obstetric X-rays and difficult deliveries go hand in hand, and none of the rival surveys had controlled either for this effect or for any later environmental influences.

"Finally, antibiotics can prevent infection deaths but not stillbirths or cot deaths, and myeloid leukemias have exceptionally short latent periods. Therefore, the answer to our original problem could be 'selective action of antibiotics on myeloid and lymphatic leukemias with fetal origins.' "

CC/NUMBER 30
JULY 27, 1981

This Week's Citation Classic

Foley G E, Lazarus H, Farber S, Uzman B G, Boone B A & McCarthy R E. Continuous culture of human lymphoblasts from peripheral blood of a child with acute leukemia. *Cancer* **18**:522-9, 1965. [Children's Cancer Res. Foundation, Boston, and Dept. Pathology, Harvard Med. Sch., Children's Hosp., Boston, MA]

This communication reports the first isolation of human lymphocytic cells in useful quantities by application of the 'population dependence phenomenon'—large inocula in small-volume substrates directly in suspension culture. Cell yield was sufficient for extensive biochemical and biological studies. [The *SCI*® indicates that this paper has been cited over 310 times since 1965.]

G.E. Foley
Sidney Farber Cancer Institute and
Department of Pathology
Harvard Medical School
Children's Hospital Medical Center
Boston, MA 02115

June 16, 1981

"In the 1950s, our cell culture laboratories became interested in the murine leukemias, and several were isolated in monolayer culture, wherein the attached cells were fibroblast-like, but when injected intraperitoneally in the mouse strain of origin, exhibited lymphocyte morphology. This led to similar experiments with human peripheral and bone marrow lymphocytes from patients with lymphocytic leukemia. These cells did not attach to any of several surfaces tried, but rather remained in suspension and appeared to 'want to grow,' but gradually died despite all nutritional and physical permutations. All attempts to cultivate these cells in suspension culture failed until it occurred to us to utilize the phenomenon of 'population dependence'[1]—by use of large inocula in small-volume primary cultures. Final success resulted in a method (at first in homemade culture apparatus) for the quantity production of these cells for biological and biochemical studies. Improved (automatic) culture apparatus increased the yield—a 15 liter vessel, for example, produced 320 x 10^8 (*ca* 20 gm ww) of cells!

"The experiments were done in the laboratories of microbiology and cell biology (which I organized in 1947), Children's Cancer Research Foundation, Boston, Massachusetts, perhaps better known as the Jimmy Fund Laboratories. The late Sidney Farber, director of the Foundation, and his clinical staff provided the clinical specimens and hematological and other relevant clinical data. Lazarus and Boone provided the priceless ingredient essential to any cell culture studies—'tender loving care' around the clock—in the beginning, seven days a week for nearly a year. Uzman provided the exquisite electron microscopy studies, and McCarthy provided the cytological studies. No particular problems were encountered, save assessment of the hazards (if any) inherent in the production and handling of these cells in huge quantities. We had no choice but to assume it was hazardous—thus strict containment facilities were built for the biochemical, animal, and large-scale culture work.

"A long series of publications from the Foundation on various aspects of the biochemistry, cytochemistry, cytology, biology, and nutrition of human leukemic cells as compared to nonleukemic lymphocytes resulted from these studies, as did the first successful heterotransplantation of human leukemia to an experimental animal (neonatal Syrian hamsters),[2] and its pathology therein,[3] as well as delineation of a fundamental nutritional difference between leukemic and nonleukemic lymphocytes.[4] However, our report attracted little attention at first—no 'awards' were received.

"We feel that our publication has become a 'classic' in its field because it indicated a direction to the isolation and cultivation of human lymphocytes which has since been modified and refined by others for many purposes. The availability of this tool, for example, enabled the development of many studies in cellular immunology."

1. **Eagle H & Piez K.** The population dependent requirements by cultured mammalian cells for metabolites which they can synthesize. *J. Exp. Med.* **116**:29-43, 1962.
2. **Adams R A, Foley G E, Uzman B G, Farber S, Lazarus H & Kleinman L.** Leukemia: serial transplantation of human leukemic lymphoblasts in the newborn Syrian hamster. *Cancer Res.* **27**:772-83, 1967.
3. **Liknaitzky D G, Takakusu A & Adams R A.** Early pathology of lymphoma developing in newborn Syrian hamsters inoculated with human leukemic lymphoblasts. *Cancer* **23**:94-100, 1969.
4. **Foley G E, Barell E F, Adams R A & Lazarus H.** Nutritional requirements of human leukemic cells. *Exp. Cell Res.* **57**:129-33, 1969.

Kay H E M, Knapton P J, O'Sullivan J P, Wells D G, Harris R F, Innes E M, Stuart J, Schwartz F C M & Thompson E N. Encephalopathy in acute leukaemia associated with methotrexate therapy. *Arch. Dis. Child.* **47**:344-54, 1972.

[Royal Marsden Hosp. and Inst. Cancer Res., Sutton; Queen Mary's Hosp. for Sick Children, Carshalton; Royal Hosp. for Sick Children, Edinburgh; Children's Hosp., Birmingham; and Welsh Natl. Sch. Med., Cardiff, UK]

Seven patients are described in whom dementia developed during treatment with methotrexate for meningeal leukaemia. The patients presented with confusion, tremor, ataxia, irritability, and somnolence and in one case there was progression to coma and death. Circumstantial evidence pointed to methotrexate as the cause. [The *SCI*® indicates that this paper has been cited in over 165 publications since 1972.]

H.E.M. Kay
Department of Haematology
Royal Marsden Hospital
London SW3 6JJ
England

January 16, 1984

"Around 1970 it seemed that acute lymphoblastic leukaemia (ALL) might be cured by more intensive therapy and that even meningeal leukaemia could be eradicated with the aid of enough methotrexate and/or radiotherapy. Indeed it can be—but in only a small proportion of cases and with a serious incidence of cerebral damage.

"At the time, the notions that methotrexate was active solely against cells during DNA-synthesis, and that the cells of the cerebral cortex were mitotically inert, made it difficult to believe that there could be a direct and selective toxicity of methotrexate on the brain. The first case at the Royal Marsden Hospital which suggested this possibility, a young man of 22 who went rapidly through a state of dementia to coma and death, was treated in collaboration with the late Gordon Hamilton Fairley (who was later tragically killed by an IRA bomb). He argued fiercely that we must just be observing an unusual manifestation of cerebral leukaemia. There was then another similar but less severe case which convinced me we were dealing with something new. When I mentioned this to members of the Medical Research Council's (MRC) Working Party, I got an immediate response. As I commented later in giving a Leukaemia Research Fund guest lecture, 'One of the criticisms levelled against clinical trials is that they do not initiate new treatments or make original contributions to knowledge of the disease. This is true only in a limited sense. A clinical trial forms an admirable seed-bed in which new ideas and observations can flourish and yield a rich harvest of information.'[1]

"In this instance other cases were at once recalled by members of the Working Party from Birmingham, Cardiff, and Edinburgh, and in a very short time it was possible to put together detailed clinical descriptions of seven similar cases. Their clinical symptoms and signs, the EEG changes, and the absence of leukaemia infiltration or virus disease pointed to a toxic cause, and the circumstantial evidence against methotrexate seemed overwhelmingly strong. So here was a new syndrome, fully described, and with a familiar but hitherto unsuspected agent as its cause. If confirmed, it was bound to be cited by those in the field.

"Subsequent evidence, notably from the St. Jude trial, Total VIII,[2] in which some histological studies were possible, amply confirmed the association. Our observations also led directly to the first major study by Eiser[3] on the effect of treatment for ALL on intellectual development, a topic which is still not fully resolved.

"Paradoxically, it was, I think, also one of the factors which led us to take a step backward in our MRC trials of ALL treatment. The avoidance of toxicity both to the central nervous system and to the immune system became a major objective in our protocols with a consequent lowering of their anti-leukaemia efficacy. Others, such as Riehm,[4] more perceptive perhaps and less influenced by our firsthand experience, pushed ahead with more intensive antileukaemic treatments and found greater success."

1. **Galton D A G & Kay H E M.** *UK leukaemia clinical trials for children and adults.* Leukaemia Research Fund Annual Guest Lecture, November 1977.
2. **Price R A & Jamieson P A.** The central nervous system in childhood leukemia. II. Subacute leukoencephalopathy. *Cancer* **35**:306-18, 1975. (Cited 235 times.)
3. **Eiser C & Lansdown R.** Retrospective study of intellectual development in children treated for acute lymphoblastic leukaemia. *Arch. Dis. Child.* **52**:525-9, 1977.
4. **Riehm H, Gadner H, Henze G, Langermann H J & Odenwald E.** The Berlin childhood acute lymphoblastic leukemia therapy study, 1970-1976. *Amer. J. Pediat. Hematol. Oncol.* **2**:299-306, 1980.

Skipper H E, Schabel F M, Jr. & Wilcox W S. Experimental evaluation of potential anticancer agents. XIII. On the criteria and kinetics associated with "curability" of experimental leukemia. *Cancer Chemother. Rep.* **35**:1-111, 1964.
[Kettering-Meyer Lab. (Affiliated with Sloan-Kettering Inst.), Southern Res. Inst., Birmingham, AL]

This paper represents a theoretical interpretation of chemotherapeutic trial results obtained in animals bearing widely different burdens of leukemia cells, and ancillary experiments showing (a) the lethality of a single viable leukemia cell, and (b) the exponential growth rate of murine leukemia cells over the range of one to almost the lethal number (ca. 10^9 in the mouse). [The ***SCI®*** **indicates that this paper has been cited over 365 times since 1964.]**

Howard E. Skipper
Kettering-Meyer Laboratory
Southern Research Institute
Birmingham, AL 35255

October 31, 1980

"The authors of this report were a diversely trained but compatible trio: a biochemist, a virologist, and a physical chemist.

"From the available data we (not I) formulated this theory: a given dose of a given drug will kill approximately the same fraction, not the same number, of widely different-sized tumor cell populations—so long as they are similarly exposed and both the growth fraction and the proportion of drug-resistant phenotypes are the same. All neoplastic cells must be eradicated to achieve cure.

"This theory is somewhat akin to one proposed around the turn of the century by Arrhenius regarding the rate of *in vitro* killing of bacterial cells by certain toxic chemicals.[1] To put it mildly, the theory of Arrhenius was not welcomed or accepted by early biologists.[2] The principal reason was lack of knowledge concerning phenomena which limit its applicability.[3]

"We first sent the subject manuscript to another journal. The editor (still a close friend) sent it back saying his reviewers thought it was an important paper and that they would be pleased to publish it *if* we would (a) delete the detailed data, (b) delete most of the charts, (c) refrain from speculation, and (d) reduce the text by about 90 percent. We declined, not out of pique, but because we thought the paper would be almost useless without documentation and charts illustrating what we thought the data implied. Parenthetically, the deletion of speculations in a theoretical paper seemed a bit much to Frank, Bill, and me!

"For some years after offering the above theory we were hard put to deduce which of several possible limitations to cure of disseminated cancers was the primary limitation in different circumstances, i.e., a low growth fraction, the presence of singly, doubly, or multidrug-resistant neoplastic cells, pharmacologic sanctuary problems, or others. Much additional experimental and clinical data, the early work of Luria and Delbrück,[4] and the mathematical model of Goldie and Coldman[5] now seem to make such deductions easier; e.g., (a) The presence or absence of drug-resistant phenotypes (tumor cells) is most often responsible for the inverse relationship between tumor cell burden and 'curability' by a drug or combination of drugs. (b) The same phenomenon (a wide variation in the proportion and absolute number of drug-resistant phenotypes) seems largely responsible for the wide variation in the degree and duration of response to chemotherapy observed in comparably staged and treated *individuals* bearing a drug-responsive neoplastic disease. Failure due to CNS disease usually is easy to determine. (c) Growth fraction differences are more apt to account for the marked differences in the initial response or lack of response to chemotherapy of different types of cancer; e.g., between different animal cancers, between different human cancers, and across species.

"It should be apparent that in some instances both of the types of tumor cell heterogeneity mentioned above may contribute to treatment failure. Local surgery or radiotherapy, when possible, will reduce the limitations to chemotherapy that result from both types of tumor cell heterogeneity."

1. **Arrhenius S.** *Quantitative laws in biological chemistry.* London: G. Bell & Sons, 1915. 164 p.
2. **Clark A J.** *The mode of action of drugs on cells.* London: Edward Arnold, 1933. 298 p.
3. **Skipper H E.** Some thoughts regarding the modes of action of drugs on cells and on application of available pharmacokinetic data (anticancer drugs). (Skipper H E, ed.) *Cancer chemotherapy.* Ann Arbor, MI: University Microfilms International, 1980. Vol. 10. (Published for the American Society of Clinical Oncology.)
4. **Luria S E & Delbrück M.** Mutation of bacteria from virus sensitivity to virus resistance. *Genetics* **28**:491-511, 1943.
5. **Goldie J H & Coldman A J.** A mathematic model for relating the drug sensitivity of tumors to their spontaneous mutation rate. *Cancer Treat. Rep.* **63**:1727-31, 1979.

This Week's Citation Classic

DeVita V T, Serpick A A & Carbone P P. Combination chemotherapy in the treatment of advanced Hodgkin's disease. *Ann. Intern. Med.* **73**: 881-95, 1970.

The paper reported two new and excitingly different results; a quadrupling of the number of patients with Hodgkin's disease who achieved complete remission (disappearance of all evidence of tumor) after treatment with a four drug combination (MOPP) (80% vs. 20% for single drug treatment). The second and most important observation reported was that over half of patients who had achieved complete remission had not developed recurrences with five years of followup after all treatment had been discontinued. It was one of the few papers in the cancer treatment field reported with sufficient follow time to give data on survival and relapse free survival, both of which were strikingly different from past experience. [The *SCI*® indicates that this paper has been cited over 390 times since 1970.]

Vincent T. DeVita, Jr.
Department of Health, Education & Welfare
National Cancer Institute
Bethesda, MD 20014

March 28, 1978

"This paper reported the results of our second attempt to develop a curative drug treatment for advanced Hodgkin's disease. This was a pilot trial to test the safety of the general approach. The second, now commonly referred to as the "MOPP" study, after the first initials of the drugs used (Nitrogen Mustard, Vincristin [Oncovin®], Prednisone and Procarbazine), was developed to incorporate new information suggesting an advantage of the then new drug, procarbazine, that led us to use it instead of an older drug methotrexate, used in the first program. In retrospect, all of us recall the trepidation with which we approached both trials. Although MOPP is now the standard drug treatment for advanced Hodgkin's disease, and used routinely as outpatient therapy, all of the groups of patients were hospitalized because of our fear of toxicity. We discussed cure as our goal, but we did so softly, since the use of the word cure in conjunction with treatment of patients with metastatic cancer was not academically acceptable in 1963 when this program was first started.

"It is worth noting how something representing as radical a departure from medical practice as MOPP got started. First, the investigators involved were relatively new in the field and not jaded by what more experienced hematologists taught was not possible. Second, the environment of the Clinical Center at the NIH, where the study was conducted, provided a buffer from the normal restraints of standard medical practice. These two facts allowed us to take advantage of principles developed in rodent tumor models and bring them rapidly to the clinic. The principles used to design MOPP were fourfold: (1) The use of individually effective non-cross-resistant drugs, in combination, in full doses, with a reasonable expectation of additive or even synergistic anti-tumor effects, (2) intermittant cycled administration of drugs at intervals calculated to match recovery of human bone marrow (laboratory data indicated marrow recovery 21-28 days after a toxic insult and MOPP was cycled at 28 days). Recovery of bone marrow turned out to be the rate limiting step for repeated cycles of drugs and the 28 day cycle still appears ideal. (3) The selection of agents with differing mechanisms of action and differing toxicities. For example, vincristine (minimally toxic to bone marrow) instead of vinblastine (marrow toxic) to minimize the side effects to the most sensitive organ, the bone marrow. (4) A long duration of treatment (6 months) as opposed to the practice at the time of treating for six week periods.

"Although it doesn't seem so now, these were all radical ideas. The intensity and duration of treatment and the use of drugs in combination were not medically sanctioned approaches to the treatment of any disease at the time. The example of the misuse of antibiotics in combination to treat infectious diseases was often cited to us as reason for not taking this approach. The results, reported in 1970, were dramatically different from those previously possible with older approaches. The article is often cited, I suppose, because the MOPP program results have since been amply confirmed and proven durable. A ten year followup report has shown that 66% of all patients who achieved remission have not developed tumor recurrences. We think these patients are rightfully considered cured of their disease. The MOPP program remains the best drug combination for treating advanced Hodgkin's disease attesting to the validity of the principles that led to its design."

CC/NUMBER 50
DECEMBER 12, 1983

This Week's Citation Classic

Carbone P P, Kaplan H S, Musshoff K, Smithers D W & Tubiana M. Report of the committee on Hodgkin's disease staging classification. *Cancer Res.* **31**:1860-1, 1971. [Natl. Cancer Inst., Bethesda, MD; Stanford Univ., CA; Roentgen-Radium-Abteilung, Freiburg, Fed. Rep. Germany; Royal Marsden Hosp., London, England; and Inst. Gustave Roussy, Villejuif, France]

The Ann Arbor staging system for Hodgkin's disease, developed in 1971, remains the currently accepted schema for comparing results on therapy and staging for most institutions treating patients with lymphoma. [The *SCI*® indicates that this paper has been cited in over 980 publications since 1971.]

Paul P. Carbone
Department of Human Oncology
Wisconsin Clinical Cancer Center
University of Wisconsin
Madison, WI 53792

July 20, 1983

"In July 1971, the American Cancer Society and the National Cancer Institute convened a meeting of investigators to update the status of Hodgkin's disease. A previous meeting held in 1965 at Rye, New York, was to be reviewed and new ideas proposed. The past six years had seen a marked change in the diagnosis and staging of Hodgkin's disease. As part of the conference, a subgroup, consisting of the authors, met to revise the Rye classification.[1] Some of the changes in Hodgkin's disease concepts of staging included the usefulness of surgical staging, including laparotomy, the more widespread use of extended field radiation therapy, and the proof that combination chemotherapy could cure Hodgkin's disease.

"At that time, some authors were reporting results where only clinical staging was used while others did an extensive surgical staging with biopsies and even laparotomy. Thus, there was no way to clarify the meaning of stage if the staging procedures were not described. Another issue revolved around the demonstration of Musshoff that apparent parenchymal involvement, such as bone and/or lung if a clear extension from adjacent lymph nodes, was treatable with X rays and had the same prognosis as nodal disease.[2] This has led to the concept of E disease and has been used extensively. While attributable to the Ann Arbor classification, the E category is implied but never mentioned.

"The second major contribution of the Ann Arbor system was to allow the characterization of surgeon staging as pathological staging (PS). Thus, one could really define patients by their clinical stage (CS) or pathological stage (PS). Results could be compared across studies on either basis. An interesting discussion occurred over the initials used to designate involvement of other organs. The 'S' category has become widely adopted. The dilemma came over the use of 'L' for lung and then what to use for liver. The designation of 'H' was suggested. In the literature, the initials, except for 'S,' are rarely used.

"The third change that occurred with this schema was the dropping of pruritus from B symptoms. This has become well accepted.

"Although the above classification was intended for Hodgkin's disease only, the same classification is regularly used in non-Hodgkin's lymphoma. There has not been any major change in the classification except that some institutions use a III and III_2 to describe the extent of disease below the diaphragm.[3] Thus, the publication is still referred to in most papers that involve Hodgkin's disease therapy or staging."[4]

1. **Rosenberg S A.** Report of the committee on the staging of Hodgkin's disease. *Cancer Res.* **26**:1310, 1966. (Cited 330 times.)
2. **Musshoff K.** Prognostic and therapeutic implications of staging in extranodal Hodgkin's disease. *Cancer Res.* **31**:1814-27, 1971.
3. **Desser R K, Golumb H M, Ultman J E, Ferguson D J, Moran E M, Griem M D, Vardiman J, Miller B, Oetzel N, Sweet D, Lester E P, Kinzie J J & Blough R.** Prognostic classification of Hodgkin's disease in pathologic stage III, based on anatomic consideration. *Blood* **49**:883-93, 1977.
4. **Aisenberg A C.** Current concepts in cancer: the staging and treatment of Hodgkin's disease. *N. Engl. J. Med.* **299**:1228-32, 1978.

CC/NUMBER 48
DECEMBER 1, 1980

This Week's Citation Classic

Gold P & Freedman S O. Specific carcinoembryonic antigens of the human digestive system. *J. Exp. Med.* **122**:467-81, 1965.
[McGill Univ. Med. Clinic, Montreal Gen. Hosp., and Dept. Physiology, McGill Univ., Montreal, Canada]

The finding of a human colon tumor-specific antigen led to a search for this material in other human tissues. This manuscript describes the presence of the same constituent in all entodermally-derived gastrointestinal cancers and in embryonic and fetal digestive tissues in the first two trimesters of gestation. The material is, therefore, designated carcinoembryonic antigen (CEA) of the human digestive system, and the genetic control of its expression is considered. [The *SCI*® indicates that this paper has been cited over 655 times since 1965.]

Phil Gold
McGill University
Montreal General Hospital
Montreal, Quebec H3G 1A4
Canada

October 28, 1980

"My colleague, Samuel Freedman, and I were delighted and flattered to learn that the second paper in the series dealing with our discovery of the carcinoembryonic antigen (CEA) as a human tumor marker[1] had achieved the designation of a *Citation Classic*. It would be very satisfying, indeed, to state that we undertook this series of investigations with clear insight into the ultimate value of the data to be obtained and the potential experimental difficulties that might be encountered. However, it is perhaps more accurate to say that any success that we achieved in the antigenic analysis of human colon cancer tissue was due at least as much to good luck as good intention, and was performed with the somewhat naive hope that the burgeoning probes of immunologic technology would provide, at once, the specificity and sensitivity that had been lacking in the tools previously employed in human cancer research.

"By the early 1960s, studies of the rejection of well-defined transplantable tumors between highly inbred animals had demonstrated the existence of tumor-specific transplantation antigens in such animal models.[2-7] Lacking a syngenic human population, to say nothing of the moral and ethical prohibitions to human tumor transplantation, we employed the techniques of antiserum absorption and immunologic tolerance to compare colon cancer tissue with normal colonic mucosa taken from the same donors. This comparison had led to the demonstration of a tumor component in the cancer tissue which we were unable to demonstrate in the corresponding normal tissue.[1] In the manuscript under consideration, then, we had gone on to show that the same cancer antigen was also present in all entodermally-derived gastrointestinal tumors and in fetal digestive organs in the first two trimesters of gestation, but in no other human tissues examined.

"The question of whether or not CEA or CEA-like substances exist in even trace quantities in other cancerous, otherwise diseased or normal tissues, remains controversial and the structure and biologic function of CEA are under continuous and active investigation in numerous laboratories including our own. We believe, however, that the frequent citation of the paper in question is most likely due to the fact that the work resulted in the development of a radioimmunoassay for CEA that presently enjoys widespread use, internationally, as a tumor marker in the management of cancer patients, both pre-operatively and post-operatively.

"It is perhaps an interesting aside that prior to submitting the initial manuscript of CEA to *The Journal of Experimental Medicine*, we had been warned by colleagues in the field that the late Peyton Rous, then on the editorial board of the journal, and presumably most involved in the evaluation of manuscripts related to cancer research in general, was not very favorably disposed toward the immunologic approach to cancer investigation. If this was, in fact, the case, we are very glad that Rous apparently relented."

1. **Gold P & Freedman S O.** Demonstration of tumor-specific antigens in human colonic carcinomata by immunological tolerance and absorption techniques. *J. Exp. Med.* **121**:439-62, 1965.
2. **Baldwin R W & Embleton M J.** Neoantigens on spontaneous and carcinogen-induced rat tumours defined by *in vitro* lymphocytotoxicity assays. *Int. J. Cancer* **13**:433-43, 1974.
3. **Baldwin R W, Embleton M J, Price M R & Robins A.** Immunity in the tumor-bearing host and its modification by serum factors. *Cancer* **34**:1452-60, 1974.
4. **Klein G.** Tumor antigens. *Annu. Rev. Microbiol.* **20**:223-52, 1966.
5. **Oettgen H F & Hellstrom K E.** Tumor immunology. (Holland J F & Frei E, eds.) *Cancer medicine.* Philadelphia: Lea and Febiger, 1973. p. 951-90.
6. **Old L J & Boyse E A.** Immunology of experimental tumors. *Annu. Rev. Med.* **15**:167-86, 1964.
7. **Smith R T.** Tumor-specific immune mechanisms. *N. Engl. J. Med.* **278**:1207-14; 1268-75; 1326-31, 1968.

CC/NUMBER 1
JANUARY 3, 1983

This Week's Citation Classic

Laurence D J R, Stevens U, Bettelheim R, Darcy D, Leese C, Turberville C, Alexander P, Johns E W & Neville A M. Role of plasma carcinoembryonic antigen in diagnosis of gastrointestinal, mammary, and bronchial carcinoma. *Brit. Med. J.* **3**:605-9, 1972.
[Royal Marsden Hospital and Chester Beatty Research Inst., London, England]

For those cancers with a relatively high incidence in the population, the carcinoembryonic antigen (CEA) has a limited role for initial detection or differential diagnosis. After therapeutic intervention, CEA testing could have value in detecting residual tumour or recurrence. [The *SCI*® indicates that this paper has been cited in over 315 publications since 1972.]

Donald J.R. Laurence
Ludwig Institute for Cancer Research
Royal Marsden Hospital
Sutton, Surrey SM2 5PX
England

November 9, 1982

"At the beginning of the 1970s, under the direction of Thomas Symington and Munro Neville, it was decided to study those cancers in man that have a high incidence of occurrence, *viz.*, cancers of the digestive tract, breast, and lung. It was intended to use existing expertise in the institute to develop the concept of functional pathology. Biochemical and immunological methods together with culture of human tumours would generate a dynamic description of tumour activity to supplement or replace the essentially static description of classical pathology. For lung cancer we had begun to develop a radioimmunoassay for ACTH but we had not yet committed ourselves to an approach to the other cancers.

"Peter Alexander returned from the first fetal antigen meeting at Oak Ridge full of enthusiasm for the way research on carcinoembryonic antigen (CEA) was developing in North America. In August 1971, I went on a tour through Duarte, California; Montreal; Boston; and Nutley, New Jersey, in order to obtain technical details of CEA production, assay, and interpretation. Charles Todd gave me a week in his laboratory at Duarte, teaching me the assay and briefing me on other aspects of the CEA scene. We came to an agreement whereby he would provide reagents so that we could start testing with established materials.

"By early September, Ulla Stevens had established an assay in London and the signal was given to start our clinical testing. A 'task force' of David Smithers and Alexander together with Cecil Leese and Radka Bettelheim toured the neighbouring hospitals, generating interest by giving seminars and receiving the willing and enthusiastic support of surgeons and histopathologists. Cooperation with more distant centers was obtained through the goodwill of Symington and Neville. Douglas Darcy used his immunological expertise to generate new anti-CEA reagents while Ernest Johns and Christopher Turberville concerned themselves with CEA production. Johns has also written a *Citation Classic* on his work on histone fractionation.[1]

"The period between September 1971 and the publication date of September 1972 was a fairly hectic one and Bettelheim remembers labelling control tubes to send to New Jersey late on a Sunday evening after a full week spent in her usual role as a histopathologist and clinical coordinator. Our results covered a wide range of tumours with a fairly intensive vertical study of the three main types of common cancer. We obtained data on the effect of tumour spread and differentiation together with the effects of inflammatory or regenerative pathology at the same sites. We used our paper to explore the general problem of use of tumour markers. Seen in retrospect, our approach seems to anticipate subsequent development of the subject[2] and this has probably encouraged others to cite our paper as an early example of their art.

"We were prepared for an application of our CEA test to population screening and Leese organised a computerized data base for this purpose. However, our results showed that this application would be of very limited benefit."

1. **Johns E W.** Studies on histones. 7. Preparative methods for histone fractions from calf thymus. *Biochemical J.* **92**:55-9, 1964. [Citation Classic. *Current Contents/Life Sciences* **22**(11):14, 12 March 1979.]
2. **Laurence D J R & Neville A M.** Biochemical tests in diagnosis and monitoring of cancer. *Clin. Biochem. Rev.* **3**:133-86, 1982.

CC/NUMBER 3
JANUARY 17, 1983

This Week's Citation Classic

Reynoso G, Chu T M, Holyoke D, Cohen E, Nemoto T, Wang J-J, Chuang J, Guinan P & Murphy G P. Carcinoembryonic antigen in patients with different cancers. *J. Amer. Med. Assn.* **220**:361-5, 1972.
[Roswell Park Memorial Inst., New York State Dept. Health, Buffalo, NY]

The paper shows that carcinoembryonic antigen (CEA) is present in normal individuals and in patients with a variety of cancers, not only gastrointestinal cancer. The paper convincingly demonstrates the positive correlation between antigenemia and clinical stage and sets the basis for the use of serial CEA measurements as monitors of therapy in cancer. [The *SCI*® indicates that this paper has been cited in over 295 publications since 1972.]

Gustavo Reynoso
Department of Pathology
Norwalk Hospital
Norwalk, CT 06856

December 16, 1982

"Cancer immunology was an exciting field of research in the late-1960s and early-1970s. The work of Sir Macfarlane Burnet[1] had led to the then widely accepted concept of immunological surveillance in cancer; alpha-feto protein had recently been discovered[2] and the Montreal group had just begun their long series of publications on the carcinoembryonic antigens (CEAs) of the human digestive tract.[3] It was believed at the time—in part because of extrapolation from animal models—that human cancer tissues contained antigens specific for malignancy and specific for the organ or site from which the antigen was isolated. Such a belief encouraged a great deal of enthusiasm in the use of tumor-specific antigens as potential laboratory tests for cancer.

"In such a climate of heightened expectations, it was important to put the ideas in perspective from a clinical point of view. To that effect, I organized a team of pathologists, clinicians, biochemists, and immunologists to study the immunological basis and the methodological limitations of measuring CEA in plasma, in the normal population and in patients with cancer of different organs, and to correlate the findings with the tumor type and the clinical stage.

"The paper, in my opinion, has been so widely cited because the results of our work provided most of the fundamentals on which later research was based. First, we demonstrated that cross-reactive antigens, immunologically and physicochemically indistinguishable from CEA, are present in normal human subjects. Second, we showed convincingly that the claimed tissue specificity of CEA is not a fundamental property of the antigen itself. Rather, methodological variability can modify the apparent specificity. When such a finding was challenged by the Montreal group, we were able to show carcinoembryonic antigenemia in patients with non-endodermally derived cancer *using their own antigen and antibody*.

"Of more importance are the positive aspects of our work. We correlated antigenemia with tumor burden and clinical stage and predicted—with clinical and experimental data—the now well-accepted use of fetal antigens as tumor markers.

"The paper and the two or three that followed[4-6] were surprisingly well received by the scientific editors even though (or perhaps because) they contradicted the cancer-specific dogma of the time. It is, I believe, the publication of this paper that led to my appointment to the task force that developed the master plan for the national cancer program and later, in the implementation phase, to several of the review committees and study sections on immunodiagnosis of the National Cancer Institute.

"A happy thought: all of the young investigators whom I invited to collaborate in my group became cancer immunologists and remain active and productive researchers in the field to this time."

1. **Burnet M.** *Immunological surveillance.* Oxford: Pergamon Press, 1970. 280 p.
2. **Abelev G I.** Production of embryonal alpha-globulin by hepatomas: review of experimental and clinical data. *Cancer Res.* **28**:1344-50, 1968.
3. **Gold P & Freedman S O.** Demonstration of tumor-specific antigens in human colonic carcinomata by immunological tolerance and absorption techniques. *J. Exp. Med.* **121**:439-59, 1968.
4. **Reynoso G, Chu T M, Guinan P & Murphy G P.** Carcinoembryonic antigen in patients with tumors of the urogenital tract. *Cancer* **30**:1-4, 1972.
5. **Chu T M, Hansen H J & Reynoso G.** Demonstration of carcinoembryonic antigen in normal human plasma. *Nature* **238**:152-3, 1972.
6. **Chu T M & Reynoso G.** Evaluation of a new radioimmunoassay method for carcinoembryonic antigen in plasma, with use of zirconyl phosphate gel. *Clin. Chem.* **18**:918-22, 1972.

CC/NUMBER 16
APRIL 20, 1981

This Week's Citation Classic

Brock D J H & Sutcliffe R G. Alpha-fetoprotein in the antenatal diagnosis of anencephaly and spina bifida. *Lancet* **2**:197-9, 1972.
[University Dept. Human Genetics, Western Gen. Hosp., Edinburgh, Scotland]

This paper showed that it was possible to make antenatal diagnoses of anencephaly and spina bifida by measurement of amniotic fluid alpha-fetoprotein concentrations. This introduced a new category of at-risk mothers to antenatal diagnosis. [The *SCI*® indicates that this paper has been cited over 310 times since 1972.]

David J.H. Brock
University Department of Human Genetics
Western General Hospital
Edinburgh EH4 2HU
Scotland

March 27, 1981

"In the early 1970s Roger Sutcliffe and I were investigating the origin of amniotic fluid protein. If most were of fetal origin we thought that it might prove useful for antenatal diagnosis. However, we were able to show fairly convincingly that the majority of protein derived from the maternal serum. The exception was alpha-fetoprotein (AFP).

"We had gone to considerable trouble to raise an antiserum against human AFP to allow us to make a series of measurements on its concentration in amniotic fluid. As we were interested in fetal abnormalities, we asked ourselves whether there were any particular disorders where one might anticipate a change in amniotic fluid AFP concentration. Once the question was posed in this way, the answer was blindingly obvious: the open neural tube defects such as spina bifida and anencephaly. The anatomical deformities in these abnormalities made it seem fairly likely to us that both fetal serum and fetal cerebrospinal fluid components passed directly into the amniotic fluid. Our reasoning suggested that we should get at least statistically significant increases in AFP, since the protein was known to be present at high levels in fetal serum.

"Fortunately we had been collecting amniotic fluids from a variety of pregnancies for a number of years. In our first experiment we set up five anencephalic amniotic fluids against five controls. The results were extraordinary. All five anencephalic fluids had such high AFP concentrations that they had gone completely off scale. My technician reported that the experiment had not worked and would have to be repeated, but both Roger and I knew that we had stumbled onto something important.

"We assembled as many other relevant amniotic fluids as we could, measured feverishly, and wrote a paper, which was accepted and published all within the space of three months. Almost as an aside, we tossed in the statement in the final paragraph that we could see no reason why this procedure should not eventually be applied to maternal blood and thus available to all pregnant women. I can't think how we arrived at that idea, which in terms of existing knowledge was absurd, but it has turned out to be exactly right.

"Within a week of the appearance of our paper a colleague had his technician in my laboratory learning the new procedure. Within a year AFP analysis was being carried out on all amniotic fluids in the United Kingdom and was an accepted part of the standard procedure of antenatal diagnosis. There were really no problems in the passage of a research technique into routine clinical usage. Recently, several articles have been published on the topic.[1-4]

"The paper was much cited in the early years because it opened up a new field of antenatal diagnosis. However, it has now become such an accepted procedure that one rarely sees 'Brock and Sutcliffe (1972).' The moral is to enjoy your moment of glory; it won't last."

1. **Brock D J H.** Prenatal diagnosis of neural tube defects. *Eur. J. Clin. Invest.* **7**:465-72, 1977.
2. ----------------. Feto-specific proteins in prenatal diagnosis. *Mol. Aspects Med.* **3**:433-553, 1980.
3. **Brock D J H, Barron L, Duncan P, Scrimgeour J B & Watt M.** Significance of elevated mid-trimester maternal plasma alpha-fetoprotein values. *Lancet* **1**:1281-2, 1979.
4. Report of the UK collaborative study on alpha-fetoprotein in relation to neural tube defects. *Lancet* **1**:1323-33, 1977.

CC/NUMBER 43
OCTOBER 24, 1983

This Week's Citation Classic

Braunstein G D, Vaitukaitis J L, Carbone P P & Ross G T. Ectopic production of human chorionic gonadotrophin by neoplasms. *Ann. Intern. Med.* **78**:39-45, 1973.
[Reproduction Research Branch, Natl. Inst. Child Health and Human Development, and Clinical Oncology Area, Natl. Cancer Inst., Natl. Insts. Health, Bethesda, MD]

Using a sensitive and specific radioimmunoassay to measure serum concentrations of human chorionic gonadotrophin (hCG), 59 percent of patients with testicular tumors and over seven percent of patients with a wide variety of non-testicular cancers were found to have immunoreactive hCG in their sera. [The *SCI®* indicates that this paper has been cited in over 330 publications since 1973.]

Glenn D. Braunstein
Department of Medicine
Cedars-Sinai Medical Center
University of California School of Medicine
Los Angeles, CA 90048

June 1, 1983

"In 1970, I had the good fortune of joining Griff Ross in his laboratory at the National Institutes of Health. Griff had received highly purified preparations of human chorionic gonadotrophin (hCG) and its alpha and beta subunits prepared by Robert Canfield at Columbia University College of Physicians & Surgeons. Griff and Judy Vaitukaitis immunized a number of rabbits with these materials in order to develop antisera that would be useful in defining the immunologic characteristics of hCG and the other glycoprotein hormones. It was known that the intact hCG molecule shared some structural characteristics with human thyroid stimulating hormone, follicle stimulating hormone, and especially luteinizing hormone (hLH). Indeed, the biologic and immunologic activity of native hCG and hLH were so similar that only elaborate chromatographic or electrophoretic methods were capable of separating these two hormones.

"Griff had predicted that antibodies generated against the purified subunits of hCG might have a greater affinity for intact hCG than hLH, and therefore would allow the development of a radioimmunoassay that could be used to distinguish serum levels of hCG from circulating hLH. His prediction was proved correct when we found that the antibodies raised against the beta subunit of hCG had relatively little cross-reactivity with hLH. We immediately recognized the potential clinical application of a radioimmunoassay using these antibodies for diagnosis of early pregnancy and for monitoring the therapy of gestational trophoblastic disease. Our paper describing this radioimmunoassay (beta hCG RIA) has recently been featured as a *Citation Classic*.[1,2]

"In initiating our clinical studies of hCG measurements with this assay, we found that we had numerous blood samples from women with gestational trophoblastic disease, but relatively few samples from men with trophoblastic testicular tumors. We learned that Paul Carbone of the National Cancer Institute had established a tumor serum bank which contained blood samples obtained from patients with testicular tumors. The serum bank contained hundreds of samples from patients with a wide variety of malignancies as well as some samples from patients with non-neoplastic disorders. We measured the immunoreactive hCG in the sera from 918 patients with cancer and 443 control patients and found that 59 percent of the patients with testicular tumors and 7.2 percent of the patients with non-trophoblastic neoplasms had immunoreactive hCG in their circulation while only 0.7 percent of the control patients had detectable hCG. Patients with carcinomas of the stomach, liver, pancreas, and breast, and with myeloma and melanoma had the highest frequency of positive responses. This was a higher frequency of hCG production by non-trophoblastic cancers than had been previously recognized.

"I feel that this study became a *Citation Classic* because it was one of the first systematic investigations of ectopic production of a hormone by tumors. The unexpectedly high frequency of hCG production by non-trophoblastic cancers stimulated a number of laboratories to study the ectopic production of hCG and other hormones by tumors.[3] Furthermore, our study suggested that hormones may be useful as objective markers for the diagnosis of cancer and for monitoring the effects of therapy."

1. **Vaitukaitis J L, Braunstein G D & Ross G T.** A radioimmunoassay which specifically measures human chorionic gonadotropin in the presence of human luteinizing hormone. *Amer. J. Obstet. Gynecol.* **113**:751-8, 1972.
2. **Vaitukaitis J L.** Citation Classic. Commentary on *Amer. J. Obstet. Gynecol.* **113**:751-8, 1972. *Current Contents/Clinical Practice* **11**(10):24, 7 March 1983.
3. **Braunstein G D.** hCG expression in trophoblastic and non-trophoblastic tumors. (Fishman W H, ed.) *Oncodevelopmental markers: biologic, diabetic and monitoring aspects, volume II.* New York: Academic Press. In press, 1983.

CC/NUMBER 29
JULY 16, 1984

This Week's Citation Classic™

Vézina J L & Sutton T J. Prolactin-secreting pituitary microadenomas: roentgenologic diagnosis. *Amer. J. Roentgenol.* **120**:46-54, 1974.
[Dept. Neuroradiol., Hôp. Notre-Dame, and Dept. Radiol., Univ. Montréal, Québec, Canada]

Criteria for the diagnosis of small pituitary adenoma in females presenting with amenorrhea, galactorrhea, and hyperprolactinemia were originally presented in the radiological literature in this article. Microsurgical removal of these small lesions resulted in restoration of normal serum prolactin values and return to fertility. [The *SCI*® indicates that this paper has been cited in over 185 publications, ranking it among the ten most-cited papers ever published in this journal.]

Jean Lorrain Vézina
Department of Radiology
Hôtel-Dieu Hospital
Montréal, Québec H2W 1T8
Canada

April 2, 1984

"Ten years ago, pathology textbooks described pituitary adenomas arising from any of three basic cells, the cellular types being the chromophobes accounting for approximately 50 percent of adenomas, the acidophils accounting for 35 percent, and the basophils accounting for the remaining 15 percent. Our article, proposing criteria for the diagnosis of prolactin-secreting pituitary adenomas, was bound to disrupt these percentages, but the impact turned out to be much greater than anticipated. In fact, during the last decade, and as a consequence of the study of large numbers of pathological specimens of the pituitary, it is now recognized that prolactinomas account for more than 50 percent of all pituitary adenomas, leaving little space for chromophobe tumors.

"The circumstances that came to favour this article were twofold. First was my privileged association with an inventive neurosurgeon, J. Hardy, who had pioneered microsurgery of the pituitary fossa by the trans-sphenoidal approach. With a binocular operative microscope, Hardy could selectively remove small pituitary adenomas while preserving the residual pituitary gland, affording cure without loss of normal pituitary functions.

"In this respect, our first radiological survey had covered a group of 80 acromegalic patients of whom 75 percent presented an enlarged sella on plain films of the skull. In the remaining 25 percent, a millimetric tomographic study of the sella revealed subtle positive changes in all cases. On this basis, we described the radiological changes of what we called 'microadenomas' and presented a classification of pituitary lesions based on sellar findings.[1] This classification is now widely used and allows medical centers around the world to compare methods and results of treatment of pituitary adenomas in their different stages.

"The concurrent development of a biochemical method to identify and accurately quantify the human serum prolactin hormone with radioimmunoassay was the second major factor leading to our publication. The new method, discovered in Montréal by Friesen,[2] focussed considerable interest on the amenorrhea-galactorrhea syndromes. This led us to investigate a group of female patients in our infertility clinic presenting hyperprolactinemia with a normal-sized sella on skull radiographs. In many of these patients, the millimetric tomographic studies showed subtle sellar changes somewhat similar to those seen in our acromegalic patients. Small adenomas were selectively removed and were confirmed as prolactin adenomas by electron microscopy. In a high percentage of these patients, we observed postoperative normalization of prolactin levels and recovery of fertility.

"This *Citation Classic* article was a first report and it was actually based on the tomographic evaluation of the sella turcica in 14 female patients presenting fine radiological changes caused by a prolactin microadenoma. These findings were presented at the Symposium Radiologicum in 1974 and they were published in *Acta Radiologica*.[3] In 1977, at the First International Symposium on Prolactin Hormone, we presented a series of 160 patients of whom 20 were males. As radiological signs had become more precise, they were proposed in a well-illustrated publication of the proceedings.[4] In that article, we reemphasized our original classification of pituitary adenomas with four stages. In 1981, we published the radiological findings and classification covering 355 prolactinomas (300 females, 55 males), introducing the new concept of a proportional relationship between the levels of serum prolactin and the size of the tumor.[5]

"The sequential articles based on the diagnostic potential of millimetric tomography have provided indirect evidence of pituitary tumors. Recent high resolution CT and NMR scanners have added a considerable dimension by showing directly the tiny intrapituitary tumor, thus confirming our original hypothesis that patients with normal-sized sellae can harbour a pituitary microadenoma leading to subtle sellar findings."

1. **Vézina J L & Maltais R.** La selle turcique dans l'acromégalie: étude radiologique. *Neurochirurgie* **19**(Suppl. 2):35-56, 1973. (Cited 30 times.)
2. **Friesen H, Webster R, Hwang P, Guyda H, Munro R E & Read L.** Prolactin synthesis and secretion in patient with Forbes-Albright syndrome. *J. Clin. Endocrinol. Metab.* **34**:192-9, 1972. (Cited 60 times.)
3. **Vézina J L, Sutton T J, Maltais R & Hardy J.** Prolactin secreting pituitary micro-adenomas. *Acta Radiol. Suppl.* **347**:561-6, 1975.
4. **Vézina J L.** Prolactin secreting pituitary adenomas: radiologic diagnosis. (Robyn C & Harter M, eds.) *Progress in prolactin physiology and pathology.* Amsterdam: Elsevier/North-Holland Biomedical Press, 1978. p. 351-61.
5. -------------. Le prolactinome: aspect radiologique de la selle turcique. *Neurochirurgie* **27**(Suppl. 1):19-29, 1981.

CC/NUMBER 31
AUGUST 1, 1983

This Week's Citation Classic

Talal N & Bunim J J. The development of malignant lymphoma in the course of Sjögren's syndrome. *Amer. J. Med.* **36**:529-40, 1964.
[Natl. Inst. Arthritis and Metabolic Diseases, Natl. Insts. Health, Bethesda, MD]

This paper was the first to relate the development of malignant lymphoma to an antecedent Sjögren's syndrome (SS). The lymphoma was either undifferentiated or associated with macroglobulinemia. We hypothesized that autoimmunity and lymphoproliferation were predisposing to malignant transformation. [The *SCI®* indicates that this paper has been cited in over 245 publications since 1964.]

Norman Talal
Department of Medicine
Division of Clinical Immunology
University of Texas Health
Science Center
San Antonio, TX 78284

May 24, 1983

"Shortly after taking up my clinical associate position at the National Institute of Arthritis and Metabolic Diseases (NIAMD) in the summer of 1962, I recall making rounds with the late Joseph Bunim. Bunim introduced me to a patient with Sjögren's syndrome (SS) of eight years duration who had developed malignant lymphoma diagnosed as reticulum cell sarcoma six months previously. I suggested to Bunim that the development of a lymphoid neoplasm in a patient with autoimmunity might imply a causal relationship. To my surprise, he informed me that he was following several other patients with SS who also had developed lymphoid malignancy.

"I was fascinated and began to review the charts and examine these other patients. I obtained serial serum samples and studied them by immunoelectrophoresis, a technique developed by Pierre Grabar that I had learned in France the year before. I observed that an initial hypergammaglobulinemia with high titers of autoantibodies progressively declined to hypogammaglobulinemia and loss of autoantibodies. Another patient had macroglobulinemia. Thus, we reported this series suggesting that autoimmunity predisposed to lymphoma which could take one of two forms, either undifferentiated or associated with IgM production (then called β_2M). I was later to substantiate this hypothesis of progressive dedifferentiation of B cells as malignancy develops in SS using tissue sections and an immunoperoxidase anti-immunoglobulin staining technique.[1]

"I believe this publication has been highly cited because it was the first to associate two disorders of immunoregulation, autoimmunity with the subsequent development of lymphoma. Future work should help explain exactly how the underlying autoimmune process may contribute to a neoplastic transformation of cells involved in that process. The original designation of 'reticulum cell sarcoma' was a misnomer for we now know on the basis of immunohistologic studies[1] and most recently chromosomal gene rearrangement studies that the malignant cell belongs to the B-cell lineage.

"Honors received for this paper and my subsequent studies on immune dysregulation and autoimmunity in patients and inbred strains of mice include the Hench Award (1975) and the Middleton Award (1980) presented by the US Veterans Administration."

1. **Zulman J, Jaffe R & Talal N.** Evidence that the malignant lymphoma of Sjögren's syndrome is a monoclonal B-cell neoplasm. *N. Engl. J. Med.* **299**:1215-20, 1978.

CC/NUMBER 26
JUNE 28, 1982

This Week's Citation Classic

Ziel H K & Finkle W D. Increased risk of endometrial carcinoma among users of conjugated estrogens. *N. Engl. J. Med.* **293**:1167-70, 1975.
[Dept. Obstet. and Gynecol., Kaiser-Permanente Med. Ctr., Los Angeles, and Dept. Med. Econ., Kaiser Foundation Health Plan, Southern California Region, CA]

Using the case-control technique, patients with endometrial cancer were compared to a twofold age-matched control group of patients from the same population. Fifty-seven percent of the patients with endometrial cancer used conjugated estrogens, whereas 15 percent of the control patients used conjugated estrogens. The risk of endometrial cancer associated with estrogen use was 7.6 times greater than without estrogen use. Risk increased with duration of exposure: from 5.6 for less than five years' use to 13.9 for greater than seven years' use. These data strongly support the association of endometrial cancer and conjugated estrogens use. [The *SCI*® indicates that this paper has been cited over 320 times since 1975.]

Harry K. Ziel
Department of Obstetrics and Gynecology
Kaiser-Permanente Medical Center
4900 Sunset Boulevard
Los Angeles, CA 90027
and
William D. Finkle
Education and Research
4747 Sunset Boulevard
Los Angeles, CA 90027

June 11, 1982

"I (Harry K. Ziel) am indeed fortunate to work with a group of gynecologic oncologists who constantly review pathologic materials from the membership of the Kaiser Foundation Health Plan of Southern California, a large prepaid health plan. In the early-1970s, we were struck with the increasing frequency with which endometrial cancer was developing. One unusual feature of this cancer epidemic was that these women did not have the usual obese habitus which one traditionally associates with endometrial cancer. Rather, these cancer patients were of average stature. Furthermore and most interesting, these normally sized women with endometrial cancer had a common denominator; most had used an estrogen, usually a conjugated estrogen, for many years.

"I remember joking about the association of estrogen with endometrial cancer at our weekly micropathologic reviews. I would quip, 'Premarin effect!' with no knowledge of the hormonal history whenever a slide of endometrial cancer was projected. Most commonly, when the drug history was recited, I was correct. Arthur Saltz, my chief at that time, goaded me more than once, saying, 'Harry, nobody will believe you until you prove it.'

"As luck would have it, I met an MIT graduate, William D. Finkle, who collaborated with me to evaluate the hypothesis totally.

"Today, 24 studies have been reported worldwide which associate estrogen use with endometrial cancer.[1,2] Cancer incidence correlates consistently with the amount of estrogen used and with duration of use in these studies. After our publication in December 1975, estrogen use abruptly fell. After estrogen use diminished, the incidence of endometrial cancer reached a plateau, then decreased.

"Our report has taken on the aura of a classic because it reversed scientific thinking on the safety of estrogen and because it established risk estimates for development of endometrial cancer following finite durations of estrogen exposure.

"No man stands alone. We owe everything to our associates. To develop a concept, we need the stimulation of both supporters and antagonists. The ingredients of a concept exist all the time. The people who receive credit for a concept are the ones who are just lucky enough to be exposed to the proper experiences and ideas, who are forced to react to them, and who then formalize a resultant concept into a report."

1. **Schwarz B E.** Does estrogen cause adenocarcinoma of the endometrium? *Clin. Obstet. Gynaecol.* **24**:243-51, 1981.
2. **Mahboubi E, Eyler N & Wynder E L.** Epidemiology of cancer of the endometrium. *Clin. Obstet. Gynaecol.* **25**:5-17, 1982.

CC/NUMBER 42
OCTOBER 18, 1982

This Week's Citation Classic

Kellermann G, Shaw C R & Luyten-Kellermann M. Aryl hydrocarbon hydroxylase inducibility and bronchogenic carcinoma. *N. Engl. J. Med.* **289**:934-7, 1973. [Sect. Med. Genetics, Dept. Biology, Univ. Texas, and M.D. Anderson Hosp. and Tumor Inst., Houston, TX]

Aryl hydrocarbon hydroxylase (AHH) is involved in the metabolism of chemical carcinogens and present in many tissues including lung and mitogen stimulated lymphocytes. Its genetic variation in normal subjects can be linked to susceptibility to bronchogenic carcinoma, thus demonstrating a close association between high levels of AHH and this particular cancer. [The *SCI*® indicates that this paper has been cited in over 345 publications since 1973.]

Gottfried Kellermann
Immuno Nuclear Corporation
P.O. Box 285
Stillwater, MN 55082

July 9, 1982

"In May 1982, it had been exactly ten years since I walked into Charles Shaw's laboratory at the M.D. Anderson Hospital and Tumor Institute in Houston, Texas, to ask him what kind of project he had in mind for me, having just received a two-year fellowship from the Deutsche Forschungsgemeinschaft. I chose to continue with the aryl hydrocarbon hydroxylase (AHH) project after D. Busbee and E. Cantrell,[1] in his laboratory, had succeeded in demonstrating the presence of the enzyme in mitogen stimulated lymphocytes.

"Using cultured lymphocytes was a very clever idea since it enabled the study of the enzyme, which is not present in the circulating blood, in virtually hundreds and thousands of individuals. All it required was five to ten milliliters of blood. The first population data were encouraging, pointing to a two- to fourfold variation of the enzyme activity in normal subjects. At the same time, I had lined up several volunteers whose 'AHH value' I would check at least twice a week for a period of 18 months. Anyone can imagine this would eventually become a very painful experience but the results were rewarding for all the sufferings. Individual AHH values were highly constant for a given subject indicating some kind of genetic control.

"A large mass of data was necessary to arrive at this conclusion because of the wide variation in culture and assay conditions. To eliminate some of the variation, my wife, Mieke, had joined me to run all these tests under highly controlled conditions. The most rewarding but also the most exhausting part of the whole research project was the family study designed to support the hypothesis of a genetic control of individual AHH values. My wife and I would drive out to the suburbs of Houston every night to draw blood samples from families, rush back to the lab, and set up cultures. Quite often it was in the early morning hours before we returned home.

"During these long rides there was always one question that kept nagging in my mind: 'What is the relationship, if any, between the enzyme activity of cultured lymphocytes and that of any other tissue such as liver or lung?' I knew the answer to this question was vital and, so to speak, the heart of the entire project. If one were able to establish a firm link between the *in vitro* activity of a certain tissue enzyme, e.g., of the liver, and that of an easily manageable culture system, it would not only allow the carrying out of large population genetic studies on otherwise inaccessible enzymes, but also help one to understand why a genetic variation could be the cause of an increased or decreased risk to contract a particular disease. Therefore, I tried to relate the *in vitro* metabolic rates of some harmless drugs to the lymphocyte AHH activity of the same individual.[2] The positive results led me to hypothesize that if this relationship between the enzyme activity of cultured lymphocytes and human liver is real, it might not be too farfetched to assume a similar relationship also for the lung. This implied that the genetic variation of AHH activity of lymphocytes reflected genetic variation of lung AHH activity. With this background I did the lung cancer study which in humans linked high AHH activity to an increased risk for lung cancer.

"The reaction and response to this study took me by surprise since I did not immediately realize its full impact in the health field. I never had planned to come up with a new biochemical marker or a test to predict individual cancer risk. To me, it just was an ideal opportunity to study how genetics and environment might interact and whether some common diseases have a genetic basis. Even after nine years the results of the cancer study are still highly controversial mainly because of experimental difficulties. However, growing evidence indicates that the original findings are valid."[3,4]

1. **Busbee D L, Shaw C R & Cantrell E T.** Aryl hydrocarbon hydroxylase induction in human leukocytes. *Science* **178**:315-16, 1972.
2. **Kellermann G, Luyten-Kellermann M, Horning M G & Stafford M.** Elimination of antipyrine and benzo[a]pyrene metabolism in cultured human lymphocytes. *Clin. Pharmacol. Ther.* **20**:72-80, 1976.
3. **Nebert D W.** The Ah locus, a gene with possible importance in cancer predictability. *Arch. Toxicol. Suppl.* **3**:195-207, 1980.
4. **Rüdiger H W, Heisig V & Hain E.** Enhanced benzo[a]pyrene metabolism and formation of DNA adducts in monocytes of patients with lung cancer. *J. Cancer Res. Clin. Oncol.* **96**:295-302, 1980.

CC/NUMBER 31
JULY 30, 1984

This Week's Citation Classic™

Bluming A Z, Vogel C L, Ziegler J L, Mody N & Kamya G. Immunological effects of BCG in malignant melanoma: two modes of administration compared. *Ann. Intern. Med.* **76**:405-11, 1972.
[Solid Tumor Ctr., Uganda Cancer Inst., and Dept. Surg., Makerere Univ. Med. Sch., Kampala, Uganda]

Two modes of administering BCG were compared for effects on immunologic reactivity and survival of malignant melanoma patients following surgical excision of clinically apparent tumor and regional lymph nodes. A nonspecific potentiating effect on cellular reactivity to both primary and recall antigens was observed in the group treated by dermal scarification. No such effect was noted in the group treated by intradermal vaccination. Significantly longer remissions were observed in the former group. [The *SCI*® indicates that this paper has been cited in over 180 publications since 1972.]

Avrum Z. Bluming
Hematology-Oncology Medical Group
of the San Fernando Valley
16311 Ventura Boulevard
Encino, CA 91436

June 28, 1984

"He was a dignified, tall, well-muscled man. Traces of gray were visible in his tightly curled, thick, black hair. Several weeks earlier, a melanoma had been widely excised from the sole of his right foot, and the light pink color around the healing lymphadenectomy incision in his right groin stood out sharply against his black skin. He was sitting in an aluminum roofed clinic in his native Uganda while ritual scarring was applied to his right upper arm in an attempt to ward off the return of the devil illness called cancer. But the healer performing the ritual was a graduate of Columbia University's College of Physicians & Surgeons sent to Uganda by the National Cancer Institute to study tumors like his, and Pasteur Institute BCG was being applied to the 5 x 5 cm grid I had raked onto his upper arm.

"In 1969, Mathé[1] reported significantly increased remission duration in ALL patients treated with Pasteur Institute BCG, applied by dermal scratching following remission induction. In 1970, Hamilton Fairley[2] reported no such benefit when Glaxo BCG was used and applied by intradermal inoculation. In order to establish a standard BCG immunotherapy regimen, Chuck Vogel, John Ziegler, and I set up a study to document the proposed nonspecific immunopotentiating effect of BCG on humoral and cellular immunity in man. Using a battery of immunologic tests, we hoped to identify the most effective BCG preparation and route of administration to be used in subsequent clinical immunotherapy trials.

"Junctional nevi are frequently found on the soles of black Ugandans with a pattern of distribution remarkably consistent among the members of each tribe. Melanomas developed commonly on the soles of this largely barefoot population in a distribution reflecting the distribution of the junctional nevi. Earlier published studies had suggested that melanoma was an immunogenic tumor and that an immune reaction to the tumor correlated with a favorable prognosis. We therefore elected to study this available patient population. Informed consent, obtained from each patient, usually required prolonged discussions in Luganda, Lango, Toro, Bunyoro, or Swahili explaining why this study, remarkably similar in outward appearance to traditional medicine man ministrations, was imported from the US.

"We were able to show: 1) a nonspecific potentiating effect on cell-mediated immunity to both primary and recall antigens in the group treated with Pasteur Institute BCG; 2) a correlation between dose of administered BCG and immune potentiation; and 3) a significant prolongation of remission duration associated with the higher dose (Pasteur Institute) BCG administered by dermal scarification. This initial result was confirmed in a follow-up report published four years later.[3]

"Our attempts to 1) provide an immunologic parameter by which the potency of nonspecific immunotherapy could be assayed, and 2) define a standard preparation and application of BCG in this setting are probably responsible for the frequent references to this article.

"Although nonspecific immunotherapy may benefit a subset of melanoma patients in remission, subsequent large-scale studies have failed to confirm a reproducibly meaningful, beneficial effect."[4]

1. **Mathé G, Amiel J L, Schwarzenberg L, Schneider M, Cattan A, Schlumberger J R, Hayat M & de Vassal F.** Active immunotherapy for acute lymphoblastic leukaemia. *Lancet* **1**:697-9, 1969. (Cited 610 times.)
2. **Hamilton Fairley G.** Immunotherapy of acute lymphoblastic leukemia. (Abstract.) *Abstracts of the XIII International Congress of Hematology, Munich, 2-8 August 1970.* Munich: Lehmann, 1970. p. 278.
3. **Bluming A Z.** Immunotherapy of cancer. (Homburger F, ed.) *The physiopathology of cancer, volume 2. Diagnosis, treatment, prevention.* Basel: Karger, 1976. p. 251-78.
4. **Veronesi U, Adamus J, Aubert C, Bajetta E, Beretta G, Bonadonna G, Bufalino R, Cascinelli N, Cocconi G, Durand J, De Marsillac J, Ikonopisov R L, Kiss B, Lejeune F, MacKie R, Madej G, Mulder H, Mechl Z, Milton G W, Morabito A, Peter H, Priario J, Paul E, Rumke P, Sertoli R & Tomin R.** A randomized trial of adjuvant chemotherapy and immunotherapy in cutaneous melanoma. *N. Engl. J. Med.* **307**:913-16, 1982.

CC/NUMBER 46
NOVEMBER 12, 1984

This Week's Citation Classic™

Salmon S E, Hamburger A W, Soehnlen B, Durie B G M, Alberts D S & Moon T E. Quantitation of differential sensitivity of human-tumor stem cells to anticancer drugs. *N. Engl. J. Med.* **298**:1321-7, 1978.
[Sect. Hematol. Oncol., Dept. Internal Med., and Cancer Ctr., Univ. Arizona, Coll. Med., Tucson, AZ]

A new *in vitro* soft agar culture system developed in our laboratory was applied to testing clonogenic tumor cells ('tumor stem cells') from patient biopsies against anticancer drugs. Unique patterns of sensitivity and resistance were documented, and good correlations were observed between *in vitro* results and clinical treatment outcome, raising the possibility of predictive cancer chemotherapy. [The *SCI*® indicates that this paper has been cited in over 465 publications since 1978.]

Sydney E. Salmon
Arizona Cancer Center
University of Arizona College of Medicine
Tucson, AZ 85724

August 1, 1984

"As an investigator interested in cancer chemotherapy, I was perplexed by the lack of predictivity of clinical response in patients with tumors of the same histopathology and stage. I suspected that intrinsic differences in drug sensitivity might be responsible for this phenomenon. I had pursued this problem unsuccessfully during the early 1970s, in part because of difficulties in cultivating human tumors *in vitro*. The first big break came when Anne Hamburger, fresh from completing a postdoctoral fellowship at the Albert Einstein College of Medicine, applied for a position, in large part because her physician-husband had been assigned to duty at a local air base. Our central focus was to develop a clonogenic assay capable of supporting human tumor growth. This approach had been used for quantitating bacterial growth and antibiotic sensitivity. It had also been successfully applied to studying growth and sensitivity of transplantable murine tumors by W.R. Bruce, Makio Ogawa, and their colleagues at the Ontario Cancer Institute. Anne tackled the tumor cultivation problem vigorously. In little more than a year, we had devised an *in vitro* soft agar culture system capable of supporting clonal growth of a variety of human tumors while suppressing normal cell proliferation.[1]

"The next step was to standardize techniques for studying cytotoxic drugs. An important early decision was to use *in vitro* drug concentrations achievable in the patient's plasma. My coauthors and I mounted a multidisciplinary effort involving cell biology, pharmacology, medical oncology, and biometry. Although our 1978 clinical report in the *New England Journal of Medicine* involved only a limited number of patients, and some of the correlations were retrospective, the results indicated the potential feasibility of applying this approach to aiding in the development of new anticancer drugs and potential individual cancer chemotherapy. We cautioned that a number of methodological problems would need to be solved before our approach could be fully tested, but concluded that the results showed sufficient promise to warrant larger-scale testing.

"The reason that our paper has been so extensively cited is that it represents the first clearly positive approach to predictive cancer chemotherapy. Since the appearance of our paper, the Arizona Cancer Center has hosted four International Tumor Cloning conferences. The monograph published from our 1984 conference[2] provides a current review of this topic.

"Many investigators now use human tumor cloning assays. Such assay systems still need further improvement as not all tumor specimens give rise to adequate colony growth *in vitro*. Correlative clinical trials from various centers have been reported and were recently reviewed,[3] including one large prospective trial.[4] Overall, *in vitro* drug sensitivity to single agents has predicted clinical response with about 60 to 70 percent accuracy, and *in vitro* resistance has predicted treatment failure with over 90 percent accuracy. Prospective randomized trials are currently under way to determine whether assay-selected treatment has any advantage over empirically selected treatment for specific tumor types. Additionally, the National Cancer Institute now employs this assay system regularly in its program to discover new anticancer drugs.[5] Insufficient time has elapsed to assess the long-term impact of our approach to anticancer drug testing on either patient survival or new drug development."

1. **Hamburger A W & Salmon S E.** Primary bioassay of human tumor stem cells. *Science* **197**:461-3, 1977. (Cited 335 times.)
2. **Salmon S E & Trent J M,** eds. *Human tumor cloning.* Orlando, FL: Grune & Stratton, 1984. 700 p.
3. **Salmon S E.** Human tumor colony assay and chemosensitivity testing. *Cancer Treat. Rep.* **68**:117-25, 1984.
4. **Von Hoff D D, Clark G M, Stogdill B J, Sarosdy M F, O'Brien M T, Casper J T, Mattox D E, Page C P, Cruz A B & Sandbach J F.** Prospective clinical trial of a human tumor cloning system. *Cancer Res.* **43**:1926-31, 1983.
5. **Shoemaker R H, Wolpert-DeFilippes M K, Melnick N, Venditti J M, Simon R M, Kern D H, Lieber M, Miller W T, Salmon S E & Von Hoff D D.** Recent results of new drug screening trials with a human tumor colony forming assay. (Salmon S E & Trent J M, eds.) *Human tumor cloning.* Orlando, FL: Grune & Stratton, 1984. p. 345-56.

CC/NUMBER 22
MAY 28, 1979

This Week's Citation Classic

Collins V P, Loeffler R K & Tivey H. Observations on growth rates of human tumors.
Amer. J. Roentgenol. **76**:988-1000, 1956.
[Baylor University College of Medicine, Department of Radiology, Houston, TX]

Linear exponential growth, determined by measurement of pulmonary metastases and expressed as 'Doubling Time,' is introduced as a characteristic of the individual cancer, governing the duration before and after diagnosis. The evidence for an age-related 'Period of Risk' for childhood tumors is a supporting application. [The *SCI*® indicates that this paper has been cited over 165 times since 1961.]

V.P. Collins
9200 Westheimer
Houston, TX 77063

July 27, 1978

"The origin of the concept of linear exponential growth as a governing characteristic of cancer cannot be recalled but the thesis was developing, and data accumulating, from 1950 on under the influence of the varied background of the authors in pathology [Collins], physics [Tivey], mathematics and bio-statistics [Loeffler]. Simply stated, the rule to be tested was that the growth of cancer was linear and exponential with a constant growth rate, as a characteristic of the individual cancer as its morphology, governing the duration of cancer before and after the time of diagnosis. With confirmation of clinical applicability, the literature has given the accolade of 'law,' better perhaps than Murphy's but not as reliable as Newton's. The ultimate acceptance must be ascribed to its simplicity and clinical applicability. Growth is a synonym for cancer. Growth is a function of time and increasing volume and both are measurable. There is a ready measure of growth rate in 'doubling time.'

"The rule explains the phenomenon of the dormant cancer; the total duration of cancer is approximately 40 doublings; three quarters of this time is in the period of silent, steady growth that occurs before the recognition of the small (but not early) cancer. It explains the phenomenon of the cancer 'that suddenly began to grow wildly;' this is the exponential upsweep after 35 to 40 doublings. It explains the paradox of earlier diagnosis and ever-improving survival rates but unrelenting mortality rates, such as characterize breast cancer. To move diagnosis to the left on the exponential curve is to start the countdown on survival at an earlier point in time, to increase survival time even without treatment, and to mask the effect of treatment with unearned credit.

"There is particular appeal in the implications for childhood tumors. The 'Period of Risk' thesis (that recurrence, if going to occur, should develop within a period equal to the age at diagnosis plus nine months) evolved in a search for justification for extrapolation of linear exponential growth back to the time of inception; several series seem to corroborate the rule. It also unmasks the error in assuming that childhood tumors are uniformly malignant and rapidly growing for lack of a sturdy host reaction. In this age group all tumors must grow rapidly; a child is not old enough for a slowly growing cancer to have reached the size of recognition; slowly growing cancers have not had time to traverse their characteristic period of silent growth when this is greater than the age of the child.

"Simplicity was the merit of the thought and the obstacle to its acceptance. On first submission for publication, it was returned with a comment to the effect that 'I have read this through twice and would not touch it because we do not accept this sort of material.'

"In the arena of cancer research the initial impact was approximately that of a presentation on fire-making with two sticks, offered at a convention of nuclear physicists. The simplicity of the hypothesis does assault the accepted infinite complexity of etiology, biochemistry and cyto-kinetics of cancer. But until nuclear physicists solve our energy problem, there is some practical application for the warmth of a small fire kindled with two sticks."

CC/NUMBER 8
FEBRUARY 22, 1982

This Week's Citation Classic

Almgård L E, Fernström I, Haverling M & Ljungqvist A. Treatment of renal adenocarcinoma by embolic occlusion of the renal circulation.
Brit. J. Urol. **45**:474-9, 1973.
[Depts. Urology, Diagnostic Radiology and Pathology, Karolinska Sjukhuset, Stockholm, Sweden]

A method is presented using autologous muscle suspension mixed with contrast medium and injected via a catheter into the renal artery. In cases of renal adenocarcinoma this will produce a reduced vascularity and widespread necrosis. Troublesome bleeding ceased and tumours were accessible for surgery. The technique was free from serious complications. [The *SCI*® indicates that this paper has been cited over 125 times since 1973.]

Lars-Erik Almgård
Department of Urology
Södersjukhuset
100 64 Stockholm
Sweden

February 3, 1982

"Renal adenocarcinoma is in many ways a peculiar disease. For instance, spontaneous regression has been reported after nephrectomy. This has been the main reason why nephrectomy is performed even in cases of metastases. The situation may also be complicated by troublesome bleeding in the urinary tract. Once I had to face a similar situation. Due to troublesome bleeding, ligation of the renal artery was recommended. From a technical point of view the operation was not at all easy. This was due to invasion of tumour tissue around the artery. Afterward, I thought that there must be some other way to stop the circulation in the kidney.

"Experience with renal transplantation and vascular studies of the kidney had taught me that the kidney has end arteries. Two reports[1,2] using muscular tissue in the treatment of arteriovenous malformations in the cerebral region influenced me to use muscular tissue to stop the renal circulation.

"Experiments on dogs and angiographic studies confirmed that small pieces of muscular tissues injected into the artery could cause an embolization. Sephadex and Spongostan were also tested for the embolization.

"After one and a half years of experiments on dogs, the first clinical case was performed. The results of the clinical trials were good and the preliminary report was presented at the French Urological Society in Paris in 1971.

"The preliminary report and the article in the *British Journal of Urology* seemed to have initiated continuous work in the field of embolization.[3,4] The technique is now used in several fields of medicine, mainly in connection with oncology. In a follow-up study on embolization, I presented the idea of combining embolization with cytotoxic therapy. A method has now been presented by colleagues in Malmö; in selected cases they use temporary occlusion combined with cytotoxic drugs. During the occlusion the cytotoxic drugs are released from the tumour tissue, thereby reducing the cytotoxic effect on bone marrow and liver.

"I believe that this publication has been highly cited mainly due to the fact that embolization facilitates surgery or offers acceptable palliation in several tumour cases."

1. **Robles C & Carrasco-Zanini J.** Treatment of cerebral arteriovenous malformations by muscle embolization. *J. Neurosurgery* **29**:603-8, 1968.
2. **Sedzimir C B & Occleshaw H V.** Treatment of carotid-cavernous fistula by muscle embolization and Jaeger's maneuver. *J. Neurosurgery* **27**:309-14, 1967.
3. **White R I.** Arterial embolization for control of renal haemorrhage. *J. Urology* **115**:121-2, 1976.
4. **Buzelin J M, Bourdon J, Mitard D, Buzelin F & Auvigne J.** L'embolisation de l'artère rénale. Étude expérimentale. Application au traitement des cancers du rein. *J. Urol. Nephrol.* **80**:541-53, 1974.

CC/NUMBER 35
AUGUST 31, 1981

This Week's Citation Classic

Gray L H, Conger A D, Ebert M, Hornsey S & Scott O C A. The concentration of oxygen dissolved in tissues at the time of irradiation as a factor in radiotherapy. *Brit. J. Radiol.* **26**:638-48, 1953.
[Radiotherapeutic Research Unit, Hammersmith Hospital, London, England]

The relationship between oxygen tension and radiosensitivity was measured, using mouse and chick cells. It was shown that oxygen might sensitize a tumour to X rays, more than the normal tissues. Oxygen had less effect on the response of cells to neutrons. [The ***SCI*®** **indicates that this paper has been cited over 240 times since 1961.]**

O.C.A. Scott
Radiotherapy Research Unit
Institute of Cancer Research
Royal Cancer Hospital
Sutton, Surrey SM2 5PX
England

July 10, 1981

"It is sad that Hal Gray is no longer with us to write his recollections of 'Gray *et al.*' His vivid personality, tremendous enthusiasm tempered by caution and humility, and his unqualified love of scientific work made the period when these investigations were carried out the most memorable in the working life of the surviving authors.

"There are some things which Gray would not have included; notably, any reference to his own modesty. He refused to be the first author, until a 'mutiny in the ship's company' forced him to put his name at the head of the list. This paper has not always been quoted correctly, and we might mention that we did not 'discover the oxygen effect,' nor were we the first to suggest the importance of oxygen in radiotherapy. We may have been the first to suggest the use of oxygen to improve the therapeutic index in radiation treatment, and this may account for the paper's frequent citation.

"The work was commenced in the autumn of 1952, to fill in gaps in existing knowledge, and was published in December 1953. Alan Conger was asked to establish the relationship between oxygen concentration and radiosensitivity for a *mammalian* cell, which he did in record time. I showed that an allogeneic tumour could be sensitized to X rays by oxygen, without obvious increase in skin reaction. An unexpected finding was the importance of tumour size. Shirley Hornsey counted degenerating cells in culture (this was the pre-Puck era!) but her data still look good. Michael Ebert's contribution from pure radiation chemistry was an example of the fruitful collaboration between chemists and biologists, which has been a feature of radiation research.

"The recent reports of randomized clinical trials with hyperbaric oxygen, which had their origin in this work, are encouraging.[1]

"Gray's outstanding ability to put together information from different sources, and build it into a logically coherent structure, provided the driving force for the team. And driving force was necessary! Our working conditions were primitive; mice, scientists, and equipment were crammed together in one small room.

"The consequences of this paper are still in evidence, not only in relation to oxygen, but also the development of hypoxic sensitizers and neutron therapy."[2]

1. **Henk J M & Smith C W.** Radiotherapy and hyperbaric oxygen in head and neck cancer. *Lancet* **2**:104-5, 1977.
2. **Adams G E.** Hypoxic cell sensitizers for radiotherapy. (Becker F F, ed.) *Cancer: a comprehensive treatise.* New York: Plenum Press, 1975. p. 181-223.

Chapter 5 Hematology

Of the 16 Citation Classics in this chapter, all but two are related to blood clotting. The exceptions pertain to hemolytic anemia and cell growth *in vitro.*

Platelets, the key cellular element in blood coagulation, serve as the focus for the first five Classics. Manual-visual counting of platelets by phase microscopic examination (p. 147) of blood that had been freed of erythrocytes by ammonium oxalate lysis is still useful unless the volume of these determinations demands an automated procedure (p. 148). The authors of these two Classics take a casual approach to their popularity. Brecher believes Citation Classic status can be achieved if one labors on a disease that has a high incidence, and Bull, in referring to the toxicity of certain chemotherapeutics, states that POMP no longer applies to administrators or MOPP to housekeepers. These acronyms refer to nitrogen *m*ustard, *O*movin[R] (vincristin), *P*rednisone, and *P*rocarbazine. Brecher and his co-authors had their report initially rejected before its publication in a second journal.

Mitchell's first sentence is better constructed than his basement laboratory that flooded when the Thames ran high. With Sharp as a co-investigator, Mitchell was able to identify that serotonin (5 hydroxytryptamine), a natural product of platelets, could aggregate platelets. ADP is another platelet autoagglutinin. These molecules explain the autocatalytic nature of platelet aggregation which continues after an initial activation from an external stimulus such as collagen.

O'Brien's paper on the toxicity of salicylates (aspirin) was one of the first to indicate that these compounds interfere with blood clotting by inhibiting normal platelet functions. As his own experimental subject, he found that aspirin in continued high doses caused a tinnitus that remained for 6 weeks after stopping the drug. Mielke's study of bleeding time as a measure of platelet function explains why biologists should do biology and not carpentry or metalwork. Cut fingers, failing templates, and unborable corks are three of the frustrations that can be avoided if this advice is followed.

Noncellular elements that participate in blood coagulation are numerous.

Variations in their name or designation have left this a confusing world for all but the coagulation hematologists. The next three "This Week's Citation Classic" (TWCC) commentaries discuss studies with Factor VIII (one labeled VIII:C) and its assay in hemophiliacs. The most common deficiency in the blood clotting cascade is that of factor VIII. The newly developed (1953) partial thromboplastin time was carefully evaluated in a 3-year in-house experience before publication (p. 152). Hardisty believes his article on factor VIII assay was more popular than an almost identical method published by a second group of investigators because of his careful statistical interpretation of the data. Platelet adhesiveness, a defect in von Willebrand's disease (Factor VIII deficiency) was first measured by determining the extent of platelet adherence to a column of glass beads (p. 154). Commercial blood collecting tubes were easily modified to include this feature so that the blood passed through a chamber filled with glass beads before entering the collecting vessel itself.

The commonly used abbreviation DIC for disseminated intravascular coagulation is used only once in the two TWCCs that highlight this phenomenon. The first description by Verstraete ascribes one cause of bleeding to a loss of blood coagulation components by virtue of DIC. Verstraete provides a scholarly commentary that makes very pleasant reading. The paper by Merskey et al. fit nicely into a Festschrift for MacFarlane, an acknowledged world leader in coagulation, whose name, surprisingly, does not appear on any of the TWCCs though he is mentioned in two of them.

Progressing from platelets through coagulation to embolism is a logical sequence, and the last of these is the topic of the next two TWCCs. The first was written by Negus, who is flattered "to find himself among scientists" by virtue of his co-authorship of an article on the deposition of ^{125}I-labeled fibrinogen in 93 patients with deep vessel thrombi or phlebitis. The location of the isotopic iodine identified the site and dimensions of the thrombus. The Citation Classic on the trapping of aggregated albumin in emboli was based on a similar methodologic approach since a radioisotopically labeled molecule was used.

Todd's two-page Citation Classic is a masterful example of how the location of a nondiffusible tissue substance could be determined by applying a little ingenuity. In his case, fibrinolytic activity was detected by imprinting the tissue onto a fibrin plate and then noting the areas of fibrin loss in comparison with tissue cytology. Bacterial fibrinolysin (streptokinase) is useful for clot dissolution in postoperative patients (p. 160) provided its proteolytic action on coagulation factors is blocked or reduced by the addition of amino caproic acid.

Genetic defects of carbohydrate metabolism are the subjects of the next two Classics. The first, on hemolytic anemia in patients with a genetic deficiency of the enzyme glucose-6-phosphate dehydrogenase, has as its biochemical explanation the need for hydrogen protons supplied by this enzyme for the maintenance of glutathione in the reduced state. Reduced glutathione is necessary for red cell membrane integrity. This research project was begun in a washroom but later moved to a laboratory with $50 worth of cabinets and workbenches! Pyruvate kinase deficiency and hemolytic anemia, though of no interest to *Science,* clearly was of interest to *Blood,* which published this Classic. Pyruvate kinase is essential to the red cell as a supplier of ATP, which, when lacking, discoordinates the ATPase ion pump, causing the red cells to swell and then rupture.

As a young postdoctoral fellow, Swift published with Hirschhorn their discovery of excessive, unrepaired chromosome breaks in persons with Fanconi's anemia. This places Fanconi's anemia with ataxia telangiectasia and xeroderma pigmentosum in which an increased sensitivity to X-ray or ultraviolet light exists. All three of these diseases are associated with an increased incidence of cancer, and this was the thrust of Swift's research idea—the association of Fanconi's anemia and cancer, rather than its etiology in unrepaired chromosome breaks.

Fracturing or distortion or erythrocytes as they pass through partially closed or abnormal blood vessels, an often ignored physical cause of anemia, and the determination of blood cell growth *in vitro* by the incorporation of tritiated thymidine are the subject of the last two Classics in this chapter.

A rich supply of source journals is available to anyone interested in the current status of hematology. The most useful of these review journals are *Clinics in Haematology* and *Seminars in Hematology.* Volume 14 of the former, published in 1985, has one issue (no. 2) entirely devoted to coagulative disorders. Three issues of the latter journal (vol. 22, 1985) contained 200 pages of review material on platelets and megakaryocytes. The following seven articles are illustrative of the coverage included in these issues.

Colvin B T. Thrombocytopenia. *Clin. Haematol.* **14:**661–81, 1985.

DeSweit M. Thromboembolism. *Clin. Haematol.* **14:**643–60, 1985.

Fass D N & Toole J J. Genetic engineering and coagulation factors. *Clin. Haematol.* **14:**547–70, 1985.

Holmberg L & Nilsson I M. von Willebrand disease. *Clin. Haematol.* **14:**461–88, 1985.

Prentice C R M. Acquired coagulation disorders. *Clin. Haematol.* **14:**411–42, 1985.

Schmaier A H. Platelet forms of platelet proteins: plasma cofactors/substrates and inhibitors contained within platelets. *Semin. Hematol.* **22:**187–202, 1985.

Walsh P N. Platelet-mediated coagulant protein interactions in hemostasis. *Semin. Hematol.* **22:**178–86, 1985.

Numerous other sources of information exist for hematologists. A few of these are *CRC Critical Reviews in Clinical Laboratory Science, CRC Critical*

Reviews in Oncology/Hematology, Advances in Internal Medicine, Annual Review of Medicine, Progress in Fibrinolysis, Progress in Haematology, and *Progress in Hemostasis and Thrombosis.* The following are recent reviews from some of these sources that apply to the subjects of this chapter.

Jackson C M. Factor X. *Prog. Hemostas. Thrombos.* **7**:55–110, 1984.

Thomas P D. Venous thrombogenesis. *Annu. Rev. Med.* **36**:39–50, 1985.

Thompson E I, Callihan T R & Mauer A M. Prophylaxis in severe granulocytopenia. *Adv. Intern. Med.* **29**:193–214, 1984.

Tiffany M L. Technical considerations for platelet aggregation and related problems. *CRC Crit. Rev. Clin. Lab. Sci.* **19**:27–69, 1983.

Whittemore A D, Couch N P & Mannick J A. Treatment of arterial occlusive disease of the lower extremities. *Annu. Rev. Med.* **36**:505–14, 1985.

This Week's Citation Classic

NUMBER 1
JANUARY 1, 1979

Brecher G, Schneiderman M & Cronkite E P. The reproducibility and constancy of the platelet count. *Amer. J. Clin. Pathol.* **23**:15-26, 1953.

In blood diluted with 1% ammonium oxalate, platelets become easily recognizable by phase microscopy. The "phase" method, based on the unequivocal identification of platelets, is highly reproducible and reflects the platelet level in the circulation. [The *SCI®* indicates that this paper was cited 282 times in the period 1961-1977.]

George Brecher
Department of Laboratory Medicine
University of California
School of Medicine
San Francisco, California 94143

February 8, 1978

"The invention of the phase microscope by Zernicke enormously facilitated the examination of living cells by revealing cellular details without stains. In 1949, during explorations of the new tool, I noticed that platelets which are smooth, round discs in the circulation sent out filamentous projection *in vitro,* depending somewhat on the anticoagulant. With ammonium oxalate, the platelets appeared as dense black bodies easily distinguished from artifacts by their characteristic processes. Red cells were hemolyzed and became invisible, so they no longer interfered with counting platelets.

"The counting methods available in 1953 gave results that differed as much as twofold. We demonstrated that the entire variability of the platelet count with the new 'phase' method was accounted for by the statistical errors of counting cells in a counting chamber. We argued that the method must, therefore, reflect the actual number of platelets in the sample because any bias would give an additional error. The argument was unconvincing to the editors of the *Journal of Laboratory and Clinical Medicine* who pointed to the many methods, some published in the *Journal of Laboratory and Clinical Medicine,* that had failed to provide reliable platelet counts. While it is pleasing that time proved our claim valid, the fact that 'phase' is still the reference method is regrettable. Our method has two drawbacks: The occasional clumping of platelets may vitiate the results and the method cannot be readily automated.

"To find oneself having written a 'Citation Classic' is pleasing to the ego. It is a sobering thought that a method paper may win these sweepstakes solely because of the frequency of the disease in which a particular measurement is useful. Thus, the frequency of citation of the phase method reflects the utility of accurate platelet counts. They are needed to quantify success of platelet transfusion and to discover mild degrees of bone marrow depression or excess platelet destruction. The physiologic message of the paper is seldom cited: platelet counts are constant for long periods in healthy individuals, but vary widely between them. The normal range is 150,000 to 450,000 platelets / mm^3. A drop from 200,000 to 100,000 is known to be medically significant. May a drop from 300,000 to 200,000 have any value in predicting impending disease, given the normal constancy of platelet levels? Generally speaking, is it valuable to know an individual's 'own' level which is much narrower for many serum constituents than the 'range of normal'?[1] These puzzling questions are still unanswered."

1. **Williams G Z.** Clinical pathology tomorrow. *Amer. J. Clin. Pathol.* **32**:121, 1962.

This Week's Citation Classic

CC/NUMBER 41
OCTOBER 13, 1980

Bull B S, Schneiderman M A & Brecher G. Platelet counts with the Coulter counter. *Amer. J. Clin. Pathol.* **44**:678-88, 1965.
[Clin. Pathol. Dept., Clin. Center and Biometry Br., Nat. Cancer Inst., Nat. Inst. Health, US Pub. Health Serv., Bethesda, MD]

A method for the machine counting of platelets in human blood is described utilizing small samples of platelet-rich plasma. The method includes correction factors by which the resultant count determined on platelet-rich plasma can be transformed into a whole blood platelet count. [The *SCI*® indicates that this paper has been cited over 300 times since 1965.]

Brian S. Bull
Department of Pathology and
Laboratory Medicine
Loma Linda University Medical Center
Loma Linda, CA 92354

July 14, 1980

"In the early 1960s at the Clinical Center of the National Institutes of Health, the concept of combination chemotherapy for leukemias and solid tumors was taking shape. POMP no longer applied only to the administrative offices nor MOPP exclusively to housekeeping! The result was a very large increase in the platelet count work load of the Clinical Center Hematology Laboratory.

"At that time, the best available method for the counting of platelets was the phase microscope technique described by the then chief of the hematology laboratory, George Brecher.[1] (The original description of this method is also a *Citation Classic.*) The accuracy of the phase count procedure was excellent, but the method was highly labor intensive. As each new chemotherapy protocol was instituted, the number of platelet counts increased in stepwise fashion, until the laboratory's future appeared to be that of a platelet counting organization that occasionally performed a few other hematologic procedures! The major problem, however, stemmed from the fact that platelet counting is an extremely tedious task and the hematology technologists, unenthusiastic at the prospect of spending ever more time counting platelets, were threatening to resign *en masse.*

"The obvious solution was to automate the procedure. Red cell counts had been successfully automated in the same laboratory only a few years before. This had occurred subsequent to a visit by Wallace Coulter, with one of the first Coulter Counters® under his arm. Despite the best efforts of the laboratory staff, however, that early Model A Coulter Counter could not reliably distinguish platelets from background noise.

"I began my career in hematology almost simultaneously with the arrival in the laboratory of a new cell counter (Model B) and was immediately assigned the task of getting it to count platelets. The task proved surprisingly easy, since the preamplifier section was now sufficiently improved so that platelet pulses could be reliably distinguished from background electronic noise. The required calculations were worked out on the back of an envelope. Only a few minor problems in diluent formulation and hematocrit correction had to be solved as the method went into routine use.

"The paper has undoubtedly been widely cited because it was a methods paper and because the method described has been widely used during the past 15 years. It has served the medical and scientific community well during this time, rendering rapid and reproducible platelet counts with a minimum of technologist involvement. The method's shortcomings have related first to the requirement of platelet-rich plasma as the starting point, and secondly to the consequent need to mathematically retransform the plasma platelet counts back into whole blood counts to render them meaningful to the practicing clinician. Both problem areas have been neatly circumvented in the very recent past by the introduction of a variety of whole blood platelet counters. Whole blood platelet counting is now the method of choice."

1. **Brecher G & Cronkite E P.** Morphology and enumeration of human blood platelets. *J. Appl. Physiol.* **3**:365-77, 1950.

This Week's Citation Classic

Mitchell J R A & Sharp A A. Platelet clumping *in vitro*.
Brit. J. Haematol. **10**:78-93, 1964.
[Departments of the Regius Professor of Medicine and Haematology,
Radcliffe Infirmary, Oxford, England]

The ability of 5HT and the adrenalines to aggregate platelets was described and the dependence of aggregation on movement and collision emphasized. The reversibility of aggregation and its relationship to calcium and magnesium ions, and therefore to the anticoagulant used, was shown, as was the affinity of polymorphs for growing platelet aggregates. Finally, the value of enzyme poisons and receptor blockers as tools in platelet research was outlined. [The *SCI*® indicates that this paper has been cited in over 295 publications since 1964.]

J.R.A. Mitchell
Department of Medicine
University Hospital
Queen's Medical Centre
Nottingham NG7 2UH
England

August 18, 1982

"An occupational disease of authors is a morbid fear that their imperishable words will never be read, so it is pleasant to find that our 1964 paper has been widely cited. It represented the second step in the recognition that some simple and universally distributed chemical substances, unrelated to blood-clotting factors, could activate platelets. The first step was the revelation by Hellem and his Oslo colleagues that ADP was an aggregating agent.[1] We asked ourselves whether the presence of large amounts of ADP in platelets provided a self-amplifying system whereby aggregation would release more ADP which would then promote further aggregation. We decided to see whether other materials stored within platelets could do the same trick and in January 1962 found that 5HT and the adrenalines were active platelet aggregating agents.

"One of our colleagues at that time was editor of the *British Journal of Haematology* so we were urged to publish our findings therein. To our dismay, we found that although we had been presenting our work at meetings, a backlog of papers meant that ours would not appear until 1964. This prevented workers who were using 5HT and the adrenalines from referring to our work. At that time we were working in the haematology department of the Radcliffe Infirmary, Oxford, with that most imaginative and creative scientist, Gwyn Macfarlane. He had come back from a Vienna congress with the news about ADP so his was the match that lit the fuse. Alan Sharp was a member of his staff, and had previously worked on platelet aggregation in response to thrombin. I was a cardiovascular physician who had been seconded from Sir George Pickering's department to undertake a massive postmortem study of vascular disease with Colin Schwartz.[2] This had shown the key role of thrombosis in stroke and heart attack, so I had moved on to work on thrombosis with Macfarlane. We worked in a basement at the Radcliffe Infirmary (which regularly flooded when the River Thames rose) with our assistants, Sheila Briers and Margaret Eggleton.

"Our work has been widely cited because, as well as the identification of 5HT and the adrenalines, it showed that aggregation was a reversible process, that the agents did not pull platelets together, but allowed them to adhere when movement produced collision, and that polymorphs adhered to platelet clumps. We also documented the crucial role of calcium and magnesium ions and of the anticoagulant chosen for studies. We did not understand the nature of the forces which produced aggregation nor how these forces could be negated to allow disaggregation. I still cannot answer these questions and I know that no one else can either. This is why, when I moved to my present position as Foundation Professor of Medicine in the new University of Nottingham Medical School in 1968, I built up an active platelet/thrombosis team headed by Stan Heptinstall, and we are still trying to answer the same questions."[3,4]

1. **Gaarder A, Jonsen J, Laland S, Hellem A J & Owren P A.** Adenosine diphosphate in red cells as a factor in the adhesiveness of human blood platelets. *Nature* **192**:531-2, 1961.
2. **Mitchell J R A & Schwartz C J.** *Arterial disease*. Oxford: Blackwell Scientific, 1965. 411 p.
3. **White A M & Heptinstall S.** Contribution of platelets to thrombus formation. *Brit. Med. Bull.* **34**:123-8, 1978.
4. **Mitchell J R A.** Prostaglandins in vascular disease; a seminal approach. *Brit. Med. J.* **282**:590-4, 1981.

CC/NUMBER 51
DECEMBER 22, 1980

This Week's Citation Classic

O'Brien J R. Effects of salicylates on human platelets. *Lancet* **1**:779-83, 1968.
[Portsmouth and Isle of Wight Area Path. Serv., Portsmouth, Hampshire, England]

When studying the aggregation of platelets, I found that the ingestion of aspirin produced an abnormal response which was dose related and lasted for days. I concluded that aspirin, possibly permanently, damages a platelet mechanism probably related to release of ADP. [The *SCI*® indicates that this paper has been cited over 375 times since 1968.]

J. R. O'Brien
Hampshire District Pathology Service
Saint Mary's Hospital
Portsmouth PO3 6AG
England

November 13, 1980

"As usual I was not really first in the field. There are few real beginnings in science. It usually grows and evolves in an appropriate climate. Mustard[1] had studied anti-inflammatory drugs in animals and Marjorie Zucker[2] had studied a normal volunteer who always had headaches and abnormal platelet responses and was a constant aspirin eater. Also, Weiss[3] had already reported some aspirin effects. The aggregometer principle applied to platelets by Born[4] and myself[5] simultaneously gave a tremendous stimulus to platelet 'phenomenology' and the aspirin effect on platelet aggregation was an early and important one. Aggregation phenomena were so exciting that I almost believe it delayed other studies of platelets *in vivo* and the search for more meaningful tests. Indeed aggregation studies still are of limited clinical application.

"Aspirin had always fascinated me. The drug has so many different effects—anti-inflammatory, analgesic, influencing red cell membranes, etc. There had to be some common factor. And now in 1968, aspirin was found to influence platelets as well and in a dose far smaller than that influencing any other identified physiological system. And aspirin was known to prolong the bleeding time. Being no chemist, I could not contribute to the unravelling of the prostaglandin story. But this paper may have helped others.

"In this paper I do not specifically discuss 'aspirin labelling' as a method of measuring the rate of platelet regeneration, but I did suggest that megakaryocytes were also damaged. Thus to an extent, the 'platelet regeneration time' (now usually monitored by the reappearance of malondialdehyde production, a biproduct of prostaglandin synthesis) may be said to have in part been initiated by this paper; however, the megakaryocyte labelling, if it occurs, is still at least a theoretical objection to this method.

"In 1963, I published a paper entitled, 'An *in vivo* trial of an anti-adhesive drug'[6] which I think was the first paper with the acknowledged aim of developing an anti-platelet drug to prevent thrombosis. So in 1968 when aspirin was known to prolong the bleeding time and to influence platelets, it was only reasonable to speculate that it might prevent thrombosis by virtue of its 'anti-platelet' activity. This was a far cry from the current complexity of platelet cyclo-oxygenase inhibition and the additional effect on vessel wall prostacyclin synthesis which may or may not be relevant to any anti-thrombotic effect which finally emerges. Nevertheless this paper contributed to the concept that anti-platelet drugs might be used to prevent thromboses.

"I am a full-time haematologist and did not carry out manually any of these experiments; S. Shoobridge, W. J. Finch, and J. Dore did all the work, but I ate much of the aspirin and salicylates—once until I got tinnitus which to my alarm continued for six weeks after stopping the drug!

"It was an exciting, happy time with new and usually quite unexplained phenomena occurring every few months. Was this the golden age for platelets? Or is this selective gilded memory looking back 12 years?"

1. **Packham M A, Warrior E S, Glynn M F, Senyi A S & Mustard J F.** Alternation of the response of platelets to surface stimuli by pyrazole compounds. *J. Exp. Med.* **126**:171-88, 1967.
2. **Zucker M B & Peterson J.** Inhibition of adenosine diphosphate-induced secondary aggregation and other platelet functions by acetylsalicylic acid ingestion. *Proc. Soc. Exp. Biol. Med.* **127**:547-51, 1968.
3. **Weiss H J & Aledort L M.** Impaired platelets/connected-tissue reaction in man after aspirin ingestion. *Lancet* **2**:495-7, 1967.
4. **Born G R V.** Aggregation of blood platelets by adenosine diphosphate and its reversal. *Nature* **194**:927-9, 1962.
5. **O'Brien J R.** Some results from a new method of study. Part II. *J. Clin. Pathol.* **15**:452-5, 1962.
6. ----------------. An *in vivo* trial of an anti-adhesive drug. *Thromb. Diath. Haemorrh.* **9**:120-5, 1963.

CC/NUMBER 6
FEBRUARY 7, 1983

This Week's Citation Classic

Mielke C H, Jr., Kaneshiro M M, Maher I A, Weiner J M & Rapaport S I. The standardized normal Ivy bleeding time and its prolongation by aspirin. *Blood* **34**:204-15, 1969. [Department of Medicine, University of Southern California School of Medicine, Los Angeles, CA]

Primary hemostasis is achieved through interaction of platelets with the vessel wall. Clinically, this can be monitored by the bleeding time, which is an *in vivo* measurement of platelet function. This paper describes a standardized technique to measure the bleeding time and its prolongation by aspirin. [The *SCI*® indicates that this paper has been cited in over 410 publications since 1969.]

C. Harold Mielke, Jr.
Medical Research Institute of San Francisco
at Pacific Medical Center
San Francisco, CA 94115

December 15, 1982

"The bleeding time is an important clinical test which is used to identify patients who are at risk for bleeding. The concept was introduced in 1910[1] and underwent several modifications over the ensuing decades.[2] However, despite these changes, the test lacked sensitivity and was poorly reproducible. In fact, many physicians stopped using the test.

"My interest in the bleeding time began in 1968 when I was a clinical fellow in hematology at the University of Southern California in Los Angeles. A patient on the surgery service had a bleeding disorder which was suspected to be secondary to a qualitative platelet dysfunction. The house staff, clinical laboratory, and surgical and hematology residents had all performed bleeding times with conflicting results. Because of my position, I was asked to unravel the mystery and make a decision concerning whether or not this patient could go to surgery. I performed the bleeding time and, to my surprise and puzzlement, failed to clarify the hematologic picture for this patient. I was rather disturbed, and that evening I reconstructed the events of the day regarding this case. Several facts emerged. First, everyone had his own variation of the bleeding time technique. They used a wide variety of punctures or incisions and performed them on different sites. Secondly, there was no control of the length or depth of the measurements. Third, everyone was trying to equate these diverse measurements to the platelets' interaction with the vessel wall. I felt that if I could control these variables and develop a standardized methodology, it would be possible to improve the precision and reliability of the bleeding time so that useful clinical information could be obtained.

"Control of the length and depth of the incision appeared to be the most important. I tried to push a #11 Bard Parker blade through a sterile cork to control the depth. This was very difficult and I cut my finger in the process. The idea of a template was developed to control the length. A heavy cardboard template was created with a center slit. Working with Melvin Kaneshiro, we launched an uncontrolled clinical trial. A reproducible incision could be made, but the trial was short-lived because we couldn't get the blades through the corks in a reproducible fashion and the cardboard template couldn't hold the force of the blade. Thus, the length of the incision was again variable.

"The idea would have died then had it not been for polystyrene. I went to the university's machine shop and they agreed to make the polystyrene blade handle and template according to my design, as well as to mill a metal gauge so that uniform control of blade depth could be achieved. We were then able to complete a clinical study to standardize the technique and at the same time to evaluate the influence of aspirin on primary hemostasis.[3]

"I believe the major reason this work has been cited so often is that it allowed the clinician a sensitive and reproducible technique to measure primary hemostasis.[4] Today the platelet is being intensively studied for its role in thrombosis and hemorrhagic diseases."

1. **Duke W W.** The relation of blood platelets to hemorrhagic disease. *J. Amer. Med. Assn.* **55**:1185-92, 1910.
2. **Ivy A C, Nelson D & Bucher G.** The standardization of certain factors in the cutaneous "venostasis" bleeding time technique. *J. Lab. Clin. Med.* **26**:1812-22, 1941.
3. **Kaneshiro M M, Mielke C H, Jr., Kasper C K & Rapaport S I.** The bleeding time after aspirin in disorders of intrinsic clotting. *N. Engl. J. Med.* **281**:1039-42, 1969.
4. **Mielke C H, Jr. & Rodvien R.** Bleeding time procedures. (Seligson D & Schmidt R M, eds.) *Clinical laboratory science, section I: hematology*. Boca Raton, FL: CRC Press, 1979. Vol. 1. p. 369-80.

This Week's Citation Classic™

CC/NUMBER 41
OCTOBER 8, 1984

Langdell R D, Wagner R H & Brinkhous K M. Effect of antihemophilic factor on one-stage clotting tests. *J. Lab. Clin. Med.* **41**:637-47, 1953.
[Department of Pathology, School of Medicine, University of North Carolina, Chapel Hill, NC]

This article describes a laboratory procedure that has been applied as a screening test for a number of hemostatic disorders and is the basis for the assay of what at the time was called the antihemophilic factor (AHF) and is now known as factor VIII:C. The principle of the bioassay has been the basis for the measurement of several other plasma coagulation factors. [The *SCI*® indicates that this paper has been cited in over 655 publications since 1955.]

Robert D. Langdell
Department of Pathology
School of Medicine
University of North Carolina
Chapel Hill, NC 27514

May 30, 1984

"At the time these studies were done, much of the research activity in the Department of Pathology at the University of North Carolina centered on a bleeding disorder that arose apparently as a mutation in a group of inbred dogs. Genetic, clinical, and coagulation studies indicated that the disorder was very similar to human hemophilia.[1] As in humans, transfusion of normal plasma corrected the clotting defect and controlled the hemorrhagic phenomena. We attributed this effect to the antihemophilic factor (AHF) that could be fractionated along with fibrinogen from normal plasma. Efforts to characterize the trace protein were impeded by the methodology for measuring AHF based on the utilization of prothrombin in clotting hemophilic blood. To simplify the measurement of AHF, we utilized an observation that in one-stage clotting tests, some extracts of normal or hemophilic tissue could compensate for the factor missing in hemophilia (complete thromboplastin), while others, such as natural or synthetic cephalins, could not (partial thromboplastin).

"The partial thromboplastin time, a new procedure based on these observations, was used in our laboratory for over three years before the article was submitted for publication. This was in part due to observations indicating that the method was sensitive to coagulation factors other than the plasma factor deficient in hemophilia, reports that other hemorrhagic states could easily be confused with hemophilia, and studies that were in progress indicating that there were mild forms of human hemophilia.[2] It was ultimately determined that the corrective effect of a test sample on canine or human hemophilic plasma used as a substrate was dependent on what is now known as factor VIII:C.

"The partial thromboplastin time is now widely used in clinical laboratories as a screening test not only for hemophilia but also for coagulation factors that were unrecognized at the time the procedure was published.[3] Although the bioassay method was developed for measuring factor VIII:C, by using plasma deficient in any one of several other clotting factors as a substrate, it is used as an assay method for other coagulation factors. The original method has been modified by a number of investigators, and reagents are now available commercially. In view of the tendency of authors to cite their own work, it is surprising that the original publication has been cited frequently.

"It is of interest that our efforts to characterize the coagulation defect in hemophilia have general applicability and have contributed to the recognition of other clotting factors and to the recently announced production of factor VIII:C through genetic splicing techniques."

1. **Graham J B, Buckwalter J A, Hartley L J & Brinkhous K M.** Canine hemophilia: observations on the course, the clotting anomaly, and the effect of blood transfusions. *J. Exp. Med.* **90**:97-111, 1949. (Cited 75 times since 1955.)
2. **Brinkhous K M, Langdell R D, Penick G D, Graham J B & Wagner R H.** Newer approaches to the study of hemophilia and hemophilioid states. *J. Amer. Med. Assn.* **154**:481-6, 1954. (Cited 90 times since 1955.)
3. **Brinkhous K M & Dombrose F A.** Partial thromboplastin time. (Schmidt R M, ed.) *CRC handbook series in clinical laboratory science. Section I: hematology.* Boca Raton, FL: CRC Press, 1980. Vol. 3. p. 221-46.

CC/NUMBER 18
MAY 4, 1981

This Week's Citation Classic

Hardisty R M & Macpherson J C. A one-stage factor VIII (antihaemophilic globulin) assay and its use on venous and capillary plasma. With a note on the calculation of confidence limits by G.I.C. Ingram.
Thromb. Diath. Haemorrhag. 7:215-29, 1962.
[Department of Haematology, Hospital for Sick Children, London, England]

The paper describes a one-stage method for the assay of factor VIII, in which contact activation is controlled by the addition of kaolin to the system. Normal range, confidence limits, and correlation with the results of a two-stage method are given. [The *SCI*® indicates that this paper has been cited over 280 times since 1962.]

R.M. Hardisty
Department of Haematology
Hospital for Sick Children
London WC1N 3JH
England

April 13, 1981

"There is nothing particularly revolutionary, or even original, about this paper. It is simply a detailed description of a method which has subsequently been widely adopted in a rapidly developing field, and has evidently stood the test of time—a contribution to technology rather than a major conceptual development. No doubt most of the citations appear in the methods section of subsequent papers: a prosaic, if honourable, way to 'classical' status.

"In the late 1950s, factor VIII (the antihaemophilic factor in plasma) was usually assayed either by two-stage methods based on the thromboplastin generation test or by one-stage methods based on the partial thromboplastin time. The latter methods, though simpler to perform, were in general less accurate and reproducible than the former. Margolis had already shown that the chief source of variability in such methods was the nature and amount of surface to which the plasma was exposed, and had devised a simple screening test for blood coagulation defects in which these were controlled by the addition of a standard amount of kaolin suspension to the test system.[1]

"The first step in the activation of the blood coagulation mechanism by such foreign surfaces had been shown to concern the Hageman factor (now called factor XII). It is therefore perhaps not surprising that the first people to adapt Margolis's test as a specific assay method should be Oscar Ratnoff (who first described Hageman and his clotting defect) and myself (who discovered the first British case of Hageman trait, and had worked with Margolis on the role of the Hageman factor in blood coagulation). Breckenridge and Ratnoff, in fact, independently arrived at a factor-VIII assay method which was almost identical to ours in every detail, and published it three months later.[2]

"Why, then, should our paper have been the one to become a *Citation Classic*? Ratnoff was kind enough to concede that our job was more thorough than theirs, thanks largely to the careful statistical evaluation carried out on our data by Ilsley Ingram. Another probable reason is that Breckenridge and Ratnoff buried their method in a paper about factor-VIII inhibitors, while the description and evaluation of the technique was the chief *raison d'être* of our paper."

1. **Margolis J.** The kaolin clotting time. A rapid one-stage method for diagnosis of coagulation defects. *J. Clin. Pathol.* **11**:406-9, 1958.
2. **Breckenridge R T & Ratnoff O D.** Studies on the nature of the circulating anticoagulant directed against antihaemophilic factor: with notes on an assay for antihaemophilic factor. *Blood* **20**:137-49, 1962.

CC/NUMBER 20
MAY 17, 1982

This Week's Citation Classic

Salzman E W. Measurement of platelet adhesiveness: a simple in vitro technique demonstrating an abnormality in von Willebrand's disease.
J. Lab. Clin. Med. **62**:724-35, 1963.
[Dept. Surg., Harvard Med. Sch., and Surg. Serv., Mass. Gen. Hosp., Boston, MA]

Passage of whole blood through a column of glass beads affords a simple measure of platelet adhesiveness, which is normal in disorders of blood coagulation and in patients receiving heparin but is deficient in thrombasthenia and in von Willebrand's disease. [The *SCI*® indicates that this paper has been cited over 590 times since 1963.]

Edwin W. Salzman
Department of Surgery
Beth Israel Hospital
Harvard Medical School
Boston, MA 02215

February 3, 1982

"Spurred by the key observation of Gaarder and associates[1] that adenosine diphosphate (ADP) was a powerful stimulus to platelet aggregation, laboratories began in the early-1960s to show increasing interest in the sticking of platelets to natural and artificial surfaces and to each other and in the importance of abnormal platelet function in bleeding and thrombosis.

"Techniques suitable for the study of these phenomena were badly needed. Hellem had described a method[2] in which anticoagulated blood was pumped slowly through a column of glass beads to measure 'platelet adhesiveness,' but the test was insensitive and did not correlate with the clinical state of patients who had hemorrhagic disorders. However, after the convenience and economy of evacuated blood collection tubes (Vacutainer®) were observed on hospital wards, it required only a simple modification of Hellem's technique to permit blood drawn by venipuncture to flow directly through a glass bead column into a Vacutainer tube containing an anticoagulant. The ratio of the platelet count in such a blood sample to that in blood without glass bead contact was for simplicity termed 'platelet adhesiveness,' although retention of platelets in the column reflected platelet aggregation as well as adhesion of platelets to the glass surfaces.

"The test proved to be a convenient bedside method for assessment of a large number and variety of patients. It was quickly found that in diseases of blood coagulation (e.g., hemophilia), retention of platelets in the column was normal, but in acquired (e.g., uremia) or inherited (e.g., Glanzmann's thrombasthenia) disorders of platelet function, the values were grossly abnormal. This also proved to be the case in von Willebrand's disease, a congenital hemorrhagic state with a long bleeding time, a low plasma level of clotting Factor VIII, and at that time a dispute about whether a vascular malformation accounted for the long bleeding time. In many respects, platelets interact with glass beads as they do with subendothelial connective tissue in hemostasis, so the test is in a sense analogous to determination of the bleeding time. Since the glass bead test was performed *ex vivo,* however, an abnormal result had to be due to defective platelet function rather than to a vascular disorder. The fault in von Willebrand's disease is now known to lie in a component of the Factor VIII molecule required for normal platelet activity.

"Though not specific, the so-called platelet adhesiveness test proved useful for screening patients with hemorrhagic disorders and a long bleeding time and also helped to identify other platelet abnormalities, e.g., during cardiopulmonary bypass. It has now given way to more specific techniques for probing the intimate details of platelet physiology.[3] In its day the test's most important contribution was probably that, by providing a simple probe of the function of blood platelets, it helped to expand the ranks of investigators attracted to the study of these interesting cellular particles."

1. **Gaarder A, Jonsen J, Laland S, Hellem A & Owren P A.** Adenosine diphosphate in red cells as a factor in the adhesiveness of human blood platelets. *Nature* **192**:531-2, 1961.
2. **Hellem A J.** The adhesiveness of human blood platelets in vitro. *Scand. J. Clin. Lab. Invest.* **12**(Suppl.):1-117, 1960.
3. **Gordon J L,** ed. *Platelets in biology and pathology.* Amsterdam: Elsevier/North-Holland, 1981. Vol. 2.

CC/NUMBER 46
NOVEMBER 14, 1983

This Week's Citation Classic

Verstraete M, Vermylen C, Vermylen J & Vandenbroucke J. Excessive consumption of blood coagulation components as cause of hemorrhagic diathesis. *Amer. J. Med.* **38**:899-908, 1965.
[Lab. Coagulation-Proteolysis, Dept. Medicine, Univ. Leuven, Belgium]

Evidence is presented that excessive consumption of certain coagulation factors may cause bleeding in the course of various diseases and unrelated syndromes, of which 12 examples are selected for discussion. The indicative value of thrombocytopenia, low fibrinogen level, and prolonged one-stage prothrombin time, mainly due to factor V depletion, is discussed. [The *SCI*® indicates that this paper has been cited in over 185 publications since 1965.]

M. Verstraete
Center for Thrombosis and
Vascular Research
Campus Gasthuisberg
University of Leuven
3000 Leuven
Belgium

August 3, 1983

"In the 1950s, I told my father, an obstetrician-gynecologist, that I deeply admired his permanent standby for unscheduled medical events but preferred to engage in haematologic research rather than succeed him. He made me promise that I should try to solve the bleeding problem associated with abruptio placentae and amniotic fluid embolism. As amniotic fluid is readily available material, I soon uncovered its thromboplastic properties and could induce fatal lung emboli or serious bleeding in dogs, depending on the perfusion rate of the phospholipid fraction of the fluid. Similar experiments with commercialized hemostatic agents, which had in common their tissue origin and clinical inefficacy, resulted in the same observation. Depending on the dose, dogs were tolerant to the infusion of this thrombin preparation, but had a gradual decrease of fibrinogen and prothrombin levels. It was therefore tempting to look for a clinical counterpart of these animal experiments. The unclottable blood of patients with abruptio placentae and those surviving amniotic fluid embolism were found to have similar characteristics as those found after thrombin or tissue thromboplastin perfusions in dogs.

"In the late 1950s and early 1960s, acquired hypofibrinogenemia was usually thought to result from proteolysis of fibrinogen by plasmin. Our concept that low fibrinogen was a consequence of its conversion by thrombin was substantiated by the corrective effect of heparin infusions in patients. This allowed the conclusion that the fibrinolytic response follows rather than causes fibrinogen depletion.

"Another reason why this article attracted attention and has been cited may be because activation or release of a coagulation promoting substance from erythrocytes, platelets, leukocytes, endothelium, complement, or from tissues was linked to intravascular coagulation and excessive consumption of hemostatic components—a common pathogenic thread in a heterogeneous group of clinical syndromes.

"Our group manifested its continued interest in the diagnosis and treatment of disseminated intravascular coagulation (DIC) by determining the survival time of radiolabeled fibrinogen, prothrombin,[1] antithrombin III, and plasminogen and by studying the effect of some drugs on the survival time of these proteins.[2,3] It was also shown by our group that complex formation of thrombin and plasmin with natural inhibitors leads to formation of neoantigens.[4,5] Specific monoclonal antibodies directed against these complexes have been produced, and clinically applicable assays are currently being developed. As the half-life of plasmin-antiplasmin and thrombin-antithrombin complexes is in the order of hours, such tests may constitute a significant improvement for the rapid and more specific detection of DIC.

"J. Vermylen and I are professors of medicine at the University of Leuven and continue in the Center for Thrombosis and Vascular Research our symbiotic scientific collaboration which has gone from strength to strength. J. Vandenbroucke retired as chairman of the department of internal medicine a few years ago; Carl Vermylen became director of the Transfusion Center of the Belgian Red Cross in Leuven, Belgium."

1. **Tytgat G N, Collen D & Verstraete M.** Metabolism of fibrinogen cirrhosis of the liver. *J. Clin. Invest.* **50**:1690-701, 1971.
2. **Verstraete M, Vermylen J & Collen D.** Intravascular coagulation in liver disease. *Annu. Rev. Med.* **25**:447-55, 1974.
3. **Collen D, Schetz J, De Cock F, Holmer E & Verstraete M.** Metabolism of antithrombin III (heparin cofactor) in man: effects of venous thrombosis and of heparin administration. *Eur. J. Clin. Invest.* 7:27-35, 1977.
4. **Collen D, De Cock F & Verstraete M.** Plasminogen turnover and plasmin-antiplasmin complex formation in clinical conditions with primary or secondary activation of the fibrinolytic system. (Paoletti R & Sherry S, eds.) *Thrombosis and urokinase*. New York: Academic Press, 1977. p. 27-41.
5. **Collen D & De Cock F.** Neoantigenic expression in enzyme-inhibitor complexes: a means to demonstrate activation of enzyme systems. *Biochim. Biophys. Acta* **525**:287-90, 1978.

This Week's Citation Classic

CC/NUMBER 31
JULY 30, 1979

Merskey C, Johnson A J, Kleiner G J & Wohl H. The defibrination syndrome: clinical features and laboratory diagnosis. *Brit J. Haematol.* **13**:528-49, 1967. [Dept. Med., Dept. Gynecol. & Obstet., and Unit for Res. in Aging, Albert Einstein Coll. Med., and Bronx Municipal Hosp.; and Dept. Med. and Amer. Nat. Red Cross Res. Lab., New York Med. Ctr., New York, NY]

This paper demonstrates that nearly all cases of defibrination syndrome are associated with evidence of intravascular coagulation. Fibrinolysis is probably a secondary phenomenon as it cannot be shown by circulating plasmin or activator in the great majority of cases. Heparin therapy is occasionally beneficial. [The *SCI®* indicates that this paper has been cited over 230 times since 1967.]

Clarence Merskey
Albert Einstein College of Medicine
Yeshiva University
Bronx, NY 10461

May 10, 1978

"In the 1950s and early 1960s hypofibrinogenemia was attributed to circulating fibrinolysis. In the 1950s in Capetown, South Africa, I remember investigating a patient with such a syndrome, with Henriette Lackner, our local fibrinolysis expert, and being very puzzled by the lack of any evidence of lytic activity. Herbert Wohl and I encountered the same situation at the Bronx Municipal Hospital Center (BMHC) in 1961. At that time we consulted with Alan Johnson of New York University who had spent many years studying fibrinolysis and had available many different tests for fibrinolytic activity, including tests for many inhibitors. Again we drew a complete blank. He and Jack Newman recommended that we treat with human fibrinogen, the approved method of therapy at that time. This was infused, but it all disappeared overnight. Meanwhile all the clotting studies we had done suggested intravascular clotting, so with much trepidation we tried an anticoagulant, heparin. To our surprise it worked, and the results of the clotting studies improved. When we stopped the heparin, to rule out coincidence, the patient deteriorated rapidly, showing symptoms suggestive of stroke. He improved when heparin therapy was resumed, convincing us that our new hypothesis was valid.

"At about this time, in John Sandson's immunology laboratory I found Joe de Vito measuring antigens with the Borden technic using formalinized, tanned red cell agglutination inhibition. I wondered whether it would work with fibrinogen as an antigen, and he thought it might. We tried it, to our joy, with success. Thus was born the tanned red cell hemagglutination inhibition immunoassay for fibrinolytic split products (TRCHII for short).

"George Kleiner and Wilma Marcus had a research laboratory in the labor ward of the BMHC, just one flight above our lab. They too were puzzled by the hypofibrinogenemia seen in obstetric patients. George visited James Pert's laboratory in Washington, DC, to learn the 'new' technic of immunoelectrophoresis. We were thus all set to study the many patients on the medical, surgical, and obstetrical services with similar disease syndromes, and the new technics at our disposal yielded positive and encouraging results.

"One day I heard from Rosemary Biggs that Gwyn MacFarlane, the doyen of the coagulation field in Great Britain, with whom I had spent an exciting two-year fellowship at the Radcliffe Infirmary, Oxford, was retiring. His colleagues were planning a *festschrift* in the *British Journal of Haematology* in his honor. Her request for a suitable paper for this special number came at the right time. By then we were assembling all our data; what better place and better occasion to publish it? Subsequent studies by ourselves and others[1] led to much better understanding of this disease syndrome and thus to more rational therapy."

1. **Merskey C, Johnson A J, Harris J U & Wang M T.** Isolation of fibrinogen-fibrin related antigen (FR-antigen) by immunoafinity chromatography from normal subjects and defibrinating patients and characterized by SDS-polyacrylamide gel electrophoresis and N-terminal analysis. *Clin. Res.* **26**:555A, 1978.

CC/NUMBER 52
DECEMBER 24-31, 1979

This Week's Citation Classic

Negus D, Pinto D J, Le Quesne L P, Brown N & Chapman M. ^{125}I-labelled fibrinogen in the diagnosis of deep-vein thrombosis and its correlation with phlebography. *Brit. J. Surg.* **55**:835-9, 1968. [Depts. Surgical Studies, Nuclear Med., and Radiology, Middlesex Hosp., London, England]

Ninety-three post-operative patients were investigated by intravenous ^{125}I-labelled fibrinogen and leg scanning. A 93% correlation with phlebography was observed in 26 legs with deep-vein thrombosis, and 100% correlation in normal veins. Most thrombi were detected within 48 hours of operation, and physical signs were present in only a few. [The *SCI*® indicates that this paper has been cited over 285 times since 1968.]

David Negus
Department of Surgery
Lewisham Hospital
London, SE13 6LH
England

September 18, 1979

"It is flattering for a surgeon to find himself among scientists, and it gives me much pleasure to be able to include some of the many people who were involved directly or indirectly in this paper. After a year's work on the post-thrombotic syndrome at St. Thomas' Hospital, I was given three opportunities: First, to remain there as a surgical registrar (resident). Second, to spend a year at the Mayo Clinic in vascular physiology, which was very tempting, but I was more interested in clinically-orientated research. I was therefore delighted with the third opportunity—to work in Professor Le Quesne's department at the Middlesex Hospital on problems related to thrombosis. My predecessor, John Ham, now in Queensland, had been interested in the relationship between platelet adhesiveness and lipoprotein lipase activity. I was encouraged to continue this and also to investigate ^{125}I-fibrinogen uptake in the diagnosis of deep vein thrombosis. This had been started by Hobbs and Davies in 1960,[1] and later developed by Atkins and Hawkins.[2] We also decided to combine these projects and to investigate platelet adhesiveness in relation to deep vein thrombosis. I was kindly allowed to investigate the patients of several surgeons and, apart from one lady who maintained that all surgical researchers were little better than murderers, these were most co-operative. Much help was also provided by Dr. (now Professor) Williams of the Nuclear Medicine Department; Nicholas Brown, medical physicist, who organised the radiation counting and suggested the useful modification of comparing 'leg counts' with 'heart counts' to compensate for biological decay; and Malcolm Chapman, consultant radiologist, whose phlebograms demonstrated that an increased isotope labelled fibrinogen uptake did accurately indicate radiologically-demonstrable thrombus.

"Atkins' and Hawkins' work at King's College Hospital, continued by Flanc and Kakkar,[3] confirmed the validity of the method. Unfortunately we were unable to demonstrate any relationship between early deep vein thrombosis and platelet adhesiveness, and the search for a simple and reliable 'early warning system' goes on. Dominic Pinto completed the work and undertook other studies with ^{125}I-fibrinogen.

"^{125}I-fibrinogen uptake has subsequently been widely used in investigating the natural history of deep vein thrombosis, and in assessing methods of prevention. Paradoxically, its extreme accuracy is its main defect in clinical research, and argument still continues as to whether these small early thrombi are 'clinically significant' or not.

"My year at Middlesex was stimulating and enjoyable, and I only regret that, by going there, I was unable to visit the Mayo Clinic. I hope to correct this deficiency in my medical and scientific education before too long."

1. **Hobbs J T & Davies J W L.** Detection of venous thrombosis with ^{125}I-labeled fibrinogen in the rabbit. *Lancet* **2**:134-5, 1960.
2. **Atkins P & Hawkins L A.** Detection of venous thrombosis in the legs. *Lancet* **2**:1217-9, 1965.
3. **Flanc C, Kakkar V V & Clarke M B.** The detection of venous thrombosis of the legs using ^{125}I-labelled fibrinogen. *Brit. J. Surg.* **55**:742-7, 1968.

CC/NUMBER 13
MARCH 31, 1980

This Week's Citation Classic

Wagner H N, Jr., Sabiston D C, Jr., McAfee J G, Tow D & Stern H S. Diagnosis of massive pulmonary embolism in man by radioisotope scanning.
N. Eng. J. Med. **271**:376-84, 1964. [Depts. Medicine, Surgery, and Radiology, Johns Hopkins Univ. Sch. Med., Baltimore, MD]

In this paper, we described the development and application of the use of radioiodine labeled macroaggregates of albumin in the diagnosis of acute pulmonary embolism. [The *SCI*® indicates that this paper has been cited over 245 times since 1964.]

H.N. Wagner
Divisions of Nuclear Medicine
and Radiation Health Sciences
Johns Hopkins Medical Institutions
Baltimore, MD 21205

February 7, 1980

"The research described in this paper is an illustration of how progress often depends on the existence of a problem. As cardiac surgery expanded in the early 1960s, attempts were made to treat patients with massive pulmonary embolism and circulatory collapse by removal of the clots from the occluded pulmonary arteries, first without, and subsequently with, cardiopulmonary bypass. This necessitated a diagnostic technique that would permit accurate diagnosis rapidly since the patients were critically ill. Pulmonary angiography was in the process of development, but was time-consuming and not widely available.

"At the same time at Johns Hopkins and in a few other institutions, research was being conducted on the use of aggregated human serum albumin to study the phagocytic process of the reticuloendothelial system. Such particles were injected intravenously and were removed by the liver and spleen where the accumulation of the radioiodine label could be imaged with the developing rectolinear scanners. These were beginning to be used to visualize organs and lesions that could not be seen with x-radiographic techniques. The albumin aggregates were prepared by heating human serum albumin under carefully controlled conditions. At times when heating was excessive, the particles became too large to pass through the pulmonary capillary bed. These could be observed to be distributed throughout the lung and it could be shown in animals that they did not enter the region of reduced pulmonary arterial blood flow associated with embolism. The first studies were a series of 42 dogs with experimentally produced emboli in which the correlation of the site of the lesions with the perfusion defects in the scans was good. The next step was to carry out toxicity studies in animals. These showed that the hemodynamic effects were negligible and the particles were not antigenic.

"The first lung scan was performed on me in September of 1963. Masahiro Iio, a research fellow and now a leading nuclear physician, injected the macroaggregates (we called them this to distinguish them from the smaller particles used to study the reticuloendothelial system), and James Langan, now our chief technologist (then our only nuclear technologist), performed the scan. The first patient with pulmonary embolism was a 75-year-old woman with a midthigh amputation and shock who was operated upon by David Sabiston at Johns Hopkins in October, 1963. The series of patients we studied subsequently formed the basis of the report.

"I think one reason for my publication being highly cited is the fact that prior to the development of a single diagnostic test, pulmonary embolism was a diagnosis usually made only at autopsy."

Todd A S. The histological localisation of fibrinolysin activator.
J. Pathol. Bacteriol. **78**:281-3, 1959.
[Dept. Pathol., Royal Victoria Infirmary, Newcastle upon Tyne, England]

A histochemical method for the study of fibrinolytic activity in tissues was devised, using a thin fibrin film as a substrate. It was shown that in human tissues most of the plasminogen activator is concentrated in the endothelium of blood vessels, especially veins. [The *SCI*® indicates that this paper has been cited over 440 times since 1961.]

A.S. Todd
Haematology Section
Department of Pathology
Ninewells Hospital and Medical School
University of Dundee
Dundee DD1 9SY
Scotland

March 30, 1981

"From 1946-1949, J.B. Duguid published his observations on the incorporation of fibrin into the walls of coronary arteries, on which he based his revival of Rokitansky's thrombogenic theory of atherosclerosis.[1] By the time I came to work in Duguid's department at Newcastle the theory had created considerable interest among those working on blood coagulation, and he himself was writing that 'in considering the aetiology of atherosclerosis attention must be turned to the blood and the factors in blood which govern thrombosis.' I saw fibrinolysis as one such factor and with Duguid's encouragement began to study fibrinolytic activity in blood. During a time of setback in this work I realised that we knew little of the role of cells and tissues in the fibrinolytic process, and that as a morphologist I was better equipped for the study of these problems than for the more orthodox biochemical approach. It was well known that plasminogen (fibrinolysin) activator was abundant in tissues, associated with the microsomal fraction of cellular homogenates, but its distribution between cells of different types was unknown.

"My approach to the problem of the cellular distribution of plasminogen activator was to scale down the classical 'fibrin plate technique' in which tissue fragments were incubated on a layer of fibrin formed in a petri dish. Instead the fibrin was deposited as a thin film on a microscope slide and the tissue was applied as a fresh frozen section.

"The first preparations were almost a failure since the sections floated off the substrate during fixation and staining so that direct correlation of areas of fibrin digestion with the structures in the section was impossible. However, the fibrinolytic activity was so intense, so focal, and distributed in such a striking pattern that it was possible to deduce that it had originated from blood vessels. The precise localisation was due to the lucky chance that the enzyme is very firmly bound to the tissues. In later preparations I was fortunate enough to see fibrinolytic activity related to cells peeling off a vein wall, thus getting a clue to the endothelial origin of the enzyme.

"It is hard to say why the paper should have been so much quoted. First, I must acknowledge the generosity of fellow writers. Secondly, the observations filled a gap between measurements of the enzyme in extracts of whole tissues or in subcellular fragments. Thirdly, the observations were visually satisfying and simple to interpret; one could see the tissues dissolving the fibrin, as they may do in life. Finally, the observations revived the view that endothelium plays an active part in the maintenance of blood fluidity, fulfilling John Hunter's prediction that '...where there is a full power of life the vessels are capable of keeping the blood in a fluid state,'[2] lending support to Copley's idea[3] of a dynamic balance between fibrin formation and dissolution at the plasma-tissue interface and providing a cellular explanation of the localised nature of the process of thrombosis. More recent work has been reported in 'Plasminogen activators—a morphologist's view.' "[4]

1. **Duguid J B.** Pathogenesis of atherosclerosis. *Lancet* **2**:925-7, 1949.
2. **Hunter J.** *A treatise on the blood, inflammation and gunshot wounds.* London: E. Cox, 1812. p. 40.
3. **Copley A L.** Fibrinolysis and atherosclerosis. *Lancet* **1**:102-3, 1957.
4. **Todd A S.** Plasminogen activators—a morphologist's view. *J. Clin. Pathol.* **33**(Suppl. 14):18-23, 1980.

CC/NUMBER 5
FEBRUARY 4, 1980

This Week's Citation Classic

Nilsson I M & Olow B. Fibrinolysis induced by streptokinase in man. *Acta Chir. Scand.* **123**:247-66, 1962.
[Dept. Surgery and Coagulation Lab., Univ. Lund, Malmö, Sweden]

The authors administered various doses of streptokinase (SK), SK plus plasminogen, and SK plus EACA in a series of 67 surgical patients. SK produced a high fibrinolytic activity, but had a significant effect on the coagulation factors. It proved possible to counteract the coagulation defect by SK combined with EACA without affecting the lysis of the clot. [The *SCI*® indicates that this paper has been cited over 240 times since 1962.]

Inga Marie Nilsson
Coagulation Laboratory
University of Lund
Allmänna Sjukhuset
214 01 Malmö
Sweden

September 20, 1979

"It was very gratifying to learn that our paper has been identified as one of the most cited articles in its field. If I ask myself why, I think it has been cited mainly because it contains detailed descriptions of various methods for assessing fibrinolysis, methods which were either not available at that time or not properly standardized. I had for some years been interested in haemophilia and von Willebrand's disease. The idea of the project was conceived at a dinner party with some colleagues in 1959. One of the guests was Bertil Olow, a skillful surgeon who had not yet received his MD. In the course of the evening it was suggested that it was about time that he thought of doing so, and I was asked to propose some suitable subject for his thesis. As he was a surgeon and I was a 'coagulationist' we thought that thrombosis would be the most suitable field.

"In 1958 Johnson and McCarty were the first to report that artificially induced thrombi in human volunteers could be lysed by infusion of purified SK preparation.[1] Such a preparation (Kabikinase) became available in Sweden in 1959. An investigation of thrombolysis by SK in man was therefore decided upon as the subject of the thesis. After some methodological studies we were able to publish methods for determining the fibrinolytic activity on fibrin plates, euglobulin clot lysis time, fibrinogen, fibrinogenolytic activity, plasminogen and the initial dose (TID) of SK. All together 93 infusions of SK were given to 67 patients. Infusion of one TID of SK produced only a brief and moderate increase of the fibrinolytic activity without any appreciable variation of the coagulation factors. The fourfold TID of SK caused an impressive rise of the fibrinolytic activity with a simultaneous clear decrease of fibrinogen, plasminogen, and factor V. Addition of plasminogen to the SK did not change the response. However, it proved possible to counteract the coagulation defect by supplementary administration of a fibrinolytic inhibitor, E-amino caproic acid (EACA), without undue depression of the thrombolytic effect. I do not think that the popularity of the article can be ascribed to the actual investigation of streptokinase, but rather to the descriptions of the methods. The results obtained hold good today. Despite the intensive research during the last ten years in this field, no agreement has been reached on the optimum dosage or duration of treatment.

"This investigation stimulated my interest in fibrinolysis, which besides von Willebrand's disease is now one of the most important research fields at our laboratory. Olow published further articles on SK.[2] After having received his MD, Olow was appointed chief surgeon at a large general hospital (Angelholm). I myself have since become a professor in coagulation research and head of the coagulation laboratory at the General Hospital in Malmö and am working full-time with coagulation and fibrinolysis."

1. **Johnson A J & McCarty W R.** Lysis of artificially induced intravascular clots in man by intravenous infusions of streptokinase. *J. Clin. Invest.* **37**:905, 1958.
2. **Olow B, Johanson C, Andersson J & Ekelöf B.** Deep venous thrombosis treated with a standard dosage of streptokinase. *Acta Chir. Scand.* **136**:181-9, 1970.

This Week's Citation Classic

NUMBER 40
OCTOBER 1, 1979

Zinkham W H & Lenhard R E, Jr. Metabolic abnormalities of erythrocytes from patients with congenital nonspherocytic hemolytic anemia. *J. Pediatrics* **55**:319-36, 1959. [Dept. Pediatrics, Johns Hopkins Sch. Med., Baltimore, MD]

Activity of glucose-6-phosphate dehydrogenase (G-6-PD) was severely reduced in red cells from four patients with a type of congenital hemolytic anemia. Although the defect was sex-linked, as in primaquine-sensitivity, the ethnic background of the patients and the extreme reduction of G-6-PD activity suggested a different genetic mutation. [The *SCI*® indicates that this paper has been cited over 155 times since 1961.]

William H. Zinkham
Children's Medical & Surgical Center
Johns Hopkins Hospital
Baltimore, MD 21205

February 22, 1978

"The early and mid-fifties in medicine heralded an amazingly rapid increase in our understanding of how abnormalities of the gene can cause human disease. Discoveries in the test tube were literally being carried to the bedside (or cribside), and conversely, patient problems were being explored in basic science laboratories. Our 1959 article is a product of these exciting times. Also, it reflects the mutual interest of clinical and basic scientists who contributed significantly to the work.

"Having finished residency and fellowship training in pediatrics and hematology, I entered the academic scene at Johns Hopkins with only a superficial knowledge of biochemistry. Jim Sidbury, working with V.A. Najjar at the Harriet Lane Home, was especially conscious of my biochemical ignorance. At his urging, I monitored courses at the Homewood campus under S.P. Colowick, E. Kaplan, A. Nason, and later C.L. Markert, and attended weekly research-journal seminars, the membership of which included basic scientists. Although never a full-fledged or even a partially knowledgeable biochemist, I now had an opportunity to exchange ideas with and learn methods from fellow faculty who were.

"The clinical problem which intrigued our group was the unique susceptibility of certain black children to the red cell destructive effects of naphthalene. Following up pioneering studies by A.S. Alving's group in Chicago (R.J. Dern, E. Beutler, P.E. Carson, and others) on primaquine-sensitivity we learned that naphthalene-induced hemolysis occurred only in children with deficient red cell G-6-PD activity.[1,2] The 1959 article represents one of a series of subsequent articles, and there are possibly two reasons for its citation frequency. In the 'Methods Section' is a detailed description of our G-6-PD assay in red cells (not entirely original but incorporating some aspects of previous methods). It was probably the reproducibility of this technique in other laboratories that attracted attention. From our point of view, the significant feature of the paper was the observation that there were going to be several mutant forms of G-6-PD, some of which may shorten red cell survival without the patient being exposed to drugs or chemicals such as naphthalene.

"The physical facilities and budgetary requirements for our research were quite modest. Beginning in a wash room of 75 square feet the activity moved to larger quarters, approximately 200 square feet, equipped with $50.00 worth of cabinets and tabletops from Sears and Roebuck, Inc. Nearby, however, both at the hospital and on the Homewood campus, were scientists interested in our work. Thus a roadway between basic and clinical research was built and during these and subsequent years was well travelled."

1. **Beutler E, Dern R J, Flanagan C L & Alving A S.** The hemolytic effect of primaquine. VII. Biochemical studies of drug-sensitive erythrocytes. *J. Lab. Clin. Med.* **45**:286-95, 1955.
2. **Flanagan C L, Schrier S L, Carson P E & Alving A S.** The hemolytic effect of primaquine. VIII. The effect of drug administration on parameters of primaquine sensitivity. *J. Lab. Clin. Med.* **51**:600-8, 1958.

This Week's Citation Classic

CC/NUMBER 2
JANUARY 11, 1982

Tanaka K R, Valentine W N & Miwa S. Pyruvate kinase (PK) deficiency hereditary nonspherocytic hemolytic anemia. *Blood* **19**:267-95, 1962. [Dept. Medicine, Univ. California Med. Ctr., and Wadsworth Hosp., Veterans Admin. Ctr., Los Angeles, CA]

The paper describes a specific deficiency of the glycolytic enzyme pyruvate kinase (PK) in the erythrocytes of seven patients with congenital nonspherocytic hemolytic anemia. Family studies indicate that PK deficiency is transmitted as an autosomal recessive trait. [The *SCI*® indicates that this paper has been cited over 265 times since 1962.]

Kouichi R. Tanaka
Division of Hematology
Department of Medicine
Harbor-UCLA Medical Center
Torrance, CA 90509

October 28, 1981

"I am indebted to William Valentine of UCLA for providing me, as a junior research hematologist, the opportunity in July 1957 of joining his laboratory located in a Quonset hut. In the early fall of 1960, we began to set up assays for each enzymatic step of the glycolytic pathway to study the nonspherocytic hemolytic anemias because (1) of Dacie's earlier report on autohemolysis,[1] (2) G6PD deficiency had been recently described as a cause of hemolytic anemia,[2] and (3) purified enzymes and substrates had become more readily available.

"In February 1961, very shortly after the PK assay had been established, I obtained a sample of blood from a 26-year-old Caucasian veteran who had been admitted to Wadsworth Hospital for investigation of his chronic anemia. Essentially no PK enzyme activity was obtained on the hemolysate of this patient; the leukocytes were found to have normal activity. We quickly found that the erythrocytes of the patient's son and daughter and parents had about half of normal activity consistent with heterozygosity for the defect. Two brothers with chronic hemolytic anemia were recalled for study and were found to be deficient in erythrocyte PK. The data on these three patients were submitted to *Science*, but the manuscript was rejected on the basis of lacking broad interest.

"Valentine wrote to the president of the Association of American Physicians, Cecil J. Watson, about our studies on the three subjects. The paper[3] was accepted for the annual session in Atlantic City on May 2, 1961, less than three months after our initial results. A total of seven patients were soon found to have a specific deficiency in the red cell glycolytic enzyme PK. This formed the basis of the manuscript published in *Blood*. Many other cases of PK deficiency were soon reported from all over the world.

"Meanwhile, I became chief of hematology at Harbor-UCLA Medical Center, and have continued to work in the field of red cell enzymology and metabolism during the past 20 years. However, I collaborated with Valentine for a number of years and we still write reviews together.[4] Miwa, who was a research fellow at the time, returned to Japan shortly thereafter and has become the leading investigator of red cell enzyme deficiency hemolytic anemias in Japan.

"The probable reasons for the frequent citation of our paper are these. Our initial brief paper on PK deficiency was published in *Transactions of the Association of American Physicians*,[3] but this is not as widely circulated as *Blood*. The paper in *Blood* defined the entity of PK deficiency hemolytic anemia, which has proven to be the first described, best studied, and most common of the hemolytic anemias resulting from an enzyme defect in the Embden-Meyerhof pathway. The discovery of PK deficiency excited interest in hereditary hemolytic anemias and led to the rapid subsequent finding of other enzyme deficiency hemolytic anemias, many in Valentine's laboratory.

"The first patient with PK deficiency hemolytic anemia has been living for a number of years in Sanger, California, where I spent the first 15 years of my life. His red cell PK enzyme was characterized recently and named PK 'Sanger.' "[5]

1. **Selwyn J G & Dacie J V.** Autohemolysis and other changes resulting from the incubation in vitro of red cells from patients with congenital hemolytic anemia. *Blood* **9**:414-38, 1954.
2. **Carson P E, Flanagan C L, Ickes C E & Alving A S.** Enzymatic deficiency in primaquine-sensitive erythrocytes. *Science* **124**:484-5, 1956.
3. **Valentine W N, Tanaka K R & Miwa S.** A specific erythrocyte enzyme defect (pyruvate kinase) in three subjects with congenital non-spherocytic hemolytic anemia. *Trans. Assn. Amer. Physicians* **74**:100-10, 1961. [The *SCI* indicates that this paper has been cited over 125 times since 1961.]
4. **Valentine W N & Tanaka K R.** Pyruvate kinase and other enzyme deficiency hereditary hemolytic anemias. (Stanbury J B, Wyngaarden J B & Fredrickson D S, eds.) *The metabolic basis of inherited disease.* New York: McGraw-Hill, 1978. p. 1410-29.
5. **Shinohara K & Tanaka K R.** Pyruvate kinase deficiency hemolytic anemia. Enzymatic characterization studies in twelve patients. *Hemoglobin* **4**:611-25, 1980.

CC/NUMBER 22
MAY 28, 1984

This Week's Citation Classic™

Swift M R & Hirschhorn K. Fanconi's anemia: inherited susceptibility to chromosome breakage in various tissues. *Ann. Intern. Med.* **65**:496-503, 1966.
[Depts. Neurology and Medicine, New York Univ. Medical Center, New York, NY]

This paper reported frequent chromosome breaks in lymphocytes, cultured skin fibroblasts, and possibly bone marrow in homozygotes with the rare autosomal recessive syndrome Fanconi anemia. It also called attention to the occurrence of two squamous cell carcinomas in one patient. [The *SCI*® indicates that this paper has been cited in over 150 publications since 1966.]

Michael Swift
Division of Medical Genetics
Department of Medicine
University of North Carolina
Chapel Hill, NC 27514

March 13, 1984

"In 1964, when I was a postdoctoral fellow in genetics with Kurt Hirschhorn in the department of medicine at New York University School of Medicine, Eleanor Ball asked me to see a patient on the dermatology service of Bellevue Hospital because a note from a previous hospitalization stated that the patient had 'wild chromosomes.'[1] This was my first encounter with a patient with Fanconi anemia (FA), which is one of a small group of rare autosomal recessive cancer-prone syndromes which are of considerable interest because of the insight they can offer into cancer predisposition and pathogenesis.

"In 1967, I was surprised when I, as a junior faculty member at NYU, was asked to discuss FA at medical grand rounds, since Hirschhorn and Fanconi himself had reviewed this rare disease very thoroughly in the previous two years. In seeking a fresh approach to this topic, I chose to explore the idea that heterozygous carriers of the FA gene, who are, according to the Hardy-Weinberg principle, common in the population, might express some of the cancer predisposition so manifest in homozygotes, and thus could constitute an important proportion of persons in the general population who are genetically cancer-prone.

"The enthusiastic response of my colleagues to this theoretical proposal led me to design a small-scale family study to see if there was indeed an excess of cancer in the families of patients with FA.[2] Even now, however, it is not clear whether or not the FA heterozygote has an excess risk of cancer at certain sites, since in 25 FA families the mortality rates for blood relatives at those sites were only slightly higher than those in the general US population, while they were substantially higher than the rates in spouse controls from the same families.[3]

"A general principle then became evident: a substantial proportion of genes predisposing to common diseases might be identified and studied through the specific rare autosomal recessive syndromes they caused in homozygotes.[4] It is surprising that this principle had not been recognized earlier, since Penrose in 1927 had proposed that the PKU heterozygote is predisposed to mental illness.[5] Hypotheses about heterozygote predisposition to common diseases can be difficult to test if there is no laboratory procedure or clinical criterion to identify the gene carriers. By studying disease incidence in families of probands with selected autosomal recessive syndromes, we have extended the methods originally used for FA to identify genes for mental retardation, birth defects, diabetes, and heart disease, as well as cancer. From an accidental encounter with a patient with this rare recessive syndrome has evolved a general approach to analyzing genes for common diseases.

"It is likely that this article has been cited frequently because it was the first to show that chromosome breakage is found in all tissues studied and therefore represents something close to the primary defect in FA. It has also been cited because it was one of the first to call attention to the occurrence of squamous cell carcinomas in FA. There are recent articles documenting how frequently such cancers occur in FA homozygotes."[6]

1. **Schroeder T M, Anschultz F & Knopp A.** Spontane Chromosomenaberrationen bei familiarer Panmyelopathie. *Humangenetik* **1**:194-6, 1964. (Cited 185 times.)
2. **Swift M.** Fanconi's anaemia in the genetics of neoplasia. *Nature* **230**:370-3, 1971. (Cited 140 times.)
3. **Swift M, Caldwell R & Chase C.** Reassessment of cancer predisposition of Fanconi anemia heterozygotes. *J. Nat. Cancer Inst.* **54**:863-7, 1980.
4. **Swift M, Cohen J & Pinkham R.** A maximum-likelihood method for estimating the disease predisposition of heterozygotes. *Amer. J. Hum. Genet.* **26**:304-17, 1974.
5. **Penrose L S.** Inheritance of phenylpyruvic amentia (phenylketonuria). *Lancet* **2**:192-4, 1935.
6. **Kennedy A W & Hart W R.** Multiple squamous-cell carcinomas in Fanconi's anemia. *Cancer* **50**:811-14, 1982.

This Week's Citation Classic

NUMBER 18
APRIL 30, 1979

Brain M C, Dacie J V & Hourihane D O'B. Microangiopathic haemolytic anaemia: a possible role of vascular lesions in pathogenesis. *Brit. J. Haematol.* **8**:358-74, 1962. [Royal Post Graduate School, London, England]

This paper postulated that the hemolytic anemia found in patients with renal failure, thrombotic thrombocytopenic purpura, or disseminated carcinoma might be due to the effect on the red blood cells or their passage through the abnormal of partially occluded blood vessels found in these patients. [The *SCI*® indicates that this paper has been cited over 325 times since 1962].

Michael C. Brain
McMaster University
Hamilton, Ontario, L8S 4J9
Canada

February 7, 1978

"When I joined Professor Dacie's department, at the Royal Post Graduate School in London,as a trainee in hematology in 1959, he suggested that I should investigate the abnormal red cell morphology he and others had observed in patients with malignant hypertension, uremia, and metastatic carcinoma. It soon became apparent that the degree of morphological abnormality did not correlate with the height of the blood urea. Before joining Dacie, I had worked at the London Hospital where Professor Clifford Wilson and his colleagues were interested in the pathogenesis of malignant hypertension. This made me aware of a highly relevant observation made there by Verel and his co-workers.[1] They had observed shortened red cell survival in a young patient with malignant hypertension with normal renal function in whom the red cell survival returned to normal when the malignant phase of hypertension had been treated. Although they did not comment upon red cell morphology, their observation suggested to me that the hemolytic anemia and the red cell fragmentation might be due to reversible arteriole necrosis. It thus seemed possible that the hemolysis in patients with malignant hypertension, the hemolytic-uremic syndrome, thrombotic thrombocytopenic purpura, and in some patients with metastatic carcinoma, might have a common pathogenesis due to microvascular disease; the association with uremia being due to renal vascular disease and not uremia per se.

"We were not the first to describe the abnormal morphology nor, indeed, did we claim credit for the suggested mechanism. In 1953, Monroe and Strauss had observed schizocytes in the blood vessels of sections obtained at necropsy from two patients who had died of thrombotic thrombocytopenic purpura.[2] These authors suggested that the abnormal blood vessels might be the site of red cell fragmentation and destruction. This perceptive observation and hypothesis was not pursued by the authors, nor did it receive the recognition it warranted.

"Our hypothesis received independent support from the observation, made at about the same time, that red cell fragmentation and hemolysis followed the insertion of prosthetic materials to correct intracardiac defects and to replace malfunctioning heart valves. More direct evidence has come from a number of experimental studies in animals undertaken by myself with various colleagues, and independently by a number of other workers.[3]

"Finally, it must be acknowledged that the initial pursuit of ideas is more dependent upon the stimulus provided in an academic environment than upon research funding; as none was sought, received, nor required for this study to be undertaken. This may serve to emphasize how important it is to encourage and support young investigators in the pursuit of their ideas, which at the outset may well make few or little demands on the resources of many academic institutions."

1. **Verel D, Turnbull A, Tudhope G R & Ross J H.** Anaemia in Bright's disease. *Quart. J. Med.* **28**:491-504,1959.
2. **Monroe W M & Strauss A F.** Intravascular hemolysis: a morphologic study of schizocytes in thrombotic purpura and other diseases. *Southern Med. J.* **46**:837-42, 1953.
3. **Brain M C.** Microangiopathic haemolytic anaemia (MHA). *Brit. J. Haematol.* **23** (Suppl.):45-52, 1972.

NUMBER 4
JANUARY 22, 1979

This Week's Citation Classic

Bond V P, Fliedner T M, Cronkite E P, Rubini J R, Brecher G & Schork P K. Proliferative potentials of bone marrow and blood cells studied by *in vitro* uptake of H^3-thymidine. *Acta Haematol.* **21**: 1-15, 1959.

In vitro **incubation with tritiated thymidine of blood from normal individuals and patients with infection and infectious mononucleosis, demonstrated the presence of small numbers of labeled large mononuclear cells of different morphological types indicating that the cells are capable of DNA synthesis and division. [The** ***SCI®*** **indicates that this paper was cited 144 times in the period 1961-1977.]**

V.P. Bond
Brookhaven National Laboratory
Upton, New York 11973

February 28, 1978

"In the years just preceding this paper, there was a great deal of work and discussion on the mechanism of protection against radiation lethality by shielding of a limb or of the spleen. There was a substantial debate as to whether the protection afforded was mediated via a humoral or a cellular factor.

"In connection with a number of shielding and cell fractionation experiments, Peggy Swift and I showed that irradiating one-half of the body followed by irradiating the other half after a brief interval afforded substantial protection compared to accomplishing the entire exposure at the same time. Nearly simultaneously, Brecher and Cronkite showed that parabiosis protected the irradiated member of the pair. Also, somewhat equivocal evidence had been available that peripheral blood might have protective action against the effects of whole body irradiation.

"These studies showed that the protective agent is produced normally and is in the blood stream. At this time no method was available that would allow us to determine directly, if cells capable of proliferation were normally in transit in the blood stream.

"Shortly thereafter Taylor and Hughes first used the specific DNA precursor tritiated thymidine and autoradiograph to study chromosome replication in plant cells. A group of us at Brookhaven (including the authors of the above publication) initiated extensive work with this new and potent tool, to study the kinetics of cell proliferation in the mammal, under normal conditions and as related to radiobiology. Although the work primarily involved studies of kinetics of cell proliferation in the bone marrow and other organs, we were also interested in using this new technique to see if under normal conditions, there were cells in the blood that were synthesizing DNA, and therefore presumably capable of proliferating in body locations distant from their origin. The experiments were not difficult to perform, and such cells were readily found.

"The finding clearly supported what had been suspected, namely that segments of a ubiquitous organ such as bone marrow are able to exchange cells, and that there is a common pool of proliferating cells available to all segments of the organ. Thus a mechanism was available for part of an organ to contribute directly to the rate of recovery of another portion of the organ that may have been damaged. Since that time a similar mechanism via the blood stream has been shown to exist in other systems, e.g., the lymphopietic system, neoplastic growth. Practical implications of the findings have been demonstrated by T. M. Fliedner and others, i.e., protection against radiation and other forms of bone marrow damage is afforded by transfusing peripheral blood leukocytes. Collection of these cells from the peripheral blood and preservation through freezing, can be used for such protection with diminution of graft versus host reactions when the circulating stem cells are largely separated from T-lymphocytes."

Chapter

6

Cardiovascular Disease

Despite the unavoidable close association of coronary heart disease, athero- and arteriosclerosis, hypertension, and blood flow, the magnitude of the popular and scientific attention to coronary heart disease is reflected here by considering it as a separate sector of this chapter. This artifice has been employed solely for organizational convenience.

Coronary Heart Disease

The "This Week's Citation Classic" (TWCC) commentaries under this subheading move through the sequence etiology, diagnosis, prevention, and treatment, with some unavoidable overlaps from dual or multiply oriented Citation Classics.

Factors that can be related to a high risk for developing coronary heart disease (CHD) are indeed numerous—cigarette smoking, stress, obesity, and improper diet are four. A 1961 analysis of these and other factors would not be expected to agree with our current evaluations, and Kannel states this in the first TWCC, which was written 17 years after an epidemiologic assessment of CHD. In his commentary, Kannel lists numerous factors considered in 1978 as predictors of CHD. The dietary influence on CHD has been studied extensively, and four of the next five articles examined this relationship. The first (p. 174) noted that potentially significant changes in retail food supplies related to CHD occurred between 1900 and 1960. During this time, the consumption of polyunsaturated fatty acids increased by 30 percent and the ratio of complex to simple carbohydrates in the diet decreased. From these data, the authors hypothesized that a balance of polyunsaturated with saturated fatty acids, and of complex with simple carbohydrates, was essential to good cardiac health. The low incidence of coronary heart disease during World War II, particularly in countries with severe food rationing, was a key to the suggestion that lipid intake was a positive correlate with CHD (p. 175). Dietary adjustment, in a cross-over experiment designed and conducted in post-war Finland, confirmed that when vegetable oils replaced dairy fat the incidence of CHD decreased. These data can now be related to the balance of high- and low-density lipoproteins in the blood (p. 176) and of cell receptors for these carriers of cholesterol. The protective role of high-density lipoproteins has not yet been explained. Oliver and his co-authors determined that an excess of fatty acids was present in blood and was associated positively with the arrythmia characteristic of patients with CHD. High-fiber diets, known to be protective against colonic cancer, also reduce the risk of ischemic heart disease (p. 178).

A two-part review on atherosclerosis written by University of Washington investigators (p. 179) sought to identify its origin more from a tissue initiation view. This presented a novel problem to the authors since the three different concepts of atherogenesis then extant had originated in their home department. Their favorite was the "response to injury" hypothesis.

A less well known associate of CHD is hemodialysis. A study of 50,000 patients (not all of whom were on maintenance dialysis, of course) confirmed that the uremic patient group on dialysis had a death rate from CHD 10 times higher than other patient groups (p. 180). Another unanticipated cause of myocardial infarcts is the drug isoproterenol. The ability of isoproterenol to induce infarcts in experimental animals in the absence of arterial obstruction suggested an ischemia relatable to reduced blood flow with intense β-adrenergic stimulation as its cause (p. 181). The article describing this was "refused by several reputable journals."

Upon turning to prognostic and diagnostic indicators of CHD, it is now clear that an abnormal heart rhythm is an early warning sign. The new syndrome of midsystolic click with late systolic murmur was described initially at Stanford University (p. 182). This condition was identified as a distinct precursor to angina, dyspnea, arrythmias, and sudden cardiac death. As young investigators, the authors were hesitant to publish their data, but the concepts they forwarded were quickly accepted. This was not the case for a parallel study by a second group that published a similar study of 90 patients with mid- and late-systolic clicks (p. 183). Two of the first manuscripts submitted by this second group were rejected, one with such acerbity that the editor apologized for the tone of the reviewer's remarks. Even the Citation Classic manuscript, apparently the third effort, was initially rejected by an American journal before becoming the second-most-cited article from the *British Heart Journal.* Weissler, Harris, and Schoenfeld attempted to reduce the use of cardiac catheterization by profiling heart function throughout the complete heart cycle. They found that the systolic time interval was clearly related to left ventricular function.

In men aged 55 to 60, EKGs revealed an incidence of 92.6 percent with cardiac rhythm abnormalities within a 6-hour test period (p. 185). Most of these men were asymptomatic, but the more frequent the arrythmia the greater the certainty of future death due to coronary disease. In his TWCC, Lown states that sudden cardiac death takes 400,000 lives each year in the United States, and the origin of this is in ventricular fibrillation. Identifying those at risk was possible by monitoring for premature ventricular beats. This is an extension of the EKG classification of heart risk patients developed in Minnesota a decade earlier (p. 187) and discussed in the paper by Weissler et al. cited above.

Robinson determined that heart rate and systolic blood pressure were the two most essential factors in determining the oxygen supply to the heart, and used the product of these as a successful predictor of angina attacks.

Arteriography as a diagnostic procedure had a mortality rate of 0.06 percent in a study of 11,402 procedures performed prior to 1963, a statistic that led to a more generalized acceptance of this procedure (p. 189). Application of this technique to 1,000 patients with CHD permitted a compilation of a massive amount of data that were summarized by Proudfit et al. One fact of interest: about one-third of these 1,000 patients with angina pectoris were found to be free of heart disease, and only 17 percent had significant lesions. Cohen's group, who examined 60 patients with CHD by arteriography, quantitated blood lactate levels and found them to be excellent predictors of persons at cardiac risk. His remarks about the Harvard undergraduate's date and her insistence on a written record of her successful treatment for arrhythmia is a humorous sidelight to their study. Bruschke's group reported on a study of 590 patients with CHD who had not received surgical treatment but who were followed for as long as 9 years. Arteriographic data were shown to be the best indicators of a second cardiac event.

The evaluation of cardiac function at the bedside (p. 193) and as a predictor of future rhythmic disturbances, chest pain, or even mortality has been of interest to several investigators. Many of these have attempted to avoid catheterization as an information source. Weissler, Harris, and Schoenfeld, in this their second Citation Classic, found the familiar systolic time interval to be the best indicator.

Electroshock treatment to alleviate tachycardia in patients who were unresponsive to drug therapy was based on the concept that an electrical incident was the initial cause of the arrythmia, and if terminated, arrythmia would not recur. The technique of cardioversion, a brief direct current applied across the chest at the proper cardiac interval, ignited the alcohol-soaked contact pads on the chest of the first patient thus aborting any further studies in that hospital. Once again, an article was refused publication initially but once published became a Citation Classic (p. 194).

Propranolol reduced the heart rate and the myocardial consumption of oxygen in 81 percent of a patient group studied, and this reduced the heart's demand for oxygen and decreased chest pain in angina pectoris. Wolfson, as a young trainee, implemented his wife's suggestion of a non-coronary disease control group to determine whether the general analgesic property of propranolol was contributory to his conclusion.

Since many victims of cardiac arrest die before medical aid can reach them, the concept of a mobile unit was conceived and put into practice in Belfast (p. 196). Within 18 months, 312 patients had been transferred via the mobile unit to a hospital without a single death in the unit itself. A portable defibrillator was determined to be the critical instrument. "In house" the intensive care unit has been demonstrated, after special training of the personnel, to reduce the mortality rate after myocardial infarct (p. 197).

Saphenous vein autografting of occluded coronary arteries as a bypass technique to repair circulation to the myocardium has achieved a remarkable popularity, far greater than one would anticipate from the 160 citations of the Citation Classic describing the procedure (p. 198).

The catheter, that invasive probe that cardiologists rely upon so heavily, is the subject of several Citation Classics, including the next, which describes an intra-aortic balloon that could be inflated and then deflated during diastole and systole to aid blood flow. This was clearly one of the first steps toward an artificial heart (p. 199). A self-guiding catheter was invented by Swan et al. to permit entrance into the right side of the heart without fluoroscopic assistance. This catheter had a sail that caught the red wind and was thus carried to the desired area.

Studies of tissue pathology following a myocardial infarct include one on the histochemical mapping of myocardial infarcts that identified the ischemic zone between the area of necrosis and normal muscle by identifying the morphology of dehydrogenase-staining areas (p. 201). Cardiogenic shock as a secondary event to myocardial infarct is detectable at autopsy by a vast necrosis of the left ventricular myocardium. Efforts to minimize this ischemic damage are an important part of the intensive care unit program (p. 202).

Other Cardiovascular Studies

The life-threatening potential of aortic aneurysms is well known. Much of the early medical knowledge about this subject was presented in the 62-page review by Hirst, Johns, and Kime published in 1958. The authors' plan to have their summary of 505 cases prepared in a year and a half was overly optimistic, as the 5-year interval before publication clearly indicates. A comparison of treatment modes for abdominal aortic aneurysm determined that surgical treatment of 248 cases extended the life expectancy of this group by twofold. Thirty-five percent of the patients in the non-surgery group (105 cases) died of vessel rupture (p. 204).

Despite the heavy emphasis on coronary heart disease in this chapter, the 55-page review on cerebral blood flow (p. 205) is one of the most heavily cited papers in this grouping. The key concept presented in this article was the autoregulation of the blood supply to the human brain to compensate for hyper- or hypotension. The sensitivity of the autoregulatory center to trauma prevented its earlier discovery by the more invasive methods used in lower animals. The relative ability of the brain to recover from ischemia *in vitro* but not *in vivo* indicated to Ames' group that, since the presence of blood was the only significant difference in the two states, blood was responsible for this difference. This conclusion was correct—when blood ceases to flow, it becomes more viscous and interferes with autoregulation. The original concept of Na^+ loss by cells as the responsible activity could not be supported.

As is true of most other tissues, heart muscle relies on glucose for energy during normal nutrition. Opie's 13-page review published in 1968 emphasized the role of oxygen in heart muscle metabolism, particularly the effect of hypoxia since this is a component of myocardial infarcts. Braunwald continued from this base with his studies and demonstrated that myocardial contractility and heart rate are determinants of oxygen consumption in the heart.

A review by Doherty on digoxin pharmacokinetics became possible because of previous experience with tritiated cholesterol.

The position of β blockers—those agents that block the activity of the β adrenergic receptors—in the treatment of heart disease stems from several early studies of which three are grouped here. As a young fellow at the National Heart Institute before its name change, Epstein used propranolol to block the β receptor so that the sympathetic contribution of cardiophysiology could be measured. Prior to that time this was not possible since both receptors were inhibited by the available drugs. Blocking only sympathetic stimulation with propranolol was found to reduce the heart rate. Two other descriptions of propranolol follow, one on the pharmacology of this drug (p. 211) and the other on its use in controlling hypertension (p. 212).

The renin-angiotensin-aldosterone triad is the subject of four Citation Classics. The first of these by Laragh et al. was instrumental in establishing the adrenal-kidney "axis" by demonstrating that the vasoconstrictor angiotensin II, the octapeptide formed by the kidney enzyme, renin, stimulated aldosterone release from the kidney. Aldosterone regulates Na^+ and K^+ exchange, particularly in the kidney. Thus a vasoconstriction-volume theory for hypertension evolved. Conn describes his personal excitement over the discovery that an adrenal tumor could cause hypertension in the absence of excess renin activity because of its ability to produce aldosterone. Examination of low-renin hypertensive patients, the same group Laragh et al. studied, resulted in the discovery that none of 59 low-renin patients had ever had a heart attack. As a consequence, blood renin analyses can be predictive of future heart disease (p. 215). Brunner, a co-author of the Citation Classic that describes this discovery, contributed also to the following one that was initially rejected by several journals (p. 216). In this second article, an inhibitor of angiotensin II formation was demonstrated to be an effective anti-hypertensive.

Alterations in the pulmonary vasculature coincident with hypertension can be graded when associated with septal defects (p. 217).

A catheterization technique to evaluate the electrical activity of the His bundle is the subject of the next Classic (p. 218). Coumel and Attuel relate bundle branch block to tachycardia in their Classic. Another "instrument article" follows (p. 220) on a blood gas calculator—a slide rule modification of an earlier nomogram—to calculate numerous parameters, not alone O_2 saturation. Now a pocket computer does it. The response of the central artery in the rabbit's ear to vasoconstrictors or dilators served as a simple method to evaluate vasoactive compounds. The "modern" technique of ultrasonography dates back to the middle 1960s and its application to the analysis of vascular disease reported by Strandness and his co-investigators.

Mason indicated that his publication on myocardial contractility was responsible for his selection as chief of cardiovascular medicine at UC-Davis and a number of subsequent awards. Mason has a prolific memory for figures and is obviously a prolific writer as well.

An early publication by DeBakey on battle injuries during World War II to arteries concludes this chapter. It is surprising that no Citation Classics on heart replacement appeared during the years from which these were selected.

Several review journals specialize in the field of cardiovascular disease. These include *Advances in Cardiology, Current Problems in Cardiology,* and *Progress in Cardiovascular Disease.* Because of the extension of cardiovascular disease into many organs or tissues, review journals in other medical specialties often contain articles pertinent to cardiologists. Familiar journals in this listing include *Advances in Drug Research, Annual Review of Medicine, Annual Review of Pharmacology and Toxicology,* and *Physiological Reviews.*

The Citation Classics in this chapter are heavily oriented toward cardiac arrhythmia, coronary heart disease, blood flow, hypertension, and cardiopharmacology. Most of these topics have remained foremost subjects for research, but even the popular medical literature has indicated the emergence of heart transplantation, pacemakers, and novel drugs as new areas of importance in cardiology. Consequently, a few articles concerned with these topics are included with those more closely related to the Citation Classics of this chapter.

Barry D I. Cerebral blood flow in hypertension. *J. Cardiovasc. Pharmacol.* 7(Suppl. 2):S94–S98, 1985.

Bjorntorp P. Obesity and the risk of cardiovascular disease. *Ann. Clin. Res.* **17**:3–9, 1985.

Bristow M R, Kantrowitz N E, Ginsberg R & Fowler M B. Beta-adrenergic function in heart muscle disease and heart failure. *J. Mol. Cell. Cardiol.* **17**(Suppl. 2):41–52, 1985.

Corwin S & Reiffel J A. Nitrate therapy for angina pectoris. Current concepts about mechanism of action and evaluation of currently available preparations. *Arch. Intern. Med.* **145:**538–43, 1985.

Dunn M. Clinical use of amiodarone. *Heart Lung* **14:**407–11, 1985.

Ergin M A, Galla J D, Lansman S & Griepp R B. Acute dissections of the aorta. Current surgical treatment. *Surg. Clin. North Am.* **65:**721–41, 1985.

Fozzard H A & Makielski J C. The electrophysiology of acute myocardial ischemia. *Annu. Rev. Med.* **36:**275–84, 1985.

Gould K L. Quantification of coronary artery stenosis *in vivo. Circ. Res.* **57:**341–53, 1985.

McCarron D A. Is calcium more important than sodium in the pathogenesis of essential hypertension? *Hypertension* **7:**607–27, 1985.

Nicholls M G. Inhibition of the renin-angiotensin system in the treatment of heart failure: why, when, and where. *J. Cardiovasc. Pharmacol.* **7**(Suppl. 4)**:**S98–S102, 1985.

Opie L H, Walpoth B & Barsacchi R. Calcium and catecholamines: relevance to cardiomyopathies and significance in therapeutic strategies. *J. Mol. Cell. Cardiol.* **17**(Suppl. 2)**:**21–34, 1985.

Singh B N, Thoden W. R & Ward A. Acebutolol: a review of its pharmacological properties and therapeutic efficacy in hypertension, angina pectoris, and arrhythmia. *Drugs* **29:**531–69, 1985.

Virmani R, Robinowitz M & McAllister H A Jr. Exercise and the heart. A review of cardiac pathology associated with physical activity. *Pathol. Annu.* **20**(Pt. 2)**:**431–62, 1985.

Weidmann P, Gerber A & Laederach K. Calcium antagonists in the treatment of hypertension: a critical overview. *Adv. Nephrol.* **14:**197–232, 1985.

This Week's Citation Classic

CC/NUMBER 29
JULY 16, 1979

Kannel W B, Dawber T R, Kagan A, Revotskie N & Stokes J. Factors of risk in the development of coronary heart disease—six-year follow-up experience. *Ann. Intern. Med.* 55:33-49, 1961. [National Heart Institute, National Institutes of Health, Dept. Health, Education, and Welfare, Bethesda, MD]

The paper reports on a six year study of a representative general population sample of men and women aged 30-59, covering factors related to the development of coronary heart disease (CHD). During the period of observation 186 men and women developed CHD. There was a 13:1 male predominance under age 45, reduced to 2:1 at ages 45-62. [The *SCI*® indicates that this paper has been cited over 350 times since 1961.]

William B. Kannel
Framingham Heart Study
Division of Heart and
Vascular Disease
National Institutes of Health
Framingham, MA 01701

March 3, 1978

"At the time of the 1961 *Annals of Internal Medicine* report, an epidemiological approach to unraveling the causes of chronic cardiovascular diseases was novel. Epidemiology has since undergone metamorphosis. The epidemiologist now explores the way morbid processes arise, evolve, and terminate fatally in relation to possible factors that may affect it, identifying highly vulnerable persons and the personal attributes and living habits which make them vulnerable.

"Since the *Annals* report in 1961, additional information has accumulated on the incidence of cardiovascular diseases, the clinical spectrum in all who have it, the identity of those vulnerable to it, its importance as a force of morbidity and mortality, and the chain of events leading to its occurrence. Numerous clues to its pathogenesis have been provided.

"Determinants of cardiovascular disease have been defined in terms of atherogenic personal attributes, living habits which affect these or precipitate attacks, early indicators of pre-clinical disease and host susceptibility to all these influences. As a consequence of the report's being so widely cited, epidemiologic investigations over the past decade have provided physicians with a broader concept of cardiovascular disease, which includes its latent or presymptomatic phase. Concepts of 'normality' have changed from usual to optimal.

"The concept of the cardiovascular risk profile has now been firmly established and validated. Nevertheless, there remain many controversial and unresolved issues. The hazards of obesity, the benefits of physical activity and the importance of most psychosocial factors are still being disputed. The hazards of the cigarette are now well established but the exact pathogenetic mechanism involved is still in contention. Coffee and alcohol appear to have been falsely indicted as contributors to atherosclerotic cardiovascular disease. The role of diet in determining serum lipid values and through them, the incidence of cardiovascular disease, is still hotly disputed.

"New concepts about the influence of serum cholesterol have evolved identifying an LDL fraction which is atherogenic and an HDL component which is protective. Since that report, triglycerides have also been indicted, but appear to have been overemphasized.

"A number of misconceptions about hypertension have been uncovered which contributed to undertreatment of this powerful promoter of cardiovascular disease. The role and mechanism of action of diabetes in cardiovascular disease clearly need further elaboration.

"Cardiovascular risk profiles which synthesize the major risk factors quantitatively into a composite risk estimate have been devised and handbooks constructed to facilitate their application. Multiple risk factor intervention trials have been undertaken using these profiles to identify high risk candidates for prophylactic intervention.

"The optimal time to begin such prophylactic endeavors against atherosclerotic disease is in dispute, but is increasingly viewed as a pediatric problem.

"There has been a recent 20% decline in cardiovascular mortality. Whatever its cause, it is clear that it is environmentally related and that the change in life-style required is neither drastic nor unacceptable. Thus, the original article back in 1961 may well have made some impact where it counts."

CC/NUMBER 17
APRIL 28, 1980

This Week's Citation Classic

Antar M A, Ohlson M A & Hodges R E. Changes in retail market food supplies in the United States in the last seventy years in relation to the incidence of coronary heart disease, with special reference to dietary carbohydrates and essential fatty acids. *Amer. J. Clin. Nutr.* **14**:169-78, 1964.
[Dept. Intern. Med., State Univ. Iowa, Iowa City, IA]

The increased incidence of coronary heart disease from 1900 to 1960 in the US cannot be attributed to a relative deficiency of dietary polyunsaturated fatty acids, since the polyunsaturated to saturated fatty acid ratio of the food supply in 1961 had increased about 30%. In contrast, the ratio of complex to simple carbohydrates had decreased to about 70%. A possible role of excess simple sugar intake, with saturated fat and concomitant low complex carbohydrates, in the development of coronary heart disease was suggested. [The *SCI*® indicates that this paper has been cited over 125 times since 1964.]

Mohamed A. Antar
Department of Nuclear Medicine
University of Connecticut Medical School
Farmington, CT 06032
and VA Medical Center
Newington, CT 06111

March 14, 1980

"It is gratifying to learn that our paper has been so frequently cited. In 1962 it was widely accepted that a high consumption of saturated fat was responsible, at least in part, for the increase of coronary heart disease in the US.

"During a three-hour wait in the rail station at Chicago, I observed the different selections made by patrons from vending machines. To my surprise, 37 people selected the highly sugared items and only one person selected an apple. This impromptu observation provoked my thoughts on the role of carbohydrates. Before 1960, little work had been carried out with dietary carbohydrates. Therefore, we studied the changes in food consumption in the US and investigated the effect of the kind of carbohydrates upon serum lipids in man.[1]

"Although as a fellow I had minimal resources to work with, I was fortunate to be able to perform my research in four different labs (those of M. Ohlson, W. Connor, G. Stearns, and M. Osborn, to whom I am most grateful). The grueling task of calculations and analysis of data was done by hand using a mechanical calculator.

"I recall distinctly how I was both surprised and pleased to observe emerging specific patterns. There was a great progressive decline (more than 55%) of complex carbohydrates with their fiber, and a concurrent dramatic increase of simple sugars (more than double) over the last 70 years. The even greater surprise was the finding that polyunsaturated fatty acids had increased by 40% while saturated acids hardly increased. The rise in dietary cholesterol was minimum. These data did not fit the hypothesis that low ratios of dietary polyunsaturated to saturated fatty acids contribute to the increase of coronary heart disease. In contrast, changes in the type of dietary carbohydrates may be a factor. Such a simple and obvious conclusion proved to my amazement not only a source of initial skepticism and controversy, but also a stimulant for research in this area. Since our initial report, hundreds of articles, several books, editorials, an Australian Academy of Science report, and two congressional Senate hearings have dealt with the subject.

"This paper is widely cited in my belief because: (a) it is one of the first comprehensive studies to offer another light on the relationship of dietary factors and coronary heart disease (carbohydrate connection) and to present a challenge to the then widely accepted hypothesis 'lack of unsaturated fat' and (b) the data were shown to have many ramifications into other fields such as dental caries, obesity, hyperinsulinemia, and cancer of the colon and rectum.

"Several years later, we found a synergistic hyperlipidemic effect between dietary simple sugars and saturated fat in patients[2] (i.e., when saturated fat levels surpassed a certain threshold, excess simple sugars with concomitant low complex carbohydrates were hyperlipidemic). These hypotheses may offer a better explanation of the problem and stimulate further research."

1. **Antar M A & Ohlson M A.** Effect of simple and complex carbohydrates upon total lipids, nonphospholipids, and different fractions of phospholipids of serum in young men and women. *J. Nutrition* **85**:329-37, 1965.
2. **Antar M A, Little J A, Lucas C, Buckley G C & Csima A.** Interrelationship between the kinds of dietary carbohydrate and fat in hyperlipoproteinemic patients. Part 3. Synergistic effect of sucrose and animal fat on serum lipids. *Atherosclerosis* **11**:191-201, 1970.

CC/NUMBER 18
MAY 5, 1980

This Week's Citation Classic

Turpeinen O, Miettinen M, Karvonen M J, Roine P, Pekkarinen M, Lehtosuo E J & Alivirta P. Dietary prevention of coronary heart disease: long-term experiment. *Amer. J. Clin. Nutr.* **21**:255-76, 1968.
[Depts. Biochem. and Physiol., Coll. Vet. Med., Helsinki; Dept. Nutr. Chem., Univ. Helsinki; Nikkilä, Kellokoski, and Koskela Hosps., Finland]

An intervention trial to test the hypothesis that the incidence of coronary heart disease could be reduced by dietary means was carried out in two mental hospitals. Practically total replacement of dairy fats by vegetable oils resulted in a substantial reduction of this disease. [The *SCI*® **indicates that this paper has been cited over 130 times since 1968.]**

Osmo Turpeinen
Department of Biochemistry
College of Veterinary Medicine
SF 00550 Helsinki 55
Finland

February 28, 1980

"The idea that coronary heart disease (CHD) might, at least partly, be a nutritional disease, and hence preventable by dietary means, presented itself soon after World War II, when it was noted that the mortality from this disease had been remarkably low in some countries during the war. These were, above all, countries which had experienced severe food rationing measures and in which, particularly, the consumption of saturated fats (dairy fats and meat fats) had greatly declined.

"The international vital statistics and certain epidemiological studies offered additional evidence on the interrelations between the consumption of saturated fats and the mortality from CHD. These two things appeared indeed to be closely correlated: high dietary intake of such fats was clearly associated with high mortality from CHD.

"These findings are of particular relevance to Finland, where the dairy fat consumption and the mortality from CHD are both very high.

"The available evidence, however, was not sufficient to establish a cause-and-effect relationship between dietary fats and CHD or to justify the conclusion that a change in the fat composition of the diet would reduce the incidence of CHD. Such problems cannot be solved by usual epidemiological studies alone. For this purpose intervention trials are required in which the diet of a population group is deliberately changed and the development of manifestations of CHD is followed over a sufficiently long period.

"In 1958 our small research group, composed of individuals interested in nutrition and preventive cardiology, decided to attempt such an intervention trial. Had we then known all that was to be written about the formidable difficulties and the deceptive pitfalls in such a study, we might have given up the whole project. Fortunately, perhaps, we were ignorant and started the trial.

"The study ran smoother than we had expected. The difficulties anticipated because of the nature of the patient material did not arise. In fact, the patients were quite cooperative, as were also the hospital staffs. The modified diet was well accepted, and very few complaints were heard. The initial financial worries were effectively dispelled by research grants from the United States National Heart Institute.

"The first part of the study lasted from 1959 to 1965. In 1965 the diets of the hospitals were reversed, and the trial was continued according to this crossover design another six years.

"This paper is an account of the first part only. The whole intervention trial has been reported in two later publications.[1,2]

"Why has this paper been frequently cited? Mainly, perhaps, because it is an attempt to solve an urgent public health problem, a try to answer the all-important question: whether the incidence of CHD can be decreased by dietary means. Intervention trials are, obviously, the best way of obtaining conclusive evidence in this sphere. Such trials, however, are laborious and costly and consequently few in number. Their relative rarity may be another reason for the frequent citation of our paper."

1. **Miettinen M, Turpeinen O, Karvonen M J, Elosuo R & Paavilainen E.** Effect of cholesterol-lowering diet on mortality from coronary heart-disease and other causes. A twelve-year clinical trial in men and women. *Lancet* **2**:835-8, 1972.
2. **Turpeinen O, Karvonen M J, Pekkarinen M, Miettinen M, Elosuo R & Paavilainen E.** Dietary prevention of coronary heart disease: the Finnish mental hospital study. *Int. J. Epidemiol.* **8**:99-118, 1979.

This Week's Citation Classic

Rhoads G G, Gulbrandsen C L & Kagan A. Serum lipoproteins and coronary heart disease in a population study of Hawaii Japanese men. *N. Engl. J. Med.* **294**:293-8, 1976. [Honolulu Heart Study, Natl. Heart and Lung Inst., Bethesda, MD]

This paper compared levels of major lipoproteins between 264 men with and 1,755 men without coronary heart disease (CHD) in a defined population of American Japanese men in Hawaii. The inverse relation between high density lipoprotein (HDL) and disease was as strong as the direct relation for low density lipoprotein (LDL). The protective effect of HDL could not be explained by other risk factors. [The *SCI*® indicates that this paper has been cited in over 470 publications since 1976.]

George G. Rhoads
Epidemiology and Biometry
Research Program
National Institute of Child Health
and Human Development
National Institutes of Health
Bethesda, MD 20205

September 8, 1982

"Following the development of Fredrickson and Levy's[1] lipoprotein phenotyping system, the National Heart, Lung, and Blood Institute undertook a major project to apply the technique to several of the population-based studies of cardiovascular disease. We benefited from the fact that the Honolulu Heart Program had the largest of the cohorts involved in this Cooperative Lipoprotein Phenotyping Study. The main purpose of the project was to look at the frequency of the various phenotypes and to see how they related to coronary heart disease (CHD) in several different clearly defined populations. High density lipoprotein (HDL) was not considered in the phenotyping criteria, but its measurement was included in the protocol as a necessary step in the quantitation of low density lipoprotein (LDL).

"Our interest in the project was largely tied to the opportunity which it provided a) to compare the distribution of lipoproteins in Japanese men in Honolulu with that in Caucasians; and b) to examine the associations of lipoproteins with CHD. The difference in HDL between cases and controls was prominent in the initial analyses, and the relative risk of CHD associated with this difference was as strong as the well-known relation of LDL to this disease. There followed some time in the library which (to our disappointment) confirmed our rediscovery. A number of case-control studies in the 1950s had reported similar findings;[2-7] and Medalie *et al.* had reported the association in their prospective study of Israeli civil servants.[8] Our contribution was mainly to show that the association was independent of other coronary risk factors. Of course the earlier reports strengthened our conviction that the association was important.

"We initially submitted the paper to the *Annals of Internal Medicine*, but in recent years the internists have not published much epidemiology. Since they recommended radical surgery for our modest manuscript, we sent it to the *New England Journal of Medicine* where a cosmetic touch-up was deemed sufficient.

"It is not clear why this report got so much attention while its predecessors got so little. Four factors which may have contributed are a) the advances in statistical methods since the 1950s which allowed us to show that the HDL association was not explained by other lipoprotein levels; b) the work of Glomset[9] and the Millers[10] which provided a possible physiological basis for the findings; c) the fact that many labs were measuring HDL as a step in the assessment of other lipoproteins; and d) the wide circulation of the *New England Journal of Medicine*."

1. **Fredrickson D S, Levy R I & Lees R S.** Fat transport in lipoproteins—an integrated approach to mechanisms and disorders. *N. Engl. J. Med.* **276**:34-44; 94-103; 148-56; 215-25; 273-81, 1967. [Citation Classic. *Current Contents* (3):11, 16 January 1978.]
2. **Barr D P, Russ E M & Eder H A.** Protein-lipid relationships in human plasma. *Amer. J. Med.* **11**:480-93, 1951.
3. **Nikkilä E.** Studies on lipid-protein relationships in normal and pathological sera and the effect of heparin on serum lipoproteins. *Scand. J. Clin. Lab. Invest.* **5**(Suppl. 8):1-101, 1953.
4. **Oliver M F & Boyd G S.** Serum lipoprotein patterns in coronary sclerosis and associated conditions. *Brit. Heart J.* **17**:299-302, 1955.
5. **Jencks W P, Hyatt M R, Jetton M R, Mattingly T W & Durrum E L.** A study of serum lipoproteins in normal and atherosclerotic patients by paper electrophoretic techniques. *J. Clin. Invest.* **35**:980-90, 1956.
6. **Brunner D & Lobl K.** Serum cholesterol, electrophoretic lipid pattern, diet and coronary artery disease: a study in coronary patients and in healthy men of different origin and occupations in Israel. *Ann. Intern. Med.* **49**:732-50, 1958.
7. **Dodds C & Mills G L.** Influence of myocardial infarction on plasma-lipoprotein concentration. *Lancet* **1**:1160-3, 1959.
8. **Medalie J H, Kahn H A, Neufeld H N, Riss E & Goldbourt U.** Five-year myocardial infarction incidence—II. Association of single variables to age and birthplace. *J. Chronic Dis.* **26**:329-49, 1973.
9. **Glomset J A.** The plasma lecithin: cholesterol acyltransferase reaction. *J. Lipid Res.* **9**:155-67, 1968.
10. **Miller G J & Miller N E.** Plasma-high-density-lipoprotein concentration and development of ischaemic heart-disease. *Lancet* **1**:16-19, 1975. [Citation Classic. *Current Contents/Life Sciences* **24**(15):21, 13 April 1981.]

CC/NUMBER 45
NOVEMBER 9, 1981

This Week's Citation Classic

Oliver M F, Kurien V A & Greenwood T W. Relation between serum-free-fatty-acids and arrhythmias and death after acute myocardial infarction. *Lancet* **1**:710-15, 1968. [Depts. Cardiology and Clinical Chemistry and Coronary Care Unit, Royal Infirmary, Edinburgh, Scotland]

Elevation of serum-free-fatty-acids (FFA) occurs during acute myocardial ischemia and, when marked, is associated with ventricular arrhythmias. This elevation results from catecholamine-induced lipolysis. Myocardial lipolysis is also increased. Metabolism of excess FFA may increase oxygen consumption in an already ischemic myocardium. [The *SCI*® indicates that this paper has been cited over 250 times since 1968.]

Michael F. Oliver
Department of Medicine
Cardiovascular Research Unit
University of Edinburgh
Edinburgh EH8 9XF
Scotland

August 20, 1981

"There were two origins to the hypothesis that an excess of free-fatty-acids (FFA) might be one of the causes of ventricular arrhythmias during acute myocardial ischemia.

"A laboratory observation made when working in the University of Edinburgh with George Boyd in the middle-1950s on paper electrophoresis of serum lipoproteins was of a fast moving, lipid-rich peak, related to the mobility of albumen, which contained no cholesterol or phospholipid. This was frequently present in patients with acute myocardial infarction (MI) and never in those with previous MI or angina pectoris. A conceptual question which later interested me was what is the relationship between available myocardial energy and the intrinsic development of ventricular arrhythmias? One possibility was that the ionic disequilibrium initiating VF is entirely related to reduced coronary blood flow and is independent of substrate availability—the arrhythmia, once initiated, would rapidly use up substrate to the point of exhaustion. The other, which formed the basis of the hypothesis, was that potentially lethal ventricular arrhythmias might be initiated and perpetuated by an uneconomic excess of one or more of the sources of myocardial energy. The obvious choice, in a situation where there is an excess of catecholamines, such as a heart attack, was FFA.

"In 1965, Abraham Kurien, who had independently been measuring 'lip-albumen,' and I showed[1] that serum FFA levels were significantly higher in patients with acute MI compared with those with acute renal colic and those with cerebral thrombosis. It was then a simple step to examine the relationship of raised serum FFA with the incidence of serious ventricular arrhythmias during an acute heart attack. The observation that arrhythmias were significantly more frequent and that there are more deaths when plasma FFA exceed a 2:1 molar binding ratio with albumen (approximately 1200 μ eq/l) is the subject of this *Citation Classic*.

"I believe that the 1968 paper has been frequently cited because it was the first that provided factual evidence pointing to a fundamental metabolic disturbance during acute myocardial ischemia in man. It also provided the basis for the subsequent hypothesis[2] that an excess of peripheral and myocardial FFA can lead to increased myocardial oxygen requirements (subsequently demonstrated)[3] and that an acute energy crisis in the ischemic myocardium can lead to the development of lethal reentry arrhythmias. Later, we showed that pharmacologic[4] reduction of peripheral and myocardial lipolysis decreased the incidence of ventricular arrhythmias in patients with MI. Lipid-free albumen reduces experimental ischemia[5] and anti-lipolytic treatment reduces the extent of myocardial ischemia in patients."[6]

1. **Oliver M F & Kurien V A.** Serum-free-fatty-acids after acute myocardial infarction and cerebral vascular occlusion. *Lancet* **2**:122-7, 1966.
2. **Kurien V A & Oliver M F.** A metabolic cause for arrhythmias during acute myocardial hypoxia. *Lancet* **1**:813-15, 1970.
3. **Mjøs O D.** Effect of free fatty acids on myocardial function and oxygen consumption in intact dogs. *J. Clin. Invest.* **50**:1386-9, 1971.
4. **Rowe M J, Neilson J M M & Oliver M F.** Control of ventricular arrhythmias during myocardial infarction by antilipolytic treatment using a nicotinic-acid analogue. *Lancet* **1**:295-300, 1975.
5. **Miller N E, Mjøs O D & Oliver M F.** Relationship of epicardial ST segment elevation to the plasma free fatty acid/albumin ratio during coronary occlusion in dogs. *Clin. Sci. Mol. Med.* **51**:209-13, 1976.
6. **Russell D C & Oliver M F.** Effect of antilipolytic therapy on ST segment elevation during myocardial ischaemia in man. *Brit. Heart J.* **40**:117-23, 1978.

CC/NUMBER 3
JANUARY 19, 1981

This Week's Citation Classic

Trowell H. Ischemic heart disease and dietary fiber.
Amer. J. Clin. Nutr. **25**:926-32, 1972.

Fiber, redefined as dietary fiber, contains hemicelluloses, cellulose, pectin, and lignin. This definition has been accepted in Europe and the United States. Lightly processed, high-fiber, high-complex carbohydrate foods protect against ischemic heart disease, the commonest cause of death in the western world. [The *SCI*® indicates that this paper has been cited over 195 times since 1972.]

Hugh Trowell
Windhover
Woodgreen, Fordingbridge
Hampshire SP6 2AZ
England

November 29, 1980

"In 1960 after teaching medicine for 30 years in East Africa I wrote a book in which a small suggestion was made that high-fiber African diets might protect against diseases of the colon, such as diverticular disease and colonic cancer.[1] Then I retired to England. In 1970 my younger surgical colleague Denis Burkitt started writing articles about fiber. Then we planned a joint article; eventually we edited a book about fiber.[2] He wrote that I must define fiber. No English or American book on nutrition or gastroenterology or food tables then even mentioned fiber. The *Index Medicus* did not have this heading until 1977. When I discovered this I was stunned; it was certainly in plant foods.

"A few animal foodstuff tables reported fiber as crude fiber, estimating it by a 150-year-old method. Plant foods were extracted by dilute acid, followed by dilute alkali; the dried residue was the crude fiber (CF). Too crude! I wanted a figure for the residue remaining after digestion by human alimentary enzymes. This I defined to be dietary fiber (DF). Wheat white flour contains CF 0.1 percent, but DF 3.4 percent. Some difference!

"Food manufacturers of animal laboratory foodstuffs had published crude fiber figures; but the authors who used these animal foods rarely reported these unimportant data in their articles. Intrigued by this simple observation I examined all animal experiments to produce atherosclerosis; many articles reported that high-fiber foodstuffs reduced serum cholesterol levels. There had been few experiments in human volunteers to test this idea.

"As ischemic heart disease is the commonest cause of death in the western world and high serum cholesterol levels are a risk factor, interest in fiber therefore grew rapidly. Subsequently no 'cures' of ischemic heart disease have been reported, but the milder form of this disease—angina—has disappeared fairly often in patients taking low-salt, high-fiber, high-complex carbohydrate, low-fat diets; they stop all drugs.[3] But then my Kikuyu patients ate this type of diet in 1930 and had virtually no ischemic heart disease."

1. **Trowell H C.** *Non-infective disease in Africa.* London: Arnold, 1960. 481 p.
2. **Burkitt D P & Trowell H C,** eds. *Refined carbohydrate foods and disease. Some implications of dietary fibre.* London: Academic Press, 1975. 370 p.
3. **Trowell H C & Burkitt D P,** eds. *Western diseases: their emergence and prevention.* London: Arnold, 1981. In press.

CC/NUMBER 34
AUGUST 23, 1982

This Week's Citation Classic

Ross R & Glomset J A. The pathogenesis of atherosclerosis. *N. Engl. J. Med.* **295**:369-77; 420-5, 1976. [Depts. Pathology, Medicine, and Biochemistry, Sch. Med., and Regional Primate Research Ctr., Univ. Washington, Seattle, WA]

The structure of the normal artery wall and data on our understanding of the cell biology of endothelium and smooth muscle *in vitro* and *in vivo* are covered. Three hypotheses of atherogenesis are discussed including the 'response to injury hypothesis,'[1] the 'monoclonal hypothesis,'[2] and the 'clonal senescence hypothesis.'[3] These are each evaluated, compared, and contrasted, and the potential role of lipids and connective tissues in atherogenesis is discussed. [The *SCI*® indicates that these papers have been cited over 880 times in 591 publications since 1976.]

Russell Ross
Department of Pathology
School of Medicine
University of Washington
Seattle, WA 98195

July 1, 1982

"The two-part paper on the pathogenesis of atherosclerosis written by John Glomset and myself began as a result of a request from the *New England Journal of Medicine* to write a review on studies that I had been pursuing on wound healing and inflammation. By the time that request had been received, John and I had, for a number of years, been very much involved in studying a number of aspects of the biology of arterial smooth muscle and endothelium and had become very much interested in the problems of atherogenesis and the state of the field. We spent many hours talking about various ideas and decided if we could convince the *New England Journal of Medicine* to change their invitation from one dealing with a review of wound healing to one dealing with atherosclerosis that we would tackle the problem of trying to put into perspective many of the ideas that we had tossed around over the preceding years, with a particular view to examining the question from the viewpoint of the cell biologist.

"One unique feature of the school of medicine at the University of Washington was the fact that at particular points in time at least three hypotheses of atherogenesis had been developed,[1-3] surprisingly, all emanating from the same department! Since all three of these hypotheses had generated a fair amount of interest, we decided that after discussing the cell biology of the problem, those notions and ideas should be related to the hypotheses at that particular state of their development, with, we must admit, some bias toward the 'response to injury hypothesis of atherosclerosis' that we had proposed to test.

"We have been fortunate to receive wide recognition for our work on the 'response to injury hypothesis.' More important, we hope that this paper served as a catalyst to help change directions in this field. Our ideas have changed quite a bit since this review was written in 1976 and although some of the notions have proved to be correct, a number of them have changed with the advent of new information concerning the biology of endothelium, smooth muscle, and, in particular, of the monocyte/macrophage and the platelet and their potential role in this entire process. Therefore, the 'response to injury hypothesis' today appears somewhat different from the one published in the cited paper and probably in another five years' time, the one that we would propose today would again appear different based on new information as it becomes available. I have recently published a paper in this field."[4]

1. **Ross R & Glomset J A.** Atherosclerosis and the arterial smooth muscle cell. *Science* **180**:1332-9, 1973.
2. **Benditt E P & Benditt J M.** Evidence for a monoclonal origin of human atherosclerotic plaques. *Proc. Nat. Acad. Sci. US* **70**:1753-6, 1973.
3. **Martin G, Ogburn C & Sprague C.** Senescence and vascular disease. (Cristafalo V J, Roberts J & Adelman R C, eds.) *Exploration in aging.* New York: Plenum Press, 1975. p. 163-93.
4. **Ross R.** George Lyman Duff Memorial Lecture. Atherosclerosis—a problem of the biology of arterial wall cells and their interaction with blood components. *Arteriosclerosis* **1**:293-311, 1981.

CC/NUMBER 52
DECEMBER 24-31, 1984

This Week's Citation Classic™

Lindner A, Charra B, Sherrard D J & Scribner B H. Accelerated atherosclerosis in prolonged maintenance hemodialysis. *N. Engl. J. Med.* **290**:697-701, 1974.
[Dept. Medicine (Nephrology), Univ. Washington Sch. Medicine, and Veterans Administration Hosp., Seattle, WA]

Life-table analysis of survival of the first 39 patients receiving maintenance hemodialysis in Seattle since 1960 revealed an inordinately high morbidity and mortality from arteriosclerotic cardiovascular complications. These findings indicated that accelerated atherosclerosis is a major risk to long-term survivors on maintenance hemodialysis. [The *SCI*® indicates that this paper has been cited in over 395 publications since 1974.]

Armando Lindner
Veterans Administration Medical Center
4435 Beacon Avenue South
Seattle, WA 98108

August 17, 1984

"In 1974, when this study was done, long-term survival on hemodialysis had become a reality for many patients with end-stage renal disease. By that time, initial assessments of life expectancy (mostly based on unsupported data) suggested that, if a patient had remained alive on dialysis for a few years, he might survive indefinitely since major complications had not been recognized. On the other hand, we and other nephrologists had observed cases of myocardial infarction, angina pectoris, and strokes, which prompted a careful statistical analysis of our patient population. Our patients were ideal for this study since they represented a homogeneous group of fairly young adult males (mean age 37 years), with no preexistent cardiovascular disease (other than hypertension in some cases) prior to the onset of dialysis treatment.

"To our surprise, life-table analysis demonstrated an inordinately high morbidity and mortality from cardiovascular complications of atherosclerosis when compared with rates for age-matched normals or hypertensive patients without renal disease.

"The implications were serious, since they indicated an increasingly higher probability of developing (and dying from) coronary heart disease after several years of dialysis. On the other hand, this study could not elucidate the causes of this phenomenon, nor the possible role of uremia *per se* in the premature production of atherosclerotic lesions.

"One factor kept us from submitting this paper for publication for about six months after its completion. Both Scribner and I agonized about the possible psychological impact of these findings, that fear of dialysis complications might deter those with end-stage renal failure from receiving this life-saving treatment. Eventually, we came to believe that our findings would stimulate others to investigate the pathogenesis of this phenomenon and to look for specific ways of preventing it.

"We think that this publication has been so highly cited for several reasons. First, it provided the first conclusive evidence of a clinical problem that could potentially shorten survival in uremic patients on long-term hemodialysis. Second, it suggested that premature atherosclerosis in uremic patients could be a model for the study of this vascular complication in the general population. Third, it provided impetus for the subsequent performance of a number of studies of this problem in many countries. Finally, even today, the conclusions of this study continue to generate controversy. Thus, a study of over 300 patients in Alabama demonstrated complication rates almost identical to ours, yet the conclusions were not alike.[1] On the other hand, the strongest confirmation of our findings came from the life-table analysis in a population of over 50,000 patients from many European countries,[2] which showed annual death rates from coronary heart disease to be more than 10 times higher among uremic patients on dialysis, particularly for the younger (15-to-34-year) age group."

1. **Rostand S G, Gretes J C, Kirk K A, Rutsky E A & Andreoli T E.** Ischemic heart disease in patients with uremia undergoing maintenance hemodialysis. *Kidney Int.* **16**:600-11, 1979.
2. **Brunner F P, Brynger H, Chantler C, Donckerwolcke R A, Hathway R A, Jacobs C, Selwood N H & Wing A J.** Combined report on regular dialysis and transplantation in Europe, IX, 1978. *Proc. Eur. Dial. Transpl. Assoc.* **16**:2-73, 1979.

CC/NUMBER 17
APRIL 27, 1981

This Week's Citation Classic

Rona G, Chappel C I, Balazs T & Gaudry R. An infarct-like myocardial lesion and other toxic manifestations produced by isoproterenol in the rat. *Arch. Pathol.* **67**:443-55, 1959.
[Research Labs., Ayerst, McKenna, and Harrison, Ltd., Montreal, Canada]

This paper reported that the synthetic catecholamine isoproterenol produced massive myocardial necrosis in rats which resembled human myocardial infarction. The fact that coronary arteries were patent suggested that a relative ischemia, elicited by exaggerated β adrenergic stimulation and reduced coronary blood flow, is responsible for the infarct-like character of the myocardial necrosis. [The *SCI*® indicates that this paper has been cited over 270 times since 1961.]

G. Rona
Department of Pathology
Pathology Institute
McGill University
Montreal, Quebec H3A 2B4
Canada

April 8, 1981

"In 1957, my wife, Agnes (also a pathologist), two young sons, and I immigrated to Canada from Budapest, Hungary, where, inspired by Joseph Baló, I had been involved in research on diabetic glomerulosclerosis. Good fortune brought me a position as head of pathology and toxicology at Ayerst Research Laboratories, Montreal, where R. Gaudry and C.I. Chappel initiated comparative studies on bronchodilators including a synthetic catecholamine in the developmental stage, CC-25. T. Balazs, who performed the subacute toxicity study, notified me of unexpected high mortality. I made the stunning discovery that the deaths appeared to be due to myocardial infarct. Previous toxicity studies in Germany made no mention of this lesion; furthermore, CC-25 was related to isoproterenol (ISO), a synthetic β adrenergic depressor catecholamine not known to have such an effect. On my recommendation, we investigated ISO under similar conditions, and to our amazement, use of a wide dose range resulted in massive infarct-like myocardial necrosis. While the pharmaceutical companies concerned were very upset, I was elated as the door opened on 20 years of rewarding research.

"Appreciation of the scientific value of our results was far from immediate; the paper cited as a classic was refused by several reputable journals including *Science* and *Lancet*. The finding that infarct-like myocardial necrosis could be produced without cutting off the blood supply to the myocardium was irreconcilable with the current medical knowledge. The only solid support came from the studies at the Büchner Institute at Freiburg im Breisgau during the 1930s which demonstrated the role of hypoxia in experimental disseminated myocardial necrosis.[1]

"On publication, our studies aroused great interest. The close correlation of dose to degree of severity offered a standardized technique for observing various interactions[2] and also the effects of drugs used to manage human myocardial disease. Among the scientists who applied our findings to basic research on cardiac metabolism and ultrastructure as well as in clinical cardiology was A. Fleckenstein, who developed a series of widely used Ca^{++} antagonistic drugs.[3]

"Our research, based at Ayerst until 1965, moved to McGill University where, assisted by a succession of brilliant research fellows, we investigated the pathogenesis of ISO-induced myocardial necrosis, particularly the role of coronary microcirculatory factors[4] in the evolution of catecholamine-induced and reperfusion injury.[5] International recognition came in 1976 when I was awarded the prestigious Arthur Weber prize. In the same year, I was elected president of the American Division of the International Society for Heart Research."

1. **Büchner F, Weber A & Haager B.** *Koronarinfarkt und Koronarinsuffizienz.* Leipzig: Georg Thieme Verlag, 1935.
2. **Rona G, Chappel C I & Kahn D S.** The significance of factors modifying the development of isoproterenol-induced myocardial necrosis. *Amer. Heart J.* **66**:389-95, 1963.
3. **Fleckenstein A.** Specific inhibitors and promotors of calcium action in the excitation-contraction coupling of heart muscle and their role in the prevention of production of myocardial lesions. (Harris P & Opie L, eds.) *Calcium and the heart.* London: Academic Press, 1971. p. 135-88.
4. **Rona G, Hüttner I & Boutet M.** Microcirculatory changes in myocardium with particular reference to catecholamine-induced cardiac muscle cell injury. (Meesen H, ed.) *Handbuch der allgemeinen Pathologie: Mikrozirkulation.* Berlin: Springer-Verlag, 1977. Vol. III, part 7. p. 791-888.
5. **Rona G, Badonnel M C, Hüttner I & Boutet M.** Reperfusion effect upon ischemic myocardial injury. *Exp. Mol. Pathol.* **31**:211-18, 1979.

CC/NUMBER 41
OCTOBER 10, 1983

This Week's Citation Classic

Hancock E W & Cohn K. The syndrome associated with midsystolic click and late systolic murmur. *Amer. J. Med.* **41**:183-96, 1966.
[Dept. Medicine, Stanford Univ. Sch. Medicine, Palo Alto, CA]

Clinical analysis of 40 patients with mid-systolic clicks, with or without associated late systolic murmur, showed that the associated features of unexplained chest pain and dyspnea, cardiac arrhythmias with potential for sudden cardiac death, familial occurrence, and the presence of other congenital anomalies indicate a somewhat characteristic syndrome which was not previously well delineated, although not rare. [The *SCI*® indicates that this paper has been cited in over 230 publications since 1966.]

E. William Hancock
Cardiology Division
Stanford University Medical Center
Stanford, CA 94305

June 9, 1983

"As a young faculty member in cardiology at Stanford University in the early 1960s, I was interested in the mid-systolic click, because of my previous work on the ejection click and because of evidence then becoming available that the mid-systolic click was probably mitral valvular in origin rather than pericardial, as had been believed by most authorities before 1960. Aided by the excellent facilities for phonocardiography that Herbert Hultgren had developed at Stanford, I began to assemble a list of patients with what I called the 'mitral-pericardial syndrome.'

"In 1965, I was visited by Norman Sissman, our pediatric cardiologist, to discuss a child he was seeing with mid-systolic click and late systolic murmur. The patient's mother, whom I had seen previously for palpitation due to multiple ventricular premature beats associated with mid-systolic click and late systolic murmur, had recently dropped dead suddenly; there was naturally a great concern about finding the same auscultatory findings in the eight-year-old child. This was my first indication that the mid-systolic click might be more important than an auscultatory curiosity. In addition, the familial occurrence seemed to be a new observation. I encouraged Keith Cohn, a fellow in cardiology, to review our collected cases to see whether any sense could be made of it. This review showed such a high prevalence of premature beats and other arrhythmias, along with other features, that we thought it was justified to describe this as a syndrome.

"The publication of our paper was not initially met with much more than polite interest. Indeed, Cohn seemed to have some reluctance to announce a new syndrome, as he felt that I should be the first author even though he had done most of the data collection and analysis. However, the concept of a click-murmur syndrome (later redefined as mitral valve prolapse after the introduction of echocardiography) was very quickly accepted, and a burgeoning literature on the subject soon developed and continues to the present.[1] In essence, a new and perhaps the most frequent form of valvular heart disease had been discovered.

"I think our paper has been frequently quoted because it was the earliest broad synthesis of previously scattered observations into the concept of a new and important cardiological syndrome. The descriptions of 1966 remain generally valid, despite the many additions later and the much continuing controversy about many aspects of this problem.

"Incidentally, the eight-year-old girl of 1965 is now a healthy young adult, and has never had any significant arrhythmia, although the click and murmur have persisted."

1. **Gravanis M B & Campbell W G, Jr.** The syndrome of prolapse of the mitral valve: an etiologic and pathogenic enigma. *Arch. Pathol. Lab. Med.* **106**:369-74, 1982.

CC/NUMBER 26
JUNE 27, 1983

This Week's Citation Classic

Barlow J B, Bosman C K, Pocock W A & Marchand P. Late systolic murmurs and non-ejection ("mid-late") systolic clicks: an analysis of 90 patients. *Brit. Heart J.* **30**:203-18, 1968. [CSIR Cardio-Pulmonary Res. Unit and Cardiovasc. Res. Unit, Depts. Med. and Thoracic Surg., Univ. Witwatersrand, and Cardiac Clinic, Gen. Hosp., Johannesburg, South Africa]

This paper reaffirmed that late systolic murmurs and mid-systolic clicks are intracardiac in origin. These auscultatory features, a characteristic electrocardiographic pattern, and billowing of the posterior mitral leaflet constitute a specific and common syndrome. Diverse etiological factors can result in mitral valve prolapse. [The *SCI*® indicates that this paper has been cited over 295 times—the second most-cited paper ever published in *Brit. Heart J.*]

J.B. Barlow
Department of Cardiology
University of the Witwatersrand
and
Johannesburg Hospital
Johannesburg 2001
South Africa

May 4, 1983

"My interest in auscultation, phonocardiography, and the effects of vasoactive maneuvers on heart sounds and murmurs was kindled in the late-1950s when I was medical registrar to John McMichael and John Shillingford at the Postgraduate Medical School in London. During that time, I observed an abnormal mitral chorda tendinea at the necropsy of a patient who had had an isolated mid-systolic click. Completely independent of that unpublished observation, my compatriot, J.V.O. Reid, postulated[1] a mitral valve origin for mid-systolic clicks and suggested that mitral regurgitation may be an associated feature.

"Using left ventricular cineangiocardiography and the effects of various vasoactive maneuvers, we concluded[2] that late systolic murmurs denoted mitral regurgitation and that mid-systolic, which I later called 'non-ejection,'[3] clicks also arose at the mitral valve. Nonetheless, an extracardiac origin for these auscultatory features had been widely accepted and when I had the opportunity, in April 1964, to address the staff of Johns Hopkins Hospital, and it was known that I intended to present additional evidence of an intracardiac origin, I was introduced by B. Tabatznik as an 'iconoclast.'[3] The cardiologists at that famous institution accepted my conclusions but I remain indebted to one of them, J.M. Criley, for correcting a serious cineangiographic misinterpretation of mine.[3] It was Criley, in fact, who subsequently introduced the term 'prolapse' to describe the mitral valve anomaly. There were important aspects of mitral valve prolapse to explore at that time and my co-worker and friend, Wendy Pocock, contributed very significantly to all of the original observations.

"All research workers appreciate the frustrations which may be encountered before publication by a prestigious journal. Neither our original paper[2] nor a later study,[4] in which we recorded potentially fatal arrhythmias after exercise, were accepted by *Circulation*. The major reason for rejecting the first paper was our 'overstated conclusion that all systolic murmurs which are mainly or exclusively in late systole are due to mitral leak.' Critiques by reviewers of the second paper were so derogatory that the editor seemed apologetic when he wrote, 'I hope that you will regard them as being objective and of having some merit.' This *Citation Classic* was also rejected by *Circulation* because the editor could not 'assign it a sufficiently high priority.' It was published by the *British Heart Journal* only after it had been considerably abbreviated. After much encouragement from T.H. Bothwell, head of the department of medicine, I submitted the detailed data to this university for my MD thesis.

"This paper has been highly cited because it was the first to review or to describe the multiple features of mitral valve prolapse in a relatively large number of subjects. It discussed many problems which are still unresolved and thus continue to arouse much interest. Jeresaty's monograph[5] remains the most comprehensive review while our own current thoughts on the significance of this frequently diagnosed condition have recently been summarized.[6]

"Although I have received no specific awards or honors, the work has resulted in international recognition including use of the eponym for the 'specific syndrome' which I had described.[3] Most rewarding for me, however, has been the consequence that cardiologists from many countries now apply to work in this department."

1. **Reid J V O.** Mid-systolic clicks. *S. Afr. Med. J.* **35**:353-5, 1961.
2. **Barlow J B, Pocock W A, Marchand P & Denny M.** The significance of late systolic murmurs. *Amer. Heart J.* **66**:443-52, 1963.
[The *SCI* indicates that this paper has been cited in over 225 publications since 1963.]
3. **Barlow J B.** Conjoint clinic on the clinical significance of late systolic murmurs and non-ejection systolic clicks. *J. Chron. Dis.* **18**:665-73, 1965.
4. **Pocock W A & Barlow J B.** Post-exercise arrhythmias in the billowing posterior mitral leaflet syndrome. *Amer. Heart J.* **80**:740-5, 1970.
[The *SCI* indicates that this paper has been cited in over 80 publications since 1970.]
5. **Jeresaty R M.** *Mitral valve prolapse*. New York: Raven Press, 1979. 251 p.
6. **Barlow J B, Pocock W A & Obel I W P.** Mitral valve prolapse: primary, secondary, both or neither? *Amer. Heart J.* **102**:140-3, 1981.

CC/NUMBER 20
MAY 16, 1983

This Week's Citation Classic

Weissler A M, Harris W S & Schoenfeld C D. Systolic time intervals in heart failure in man. *Circulation* **37**:149-59, 1968.
[Dept. Medicine, Ohio State Univ. College of Medicine, Columbus, OH]

The systolic time intervals constituted the first contemporary quantitative noninvasive measure of global left ventricular performance in man. In this investigation, normative data were established and the pattern of change in left ventricular decompensation was documented. [The *SCI*® indicates that this paper has been cited in over 700 publications since 1968.]

Arnold M. Weissler
Department of Medicine
Rose Medical Center
Denver, CO 80220

March 28, 1983

"In the mid-1960s, technical developments in cardiac catheterization had emerged to the point where virtually all hemodynamic measures characterizing the performance of the cardiac chambers could be determined in patients with cardiovascular disease. With the escalating cost of cardiac catheterization and knowledge that vast numbers of patients required cardiac evaluation, it soon became evident that newer, less expensive, and less intrusive diagnostic methods were needed. It was at this time that I promoted the view that valid quantitative physiologic measures of the performance of the heart could be derived by methods which involved only the recording of potentials and pulsations at the body's surface. Adding to the advantage of modifying and reducing the use of invasive diagnostic modalities, such methods offered the benefits of reduced risk, less discomfort, and a potential for diminished expense in medical care.

"In conceptualizing such methods, it became apparent that of the various measures of cardiac performance conventionally applied, the determination of the duration of the events of the cardiac cycle was the most neglected. I hypothesized that the heart must be regulated relative to the timing of its performance. Thus, just as alterations in chamber pressure, volume, and output occurred in left ventricular decompensation, the time intervals of the contractile cycle might also change in a predictable fashion.

"In this paper, my colleagues, W.S. Harris and C.D. Schoenfeld, and I established the normal linear regression relationships between heart rate and the duration of the systolic time intervals among 121 normal male and 90 normal female subjects in the age range of 19-65 years. These normative data were the first to be established by modern methods. They served as a basis for comparison with patients with cardiovascular disease. In order to focus on the effects of left ventricular decompensation on systolic intervals, studies were performed on cardiac patients in sinus rhythm who retained normal ventricular depolarization, and who were receiving no digitalis or antihypertensive medication. The studies demonstrated that the failing left ventricle is characterized by the presence of a prolonged systolic pre-ejection period (PEP) and an abbreviated left ventricular ejection time (LVET) while total electromechanical systole remains within normal limits. Both subcomponents of the PEP, the Q-1 interval and the isovolumic contraction time, were found to be prolonged. Since this study was performed prior to the availability of ejection fraction measurements, the alterations in systolic time intervals were related to the left ventricular stroke volume and the cardiac output as measured by the indicator dilution technique. It was demonstrated that the prolongation in the PEP and the abbreviation in the LVET were well correlated with the reduced stroke volume and cardiac output. In addition, it was shown that when arterial diastolic pressure exceeded 100 mm Hg, there was independent prolongation of the PEP with no influence on the LVET.

"This study was the first to establish the consistent pattern of alterations in systolic time intervals in patients with left ventricular decompensation. It provided a new dimension of left ventricular function which could be added to conventional expressions for quantitating left ventricular decompensation. The systolic time interval measurement offered the special advantage that it could be obtained by entirely noninvasive methods. Indeed, the systolic time intervals constituted the first measure of left ventricular performance to which the term noninvasive was applied. Numerous papers on the application of systolic time intervals followed.[1] In subsequent years the use of echocardiography and radioisotopic methods for determining the extent and rate of left ventricular chamber contraction were added as useful noninvasive modalities."

1. **Weissler A M, Lewis R P & Boudoulas H.** Key references, systolic time intervals. *Circulation* **64**:862-7, 1981.

CC/NUMBER 22
MAY 30, 1983

This Week's Citation Classic

Hinkle L E, Jr., Carver S T & Stevens M. The frequency of asymptomatic disturbances of cardiac rhythm and conduction in middle-aged men. *Amer. J. Cardiol.* **24**:629-50, 1969.
[Div. Human Ecology, Depts. Medicine and Psychiatry, Cornell Univ. Med. Coll., New York, NY]

The electrocardiograms (ECGs) of a random sample of 301 men aged 55-60 were recorded during six hours of standardized activity. Asymptomatic abnormalities of rate, rhythm, or conduction were found in 92.6 percent. Men with frequent ventricular dysrhythmias or conduction abnormalities had significantly more coronary deaths within five years. [The *SCI*® indicates that this paper has been cited in over 290 publications since 1969.]

Lawrence E. Hinkle, Jr.
Department of Medicine
Division of Human Ecology
New York Hospital—
Cornell Medical Center
New York, NY 10021

March 31, 1983

"In the early-1960s, I was seeking a method for recording the ECGs of active people over long periods to investigate the hypothesis that many out-of-hospital sudden deaths were caused by cardiac arrhythmias. Learning that Norman J. Holter had developed a recorder, I flew to his laboratory in Helena, Montana, and borrowed one. It proved able to do the job, but what was 'normal' and what was 'abnormal' for ECG recordings obtained with these devices was not evident.

"With Jerome Meyer, we first determined the electronic and mechanical characteristics of the recorders that might affect the form of the ECG signal, and we developed a method for obtaining accurate hard copy write-outs of ECGs using a photographic rapid-writer with a wide frequency range.[1] My colleague, Susan T. Carver, developed a standard protocol of recording, designed to demonstrate the effects of position of the body, physical activity, intake of food and fluids, digestion, cigarette smoking, and mild anxiety. She and I together developed a protocol for analyzing the ECG data for abnormalities of rate, rhythm, conduction, and repolarization. Michael Stevens, working with us, learned how to recognize the waveforms in the recordings. Over the course of four years, he laboriously investigated every area of potential abnormality that appeared in the photographic write-outs, which Carver and I then reviewed independently.

"To obtain a sample of 'normal men' we utilized the nationwide population of 260,000 men in the Bell Telephone System, which had known demographic characteristics and rates of coronary heart disease and sudden deaths similar to those of all American men. We drew a random sample of 356 men aged 55-60 from all those on the payroll in New Jersey and then traveled to cities, towns, and rural areas throughout the state persuading the designated men to come to New York and spend a day having their ECGs recorded. All of the 301 who did so were followed thereafter for ten years.

"I believe that the report of this research has been cited so widely because it was influential in establishing long-term recording of the ECGs of active people as a valuable diagnostic procedure. It demonstrated that a large proportion of ostensibly healthy American men had disorders of their cardiac rate, rhythm, conduction, and repolarization, most of which were asymptomatic; and that the risk of death was greater among the men who had many ventricular dysrhythmias or major disorders of conduction. The report stimulated the widespread use of Holter's recorder. Ultimately, it helped to provide a basis for the present efforts to prevent sudden death by controlling ventricular dysrhythmias and disorders of conduction.

"This research was carried out by the Division of Human Ecology in the department of medicine at the Cornell University Medical College. I was associate professor of medicine, Carver was assistant professor of medicine, and Stevens was research assistant to Carver and me.

"For recent summaries of work in this field, see references 2 and 3."

1. **Hinkle L E, Jr., Meyer J, Stevens M & Carver S T.** Tape recordings of the ECG of active men: limitations and advantages of the Holter-Avionics instruments. *Circulation* **36**:752-65, 1967.
2. **Wenger N K, Mock M B & Ringqvist I,** eds. *Ambulatory electrocardiographic recording*. Chicago: Yearbook Medical Publishers, 1981. 456 p.
3. **Hinkle L E, Jr.** The immediate antecedents of sudden death. *Acta Med. Scand.* **210**(Suppl. 651):207-17, 1981.

CC/NUMBER 50
DECEMBER 13, 1982

This Week's Citation Classic

Lown B & Wolf M. Approaches to sudden death from coronary heart disease. *Circulation* **44**:130-42, 1971.
[Cardiovascular Res. Labs., Dept. Nutrition, Harvard Sch. Public Health, and Levine Cardiac Unit, Cardiovascular Div., Dept. Med., Peter Bent Brigham Hosp., Boston, MA]

Sudden cardiac death (SCD) claims over 400,000 lives annually in the US. If they are to be saved, the victims need to be identified prior to the fatal event. The presence of certain types of ventricular extrasystoles exposed by monitoring and exercise stress testing is an indicator of risk for SCD. [The *SCI*® indicates that this paper has been cited in over 415 publications since 1971.]

Bernard Lown
Department of Nutrition
Harvard University School of Public Health
Boston, MA 02115

October 19, 1982

"The article was based on the Lewis A. Conner Memorial Lecture delivered at the Annual Scientific Session of the American Heart Association in 1970 before more than 7,000 physicians. It represented a review of ten years of work in my laboratory at the Harvard University School of Public Health and the Peter Bent Brigham Hospital. The research concerned the problem of sudden cardiac death, the leading cause of fatality in the industrially developed world. In the US alone it claims over 400,000 lives annually. Yet, the medical profession remained largely indifferent to this enormous challenge. The reasons related to the facts that sudden death was unexpected, occurred in seemingly healthy individuals outside the hospital without prodromes, and appeared as an act of God for which no remedy was in sight. The underlying mechanism was established to be ventricular fibrillation (VF), which represented an electrical disorganization of the heartbeat. Our early work indicated that this was a reversible and preventable electrical accident.[1] In the coronary care unit, the patient who develops VF can be promptly reverted electrically to a normal rhythm.[2] But how is the individual at risk to be identified. None of the usual risk factors such as smoking, high cholesterol, hypertension, or sedentary habits distinguished the individual prone to sudden death.

"Our hypothesis was that the occurrence of ventricular premature beats (VPBs) is associated with sudden death. This was a wild but not illogical conjecture. VPBs were ubiquitous and demonstrable among nearly 90 percent of patients with coronary heart disease. Therefore, it seemed unlikely that they could discriminate risk for fatality. However, VPBs are differentiated by attributes of frequency, by varying morphologies, by differed sites of origin within the heart, by occurring singly or in salvos, by their degree of prematurity, etc. Which of these attributes were of importance?

"To catapult the heart into VF requires that a strong electric current be delivered in the vulnerable period of the cardiac cycle. Thus, markedly premature VPBs were likely to discharge in their vulnerable period. But the energy content of VPBs was but one micro joule while it required 50,000 micro joules to induce VF. We solved this riddle by demonstrating that a sequence of closely coupled VPBs lowers the threshold for VF. And in the ischemic heart, a sequence of three early premature beats may prove sufficient to provoke VF. On the basis of these physiological observations, a grading system for VPBs, in relation to the risk of sudden death, was first proposed. By utilizing Holter monitoring and exercise stress testing, advanced grades of VPBs could be exposed. We also provided data showing that in the experimental animal sudden death could be prevented by the use of appropriate antiarrhythmic drugs. The VPB hypothesis has since been amply confirmed.[3]

"The importance of this work and the reason that it is highly cited is that for the first time it provided the clinician with an approach to the patient threatened with sudden death. The grading system for VPBs proposed in this communication continues to be employed worldwide to stratify patients at risk or to assess the efficacy of antiarrhythmic drug therapy."

1. **Lown B, Fakhro A M, Hood W B, Jr. & Thorn G W.** The coronary care unit: new perspectives and directions. *J. Amer. Med. Assn.* **199**:188-98, 1967.
2. **Lown B, Amarasingham R & Neuman J.** New method for terminating cardiac arrhythmias: use of synchronized capacitor discharge. *J. Amer. Med. Assn.* **182**:548-55, 1962.
[Citation Classic. *Current Contents/Clinical Practice* 7(17):18, 23 April 1979.]
3. **Ruberman W, Weinblatt E, Goldberg J D, Frank C W & Shapiro S.** Ventricular premature beats and mortality after myocardial infarction. *N. Engl. J. Med.* **297**:750-7, 1977.

This Week's Citation Classic

Blackburn H, Keys A, Simonson E, Rautaharju P & Punsar S. The electrocardiogram in population studies: a classification system. *Circulation* **21**:1160-75, 1960.
[Lab. Physiol. Hygiene, Univ. Minnesota, Minneapolis, MN]

The Minnesota Code meets a need in population studies and clinical trials for discrete, quantitative criteria, numerical codes, and detailed procedures for classification, training, and quality control. It is based on validated clinical-pathological criteria for electrocardiogram (ECG) items related to major cardiac conditions. [The *SCI*® indicates that this paper has been cited over 405 times since 1961.]

Henry Blackburn
Laboratory of Physiological Hygiene
University of Minnesota
Minneapolis, MN 55455

September 28, 1981

"In the 1950s, systematic population studies began on heart disease. They eventually demonstrated large population differences in the frequency of coronary and other major cardiovascular diseases. They established the influence of personal behavior and characteristics on future risk. Fresh from a residency in internal medicine, I joined the group of Ancel Keys and the laboratory of physiological hygiene at Minnesota. An immediate research need was to compare disease rates in populations and I was charged with development of clinical criteria and procedures to reduce random and systematic error in cardiac diagnoses. The ECG suggested obvious advantages for objective population comparisons. It represents relevant endpoints of ischemia, infarction, hypertrophy, and arrhythmia and is independent of other measures. In graphic form, it is amenable to standardized acquisition and bias-free measurement and classification. It is simple, inexpensive, and feasible for population studies and clinical trials. But nowhere to be found were agreed upon ECG criteria or any format for quantitative classification and coding. I thus set about to assemble the best criteria available and, where not available, worked with Ernst Simonson, Pentti Rautaharju, Gunnar Blomqvist, and Sven Punsar to develop and test sensitivity and specificity of new criteria among defined populations.

"The goal was to avoid impressionism and terminology—to stay strictly descriptive and quantitative. Findings were assembled according to Q-waves, representing scar, axis, and wave amplitudes reflecting hypertrophy, ST segment and T-wave findings reflecting ischemia, atrioventricular conduction defects, and arrhythmias. Within items, findings were arranged by magnitude, but without probability labels and were tested anew in independent populations. Finally, criteria were circulated among cardiological and epidemiological experts for use and criticism. The whole was assembled in the late-1950s, assigned codes, and published in the *Circulation* reference cited. Within days it happily became known as the Minnesota Code, reflecting well the far-flung collaborative researches of this laboratory.

"Designed primarily for our own comparisons of disease prevalence, the Minnesota Code showed considerable systematic and random variation in others' hands. So we set about to develop standard procedures, training, testing, and quality control. And we found, simultaneously with Geoffrey Rose at the University of London, that students and technicians could be trained to code ECGs routinely as reliably, and with greater incentive, than young physicians.

"Over the years, the need for ECG coding has increased for longitudinal population studies, and for objective classification of events and serial records in clinical and preventive trials. The needed modifications were first published in the manual *Cardiovascular Survey Methods*,[1] then for the Coronary Drug Project Trial,[2] and finally as a complete training and testing manual prepared by Ronald Prineas and Richard Crow of this laboratory.[3]

"The Minnesota Code met a need at a propitious time in the expansion of major population studies and preventive trials in cardiovascular diseases, and met further notoriety by WHO endorsement and publication. More sophisticated computerized ECG systems are now available and we are collaborating in this development to replace the Minnesota Code. But the economics of small studies, the necessity for comparison with past studies, and the persistent absence of an internationally agreed upon diagnostic computer ECG program have resulted in continued use of the Minnesota Code as the standard manual-visual ECG system for population studies.[4] It is not, however, recommended by us for clinical diagnostic use."

1. **Rose G A & Blackburn H.** *Cardiovascular survey methods.* Geneva: World Health Organization, 1968. p. 98-105; 137-54.
2. Selected CDP study forms. (Coronary Drug Project Research Group) *The coronary drug project: design, methods, and baseline results.* New York: American Heart Association, 1973. p. I-50-I-79.
3. **Prineas R, Crow R & Blackburn H.** *The Minnesota Code manual: procedures for measurement and classification of electrocardiographic findings in clinical trials and population studies.* Littleton: Wright-PSG. To be published, 1982.
4. **Prineas R & Blackburn H.** The resting electrocardiogram in epidemiological studies. Description and prediction. (van Bemmel J H & Willems J L, eds.) *Trends in computer-processed electrocardiograms.* Amsterdam: North-Holland, 1977. p. 339-44.

CC/NUMBER 31
AUGUST 3, 1981

This Week's Citation Classic

Robinson B F. Relation of heart rate and systolic blood pressure to the onset of pain in angina pectoris. *Circulation* **35**:1073-83, 1967.
[Dept. Medicine, St. George's Hospital Medical School, London, England]

Studies in patients with angina pectoris showed that the onset of pain under varying conditions could be consistently related to the level achieved by the product of heart rate and systolic arterial pressure. The rate-pressure product provides a useful clinical index of myocardial work. [The *SCI*® indicates that this paper has been cited over 295 times since 1967.]

Brian F. Robinson
Department of Pharmacology
St. George's Hospital Medical School
Cranmer Terrace
London SW17 0RE
England

June 15, 1981

"The early 1960s saw a sudden surge of interest in angina pectoris with the development of coronary arteriography by Mason Sones[1] and the emergence of the first β-adrenoceptor antagonist, pronethalol. I was fortunate to be involved through A.C. Dornhorst in the early clinical studies with pronethalol. The β-adrenoceptor antagonists had been the brainchild of J.W. Black[2] (since knighted by the Queen for his remarkable contributions to pharmacology) and he had been led to develop this new class of compound by the thought that selective inhibition of the effects of catecholamines upon the heart might provide a useful means of controlling the work and oxygen requirements of the myocardium in patients with angina pectoris. The role of the myocardial work load in determining the onset of angina was at that time far from clear (many problems remain today!) and this suggested to me the idea of investigating the relation between the two. Review of the physiological literature indicated that the heart rate and systolic pressure were probably the most important variables determining changes in myocardial oxygen consumption between rest and exercise and I therefore chose to use the product of the two as an index of myocardial work.

"The experimental work was carried out in the course of 1963 on the one day a week that I could keep relatively free for research. Each study involved continuous recording of intraarterial pressure during repeated bouts of exercise and other types of stress. The results led to the conclusion that the precipitation of angina normally resulted from an increase in the work of the myocardium, as measured by the rate-pressure product, to a critical level that was essentially fixed in each patient.

"It is pleasing to know that work I carried out nearly 20 years ago with a view to obtaining my MD has been accepted and is still referred to. The concept it put forward undoubtedly represents an oversimplification of the complex circulatory disturbances that lead to the onset of angina, but I hope, nevertheless, that it has proved useful as a way of thinking about the problem. Why has the paper been so frequently cited? Largely, I think, as a reference for the use of the rate-pressure product as a clinical index of myocardial work. When I originally decided upon these variables for my measure of myocardial work, I was strongly influenced by the fact that they could at least be easily measured and I had some reservations as to whether they provided the best available index. It was therefore with delight (and some relief!) that I learned that more recent work involving direct measurement of myocardial oxygen uptake in normal subjects had shown that the rate-pressure product is not only a valid index of oxygen consumption, but is a better predictor than some other indices that have been proposed."[3]

1. **Sones F M, Jr. & Shirey E K.** Cine coronary arteriography. *Mod. Conc. Cardiovasc. Dis.* **31**:735-8, 1962.
2. **Black J W & Stephenson J S.** Pharmacology of a new adrenergic beta-receptor-blocking compound (nethalide). *Lancet* **2**:311-14, 1962.
3. **Nelson R R, Gobel F L, Jorgensen C R, Wang K, Wang Y & Taylor H L.** Hemodynamic predictors of myocardial oxygen consumption during static and dynamic exercise. *Circulation* **50**:1179-89, 1974.

CC/NUMBER 19
MAY 7, 1979

This Week's Citation Classic

Lang E. A survey of complications of percutaneous retrograde arteriography (Seldinger Technique). *Radiology* **81**:257-63, 1963.
[Department of Radiology, Methodist Hospital, Indianapolis, IN]

The incidence of complications attendant to percutaneous retrograde arteriography is established on the basis of a survey tabulating 11,402 procedures. Contributing factors and underlying cause for the principal serious complications are identified, and potential modes for prevention or management of complications delineated. [The *SCI*® indicates that this paper has been cited over 185 times since 1963.]

Erich K. Lang
Department of Radiology
Louisiana State University
Medical Center
New Orleans, LA 70112

March 22, 1978

"The frequency of citation of this paper may well reflect its impact on wide acceptance of percutaneous retrograde arteriography in today's medical practice. While the diagnostic value of arteriography had been duly recognized for some time, the complexity of this procedure, and its attendant high rate of complication, had curtailed widespread use of this technique. Retrograde percutaneous arteriography offered for the first time a technically simple procedure to obtain this goal. Initially, however, acceptance of this valuable technique was restrained by the then unknown but often overestimated incidence of complication accompanying this procedure.

"On the basis of a large survey, the above treatise established in an authoritative fashion the true incidence of complications attendant retrograde percutaneous arteriography. The surveyed institutions represented a wide cross section of types of medical practice in this country and Canada. The established rate of mortality of 0.06% and of major complications of 0.7%, once forever, laid to rest apprehensions of a prohibitively high and hence unacceptable complication rate.

"With this restriction removed, the use and deployment of percutaneous retrograde arteriography experienced an unprecedented increase. The procedure, formerly primarily available in tertiary care centers, became now widely practiced in all community hospitals. The resultant enormous numerical experience identified new applications for this valuable technique. The facility for selective engagement of subsegmental vessels of deep seated organ systems suggested use as a therapeutic pathway to such remote segments. Selective perfusion with chemotherapeutic agents, selective embolization with radioactive infarct particles or embolization with inert material to curtail hemorrhage, all via a transcatheteral route, were added to the well established diagnostic applications of retrograde percutaneous arteriography.

"Much of the credit for acceptance of percutaneous retrograde arteriography for diagnostic and now therapeutic purposes, however, must be given to the authoritative and meticulous treatise establishing the safety of this technique at a time of early fields trials in their infancy."

CC/NUMBER 46
NOVEMBER 16, 1981

This Week's Citation Classic

Proudfit W L, Shirey E K & Sones F M, Jr. Selective cine coronary arteriography: correlation with clinical findings in 1,000 patients. *Circulation* **33**:901-10, 1966. [Depts. Cardiovascular Disease and Pediatric Cardiology and Cardiac Lab., Cleveland Clinic Foundation, Cleveland, OH]

Selective coronary arteriographic findings and clinical diagnoses were correlated in 1,000 patients. Of 300 thought to have no coronary disease clinically, only 17 percent had significant lesions. Almost all who had angina pectoris or myocardial infarction had arterial obstruction. [The *SCI®* indicates that this paper has been cited over 285 times since 1966.]

William L. Proudfit
Department of Cardiology
Cleveland Clinic Foundation
Cleveland, OH 44106

August 31, 1981

"Selective coronary arteriography was performed first by Sones in 1959. Sones was cautious about initiating clinical correlative studies, fearing misinterpretation of the arteriograms in early experience with a new technic. By 1961, he and Shirey had accumulated sufficient confidence that they were willing to permit me, whom they considered a clinical skeptic, to start such a study on 1,000 consecutive patients, except one patient was excluded because the left coronary artery was not visualized adequately. Most patients had ventriculography as well. Criteria for clinical and arteriographic diagnosis were developed and have been used with little modification since. Rigid definitions are required if correlations are to be meaningful.

"All patients had been suspected to have coronary disease by at least one physician. Although 300 were thought not to have significant coronary disease prior to catheterization, many of this group were convinced that they suffered from serious conditions, believed to limit life expectancy. Only 17 percent were shown to have significant disease, despite the fact that most were of an age that many physicians considered indicative of almost universal coronary disease. About one third of the 1,000 patients had no appreciable disease demonstrated, and approximately 60 percent had severe disease. A relatively small number had pain considered to be typical of severe angina pectoris, but no disease was found. Dramatic symptoms tend to occur in conversion neurosis and the text of the submitted manuscript referred to this fact as an explanation for the extreme symptoms in this subset. The editor wished rewording of the sentence in the proofs, so it was changed to, 'The neurotic with conversion obtains secondary gain by having the most severe and disabling symptoms.' The printer changed 'conversion' to 'convulsion'—a wording that must have mystified many.

"If coronary arteriography is a sensitive test, it should be possible to demonstrate severe coronary disease in almost all patients who have typical angina pectoris or myocardial infarction, the two best-defined clinical syndromes. Serious coronary obstructions were shown in 93 and 98 percent of such patients, respectively. Other clinical syndromes caused by coronary disease are less well defined, so correlation with the presence of severe coronary lesions would be expected to be lower, and it was. Later, the distribution of coronary lesions in this same group of 1,000 patients was reported.[1]

"This paper may be cited frequently because it confirmed objectively opinions held by many clinicians since the introduction of postmortem injection studies of the coronary arteries. Coronary arteriography is so simple and safe and the results so clear that correlation with defined clinical diagnoses is easy to understand and accept. The earliest beneficial effect was increased caution subsequently in the clinical diagnosis of coronary disease without adequate basis. Finally, it formed a rational foundation for later prognostic studies. The conclusions of this paper have been confirmed in a recent review."[2]

1. **Proudfit W L, Shirey E K & Sones F M.** Distribution of arterial lesions demonstrated by selective cinecoronary arteriography. *Circulation* **36**:54-62, 1967.
2. **Chaitman B R, Bourassa M G, Davis K, Rogers W J, Tyras D H, Berger R, Kennedy J W, Fisher L, Judkins M P, Mock M B & Killip T.** Angiographic prevalence of high-risk coronary artery disease in patient subsets (CASS). *Circulation* **64**:360-7, 1981.

NUMBER 7
FEBRUARY 12, 1979

This Week's Citation Classic

Cohen L S, Elliott W C, Klein M D & Gorlin R. Coronary heart disease: clinical, cinearteriographic and metabolic correlations. *Amer. J. Cardiol.* **17**:153-68, 1966.

Sixty patients with coronary artery disease were studied by selective coronary cinearteriography and coronary sinus catheterization, with measurement of coronary flow, oxygen and lactate extraction at rest and during a stressful state. Coronary flow and coronary oxygen extraction patterns did not distinguish patients with coronary artery disease from normal subjects, whereas myocardial lactate production was seen as a hallmark of coronary artery disease in 73% of subjects. [The *SCI*® indicates that this paper has been cited 188 times since 1966.]

Lawrence S. Cohen
Yale University School of Medicine
New Haven, CT 06510

January 24, 1978

"The technique of selective coronary arteriography was introduced in the United States in the early 1960s. William C. Elliott and I joined Richard Gorlin's laboratory, Peter Bent Brigham Hospital and Harvard Medical School, in 1962 as research fellows. I recall the very first selective coronary arteriogram performed in that laboratory, as it took place in the fall of 1962, soon after we started the fellowship. Elaborate precautions were taken, incuding having a cardiac surgeon available should any mishap occur. The procedure went smoothly, however, and it launched an investigation over the next two years in which a series of patients with coronary heart disease were studied. Gorlin's leadership in the laboratory moved us toward investigating not only the arteriographic profile of the coronary arteries but also correlating these changes with simultaneous hemodynamic, and biochemical data from the patient. It was not unusual for a catheterization to take upwards of four hours in those early days.

"By 1964 we had studied over 50 patients, and it appeared worthwhile to collate these data to determine what some of the clinical, electrocardiographic, hemodynamic, and biochemical correlations were. The observation that lactate production by the myocardium was the hallmark of the ischemic myocardium is an observation which has stood the test of time.

"One amusing memory of this investigation will never be forgotten. It was 1965, and I had left the laboratory to join the National Heart Institute. Elliott remained in the laboratory to spend a third year and was working at the Harvard Student Infirmary on a Saturday afternoon. I travelled to Boston that weekend, and Gorlin, Elliott and I were writing the paper in the infirmary. A Harvard undergraduate's weekend date came into the infirmary with a rapid heart arrhythmia. She did not know who the doctors treating her were and after her heart had gone back to a normal rhythm, she asked us to please write down what we had done for her so that she might check it out with her own doctor to make certain she had received the correct therapy.

"I know that my associates in this collaborative effort feel equally pleased to see this early work cited for review."

CC/NUMBER 51
DECEMBER 20, 1982

This Week's Citation Classic

Bruschke A V G, Proudfit W L & Sones F M, Jr. Progress study of 590 consecutive nonsurgical cases of coronary disease followed 5-9 years. I. Arteriographic correlations. II. Ventriculographic and other correlations. *Circulation* **47**:1147-53; 1154-63, 1973. [Depts. Clin. Cardiol. and Cardiovasc. Dis., Cleveland Clinic Foundation and Cleveland Clinic Educ. Foundation, OH]

Mortality and the occurrence of myocardial infarction were the main end points considered in a follow-up study on 590 patients with coronary artery disease documented by angiography. The angiographic findings proved to be of high predictive value, exceeding that of any of the other available clinical data. [The *SCI*® indicates that these papers have been cited over 595 times in 487 publications since 1973.]

Albert V.G. Bruschke
Department of Cardiology
St. Antonius Hospital
3500 CJ Utrecht
The Netherlands

October 26, 1982

"At conferences during the early days of coronary surgery, it often happened that a thoracic surgeon showed beautiful angiographic evidence of a successful surgical intervention and subsequently claimed that that patient would certainly have died if it had not been for his prompt and adequate action. This never failed to leave the audience with mixed feelings and more often than not a fruitless debate ensued between those who agreed with the surgeon's point of view and those who stated that the main effect of surgery had been an acceleration of the disease. The arguments used were more of an emotional than a rational nature, which was understandable because in the first place little was known about what would have happened without surgery. Obviously, data on nonoperated patients were needed.

"As in the surgical decision making process, the angiographic findings were (and still are) of primary importance; somehow the clinical follow-up had to be related to angiographic findings. Today, this may appear obvious but at the time we started the study, few people believed that the angiographic findings, which after all only reflect a momentary stage in the disease process, could have much prognostic value. The enthusiasm for surgical intervention, stimulated by improving results, made it difficult to obtain data on nonoperated patients. To start a prospective (randomized) study seemed ethically difficult to justify and could hardly be expected to be successful. Moreover, because of the chronic nature of coronary artery disease it would take many years before results would become available, and data were urgently needed. What then was more logical than to return to the source, namely, the Cleveland Clinic, where F. Mason Sones had established the foundation for surgery by developing coronary angiography to a safe and reliable diagnostic technique?

"The Cleveland Clinic was the only place where excellent angiographic data were available on a large number of patients who were examined during a period when selection for surgery still played a minor role. When we discussed this during one of my regular visits to the Cleveland Clinic, it appeared that a few colleagues from the clinic had been working on the subject, but mainly restricted it to selected groups of patients. Soon arrangements were made to begin the study. During the study, I had invaluable help from the cardiology staff of the Cleveland Clinic, particularly from William L. Proudfit, who later extended the follow-up and further improved the study.[1-3] Apart from the difficulty in tracing the patients (occasionally I felt more like a detective than a cardiologist) and establishing causes of death, there were no particular problems.

"The fact that this study has been cited so often can easily be explained by the uniqueness of the available data and their practical significance. This study has influenced the management of so many patients that it illustrates clearly that clinical investigators have a tremendous responsibility to present unconditionally reliable data. I am grateful for having had access to such excellent material."

1. **Proudfit W L, Bruschke A V G & Sones F M, Jr.** Natural history of obstructive coronary artery disease: ten-year study of 601 nonsurgical cases. *Progr. Cardiovasc. Dis.* **21**:53-78, 1978.
2. --. Survival and ischemic events in nonoperated patients. (Bruschke A V G, van Herpen G & Vermeulen F E E, eds.) *Coronary artery disease today: diagnosis, surgery, and prognosis. Proceedings of an international symposium, 25-27 May 1981, Utrecht, The Netherlands.* Amsterdam: Excerpta Medica, 1982. p. 31-8.
3. --. Prognosis of stable angina pectoris. (Mason D T & Collins J J, eds.) *Myocardial revascularization.* New York: Yorke Medical Books, 1981. p. 1-20.

CC/NUMBER 8
FEBRUARY 23, 1981

This Week's Citation Classic

Weissler A M, Harris W S & Schoenfeld C D. Bedside technics for the evaluation of ventricular function in man. *Amer. J. Cardiol.* **23**:577-83, 1969. [Dept. Med., Ohio State Univ. Coll. Med., Columbus, OH]

This investigation documented a distinct pattern of change in the systolic time intervals in left ventricular decompensation. The ease with which these measures can be obtained prompted their use as quantitative noninvasive measures of cardiac performance in man. [The *SCI*® indicates that this paper has been cited over 385 times since 1969.]

Arnold M. Weissler
Department of Medicine
Wayne State University
Detroit, MI 48201

February 9, 1981

"During the 1960s cardiac catheterization emerged as the dominant, and in the minds of many, the only definitive diagnostic modality in cardiovascular medicine. Technology had advanced to the point that virtually every hemodynamic measure characterizing the performance of the cardiac chambers could now be determined. So readily available and specific was the physiologic data that few cardiologists raised objection to the inconvenience, discomfort, risk, and expense imposed upon our patients by cardiac catheterization. It was in this setting that I introduced the view that valid quantitative physiologic measures of cardiac performance could be derived from recordings of potentials and pulsations at the body's surface. Such an approach could offer many unique clinical advantages and could potentially augment and/or replace some cardiac catheterization methods.

"It was at this time that I discovered that of the various measures of cardiac performance the one most often neglected was the determination of the duration of the events of the cardiac cycle. Since the studies of Carl Ludwig, the performance characteristics of the heart had been described relative to a constant time base.[1] Time remained the independent variable relative to which measures of pressure, volume, and flow were determined. I hypothesized that in order to maintain adequate performance through a wide range of heart rate and loading conditions, the heart, a reciprocating pump, must have time to fill and time to empty. Thus, just as alterations in chamber pressure, contractile volume, and blood flow occur in left ventricular decompensation, the time intervals of the contractile cycle might change as well. That such changes may reflect alterations in cardiac performance was postulated by earlier investigators including Bowen,[2] Lombard and Cope,[3] Katz and Feil,[4] and Blumberger.[5] It had not been established, however, that changes in the temporal dynamics of the cardiac cycle paralleled other hemodynamic consequences of left ventricular decompensation or retained any quantitative relationship to ventricular performance.

"The present paper was based on our previous studies[6] documenting that prolongation of the preejection phase (PEP) and shortening of the ejection time (LVET) in cardiac decompensation was closely related to abnormalities in other measures of cardiac performance. In this work my colleagues Willard S. Harris, Clyde D. Schoenfeld, and I proposed the use of the ratio PEP/LVET, as a convenient quantitative expression of the overall changes in systolic intervals accompanying left ventricular decompensation. This PEP/LVET ratio is now the most commonly applied measure of systolic time intervals for the evaluation of global left ventricular function in man. It was in this paper, too, that we coined the currently popular term 'noninvasive' as a general expression of this diagnostic concept. This paper prompted several later investigations which verified the close relationship between the systolic time intervals and other measures of cardiac chamber performance obtained by cardiac catheterization.

"In perspective, the systolic time intervals constituted an initial attempt to quantitate altered ventricular performance in cardiovascular disease by noninvasive technics. Almost simultaneous with their development, the echocardiographic approach to noninvasive diagnosis emerged and, soon thereafter, nuclear methods for defining altered ventricular contractile performance were introduced. These three independent approaches now stand as prototypes for the development of the new discipline of noninvasive cardiovascular medicine, one which promises to add significantly to our knowledge of the physiologic disorders which accompany cardiovascular disease and will lend a more scientific and critical approach to the clinical management of cardiovascular disease. I published a more recent review of the subject in the *New England Journal of Medicine*."[7]

1. **Ludwig C.** *Arch. Anat. Physiol. Wiss. Med.* **1847**:242, 1847.
2. **Bowen W P.** *Amer. J. Physiol.* **11**:59-77, 1904.
3. **Lombard W P & Cope O M.** *Amer. J. Physiol.* **77**:263-95, 1926.
4. **Katz L N & Feil H S.** *Arch. Intern. Med.* **32**:672-92, 1923.
5. **Blumberger K.** *Ergeb. Inn. Med. Kinderheilk.* **62**:424-531, 1942.
6. **Weissler A M, Harris W S & Schoenfeld C D.** *Circulation* **37**: 149-59, 1968.
7. **Weissler A M.** *N. Engl. J. Med.* **296**:321, 1977.

NUMBER 17
APRIL 23, 1979

This Week's Citation Classic

Lown B, Amarasingham R & Neumann J. A new method for terminating cardiac arrhythmias. *J. Amer. Med. Ass.* **182**:548-55, 1962.
[Harvard School of Public Health Cambridge, MA and Peter Bent Brigham Hospital, Boston MA.]

The authors introduce an entirely new concept for treatment of attacks of rapid heart action, as well as a new method involving use of a brief electrical pulse across the chest wall to abolish the tachycardia. The electric pulse is delivered within a safe part of the cardiac cycle. [The *SCI*® indicates that this paper has been cited over 300 times since 1962.]

Bernard Lown
Professor of Cardiology
Harvard School of Public Health
Boston, MA 02115

January 24, 1978

"Perhaps the seed of the idea to develop a new approach for controlling tachycardias of all types was planted during the many night vigils with patients afflicted with these cardiac disorders who did not respond to diverse drugs. But like most novel ideas, it was based on an unproved hypothesis. I surmised that the abnormal mechanism was the result of an electrical accident which, if once terminated, was unlikely to recur. The arrhythmia was maintained by a recirculating wave of excitation. This possibility had already been demonstrated in the medusa at the turn of the century by the American marine biologist A. G. Mayer.[1] My idea was simplicity itself, namely: to block passage of the depolarizing electrical wave by making cardiac fibers refractory. This could be achieved by an externally delivered electrical pulse across the intact chest.

"While the concept was straightforward, its implementation was complex. It was well known that electricity could injure as well as stop the heart entirely. The question therefore was not only whether the concept was correct but how to make electricity safe for human use. After a year of arduous effort, we found that an underdamped sine wave was effective in animal models and caused but minimal heart damage. Further experimentation demonstrated that if electrical shock was synchronized to discharge outside the brief ventricular vulnerable period following each heart beat, electrical pulses could be administered with great safety. This method of delivering a synchronized DC pulse across the chest has been designated cardioversion. The application of this method is worldwide; its prompt acceptance and incorporation into routine clinical practice testifies to the fact that a therapeutic need has been met.

"Yet implementing this idea was by no means simple. The early experience brings a flood of memories that will provoke unease. No one was initially willing to submit patients to this procedure. The authorities of my hospital discouraged its use. The first patient subjected to this procedure was in a small outlying hospital following a mitral valve operation. As soon as the thoracotomy incision was closed, the surgeon applied the electrode paddles to the chest wall. As I pressed the button on the primitive cardioverter, there was an enormous explosion. A fire started in the operating room. What had happened was that without my knowledge, the surgeon had placed an alcohol soaked sponge on the patient's chest beneath each elecrode paddle to obtain a better electrical contact. The 3000 volt discharge ignited the alcohol, causing a fire. Needless to say, I was never invited back to that hospital.

"There were other difficulties. Research grants were not forthcoming, as the idea was assessed as outlandish. Furthermore, my credentials were deemed inadequate in the field of bioengineering. Private funds provided by Dr. Fredrick Stare, chairman of my department at the Harvard School of Public Health, permitted this work to be carried out. In retrospect, it is ironic that the report of this investigation was refused publication because the reviewer felt that it had little relevance. However, it was accepted for presentation at the annual meeting of the Society for Clinical Investigation and reached the medical and scientific community through the mass media.

"Like the proverbial pebble cast in the water, the ripple effect of this work has been profound. It directly influenced the development of demand pacemakers; it contributed to the emergence of the coronary care unit; and helped focus attention on the formidable, out-of-hospital problem of sudden death, claiming over 400,000 lives annually in the USA."

1. **Mayer A G.** *Medusae of the world.* Washington, DC: Carnegie Institution, 1910. 3 vols.

CC/NUMBER 19
MAY 7, 1984

This Week's Citation Classic™

Wolfson S, Heinle R A, Herman M V, Kemp H G, Sullivan J M & Gorlin R. Propranolol and angina pectoris. *Amer. J. Cardiol.* **18**:345-53, 1966.
[Cardiovascular Res. Lab., Dept. Medicine, Harvard Med. Sch. and Peter Bent Brigham Hosp., Boston, MA]

Propranolol was administered orally to 37 patients with severe angina pectoris, producing a favorable clinical response in 81 percent. The mechanism of action of the drug was studied at the time of diagnostic catheterization in 13 patients. Propranolol induced reductions in heart rate and indices of left ventricular mechanics, with an accompanying reduction in coronary blood flow and myocardial oxygen consumption. No clinical effect was demonstrable when propranolol was given orally to patients with noncoronary chest pain syndromes. [The *SCI*® indicates that this paper has been cited in over 190 publications since 1966.]

Steven Wolfson
Cardiology Associates of New Haven, P.C.
60 Temple Street
New Haven, CT 06510

February 14, 1984

"The cited paper reported the first study in the US of a beta-adrenergic blocking agent as an anti-anginal drug. It presented a combination of a clinical study and a basic evaluation of the effects of intravenous propranolol upon hemodynamics, coronary flow, and myocardial oxygen consumption in patients during the course of cardiac catheterization. These data were then integrated into a hypothesis which attempted to explain how such agents might be of benefit to patients with coronary artery disease.

"This paper laid the groundwork for much of the subsequent work both with adrenergic blocking agents and other approaches to angina pectoris by the avenue of decreasing myocardial oxygen demand. A recent review has discussed the extension of this approach to the prevention of infarction.[1] The study was successful because of a combination of hard work, the foresight of my mentor, Richard Gorlin, and the timing of the first international symposium on propranolol in November 1965. I arrived in Gorlin's laboratory as a cardiology fellow in July 1965, with the background of having performed a study of pronetholol (a precursor of propranolol) for the treatment of cardiac arrhythmias during my internship and junior residency.[2] The Gorlin laboratory had in the years previous to this developed techniques for studying coronary blood flow, hemodynamics, and myocardial metabolism.[3] Gorlin foresaw the utility of the beta-adrenergic blocking agents for the treatment of angina pectoris, and saw in me a trainee with great reserves of energy. July and August 1965 became a blur of activity. Nearly every patient catheterized for diagnostic purposes received propranolol as an investigative tool. As a result, when an invitation was received to present data at the symposium in November, to be held in Great Britain, we had already accumulated a considerable amount of clinical and basic data. These were then included in a symposium issue of the *American Journal of Cardiology* the following year.

"The work was the result of an effort coordinated by Gorlin which included the fellowship cadre at that time, the entire laboratory staff, and even extended to my family. One question which we considered was the possibility that propranolol, which had local anesthetic properties, might ameliorate anginal symptoms because of analgesic effects. When discussing this question at home one evening, my wife suggested that we try the drug in patients who had pain syndromes that were not related to coronary artery disease. As I brought this suggestion to Gorlin the following morning, his reply was to set up a controlled trial in patients with chest pain syndromes but normal coronary arteries. The group of subjects became known in the laboratory as the 'Susan Wolfson Series.' The results were edifying because the great majority of patients with coronary artery disease encountered relief of their anginal symptoms with the drug. Very few of the patients with chest pain syndromes and normal coronary arteries had any clinical effect from propranolol.

"As I look back on the two years that I spent with Gorlin, they glow in recollection. He was a stimulating, exciting, coordinating force in directing our research and our education. I have seldom met a more dedicated, brilliant, supportive, and cooperative group of men than my fellow trainees in that laboratory. These factors and the good fortune which dictated that they came together at the right time led, I believe, to the development of a *Citation Classic*."

1. **Braunwald E, Muller J E, Kloner R A & Maroko P R.** Role of beta-adrenergic blockade in the therapy of patients with myocardial infarction. *Amer. J. Med.* **74**:113-23, 1983.
2. **Wolfson S, Robbins S I & Krasnow N.** Treatment of cardiac arrhythmias with beta-adrenergic blocking agents. *Amer. Heart J.* **72**:177-87, 1966.
3. **Krasnow N, Neill W A, Messer J V & Gorlin R.** Myocardial lactate and pyruvate metabolism. *J. Clin. Invest.* **41**:2075-83, 1962. (Cited 135 times.)

CC/NUMBER 9
MARCH 2, 1981

This Week's Citation Classic

Pantridge J F & Geddes J S. A mobile intensive-care unit in the management of myocardial infarction. *Lancet* **2**:271-3, 1967.
[Cardiac Dept., Royal Victoria Hosp., Belfast, Northern Ireland]

This article describes 18 month's experience of the operation of the first mobile coronary care unit. In that period, 312 patients were managed by the unit. There were no deaths during transport. The first successful correction of cardiac arrest outside the hospital was recorded and it was shown for the first time that successful resuscitation outside the hospital is a practical proposition. [The *SCI*® indicates that this paper has been cited over 260 times since 1967.]

J.F. Pantridge
Regional Medical Cardiology Centre
Royal Victoria Hospital
Belfast BT12 6BA
Northern Ireland

February 3, 1981

"The article records the experience of the use of the portable defibrillator introduced by us[1] in 1966 and describes the organisation of a mobile coronary care unit at the Royal Victoria Hospital in Belfast. The article points out that the majority of the deaths from heart attacks are sudden, occur outside a hospital, and result from an electrical disturbance of the heart muscle and that, since this can be easily corrected, the deaths are unnecessary. The last sentence of the summary of the article states, 'It has been shown perhaps for the first time that the correction of cardiac arrest outside hospital is a practical proposition.' This statement proved to be erroneous. It was pointed out that cardiac arrest had been corrected in 1775, since in that year Abildgaard had 'shocked a single chicken into lifelessness, and upon repeating the shock, the bird took off and eluded further experimentation.'[2]

"It has been stated that the introduction of the portable defibrillator and the mobile coronary care unit described in the article has 'revolutionised emergency medicine and led to a proliferation of pre-hospital coronary care schemes notably in the U.S.A.'[3] Pre-hospital coronary care units equipped with portable defibrillators have saved countless thousands of lives throughout the world. The article is frequently cited because coronary heart disease is the major cause of premature death in the Western World. It is estimated that nearly 1,000 Americans die each day from acute heart attacks outside the hospital and that more than two-thirds of all coronary deaths are sudden.

"It has also been said that the spin-off from the operation of the pioneer mobile pre-hospital coronary care unit initiated in Belfast in 1966 has been as significant as its introduction. The Belfast workers quickly demonstrated that 90 percent of sudden coronary deaths resulted from ventricular fibrillation, an electrical disturbance readily corrected by the portable defibrillator. The mobile unit also enabled detailed observation of patients in the very acute phase of the heart attack and showed that early intensive care may limit the amount of heart muscle destroyed and thus reduce the incidence of shock and improve the long term outlook.

"The demonstration of the importance of the portable defibrillator has led to much research and development directed towards a reduction in size, weight, and portability of the apparatus. The initial 'portable' defibrillator weighed 60 kilos. A machine weighing less than 3 kilos is now available."

1. **Pantridge J F & Geddes J S.** Cardiac arrest after myocardial infarction. *Lancet* **1**:807-8, 1966.
2. **Abildgaard P C.** Tentamina electrica in animalibus instituta. *Societatis Medicae Havniensis Collectanae* **2**: 157-61, 1775.
3. Editorial: Ventricular fibrillation outside hospital. *Lancet* **2**:508-9, 1979.

CC/NUMBER 32
AUGUST 9, 1982

This Week's Citation Classic

Killip T & Kimball J T. Treatment of myocardial infarction in a coronary care unit: a two year experience with 250 patients. *Amer. J. Cardiol.* **20**:457-64, 1967. [Dept. Medicine, Cornell Univ. Medical Coll., New York, NY]

This paper describes the results of treatment of 250 consecutive patients with acute myocardial infarction in a coronary care unit (CCU). Criteria for diagnosis are carefully defined. A classification of functional severity based on clinical evidence of heart failure presented. Morbidity and mortality are related to severity of illness according to the classification. Mortality in the CCU improved compared to regular care only after nurses were trained and given authority to recognize and treat arrhythmia and initiate resuscitation including defibrillation. [The *SCI*® indicates that this paper has been cited in over 315 publications since 1967.]

Thomas Killip
Department of Medicine
Henry Ford Hospital
Detroit, MI 48202
and
Department of Medicine
University of Michigan
Ann Arbor, MI 48104

May 26, 1982

"In the 1960s, academic medicine 'discovered' that patients with ischemic heart disease faced a high mortality and were sitting in large numbers in every hospital. Few clinical or experimental papers were being published on coronary artery disease, the leading cause of death in the Western world. In 1960, H.W. Day, working in a nonteaching community hospital, found that the care of patients with myocardial infarction was facilitated if they were clustered in a special unit during the first few days of their illness.[1] Closed chest cardiac resuscitation, defibrillation, and oscillographic monitoring of the electrocardiogram had been recently developed thus making the coronary care unit (CCU) feasible.[2]

"In 1961, I returned from a special fellowship at the Karolinska Institute to become chief of the division of cardiology at Cornell University Medical College. Our group quickly developed an interest in the problems of coronary artery disease. We developed a four-bed experimental CCU at the New York Hospital-Cornell Medical Center. John Kimball joined our group as a clinical fellow, and subsequently became a member of the faculty as we collaborated for several years.

"Does the CCU save lives? Our initial experience with 100 consecutive cases did not show improved survival. We then trained nurses to recognize arrhythmias, initiate therapy, and defibrillate if cardiac arrest occurred. The gratifying results of our experience were published in the article cited.

"I have long had an interest in the quantification of clinical events so that the physician can measure severity of illness or effect of treatment. Myocardial infarction alters function of the heart as a pump. An important index of the severity is the degree of heart failure. Prognostic indices had been devised by others[3] but Kimball and I focused on the degree of clinical heart failure as reflecting left ventricular function and, hence, damage. We devised a classification of severity based on presence or absence of signs of heart failure or shock for patients in the CCU with myocardial infarction.

"It is the clinical classification which we proposed which has led to the frequent citing of this article. We showed that mortality is directly related to the bedside estimation of the severity or class of heart failure. Later, several clinical centers, including Cornell, were awarded NIH grants to support myocardial infarction research units (MIRU). Our classification was adopted by the MIRUs and used in a number of papers emanating from that program.

"Determination of a patient's clinical class depends upon serial bedside examination by the physician or nurse. The classification provides a good guide to prognosis, permits comparison of clinical results between institutions, is an index of ventricular damage, and offers a degree of objectivity to the bedside evaluation of a common disease. This is why it has been widely used.

"I have been surprised by the popularity of this paper. Requests for reprints still arrive from all over the world. It is certainly not my most profound publication. What Kimball and I showed was that a classification of clinical severity based upon simple bedside observations could be related to outcome and is a useful guide to the effectiveness of therapy in patients with myocardial infarction."

1. **Day H W.** An intensive coronary care area. *Dis. Chest* **44**:423-7, 1963.
2. **Jude J R, Kouwenhoven W B & Knickerbocker G G.** Cardiac arrest: report of application of external cardiac massage on 118 patients. *J. Amer. Med. Assn.* **178**:1063-70, 1961.
3. **Peel A A F, Semple T, Wang I, Lancaster W M & Dall J L G.** A coronary prognostic index for grading the severity of infarction. *Brit. Heart J.* **24**:745-60, 1962.

CC/NUMBER 32
AUGUST 10, 1981

This Week's Citation Classic

Favaloro R G. Saphenous vein autograft replacement of severe segmental coronary artery occlusion. Operative technique.
Ann. Thorac. Surg. 5:334-9, 1968.
[Dept. Thoracic and Cardiovascular Surgery, Cleveland Clinic Foundation, Cleveland, OH]

This paper presents our early effort to reconstruct the coronary circulation impaired by arteriosclerosis. The operative technique of replacing a segment of the coronary artery tree is described in detail. Early, pre-, and postoperative cine coronary angiograms are shown, including the first patient, a 55-year-old woman operated upon in May 1967. [The *SCI*® indicates that this paper has been cited over 160 times since 1968.]

René G. Favaloro
Departamento de Diagnostico
y Tratamiento
de Enfermedades Toracicas
y Cardiovasculares
Sanatorio Güemes
Córdoba 3933
1188 Buenos Aires
Republic of Argentina

June 30, 1981

"The utilization of the saphenous vein was the result of our previous work with pericardial patch graft repair in segmental localized obstructions mainly of the right coronary artery. The saphenous vein had been previously used on peripheral artery (femoropopliteal) bypasses and on renal artery reconstruction with excellent clinical results. It was logical to think that the same technique could be applied to the coronary circulation.

"At the beginning, long obstructed segments of the coronary arteries were replaced with portions of saphenous veins with two end-to-end anastomosis. Very early in our experience we realized the limitations of this technique, mainly among patients with proximal obstructions, and bypasses from the anterolateral wall of the aorta were performed (the first patient is mentioned on page 337).

"With more clinical application the bypass operation became the routine procedure. Encouraged by the postoperative angiograms performed by F. Mason Sones, Jr., and his associates at the Cleveland Clinic, we followed a steady effort to develop a routine surgical technique for the right and left coronary artery.[1] In May 1968 we applied for the first time the same approach to patients with preinfarction angina and even with acute infarction.[2] At the beginning, it was difficult to convince our medical colleagues, and even some of our surgical colleagues, that we had a simple operative procedure which was able to immediately restore myocardial perfusion.

"The World Congress of Cardiology held in London in 1970 set a significant landmark in the acceptance of this surgical approach after my debate with Charles Friedberg. In 1970, I published a monograph[3] which summarizes our work performed at the Cleveland Clinic under the leadership of Sones, Donald B. Effler, and William L. Proudfit. At present, this operation is applied all over the world and more than 2,000 papers have been published on the subject.

"We can conclude that the quality of life is enhanced and life expectancy improved in properly selected patients. I had the opportunity to summarize the first ten years of clinical experience when I gave the Bishop Lecture[4] at the annual meeting of the American College of Cardiology in 1978.

"This paper has been highly cited because it deals with the number one epidemic of our time: coronary arteriosclerosis. Indeed, this publication started a new life for me. Since then, with my colleague and good friend Sones, I often toured different cardiovascular centers in the United States and traveled abroad engaged in a teaching career which has been highly rewarding. Not only have we been able to help thousands of patients—the main reason of our daily practice—but more than that we have strengthened our friendship with cardiologists and cardiovascular surgeons with whom we have had discussions—learning and teaching at the same time—in an atmosphere of scientific freedom and respect."

1. **Favaloro R G, Effler D B, Groves L K, Sheldon W C, Shirey E K & Sones F M, Jr.** Severe segmental obstruction of the left main coronary artery and its divisions. Surgical treatment by the saphenous vein graft technique. *J. Thorac. Cardiovasc. Surg.* **60**:469-82, 1970.
2. **Favaloro R G, Effler D B, Cheanvechai C, Quint R A & Sones F M, Jr.** Acute coronary insufficiency (impending myocardial infarction and myocardial infarction). Surgical treatment by the saphenous vein graft technique. *Amer. J. Cardiol.* **28**:598-607, 1971.
3. **Favaloro R G.** *Surgical treatment of coronary arteriosclerosis.* Baltimore, MD: Williams and Wilkins, 1970. 132 p.
4. ------------------. Direct myocardial revascularization: a ten year journey. Myths and realities. *Amer. J. Cardiol.* **43**:109-30, 1979.

CC/NUMBER 8
FEBRUARY 20, 1984

This Week's Citation Classic™

Moulopoulos S D, Topaz S & Kolff W J. Diastolic balloon pumping (with carbon dioxide) in the aorta—a mechanical assistance to the failing circulation. *Amer. Heart J.* **63**:669-75, 1962.
[Dept. Artif. Organs, Cleveland Clinic Fndn. and Frank E. Bunts Educ. Inst., Cleveland, OH]

This paper presents a method based on the principle of counterpulsation to assist the blood circulation when the heart is unable to maintain it. It consists of inflating during ventricular diastole and deflating during systole an elongated balloon introduced into the descending aorta. [The *SCI*® indicates that this paper has been cited in over 205 publications since 1962.]

Spyridon D. Moulopoulos
Department of Clinical Therapeutics
School of Medicine
University of Athens
Athens, Greece

January 8, 1984

"When I started working at the Cleveland Clinic in December 1960, Willem Kolff had already embarked upon the project of making an 'artificial heart' to replace the irreparably ailing human heart. To the scientific community at that time, the effort appeared Utopian. To me, it represented an extremely interesting but long jump in that line of research, so I tried to find a way to assist the heart until Kolff was successful in replacing it, which he did 22 years later.

"Several cardiac assistance techniques were then already in existence, but most were handling blood outside the body. The intra-aortic balloon did not require an extracorporeal blood circuit. Instead of drawing the blood outside the body during ventricular systole and pumping it back during diastole, as was done by Harken, we introduced a long polyurethane balloon, mounted on a catheter, into the descending aorta and pumped the blood 'intra-aortally' toward the peripheral (and coronary) vessels during diastole, while deflating it during systole. Thus, peripheral resistance to the heart was reduced without reducing perfusion pressure to the tissues. The device, operating with an inexpensive solenoid valve and a delay circuit triggered from the R-wave of the electrocardiogram, was tested in mock circulation in dogs and in a human cadaver.

"There were practically no obstacles in the realization of the project. The equipment needed was available, the laboratory offered all facilities, but, mostly, the unique experience of Kolff in the field of artificial organs helped in quickly solving all emerging problems. The contribution of the engineer, Topaz, in setting and testing the equipment was valuable.

"The clinical application of the device started in 1967, when Adrian Kantrowitz used it in a number of patients.[1] The method has since been used all over the world to provide lifesaving temporary assistance, mainly in cases of post open-heart surgery when the patient cannot be 'weaned' from the extracorporeal heart-lung machine. It is also used in cardiogenic shock after acute myocardial infarction, in unstable angina or in pericardial tamponade in preparation for surgery, in rupture of the intraventricular septum, in irreversible ventricular tachycardia, etc.

"The method was presented for the first time at an American Society for Artificial Internal Organs meeting.[2] A comprehensive review of circulatory assistance techniques appeared in 1969.[3] The most recent review, with emphasis on intra-aortic balloon pumping, can be found in *Clinical Essays on the Heart*.[4] Further developments in the same field can be found in two other recent publications.[5,6]

"The paper is frequently cited because the method reported therein has been widely used in several experimental settings in order to investigate its peculiar effects on the circulation, as well as in patients for the treatment of various clinical syndromes. It made mechanical assistance practical, divulged the principle of counterpulsation, and pointed out the effectiveness of optimally timed interventions within a cardiac cycle.

"There is evidence that this work contributed significantly to the award of an honorary degree (Doctor of Science) to me by the University of Utah in 1983."

1. **Kantrowitz A, Tjonneland S, Krakauer J, Butner A N, Phillips S J, Yahr W Z, Shapiro M, Freed P S, Jaron D & Sherman J L, Jr.** Clinical experience with cardiac assistance by means of intraaortic phase-shift balloon pumping. *Trans. Amer. Soc. Artif. Intern. Org.* **14**:344, 1968.
2. **Moulopoulos S, Topaz S & Kolff W.** Extracorporeal assistance to the circulation and intraaortic balloon pumping. *Trans. Amer. Soc. Artif. Intern. Org.* **8**:85-8, 1962.
3. **Kolff W, Moulopoulos S, Kwan-Gett C & Kralios A.** Mechanical assistance to the circulation: the principle and the methods. *Progr. Cardiovasc. Dis.* **12**:243-70, 1969.
4. **Moulopoulos S.** Mechanical cardiac assistance. (Hurst J W, ed.) *Clinical essays on the heart.* New York: McGraw-Hill, 1983. p. 233-47.
5. **Moulopoulos S, Stamatelopoulos S, Petrou P, Saridakis N, Yannopoulos N & Jarvick R.** Left intraventricular "pseudoaugmentation." A new principle of mechanical assistance. *Trans. Amer. Soc. Artif. Intern. Org.* **27**:588-91, 1981.
6. **Sideris D, Nanas J, Chrysos D & Moulopoulos S.** Intra-aortic balloon assistance without a pump. *Eur. Heart J.* **4**:536-46, 1983.

CC/NUMBER 1
JANUARY 4, 1982

This Week's Citation Classic

Swan H J C, Ganz W, Forrester J, Marcus H, Diamond G & Chonette D. Catheterization of the heart in man with use of a flow-directed balloon-tipped catheter. *N. Engl. J. Med.* **283**:447-51, 1970.
[Dept. Cardiology, Cedars-Sinai Medical Ctr., and Dept. Medicine, Univ. California, Los Angeles, CA]

A self-guiding flow-directed catheter was developed which permitted catheterization of the right side of the heart and pulmonary artery without the use of fluoroscopy and with minimal complications. The addition of multiple sensors has allowed for the quantitative measurement of cardiac function. This development has permitted the application of quantitative cardiac catheterization procedures to the management of the critically ill. [The *SCI®* indicates that this paper has been cited over 610 times since 1970.]

H.J.C. Swan
Department of Cardiology
Cedars-Sinai Medical Center
and
Department of Medicine
University of California
School of Medicine
Los Angeles, CA 90024

November 9, 1981

"In the two decades following World War II, the newly developed technique of cardiac catheterization allowed application of basic physiologic principles to clinical diagnosis and made the development of a cardiac surgical treatment of congenital and valvar heart disease possible. My training in the early-1950s at the Mayo Clinic with Earl H. Wood—a true pioneer in the development of cardiac catheterization—established a strong basis for my own career in investigative cardiology. In 1965, I left the Mayo Clinic, a major referral center, to direct cardiology at Cedars of Lebanon Hospital, a community institution. I was amazed by the paucity of knowledge of the hemodynamics of ischemic heart disease and, in particular, of acute myocardial infarction, which then carried a mortality of 20-25 percent. Empirical approaches to treatment appeared to be remarkably ineffective, if not positively harmful. It appeared essential to obtain hemodynamic measurements at the bedside if these clinical syndromes were to be understood. However, my interactions with Wood and John Kirklin convinced me that standard cardiac catheterization techniques could not be applied in the usual clinical setting. Therefore, the techniques would have to be modified.

"In the fall of 1966, I was watching the sailboats in Santa Monica Bay and conceived the idea that a sail or parachute combined with a highly flexible catheter would be the ideal mechanism to flow-guide a catheter into the central circulation. In discussing the potential fabrication of such a device, the experience of Edwards Labs with the Fogarty embolectomy catheter provided a solution, although, in retrospect, a parachute type device could have had important advantages. When the first batch of catheters actually arrived, I brought them over to my animal laboratory, where my most recent recruit to the then infant division of cardiology, William Ganz, was finishing an experiment on the measurement of ventricular volume, using the dilution principle. I placed the first of the flotation catheters in the right atrium of a dog and inflated the guidance balloon, whereupon the catheter and the balloon immediately disappeared from the field of view. After recognizing that the balloon had not burst, we were able to demonstrate consistent passage to the pulmonary artery within one to two beats after inflation of the guidance balloon. The device worked. The point was proven.

"From there, we took it to the catheterization laboratory and then to the CCU, where the contributions of many, including a then resident in medicine, George Diamond, allowed us to report on the first 100 bedside catheterizations in August 1970. The addition of multiple pressure ports, a thermistor for measurement of cardiac output by the thermodilution principle, and electrodes for atrial and ventricular sensing and pacing represented a natural series of additional applications.

"In 1970, my colleagues and I developed the balloon flotation catheter to investigate the clinical syndromes of ischemic heart disease. The broad application in the field of hemodynamic monitoring and the management of hundreds of thousands or, now, millions of critically ill patients was a secondary objective. The frequency of citation is related to the wide acceptance of a practical technique which permits the measurement of basic physiological data in a clinical setting. Recent work in this field has been published by me and N.L. Pace."[1,2]

1. **Swan H J C.** The role of hemodynamic monitoring in the management of the critically ill. *Crit. Care Med.* 3:83-9, 1975.
2. **Pace N L.** A critique of flow-directed pulmonary arterial catheterization. *Anesthesiology* **47**:455-65, 1977.

CC/NUMBER 16
APRIL 16, 1984

This Week's Citation Classic™

Cox J L, McLaughlin V W, Flowers N C & Horan L G. The ischemic zone surrounding acute myocardial infarction. Its morphology as detected by dehydrogenase staining. *Amer. Heart J.* **76**:650-9, 1968.
[Sect. Cardiology, Dept. Medicine, Univ. Tennessee, Memphis, TN]

This article offers the first pathologic description of the so-called 'twilight zone' of intermediate cellular injury located at the periphery of an acute myocardial infarction. The presence of this twilight zone served as the stimulus for the evaluation of much of the pharmacologic and mechanical therapy subsequently introduced for the treatment of acute myocardial ischemic injury and is believed to be the site of origin of reentrant ventricular tachyarrhythmias associated with coronary artery disease. [The *SCI*® indicates that this paper has been cited in over 235 publications since 1968.]

James L. Cox
Division of Cardiothoracic Surgery
Washington University School of Medicine
St. Louis, MO 63110

February 22, 1984

"Prior to the mid-1960s, the general concept of an acute myocardial infarction was that the tissue injury that followed acute coronary artery occlusion was most likely nonuniform. However, this nonuniformity of tissue injury had never been demonstrated, and thus, from a diagnostic and therapeutic standpoint, an acute myocardial infarction was perceived as being a single event that resulted in tissue death within a predetermined region of myocardium. The likelihood of altering the course of tissue death following acute coronary artery occlusion was, therefore, considered remote because therapeutic interventions could be applied only after the fact.

"In the spring of 1965, as a sophomore medical student at the University of Tennessee Medical School in Memphis, I was given the opportunity to work in the research laboratory of Leo G. Horan and Nancy C. Flowers, both cardiac electrophysiologists. We felt that it might be possible to demonstrate by histochemical techniques that tissue injury in acute myocardial infarction was nonuniform and that the progression of injury during the first several hours following coronary occlusion was a dynamic process amenable to potentially beneficial therapeutic intervention. I was given a copy of A.G.E. Pearse's histochemistry textbook,[1,2] a small laboratory, a certain amount of research funds, and a great deal of encouragement to document our hypothesis pathologically. After an entire year of literally hundreds of failures, I adjusted the pH of the tissue incubating solution incorrectly in one experiment and, as a result, was able to document quite clearly for the first time the nonuniformity of injury in acute myocardial infarction. My expletive at seeing this zone for the first time must be deleted.

"Within a few months, I was joined by Victor W. McLaughlin, a medical intern, and together we were able to reconstruct two-dimensional, then three-dimensional, 'histochemical maps' of acute myocardial infarctions that clearly documented the presence of an ischemic but viable zone of tissue separating the central zone of progressive necrosis from surrounding normal myocardium. I presented this work at the American Heart Association meeting in New York City in October 1966,[3] and subsequently published it in the *American Heart Journal* **in November 1968. The ischemic zone that we identified has frequently been referred to as the 'twilight zone' of injury in acute myocardial infarction. Although subsequent, more sophisticated pathologic studies have questioned the existence of such an intermediate zone of ischemic injury,[4] much of the pharmacologic and mechanical (i.e., intra-aortic balloon pumping) therapy introduced for the treatment of myocardial ischemic injury in the past 15 years has been based on the presence of such a zone. In addition, most investigators feel that this twilight zone is the site of origin of reentrant ventricular tachyarrhythmias associated with coronary artery disease.**

"I believe this work has been cited often for two reasons: 1) it formed the basis for rational efforts to decrease the size of an acute myocardial infarction by therapeutic intervention, and 2) it established the anatomic basis of ischemic ventricular tachyarrhythmias that led to the development of direct endocardial surgical techniques that are now being applied widely for the treatment of refractory ventricular tachycardia associated with coronary artery disease."[4]

1. **Pearse A G E.** *Histochemistry: theoretical and applied.* London: Churchill, 1960. 998 p.
2. ------------------. Citation Classic. Commentary on *Histochemistry: theoretical and applied. Current Contents/Life Sciences* **24**(32):17, 10 August 1981.
3. **Cox J L, McLaughlin V W, Flowers N C & Horan L G.** Changes in cellular dehydrogenase enzymes in acute myocardial infarction. *Circulation* **34**:III-80, 1966.
4. **Cox J L.** Anatomic-electrophysiologic basis for the surgical treatment of refractory ischemic ventricular tachycardia. *Ann. Surg.* **198**:119-29, 1983.

This Week's Citation Classic™

Page D L, Caulfield J B, Kastor J A, DeSanctis R W & Sanders C A. Myocardial changes associated with cardiogenic shock. *N. Engl. J. Med.* **285**:133-7, 1971.
[Depts. Pathology and Medicine, Massachusetts General Hosp. and Harvard Medical Sch., Boston, MA]

Patients dying with cardiogenic shock secondary to myocardial infarction had necrosis of at least 40 percent of the left ventricular myocardium demonstrated at necropsy. All patients dying with myocardial infarction without shock (with one exception) had lost 35 percent or less of the left ventricular muscle. [The *SCI*® indicates that this paper has been cited in over 410 publications since 1971.]

David L. Page
Department of Pathology
School of Medicine
Vanderbilt University
Nashville, TN 37232

December 16, 1983

"This paper was the result of a collaborative effort among basic scientists, cardiologists, and anatomic pathologists. The project had its inception in the establishment of the Myocardial Infarction Research Unit at the Massachusetts General Hospital in 1967. This sponsored program was begun at the initiation of the National Heart Institute in order to foster research in myocardial infarction. The original proposal, with Charles Sanders as the principal investigator, included a request to study the syndrome of cardiogenic shock. This portion of the proposal was written by J.B. Caulfield, who had described the ultrastructure of ischemic myocardium in 1959.[1] As a resident in pathology, I performed the necropsy examinations on these patients so that they might all be done in a uniform and prospective manner. With the considerable aid of a research technician and support from a superb departmental photography unit, the studies could be done with care using a technique developed by D.B. Hackel of Duke University.[2]

"Close correlation between anatomic findings and clinical events was guaranteed by frequent meetings between cardiologists and pathologists. Our demonstration that anatomic events within the coronary arterial tree were the same in patients dying of myocardial infarction with and without cardiogenic shock, combined with our demonstration that the quantity of injured myocardium was different, led us to conclude that loss of more than approximately 40 percent of the left ventricular myocardium produced irreversible pump failure. We also demonstrated that the pattern of myocardial injury in shock secondary to noncardiac events was quite different from that found in the other patients, completing our attempt at understanding the correlation of clinical, coronary arterial, and myocardial events.

"Our conclusions were first published in 1970[3] and were supported almost simultaneously by a British study,[4] and confirmed by a similarly conducted study reported from Cornell University in 1973.[5]

"The demonstration that the quantity of myocardial necrosis is central to the production of cardiogenic shock has led to a great deal of study,[6] much of it aimed at preservation of ischemic and sublethally damaged myocardium.

"This study was also important in demonstrating the heterogeneity of clinical and pathophysiologic events in ischemic heart disease. Caulfield *et al.* later suggested therapeutic implications of rapid *versus* delayed onset of shock after myocardial infarction.[7] These studies, based on data obtained from clinicopathologic correlation at time of autopsy, illustrate the current usefulness of such studies. Clinically relevant observations and new concepts are still coming from the autopsy room as evidenced by the interest in infarct extension as opposed to infarct expansion as proposed by Hutchins and Bulkley."[8]

1. **Caulfield J & Klionsky B.** Myocardial ischemia and early infarction: an electron microscopic study. *Amer. J. Pathol.* **35**:489-535, 1959. (Cited 175 times since 1959.)
2. **Hackel D B.** A technic to estimate the quantity of infarcted myocardium post mortem. *Amer. J. Clin. Pathol.* **61**:242-6, 1974.
3. **Page D L, Caulfield J B, Kastor J A, DeSanctis R W & Sanders C A.** Myocardial changes associated with cardiogenic shock. *Proceedings of the Second Annual Meeting. International Study Group for Research in Cardiac Metabolism.* Pavia, Italy: Editrice Fucc. Fusi, 1970. p. 265-81.
4. **Harnarayon C, Bennett M A, Pentecost B L & Brewer D B.** Quantitative study of infarcted myocardium in cardiogenic shock. *Brit. Heart J.* **32**:728-32, 1970. (Cited 180 times.)
5. **Alonso D R, Scheidt S, Post M & Killip T.** Pathophysiology of cardiogenic shock. *Circulation* **48**:588-96, 1973. (Cited 135 times.)
6. **Reimer K A.** Myocardial infarct size. *Arch. Pathol. Lab. Med.* **104**:225-30, 1980.
7. **Caulfield J B, Leinbach R & Gold H.** The relationship of myocardial infarct size and prognosis. *Circulation* **53**(Suppl. I):141-4, 1976.
8. **Bulkley B & Hutchins G.** Infarct expansion versus extension: two different complications of acute myocardial infarction. *Amer. J. Cardiol.* **41**:1127-32, 1978.

This Week's Citation Classic

Hirst A E, Jr., Johns V J, Jr. & Kime S W, Jr. Dissecting aneurysm of the aorta: a review of 505 cases. *Medicine* **37**:217-79, 1958.
[Depts. Pathology and Medicine, College of Medical Evangelists, Los Angeles, CA]

This is a collective review of 505 cases of dissecting aneurysm of the aorta published in English literature during the years 1934 to 1954, emphasizing historical aspects, clinical pathologic correlations, unusual manifestations, course, and treatment of the disease. [The *SCI®* indicates that this paper has been cited over 285 times since 1961.]

Albert E. Hirst
Department of Pathology
School of Medicine
Loma Linda University
Loma Linda, CA 92350

June 17, 1981

"In 1950, three authors—one pathologist, one internist, and a junior medical student—decided to collaborate on a review of published information on dissecting aneurysm of the aorta in English literature, emphasizing the contributions made since the classical monograph of Shennan was published in 1934.[1]

"To assure ourselves of interest in such a manuscript, we wrote John H. Talbott, who was then editor of *Medicine*, a journal catering to review articles, regarding his interest in the topic. In his cryptic reply he indicated that he was 'always interested in reviewing a good manuscript'—a reply that was encouraging enough for us to initiate the effort but permitted him the latitude to reject our manuscript if he considered it unsuitable for publication. We indicated that we expected to complete the manuscript in about a year and a half.

"Six years (and several revisions) later, the article was ready to submit. Our junior coauthor's contribution consisted largely of a summer vacation spent reviewing articles for the compilation. At that time, tabulation of data was tedious since there were over 400 articles on the subject and inexpensive duplicating techniques were not generally available. The articles were abstracted by hand, and many had to be obtained on interlibrary loans. We are greatly indebted to our two secretaries, Ardyce Koobs and Wanda Rice, for their patience in retyping the manuscript. Our opus was submitted in the spring of 1957, but we had not received any word of its acceptance by fall. Suspecting no news was bad news, we wrote Talbott, who informed us that his editorial board had been on vacation and had not had time to read the manuscript. It was an exciting day when we received the letter of acceptance, with publication scheduled for September 1958. Our 62 page review included information on 505 cases and included 346 references. No doubt the exhaustive review of this large series of dissecting aneurysms is responsible for this article being so frequently cited.

"A brief historical account was followed by a discussion of the causes and mechanisms of development of dissecting aneurysm of the aorta. When possible, an attempt was made to correlate symptoms and signs with the underlying pathologic process. We particularly searched for unusual findings on physical examination, x-rays, or laboratory studies which provided diagnostic clues that would prove helpful in recognition of the disease.

"A resurgence of interest in dissecting aneurysm occurred early in the 1950s with the development of effective surgical procedures by De Bakey and associates[2] and more recently by the development of encouraging medical regimens by Wheat *et al.*[3] Despite these signal advances, the mortality from the disease remains distressingly high, indicating that there is still much to be learned about this catastrophic disease.

"A recent, comprehensive, although less detailed, study of the disease is found in *Acute Aortic Dissections* by C. E. Anagnostopoulos."[4]

1. **Shennan T.** *Dissecting aneurysms.* London: His Majesty's Stationery Office, 1934. 138 p. MRC Special Report No. 193.
2. **De Bakey M E, Cooley D A & Creech O, Jr.** Surgical considerations of dissecting aneurysm. *Ann. Surg.* **142**:586-612, 1955.
3. **Wheat M W, Jr., Harris P D, Malm J R, Kaiser G, Bowman F O, Jr. & Palmer R F.** Acute dissecting aneurysms of the aorta: treatment and results in 64 patients. *J. Thorac. Cardiovasc. Surg.* **58**:344-51, 1969.
4. **Anagnostopoulos C E.** *Acute aortic dissections.* Baltimore, MD: University Park Press, 1975. 255 p.

CC/NUMBER 27
JULY 2, 1984

This Week's Citation Classic™

Szilagyi D E, Smith R F, DeRusso F J, Elliott J P & Sherrin F W. Contribution of abdominal aortic aneurysmectomy to prolongation of life.
Ann. Surg. **164**:678-99, 1966.
[Department of Surgery, Henry Ford Hospital, Detroit, MI]

This was a retrospective study of the survival experience of two nonsynchronous groups of patients with the diagnosis of abdominal aortic aneurysms, one group (248 cases) with, the other (105 cases) without, surgical correction, appropriately standardized for comparison. The surgically treated patients doubled their life expectancy. Thirty-five percent of the surgically untreated cases died of rupture. [The *SCI*® indicates that this paper has been cited in over 170 publications since 1966.]

D. Emerick Szilagyi
Division of Vascular Surgery
Department of Surgery
Henry Ford Hospital
Detroit, MI 48202

February 9, 1984

"Because of a number of easily observable clinical features of abdominal aortic aneurysms, surgeons intuitively adopted an aggressive attitude in their management as soon as the technique of aneurysmectomy became available (in 1951). The early operative mortality rate was rather high, however, and soon questions were raised whether the surgical treatment of any but the largest aneurysms of the abdominal aorta was justified. To decide this issue, there were a number of practical reasons that made a clinical controlled study unfeasible. The great benefit of the surgical treatment in many cases was obvious and its denial to randomly selected patients seemed ethically unjustified. In the Henry Ford Hospital, a fortuitous and fortunate situation existed that made it possible to construct two cohorts of patients with abdominal aortic aneurysms, the study of which could be expected to supply an answer to the question of what the actual benefit of surgical treatment was.

"Our internists were particularly conservative in managing abdominal aortic aneurysms, and during the 1950s seldom referred patients to the surgeon. When we became interested in the problem of the evaluation of the worth of abdominal aortic aneurysmectomy, we were pleasantly surprised to find that a relatively large group of patients (223 cases) who had not received surgical treatment was available. Since the group of nonsurgical cases was not strictly comparable to the surgical group, primarily because it contained cases that had been deemed to be unsuitable for surgical treatment owing to risk factors, a method had to be devised to reduce the disparity of the two groups. We achieved this by excluding from the groups we compared all those whose principal risk factors exceeded certain predetermined limits.

"Having overcome the main statistical difficulty, our next problem was to find a suitable method for determining survival experience. Since the life-table method of analysis now universally used was not at that time available, we worked out a method of our own which allowed the comparison of the survival experience of the two groups in spite of the differences in the length of survival of the patients and the variations in the time of their entry into the study. Later recalculation of the data with standard life-table methods yielded almost identical results.

"An important aspect of this study was the demonstration that while the rupture of the untreated aneurysm was by far the most common cause of death in untreated cases (34.9 percent), the ravages of coronary atherosclerosis were only second in importance (having been the cause of death in 17 percent of the two groups). The study also brought forth that, even in the cases with the aortic aneurysm removed, coronary atherosclerosis remained an important factor of mortality and eventually led to the death of 12 percent of the survivors of the operation. In subsequent years, the considerable operative mortality of 13.6 percent was reduced dramatically (to around three percent), further enhancing the value of surgical treatment.

"Our study remained the only large survey of this problem simply because the necessary clinical material either was not available or was not recognized in other centers. As more and more patients with abdominal aneurysms were subjected to surgical treatment, the opportunity for such a study completely disappeared. Our demonstration of the value of surgical treatment undoubtedly had an important role in the general acceptance of the current approach to the treatment of these lesions. See reference 1 for a recent publication in this field."

1. **Szilagyi D E.** Abdominal aortic aneurysms: natural history and operative indications. (Stipa S & Cavallaro A, eds.) *Peripheral arterial diseases: medical and surgical problems.* London: Academic Press, 1982. p. 27-37.

This Week's Citation Classic

CC/NUMBER 10
MARCH 10, 1980

Lassen N A. Cerebral blood flow and oxygen consumption in man. *Physiol. Rev.* **39**:183-238, 1959.
[Lab. Clin. Sci., National Institute of Mental Health, National Institutes of Health, Bethesda, MD]

The concept of autoregulation of cerebral blood flow was presented in detail for the first time. The paper also summarizes the field in general and contains a thorough discussion of the methods that, at that time, were available to study CBF and CMRO$_2$ in man. [The *SCI*® indicates that this paper has been cited over 480 times since 1961.]

Niels A. Lassen
Department of Clinical Physiology
Bispebjerg Hospital
2400-Copenhagen NV
Denmark

January 4, 1980

"This review's most lasting contribution to the understanding of cerebral circulation, and the reason for its frequent citation, is perhaps the section on *autoregulation of cerebral blood flow:* the fact that normally the cerebral vessels constrict when the blood pressure increases and dilate when the pressure decreases. Basic animal experiments showing this regulatory mechanism had been made by Mogens Fog in the 1930s.[1] However, undoubtedly due to the ease with which the autoregulation is abolished by trauma or transient hypoxia, many other workers had been unable to demonstrate it. In my article, support for the autoregulation of CBF was adduced by collecting several series of studies of induced hyper- and hypotension in man, showing that within limits (and with unchanged arterial pCO$_2$) CBF was in fact unchanged. Why were the studies in man so uniformly effective in showing the autoregulation? I think the answer is simply that in man you must employ techniques that are essentially atraumatic.

"The data collected in the 1959 review also included several series of studies in patients with *essential hypertension.* They were interpreted to suggest that in this disease the autoregulatory plateau—the limits of pressures between which flow is maintained constant—is shifted toward higher pressures. The cerebral resistance vessels appeared to be adapted (hypertrophied?) to the higher pressure.

"Since then we have come to know much more about the cerebral autoregulation. Its shift in chronic hypertension has been seen quite clearly, and there has been presented evidence suggesting that it may return to the normal pressure range after prolonged effective treatment.[2] Of special interest is the finding of a flow increase with more marked hypertension to pressures above the 'upper limit' of autoregulation.[3] This flow increase and the concomitant abnormal protein permeability of the blood brain barrier is probably an initiating event in *acute hypertensive encephalopathy.*

"Recently it has been demonstrated that in severe cases of traumatic brain tissue injury with edema as well as in cases of brain edema induced experimentally by cold or associated with brain tumors autoregulation of CBF is present![4,5] This is so, even though we know that with milder degrees of the same noxious stimuli the mechanism is indeed abolished! This paradox was first thought to be caused by a massive variation in intracranial pressure in the 'worst' cases. Now it appears that this is not always the case and local variations in brain tissue pressure are then invoked to explain the 'false autoregulation.' Perhaps this is so. But no proof of the tissue pressure hypothesis is yet at hand.

"Many other aspects of this article's concepts and facts continue to be elaborated in current research. What was then (and is now) called the metabolic regulation of cerebral blood flow is fertile ground. One can by measuring blood flow in a given area reveal *if it is active or inactive.* We can map the areas of the brain in animals or in man during sensory perception movements, vocalization, etc., as reviewed by Lassen, Ingvar, and Skinhoj in 1978."[6]

1. **Fog M.** The relationship between the blood pressure and the tonic regulation of the pial arteries. *J. Neurol. Psychiat.* **1**:187-97, 1938.
2. **Strandgaard S.** Autoregulation of cerebral blood flow in hypertensive patients. The modifying influence of prolonged antihypertensive treatment on the tolerance to acute, drug-induced hypotension. *Circulation* **53**:720-7, 1976.
3. **Strandgaard S, MacKenzie E T, Sengupta D, Rowan J O, Lassen N A & Harper A M.** Upper limit of autoregulation of cerebral blood flow in the baboon. *Circ. Res.* **34**:435-40, 1974.
4. **Enevoldsen E M & Taagehøj-Jensen F.** Autoregulation and CO$_2$ responses of cerebral blood flow in patients with acute severe head injury. *J. Neurosurgery* **48**:689-703, 1978.
5. **Palvölgyi R.** Regional cerebral blood flow in patients with intracranial tumors. *J. Neurosurgery* **31**:149-63, 1969.
6. **Lassen N A, Ingvar D H & Skinhøj E.** Brain function and blood flow. Changes in the amount of blood flowing in areas of the human cerebral cortex, reflecting changes in the activity of those areas, are graphically revealed with the aid of a radioactive isotope. *Sci. Amer.* **239**:62-71, 1978.

CC/NUMBER 33
AUGUST 18, 1980

This Week's Citation Classic

Ames A, III, Wright R L, Kowada M, Thurston J M & Majno G. Cerebral ischemia. II. The no-reflow phenomenon. *Amer. J. Pathol.* **52**:437-53, 1968. [Neurosurgical Serv., Mass. Gen. Hosp., and Dept. Pathol., Harvard Med. Sch., Boston, MA]

After seven minutes of circulatory arrest, it became increasingly difficult to fill rabbits' cerebral vessels with a carbon black suspension or to wash out the blood with Ringer's solution. If the blood had been displaced prior to the arrest, reperfusion with carbon black was complete. [The *SCI*® indicates that this paper has been cited over 320 times since 1968.]

Adelbert Ames III
Neurosurgical Service
Massachusetts General Hospital
Boston, MA 02114

July 10, 1980

"This study was a novel experience for me. Experiments designed to test a rather adventurous hypothesis provided support for each aspect of it—or so it appeared.

"We had previously found, to our surprise, that central nervous tissue maintained *in vitro* could recover from 20 minutes of ischemia, and we were trying to reconcile this observation with conventional wisdom that brain *in situ* is severely damaged after seven minutes of circulatory arrest. An important difference between the two situations is the dependence of the brain *in situ* on resumption of blood flow. There might be some difficulty, we postulated, on reestablishing flow. If ischemia stopped the active transport of Na^+ out of the cells, they would swell with fluid from the interstitial spaces and capillaries until the latter became too narrow to permit passage of the formed elements in the blood. At this point the situation would become irreversible, though the cells themselves were still viable. That was the hypothesis.

"Reversible ischemia was produced by the neurosurgical skills of Wright and Kowada, and the brains were examined in the pathology laboratories of Majno and Thurston. The experiments demonstrated an impairment of reperfusion following stasis that was not prevented by anticoagulants. Separate studies showed swelling of perivascular cells, with luminal narrowing, and protection by osmotic agents added to the blood. Q.E.D. (we thought).

"Experiments we have performed since then have confirmed the difficulty with reperfusion, but have not confirmed the mechanism proposed for it. There is now good evidence that the main problem is a progressive increase in the viscosity of the immobilized blood, compounded by a loss of autoregulation and neurogenic hypotension.[1] Osmotic agents protect by lowering blood viscosity rather than by preventing cell swelling, which is not marked until later. So it is now apparent that our original hypothesis only partially survived experimentation.

"The paper received little attention at first. Few laboratories were studying ischemia at that time. There was an aura of inevitability about ischemic cell death that discouraged investigation. But with the concept that survival may be determined by factors that can be defined and perhaps controlled there has been a rapidly increasing interest in the subject. I believe our paper has contributed to this.

"Studies of reperfusion following ischemia have now been reported by many investigators working with a variety of tissues. The phrase 'no-reflow phenomenon' has come into rather common usage, which is flattering but also unfortunate since it is now evident that the all-or-none connotation is inappropriate. The circumstances under which impaired reperfusion contributes to cell death from ischemia have not been fully defined and remain the subject of a healthy controversy."

1. **Fischer E G, Ames A, III & Lorenzo A V.** Cerebral blood flow immediately following brief circulatory arrest. *Stroke* **10**:423-7, 1979.

CC/NUMBER 18
APRIL 30, 1984

This Week's Citation Classic™

Opie L H. Metabolism of the heart in health and disease. Part I. *Amer. Heart J.* **76**:685-98, 1968.
[MRC Metabolic Reactions Research Unit, Department of Biochemistry, Imperial College, London, England]

The major fuels for the normal human heart are free fatty acids in the fasted state and glucose in the fed state. During hypoxia, glucose metabolism is accelerated with the production of lactate (anaerobic glycolysis). When lactate accumulates or when the intracellular pH falls, glycolysis may be limited. During hypoxia, products of lipid metabolism, such as triglycerides, accumulate and these might have harmful effects. The state of oxygenation therefore profoundly affects myocardial metabolism. [The *SCI*® indicates that this paper has been cited in over 220 publications since 1968.]

Lionel H. Opie
Division of Cardiology
Department of Medicine
Stanford University Medical Center
Stanford, CA 94305

March 23, 1984

"My interest in myocardial metabolism was awakened by Sir John McMichael, previous director of the department of medicine at the Hammersmith Royal Postgraduate Medical School, in 1959. He pointed out: 'When the heart fails, the anatomy looks the same, but something has gone wrong with the chemistry.' In a flash of enthusiasm I realized that not only congestive heart failure, but drug action and many clinical aspects of heart function were ultimately going to be explained by myocardial metabolism. I avidly began to read about the subject but could find no suitable review reference material except for two: Olson and Schwartz reviewed basic science in *Medicine* in 1951,[1] and Richard Bing described human heart metabolism in *Circulation* in 1955.[2] The field was clearly developing, as shown by Bing's Harverian Oration to the New York Academy of Sciences in 1946, so it seemed to me before any extensive research work should be undertaken that existing knowledge required gathering and analysis. That decision was made in 1960 when I was a research fellow at Harvard Medical School.

"The review took much longer to write than I had anticipated, and it only began to look like something reasonable in 1966 while I was working with Sir Hans Krebs in biochemistry at Oxford University, England. However, Sir Hans pointed out that the review was still not ready and required even more work. Consequently, I had grave doubts about the academic quality of the proposed publication, which was not completed until I was working with Sir Ernst Chain (like Krebs, also a refugee from Nazi Germany and, like Krebs, also a Nobel prizewinner). By now the review was becoming more solid and Chain encouraged me to proceed. The *American Heart Journal* accepted it at once.

"I believe the article was a success for four reasons. First, my article was among those which led clinical cardiologists to see, as Sir John had emphasized, that the way the heart muscle functioned was more important than the way it looked. Secondly, it was written at a time when there was an enormous amount of new work in the area of human heart metabolism (Bing at Detroit)[2] and in glucose and fatty acid metabolism of the heart, coming especially from the units of Howard Morgan[3] at Nashville and Philip Randle[4] at Cambridge. Thirdly, because of the very high standards of Krebs and Chain, I had to go to great lengths to establish that the article was of the highest possible academic standard. The ultimate product was therefore accepted not only by cardiologists but also by biochemists and physiologists as a standard reference. I should add a fourth reason for the success of the article—namely, that the *American Heart Journal* had the foresight to publish what was basically an *avant-garde* subject at that time and thereby brought the subject of myocardial metabolism to the attention of the cardiological community as a whole.

"My interest in myocardial metabolism has served as a basis for my forthcoming book entitled *The Heart: Physiology, Metabolism and Pharmacology*.[5] The fascinating relationship between cardiac metabolism and mechanics is well explored in the book *Cardiac Metabolism*,[6] edited by Angela Drake-Holland and Mark Noble. Myocardial metabolism is now largely concerned with the regulation of calcium ion movements and, therefore, with contractility; hence, it is a subject that continues to be fundamental to modern cardiology."

1. **Olson R E & Schwartz W B.** Myocardial metabolism in congestive heart failure. *Medicine* **30**:21-41, 1951.
2. **Bing R J.** Metabolism of the human heart. *Circulation* **12**:635-47, 1955.
3. **Morgan H E, Henderson M J, Regan D M & Park C R.** Regulation of glucose uptake in muscle. *J. Biol. Chem.* **236**:253-61, 1961. (Cited 510 times.)
4. **Randle P J, Newsholme E A & Garland P B.** Regulation of glucose uptake by muscle. *Biochemical J.* **93**:652-65, 1964. (Cited 260 times.)
5. **Opie L H.** *The heart: physiology, metabolism and pharmacology.* New York: Grune & Stratton. To be published, 1984.
6. **Drake-Holland A J & Noble M I M,** eds. *Cardiac metabolism.* New York: Wiley, 1983. 544 p.

CC/NUMBER 1
JANUARY 2, 1984

This Week's Citation Classic™

Braunwald E. Control of myocardial oxygen consumption: physiologic and clinical considerations. *Amer. J. Cardiol.* **27**:416-32, 1971.
[Department of Medicine, School of Medicine, University of California, La Jolla, CA]

This paper summarizes experiments carried out in the dog heart and cat papillary muscle designed to elucidate the determinants of the heart's requirements for O_2. The basal O_2 consumption of the heart and the O_2 cost of depolarization were relatively small. The oxygen cost of 'pressure work' was found to be far greater than 'flow work,' and a close relation was found between the area beneath the left ventricular pressure curve and myocardial oxygen consumption. Myocardial contractility, as reflected in the maximal velocity of isotonic shortening, and heart rate were found to be additional major determinants of myocardial oxygen consumption. [The *SCI*® indicates that this paper has been cited in over 455 publications since 1971.]

Eugene Braunwald
Department of Medicine
Harvard Medical School
Boston, MA 02115

October 31, 1983

"This paper represents the culmination of experimental work which my colleagues and I carried out during a 13-year period at the National Institutes of Health, begun during my postdoctoral fellowship in S.J. Sarnoff's laboratory and continued in my own laboratory. This effort involved many talented scientists, including Sarnoff, R.B. Case, J. Ross, and E.H. Sonnenblick.

"The experiments summarized in this paper depended on the development of techniques for independently regulating aortic pressure, stroke volume, and heart rate. The preparation employed was an isolated heart from which the coronary venous return was directed to the jugular veins of a second (support) dog, which renewed the isolated heart circuit with fresh arterialized blood[1] permitting the preparation to exhibit stable performance for hours. We found that the myocardial oxygen consumption ($M\dot{V}O_2$) per beat was closely related to what we termed the tension-time index, i.e., the area under the left ventricular pressure curve. Thus, it is *not* possible to estimate the energy needs of the heart from the external work when the latter is calculated as the product of developed pressure and stroke volume. External myocardial efficiency, i.e., the ratio of external work performed to the oxygen consumed, varies widely depending on the hemodynamic conditions. In addition to the tension-time index, heart rate emerged as a second major determinant of $M\dot{V}O_2$. In closely related studies, we found that $M\dot{V}O_2$ is a major determinant of coronary blood flow.[2]

"Six years after the completion of these experiments, we were working on the technique of paired electrical pacing[3] by which we hoped to slow heart rate and thereby reduce $M\dot{V}O_2$. To our surprise, paired pacing *increased*, not reduced, $M\dot{V}O_2$, even though the heart rate decreased. Since paired pacing increases contractility, we reasoned that in addition to the tension-time index and heart rate, myocardial contractility must be another major determinant of $M\dot{V}O_2$. This was soon confirmed using other interventions which stimulated or depressed contractility while heart rate and tension-time index were held constant.[4]

"Subsequently, we used the results in a long series of experiments—still ongoing—designed to reduce the size of myocardial infarction following coronary occlusion.[5] Since myocardial ischemia and ultimately myocardial necrosis depend on an imbalance between myocardial O_2 supply and demand, interventions which reduce demand (by lowering the tension-time index, heart rate, and/or contractility) reduce infarct size. It was found that they do so in experimental animals and in patients as well, if $M\dot{V}O_2$ can be reduced immediately following coronary occlusion.

"This paper has been widely quoted because it was published at a time when interest in the treatment of myocardial ischemia became intense. Manipulations to reduce $M\dot{V}O_2$, such as beta adrenergic blockade and balloon counterpulsation, were becoming available for clinical use. Methods to challenge coronary reserve, such as electrical stimulation of heart rate, were being used in cardiac diagnostic laboratories. An understanding of the mechanism of producing myocardial ischemia in the face of a restricted coronary vascular reserve, of the amelioration of ischemia, and of the prevention of necrosis all require knowledge of the factors that regulate $M\dot{V}O_2$; these factors and their relative importance and interactions were summarized in this paper. Early in 1983, I reviewed more recent experimental work on the determinants of myocardial oxygen consumption, and related the results of these physiological studies to clinical problems in ischemic heart disease.[6]

"This work on $M\dot{V}O_2$ resulted in my receiving the Research Achievement Award of the American Heart Association in 1972."

1. **Sarnoff S J, Braunwald E, Welch G H, Jr., Case R B, Stainsby W N & Macruz R.** Hemodynamic determinants of oxygen consumption of the heart with special reference to the tension-time index. *Amer. J. Physiol.* **192**:148-56, 1958. (Cited 1,140 times since 1958.)
2. **Braunwald E, Sarnoff S J, Case R B, Stainsby W N & Welch G H, Jr.** Hemodynamic determinants of coronary flow: effect of changes in aortic pressure and cardiac output on the relationship between myocardial oxygen consumption and coronary flow. *Amer. J. Physiol.* **192**:157-63, 1958.
3. **Braunwald E, Ross J, Jr., Frommer P L, William J F, Jr., Sonnenblick E H & Gault J H.** Clinical observations on paired electrical stimulation of the heart: effects on ventricular performance and heart rate. *Amer. J. Med.* **37**:700-11, 1964.
4. **Sonnenblick E H, Ross J, Jr., Covell J W, Kaiser G A & Braunwald E.** Velocity of contraction as a determinant of myocardial oxygen consumption. *Amer. J. Physiol.* **209**:919-27, 1965. (Cited 325 times.)
5. **Rude R E, Muller J E & Braunwald E.** Efforts to limit the size of myocardial infarcts. *Ann. Intern. Med.* **95**:736-61, 1981.
6. **Braunwald E & Sobel B E.** Control of myocardial oxygen consumption. (Braunwald E, ed.) *Heart disease.* Philadelphia: W. B. Saunders, 1983. p. 1235-57.

This Week's Citation Classic

NUMBER 42
OCTOBER 15, 1979

Doherty J E. The clinical pharmacology of digitalis glycosides: a review.
Amer. J. Med. Sci. **255**:382-414, 1968.
[Univ. Arkansas Sch. Med., Dept. Med. & Med. Serv., Little Rock Vet. Admin. Hosp. Little Rock, AR]

The biologic half-times and pharmacokinetic behavior of the important digitalis glycosides are reviewed. Digoxin is excreted primarily in the urine as the unchanged glycoside and T½ is prolonged by renal failure. Digitalis resistance is noted in thyrotoxicosis; sensitivity in myxedema, and pulmonary disease. A plea is made for smaller doses to avoid toxicity. [The *SCI*® indicates that this paper has been cited over 180 times since 1968.]

James E. Doherty
College of Medicine
University of Arkansas
Little Rock, AR 72201
and
Veterans Administration
Hospital, Little Rock, AR 72206

February 22, 1978

"I was surprised to receive this invitation. This paper is a review. I suppose one of the major reasons it was so popular was because it was timely. This places most of the credit on Arnold Weissler, the editor of the *Journal* at the time, who asked me to prepare the manuscript.

"The review was based upon a paper I read at an American Heart Association meeting a year or so before for a panel discussion on the digitalis glycosides. I suppose that one of the reasons for its 'citation' popularity was its emphasis on pharmacokinetics. It was the first review of digitalis to emphasize this discipline and to focus on the special contribution of the post World War II tracer isotope turnover studies to this part of clinical management of patients who required this medication. Digoxin was the fourth most frequently prescribed drug by physicians in 1971 and continues to be near the 'top-of-the-line' today.

"Our group in Little Rock was fortunate enough to have had a major role in these studies, having conceived and contracted for a tritium label of digoxin after earlier studies with tritiated cholesterol, a compound of similar chemical structure, demonstrated this was feasible.[1] The experience we gained with this work assisted us in experimental design and techniques used in human tracer turnover studies essential to success of the experiments which led to publication and later to the review.

"I recall vividly the quiet excitement of the late Bill Perkins, my nuclear medicine associate, when we began this work. Ours was a small operation and the opportunity to 'scoop' was a very compelling reason to push ahead. We knew that studies with tritium labeled digoxin would provide significant new knowledge, immediately visible and important to the clinical use of this popular glycoside. We ultimately published about fifty papers related to tritiated digoxin, including this review.

"A review of clinical pharmacologic studies appeals to physician-readers because of the clinical application that is more often apparent in a review than in original publications. In addition, there is opportunity to link the more basic studies to clinical practice, as well as providing subsequent authors with a single reference, rather than multiple reference sources.

"Due credit is acknowledged and given to cooperative patients, dedicated technicians, house staff, professional associates, as well as our students, who continue to inspire us."

1. **Doherty J E, Perkins W H, Shapiro J & Dodd C.** Radiocarbon and tritium labeled cholesterol in alpha and beta lipoproteins after oral administration to human subjects. *J. Lab. Clin. Med.* **59**:550-7, 1962.

This Week's Citation Classic

CC/NUMBER 20
MAY 19, 1980

Epstein S E, Robinson B F, Kahler R L & Braunwald E. Effects of beta-adrenergic blockade on the cardiac response to maximal and submaximal exercise in man. *J. Clin. Invest.* **44**:1745-53, 1965.
[Cardiology Branch, National Heart Institute, Bethesda, MD]

The sympathetic contribution to the cardiac response to exercise was determined in man using propranolol, a beta-adrenergic blocking agent. Blocking sympathetic stimulation reduced heart rate, cardiac output, and mean arterial pressure during submaximal and maximal exercise, and diminished both maximum VO_2 and capacity for strenuous exertion. [The *SCI*® indicates that this paper has been cited over 305 times since 1965.]

Stephen E. Epstein
Cardiology Branch
National Heart, Lung,
and Blood Institute
National Institutes of Health
Bethesda, MD 20205

April 29, 1980

"Eugene Braunwald and Richard L. Kahler had performed some interesting preliminary work in the early 1960s on oxygen debt occurring during strenuous exercise in patients with heart disease.[1] I joined Braunwald and Kahler in July, 1963 and Brian Robinson, from St. George's Hospital in London, began a two year fellowship with us later that year.

"As a result of the initial work, the four of us undertook a more systematic investigation of oxygen debt in an attempt to develop a reliable index of circulatory impairment, as well as a means of documenting therapeutic efficacy of various cardiovascular interventions. Over the next year we delved into the intricacies of exercise testing in normal subjects and in patients with heart disease. It soon became apparent that oxygen debt was neither a reliable means of assessing cardiovascular dysfunction nor of ascertaining the response of the cardiovascular system to interventions. Although our original goals seemed thwarted, in the process we gained a considerable amount of expertise in exercise physiology. We also developed a deep interest in the mechanisms responsible for the profound circulatory changes occurring during exercise.

"There had been a great deal of interest in the role of the sympathetic nervous system in modulating this response. However, definitive studies were impossible to perform because of the inability to isolate the sympathetic component of the response. For example, most blocking drugs available had both anti-adrenergic and anti-parasympathetic effects. It so happened that Robinson, while in England, had worked with pronethalol, the first specific beta-adrenergic blocking agent developed. Shortly thereafter, propranolol, the successor to pronethalol, had become available. Thus, by mid-1964, we were in a fortunate situation: the laboratory had an intense interest in exercise physiology, and especially in the sympathetic component of the cardiovascular response to exercise; a specific beta-adrenergic blocking drug had recently been developed; and a large scale exercise-related effort the laboratory was engaged in had floundered, creating the time necessary to initiate what ultimately proved to be a fruitful investigation.

"The manuscript resulting from this study has been frequently cited mainly, I believe, for two reasons. First, the investigation was of interest to the physiologist exploring the basic mechanisms responsible for modulating the circulatory response to exercise. Second, beta-adrenergic blocking drugs were soon to become one of the more frequently used drugs in the therapy of various types of cardiovascular disorders. Clinicians and clinically oriented investigators therefore became vitally interested in the cardiovascular effects of beta-blocking agents and the effects these drugs have on exercise capacity."

1. **Kahler R L, Thompson R H, Buskirk E R, Frye R L & Braunwald E.** Studies on digitalis. VI. Reduction of the oxygen debt after exercise with digoxin in cardiac patients without heart failure. *Circulation* **27**:397-413, 1963.

CC/NUMBER 9
MARCH 1, 1982

This Week's Citation Classic

Paterson J W, Conolly M E, Dollery C T, Hayes A & Cooper R G.
The pharmacodynamics and metabolism of propranolol in man.
Pharmacologia Clinica **2**:127-33, 1970.
[Dept. Clin. Pharmacol., Royal Postgrad. Med. Sch., London, and Dept. Biochem., Imperial Chem. Industries, Macclesfield, Cheshire, England]

This paper was the first full study of the pharmacokinetics of propranolol after both intravenous and oral administration in man. It also described a method for quantifying the pharmacological response to propranolol using intravenous isoprenaline. The method was used to correlate pharmacodynamics with pharmacokinetics following administration of propranolol in man. [The ***SCI*®** **indicates that this paper has been cited over 245 times since 1970.]**

J.W. Paterson
Department of Pharmacology
Queen Elizabeth II Medical Centre
University of Western Australia
Nedlands 6009
Western Australia

December 11, 1981

"At the time this project was conceived, I was working as a Wellcome Fellow in clinical pharmacology with Colin Dollery at the Royal Postgraduate Medical School. We were concerned with the pharmacology of beta adrenoceptor antagonists in man as there was then considerable controversy about the mechanism of action of propranolol in the treatment of angina, hypertension, and arrhythmias. The problem was handicapped by the lack of adequate kinetic data in man and the lack of a suitable method of quantifying beta blockade in human subjects. At that time, beta blockade was measured in man by using a dose of isoprenaline sufficient to cause a pulse rate rise of up to 40 beats per minute and then finding the dose of propranolol to prevent this tachycardia. This dose was then defined as the 'beta blocking dose.' The doses of propranolol used in therapy were larger than these, and so other properties of the drug were proposed to explain the therapeutic effect. As propranolol had been shown to be a competitive beta blocker in the laboratory, it appeared to us that the concept of a 'beta blocking dose' was erroneous. It also seemed unreasonable to comment on the variation in dose required to give a therapeutic effect without adequate kinetic data. Fortunately, Alan Hayes of Imperial Chemical Industries was concerned about obtaining accurate kinetic data in man. Previous studies with conventional assay techniques using nonradioactive material were difficult to interpret as the blood levels seen in man at therapeutic doses were near the lower limits of assay sensitivity. We thus set up a joint study to explore the concept of the 'beta blocking dose' and the kinetics of propranolol using ^{14}C labelled drugs. This was an exciting project in which the expertise and resources of the academic department at the Royal Postgraduate Medical School and the industrial laboratory at Imperial Chemical Industries produced very fruitful results. I well remember carrying out the initial studies on myself as subject, and Figures 2 and 3 in the paper show that data. These studies showed that in man, propranolol exhibited the characteristics of competitive receptor blockade and that the concept of complete beta-receptor blockade was not tenable.

"The kinetic data demonstrated that after oral administration the drug was completely absorbed, and that peak blood levels of propranolol and 4-hydroxy propranolol (a metabolite with beta blocking properties) were seen 1¼ hours after administration. The isoprenaline dose-response studies confirmed that the maximum degree of beta blockade occurred at the same time. No 4-hydroxy propranolol was seen after intravenous administration and so we correlated plasma levels of propranolol given intravenously with the degree of beta blockade measured with isoprenaline. This was the first demonstration that the degree of beta blockade was related to the plasma level of propranolol.

"I believe that the paper is frequently cited for two main reasons. First, it completely changed clinical thinking on the meaning of beta blockade in man and on the techniques which should be used in its assessment. For a recent review of this problem see McDevitt.[1] Secondly, it was the first adequate kinetic study in man and demonstrated the formation of an active metabolite after oral but not intravenous administration. For a recent review of the kinetics of propranolol see Routledge and Shand."[2]

1. **McDevitt D G.** The assessment of beta-adrenoceptor blocking drugs in man. *Brit. J. Clin. Pharmacol.* **4**:413-25, 1977.
2. **Routledge P A & Shand D G.** Clinical pharmacokinetics of propranolol. *Clin. Pharmacokinet.* **4**:73-90, 1979.

CC/NUMBER 28
JULY 11, 1983

This Week's Citation Classic

Zacharias F J, Cowen K J, Prestt J, Vickers J & Wall B G. Propranolol in hypertension: a study of long-term therapy, 1964-1970.
Amer. Heart J. **83**:755-61, 1972.
[Clatterbridge General Hospital, Bebington, Wirral, Cheshire, England]

This paper reviews the use of propranolol in 300 hypertensive patients of all grades of severity over a six-year period. Data are provided about the effectiveness of propranolol as a first line antihypertensive drug, both alone and in combination with other remedies, and about its dose range and its profile of adverse effects. [The *SCI*® indicates that this paper has been cited in over 245 publications since 1972.]

F.J. Zacharias
Hypertension Unit
Clatterbridge General Hospital
Wirral, Cheshire
England

May 5, 1983

"In 1950, when I first became interested in the management of hypertension, the available drugs were few in number, unpleasant to take, and unpredictable in their effects.

"Then, following Ahlquist's original paper,[1] and before the first beta blockers were produced, Black correctly predicted that they would be of great value in the treatment of cardiovascular disease, especially angina.[2] What nobody predicted was their outstanding value as antihypertensives.

"My confidence in beta blockers in those days was no more than a hunch, but it was founded on two vital clinical observations by Brian Prichard on patients whom he was treating with propranolol and sotalol and who also happened to have raised blood pressures. Prichard said two things: that beta blockers did lower blood pressure, and that the response of the blood pressure was dose-dependent.[3,4] Both observations met with indifference and the second was widely disbelieved.

"I have always believed that unless hypertension could be managed in ordinary district general hospitals without special human or financial resources, we should never do more than scratch the surface of the problem. Such departments as the Hypertension Unit at Clatterbridge, involving three clinics five days a week, could, I hoped, deal with long-term studies involving large numbers, and, staffed largely by selected general practitioners, could also help by example to spread the gospel of good management.

"In a sense, therefore, this work was the logical outcome of my philosophy of management, which recognised that the family practitioner had to do most of the work and that the ultimate aim of the hospital physician should be to improve the standard of treatment in general practice.

"The propranolol paper was the preliminary report of a long-term study intended to answer questions of efficacy and safety and also the place of beta blockers in the therapeutic spectrum. It was the first of several such studies involving practolol, atenolol, sotalol, and others. These studies are tedious but if anyone doubts their necessity they have only to recall the practolol saga, in which I was intimately involved. We had 167 patients on practolol under observation for a period of six years, with ultimately more than 40 cases of the oculomucocutaneous syndrome.

"Just after the publication of this paper we started to look at atenolol, a drug specifically designed for hypertension, and which after ten years of observation and more than 1,400 patients, I regard as the most satisfactory antihypertensive beta blocker yet produced.

"Several factors may have contributed to the frequent citation of this paper: we had great latitude in the design and development of our study; we had a great range of tablets provided by the pharmaceutical industry; we had a unit of unusual functional design which enabled us to study very large numbers of patients over a very long period of time. These factors helped us to exploit the full potential of this treatment in a way that other investigators could not readily do.

"For a recent review publication in this field, see the proceedings of the symposium at Monte Carlo in 1982 and in particular the opening paper by J.I.S. Robertson."[5,6]

1. **Ahlquist R P.** A study of the adrenotropic receptors. *Amer. J. Physiol.* **153**:586-600, 1948.
2. **Black J W.** The predictive value of animal tests in relation to drugs affecting the cardiovascular system of man. (Wolstenholme G E & Porter R, eds.) *Drug responses in man.* London: Churchill, 1967. p. 111-18.
3. **Prichard B N C & Gillam P M S.** Use of propranolol (Inderal) in treatment of hypertension. *Brit. Med. J.* **2**:725-7, 1964.
4. ---------------------------------------. Treatment of hypertension with propranolol. *Brit. Med. J.* **1**:7-16, 1969.
5. **Robertson J I S, Kaplan N M, Caldwell A D S & Speight T M,** eds. Symposium on β-blockers in the 1980s: focus on atenolol. (Whole issue.) *Drugs* **25**(Suppl. 2), 1983. 346 p.
6. **Robertson J I S.** State-of-the-art review: β-blockade and the treatment of hypertension. *Drugs* **25**(Suppl. 2):5-11, 1983.

This Week's Citation Classic

CC/NUMBER 35
AUGUST 27, 1979

Laragh J H, Angers M, Kelly W G & Lieberman S. Hypotensive agents and pressor substances: the effect of epinephrine, norepinephrine, angiotensin II, and others on the secretory rate of aldosterone in man.
J. Amer. Med. Ass. **174**:234-40, 1960.
[Depts. Med., Obstet., and Gynecol. and Biochem., College of Physicians and Surgeons, Columbia Univ. & Presbyterian Hosp., NY]

Of a number of vasoconstrictors infused into volunteers, only angiotensin (the substance released by the kidney enzyme renin) stimulated aldosterone secretion. This revealed a kidney-adrenal biochemical 'axis' for control of sodium and potassium balance and blood pressure, and indicated that its derangement can cause malignant hypertension, with aldosterone excess and hypokalemia. [The *SCI*® indicates that this paper has been cited over 385 times since 1961.]

John H. Laragh
Cardiovascular Center
Cornell University Medical College
New York, NY 10021

March 21, 1978

"This paper, demonstrating the chemical interaction between the kidney and the adrenal cortex, was a keystone in the research journey that first exposed the renin-angiotensin-aldosterone hormonal 'axis' as a true biological control system for regulating simultaneously sodium and potassium homeostasis and blood pressure and tissue perfusion. The paper then showed its involvement in hypertensive diseases. We focused on how aldosterone regulates the amount of body sodium and water and had demonstrated that plasma potassium levels regulate aldosterone secretion. Observing hypokalemia in patients with malignant hypertension, we showed it was due to massive oversecretion of aldosterone. This was the first biochemical abnormality of causal relevance to be revealed in human hypertensive disease. We reasoned that the aldosterone excess might be caused by damaged kidneys. The renal enzyme, renin, was in disrepute as a biologically relevant substance. But its active product, angiotensin, had recently been synthesized, so we decided to see if it could affect aldosterone. By infusing angiotensin into volunteers, we demonstrated that angiotensin II, unlike other pressor agents, sharply stimulated aldosterone secretion. Thus, a new hormonal link was established, with angiotensin (like $K+$) emerging as the second major stimulus for aldosterone secretion. The outlines of a new control system became apparent and we proposed that a disorder of it, with excesses of renin and aldosterone, caused malignant hypertension.

"Reasoning teleologically (i.e., if this is an organized system what are its purposes?) we detailed the normal, coherent regulation of sodium and potassium balance, arterial pressure, and tissue flow by the renin axis. We showed that derangements of the system either cause, sustain, or react to all naturally-occurring hypertensive disorders.

"Using the plasma renin activity, indexed against the 24 hour excreted sodium (renin profiling), derangements of the renin axis were defined in malignant hypertension, primary aldosteronism, oral contraceptive hypertension, and renovascular hypertension. We then showed that essential hypertension is not all alike, its different renin profiles expressing different mechanisms that respond to different treatments. In parallel, using pharmacologic probes, renin activity was shown to sustain part or all of the high blood pressure in some 70% (high and 'normal' renin forms) while its activity is virtually absent in another 30% with low-renin disease. This provided the basis for an all-encompassing vasoconstriction-volume hypothesis, viewing all hypertension as a spectrum ranging between excess vasoconstriction and excess volume. Renin profiling differentiates patients diagnostically and allows selection of lesion specific therapy. This research laid the foundation for the modern analysis and treatment of one of man's most life-limiting disorders.

"To me the three essential ingredients for such discoveries are a capacity to (1) recognize unusual clinical phenomena, (2) develop an hypothesis to explain the anomaly and design studies to test it, using (3) technically impeccable measurements. Without all three, discovery is unlikely."

This Week's Citation Classic

Conn J W, Cohen E L & Rovner D R. Suppression of plasma renin activity in primary aldosteronism; distinguishing primary from secondary aldosteronism in hypertensive disease. *J. Amer. Med. Ass.* **190:**213-21, 1964.

Hypertension associated with overproduction of aldosterone, the salt-active adrenal hormone, results from either an abnormality of the adrenal gland itself or a circulatory deficiency of the kidney. This paper demonstrates that these two causes of hypertension can be distinguished functionally by measuring the level of plasma renin activity, subnormal in adrenal cases and supernormal in renovascular cases. [The *SCI*® indicates that this paper has been cited 276 times since 1964.]

Jerome W. Conn
Admiralty Point
2369 Gulf Shore Blvd., North
Naples, FL 33940

January 23, 1978

"We are delighted that one of our publications is included on the list of 'most cited papers.' Its review has awakened memories of excitement that my collaborators and I experienced as the data accumulated. It also recalled exciting earlier work which constituted the impetus for the 'most cited paper.'

"In 1954, after eight months of continuous and intensive study of a single patient, I had come to a novel conclusion: this hypertensive patient was suffering from a hitherto unrecognized disease due to excessive production of a then recently discovered hormone, aldosterone. I now faced two immediate problems: (1) to advise the patient to undergo surgical adrenal exploration and (2) to persuade a surgeon to do the operation. This kind of surgery had always been done for other purposes and with an entirely different constellation of biochemical indications. 'Can you justify this approach to the treatment of your patient? Is this an experiment?' asked the surgeon. I was floored, but I explained patiently again the important aspects of my data.

"In the operating room I watched as the surgeon, through a deep incision, was palpating the right adrenal gland. He turned and said quietly, 'I can feel a small tumor in the gland and it bulges on the surface.' I stepped off my lift, aware that my head was suddenly full and pounding. I recall thinking, 'This will not be the last one.' Two weeks later my patient was cured. I called the disease Primary Aldosteronism (PA). Since then, thousands of such patients throughout the world have undergone similar operations.

"Now back to the 'most cited paper.' By 1961 the renin-angiotensin system had been linked to aldosterone production. Renovascular hypertension (RVH), associated with aldosteronism, now had a clear explanation: excessive renin-angiotensin production with stimulation of too much aldosterone from *normal* adrenals (secondary aldosteronism). How could we distinguish between these two forms of hypertension, each associated with excessive production of aldosterone? I was aware of a 1957 report by F.W. Dunihue and W.V.B. Robertson demonstrating atrophy of renal juxtaglomerular cells (site of renin production) following administration of desoxycorticosterone, a steroid with properties similar to those of aldosterone.[1] This proved to be the key. It suggested that renin production might be very low in PA and, indeed, it was. By a then crude bioassay we could measure the range of renin activity in normal people and the very high levels in RVH. But we could detect none in PA. A clear functional distinction was now established. It was evident also that angiotensin was not involved in the genesis of the hypertension of PA. We now recognized low-renin and high-renin forms of human hypertension. The need for hypertension researchers to study the low end of the renin scale, as well as the high, became evident."

REFERENCE

1. **Dunihue F W & Robertson W V B.** Effect of desoxycorticosterone acetate and of sodium on juxtaglomerular apparatus. *Endocrinol.* **61**:293-7, 1957.

This Week's Citation Classic

Brunner H R, Laragh J H, Baer L, Newton M A, Goodwin F T, Krakoff L R, Bard R H & Bühler F R. Essential hypertension: renin and aldosterone, heart attack and stroke. *N. Engl. J. Med.* **286**:441-9, 1972.
[Dept. Med., Coll. Physicians and Surgeons, Columbia Univ., and Presbyterian Hosp., New York, NY]

In a retrospective analysis of 219 patients with essential hypertension, heart attacks and strokes were observed when plasma renin activity was normal or high, but in no instance when it was low. It was concluded that renin may be a risk factor in these patients. [The *SCI*® indicates that this paper has been cited in over 465 publications since 1972.]

Hans R. Brunner
Département de Médecine Interne
Centre Hospitalier
Universitaire Vaudois
CH-1011 Lausanne
Switzerland

September 15, 1982

"Essential hypertension has long presented a puzzle to investigators. First results of measurements of plasma renin activity in these patients had been a disappointment insofar as they were rarely elevated.[1] Indeed most patients had seemingly normal, and a sizable fraction even subnormal, levels. However, those patients with low renin levels were most intriguing to us. We were convinced that widely varying renin levels must reflect basic differences among the patients and therefore we decided to review retrospectively all hypertensive patients who had been studied by J.H. Laragh's group at the Columbia-Presbyterian Medical Center during the years before renin measurements had become possible.

"After months of searching through charts and compiling data, I stumbled over the fact that none of the 59 low renin patients had suffered a severe cardiovascular complication such as heart attack or stroke. Since angiotensin, the vasoactive hormone produced by renin, had previously been shown experimentally to elicit vasculotoxic effects, it seemed to make sense that the level of renin measured in hypertensive patients had some prognostic value. Together with Laragh, who happened to come by that Saturday morning, we were very excited about this observation and new concept.

"During the weeks that followed, while the manuscript was prepared, submitted to the *New England Journal of Medicine*, and finally in press, we were concerned that many other investigators may have made the same, what by then seemed to us obvious, observation and that the reaction at the time of publication would be, 'We have known this for a long time.' Our worries proved completely unnecessary, since the reaction of our peers was rather one of disbelief and eagerness to prove that we were wrong. Conceivably, it is largely based on this negative reaction that the paper has become a *Citation Classic*. Thus, I fear that if one analysed all individual citations, one would find that a large majority have referred to the paper in disbelief.

"The study was carried out retrospectively as were most of the studies which followed attempting to disprove the concept that renin may be a risk factor in patients with essential hypertension. Ten years later, the decisive prospective study still does not exist. Over the years, while many have challenged the idea, there has also been increasing support coming from experimental and clinical studies.[2] Perhaps more importantly, the provocative nature of our findings had triggered at the time a lot of new interest and research, trying to elucidate the role of the renin system in essential hypertension. This has, among other results, produced a new specific treatment for the disease by the development of inhibitors of the renin system."[3]

1. **Helmer O M.** Renin activity in blood from patients with hypertension. *Can. Med. Ass. J.* **90**:221-5, 1964.
2. **Gavras H, Brunner H R & Laragh J H.** Renin and aldosterone and the pathogenesis of hypertensive vascular damage. *Progr. Cardiovasc. Dis.* **17**:39-49, 1974.
3. **Ondetti M A, Rubin B & Cushman D W.** Design of specific inhibitors of angiotensin-converting enzyme: new class of orally active antihypertensive agents. *Science* **196**:441-4, 1977.

CC/NUMBER 42
OCTOBER 15, 1984

This Week's Citation Classic™

Gavras H, Brunner H R, Turini G A, Kershaw G R, Tifft C P, Cuttelod S, Gavras I, Vukovich R A & McKinstry D N. Antihypertensive effect of the oral angiotensin converting-enzyme inhibitor SQ 14225 in man. *N. Engl. J. Med.* **298**:991-5, 1978.
[Dept. Med. and Thorndike Res. Inst., Boston Univ. Med. Ctr., MA; Dept. Med., Hôp. Cantonal Universitaire, Lausanne, Switzerland; and Squibb Res. Inst., Princeton, NJ]

The antihypertensive effects of an inhibitor of the potent pressor hormone angiotensin II were described in patients with severe hypertension refractory to conventional medications. This study demonstrated the value of this novel therapeutic modality that has since become established treatment for hypertension and congestive heart failure. [The *SCI*® indicates that this paper has been cited in over 440 publications since 1978.]

Haralambos Gavras
Department of Medicine
Boston University School of Medicine
Boston, MA 02118

June 29, 1984

"The contribution of the renin-angiotensin system in the development and maintenance of high blood pressure had been a matter of controversy despite extensive investigation for many years. While studying a Brazilian snake venom extract, Ferreira[1] discovered a number of polypeptides that, among other actions, could inhibit the formation of angiotensin II and that were shown by Krieger *et al.*[2] to have an important antihypertensive effect in animals. I had been interested for many years in the role of angiotensin in hypertension and cardiac function. When a derivative of these snake venom extracts was synthesized at Squibb[3] and purified for human use, I saw the opportunity to test my theories regarding the relationship of renin and sodium in blood pressure maintenance in man.

"This work was an example of how intensive research in the pathophysiology of hypertension over several years finally culminated in the development of a new potentially lifesaving therapeutic concept. A parallel study describing for the first time the use of angiotensin blockade in congestive heart failure was first greeted with skepticism and, in fact, was rejected by several British and American journals before it was accepted by *Circulation*.[4] Both papers were followed by a flurry of clinical research activity by investigators in several countries, which eventually established the advantages of this approach in the treatment of both hypertension and congestive heart failure. Three years later, the compound (Captopril) received FDA approval and has since come into increasingly wide use as treatment for these conditions.[5,6] Furthermore, a number of second-generation converting-enzyme inhibitors have been developed and tested since then for possibly higher potency, longer duration of action, and fewer adverse reactions. I believe the wide practical applications and the large number of clinical studies spurred by the original observations described in our paper are the reasons that this paper has become a *Citation Classic*."

1. **Ferreira S H.** A bradykinin-potentiating factor (BPF) present in the venom of *Bothrops jararaca*. *Brit. J. Pharmacol.* **24**:163-9, 1965. (Cited 175 times.)
2. **Krieger E M, Salgado H C, Assan C J, Greene L L J & Ferreira S H.** Potential screening test for detection of overactivity of renin-angiotensin system. *Lancet* **1**:269-71, 1971. (Cited 110 times.)
3. **Ondetti M A, Rubin B & Cushman D W.** Design of specific inhibitors of angiotensin converting enzyme: new class of orally active antihypertensive agents. *Science* **196**:441-4, 1977. (Cited 530 times.)
4. **Gavras H, Faxon D P, Berkoben J, Brunner H R & Ryan T J.** Angiotensin converting enzyme inhibition in patients with congestive heart failure. *Circulation* **58**:770-6, 1978. (Cited 105 times.)
5. **Gavras H, Brunner H R & Gavras I.** Captopril in the treatment of hypertension. *Ann. Intern. Med.* **95**:505-6, 1981.
6. **Gavras H.** Hypertension and congestive heart failure: benefits of converting enzyme inhibition (Captopril). *J. Amer. Coll. Cardiol.* **1**:518-20, 1983.

CC/NUMBER 31
AUGUST 4, 1980

This Week's Citation Classic

Heath D & Edwards J E. The pathology of hypertensive pulmonary vascular disease. A description of six grades of structural changes in the pulmonary arteries with special reference to congenital cardiac septal defects. *Circulation* **18**:533-47, 1958.
[Mayo Clinic; and Mayo Foundation, Univ. Minnesota, Rochester, MN]

Progressive histological changes occur in the small pulmonary blood vessels as an association of the chronic pulmonary hypertension complicating many congenital cardiac septal defects. This progression is so stereotyped as to allow the recognition of six grades of change. [The ***SCI***® **indicates that this paper has been cited over 300 times since 1961.]**

Donald Heath
Department of Pathology
Duncan Building
Royal Liverpool Hospital
Liverpool L69 3BX
England

June 9, 1980

"The advent of cardiac surgery in the early 1950s brought with it an urgent and unexpected demand for a comprehensive understanding of the pathology of an area virtually previously ignored by morbid anatomists, namely, the pulmonary circulation. It became vital to know the pathology of the pulmonary hypertension which complicated many of the congenital cardiac anomalies coming to surgery and in particular to know if the altered pulmonary haemodynamics and vascular lesions were reversible or not. The only information available at that time was the data gathered in the US in the thirties by a British cardiologist, Oscar Brenner,[1] who had published five papers on the histology of the pulmonary vasculature. He told me in later years that he had had the greatest difficulty in publishing these articles which subsequently became classics, the reason given being that the subject was of no interest to doctors.

"In the 1950s I held a junior training post in cardiology in Sheffield in the north of England working in the field of congenital heart disease under James W. Brown and William Whitaker. It became increasingly apparent to us that pulmonary hypertension was exerting great influence on the clinical picture of our patients, but we were totally ignorant of the underlying pathology of the pulmonary circulation. I forsook cardiology for pathology, I thought then temporarily, to work for a year at the Mayo Clinic as a Rockefeller Fellow to study the pathology of pulmonary hypertension with Jesse E. Edwards, a world authority on cardiac pathology.

"Here it proved possible to show that the pathological changes in the pulmonary arteries in congenital cardiac shunts followed a stereotyped pattern in which distinct grades could be recognised. The significance of this paper was that it was followed by two others[2,3] showing that each of these succeeding histological grades had close physiological relationships so it became possible for the first time to look at sections of lung and interpret the appearances in haemodynamic terms. This later was shown to have great relevance to the reversibility of pulmonary hypertension following surgical correction of defects. This work was possible at the Mayo Clinic because of the wonderful spirit of friendliness and cooperation there that allowed me to wander at will through the files of the departments of pathology and physiology and so put the whole story together. This was an exhilirating experience for a young man trained in the more traditional approach of British morbid anatomy. Indeed this very functional approach to histopathology learned at the Clinic has remained with me ever since and has not met favour in some quarters.

"In 1953 I said to Bill Whitaker, 'Do you think there is enough in the pathology of pulmonary hypertension to make an MD thesis?' Some 30 years later I can look back over five books and 200 papers on the subject and smile at the question. I never found my way back to cardiology. This paper proved to be a gateway to a professorship in pathology, a doctorate of science, and a lifetime spent in asking and answering questions about the pathology of the pulmonary circulation."

1. **Brenner O.** Pathology of the vessels of the pulmonary circulation. *Arch. Intern. Med.* **56**:211-37, 1935.
2. **Heath D, Helmholz H F, Jr., Burchell H B, DuShane J W & Edwards J E.** Graded pulmonary vascular changes and hemodynamic findings in cases of atrial and ventricular septal defect and patent ductus arteriosus. *Circulation* **18**:1155-66, 1958.
3. **Heath D, Helmholz H F, Jr., Burchell H B, DuShane J W, Kirklin J W & Edwards J E.** Relation between structural changes in the small pulmonary arteries and the immediate reversibility of pulmonary hypertension following closure of ventricular and atrial septal defects. *Circulation* **18**:1167-74, 1958.

This Week's Citation Classic

CC/NUMBER 21
MAY 26, 1980

Scherlag B J, Lau S H, Helfant R H, Berkowitz W D, Stein E & Damato A N. Catheter technique for recording His bundle activity in man. *Circulation* **39**:13-8, 1969. [Cardiopulmonary Lab., US Public Health Service Hosp., Staten Island, NY]

A clinical technique is described for recording electrical activity from a specialized conducting fascicle, the His bundle, within the heart. The His bundle electrogram allows a more accurate determination of the site and degree of conduction delay or heart block than the electrocardiogram alone. [The *SCI*® **indicates that this paper has been cited over 720 times since 1969.]**

Benjamin J. Scherlag
Department of Medicine
University of Oklahoma
Health Sciences Center
Oklahoma City, OK 73104

December 10, 1979

"Hoffman and his associates in the early 1960s published an excellent series of studies in which recordings were made from the His bundle and bundle branches of the dog heart after cardiotomy and cardiopulmonary bypass.[1,2] In 1965, as Hoffman's postdoctoral student, I was involved in a project requiring the surgical induction of complete heart block in the experimental animal. In the anesthetized dog subjected to thoracotomy, I was able to locally inject the area of the His bundle with formaldehyde to induce complete heart block without cardiotomy or cardiopulmonary bypass. When I arrived at my first 'real' job at the Staten Island US Public Health Service Hospital in 1965, I realized my injection technique to destroy the His bundle could be used just as easily to record its electrical activity. By threading two Teflon-coated stainless steel wires into a hypodermic needle, the wires could be 'injected' into the His bundle region to record bipolar electrograms. Also, selective electrical pacing from the His bundle could be achieved through the same wires.[3]

"The next objective was to record and electrically pace from the His bundle without thoracotomy. John Lister, a colleague, had written a grant proposal before leaving Staten Island for Miami. In it he proposed to map the right heart using an electrode catheter with as many as six bipolar pairs on it. With the objective of recording electrical activity from the His bundle, Richard Helfant and I developed a technique by which a standard bipolar pacing catheter (2 electrode rings 1 cm apart) was passed via a femoral vein into the right heart of the dog. By monitoring the electrical activity we were able to position the electrode tip in apposition to the His bundle and record its electrical activation during the P-R segment of the simultaneously recorded electrocardiogram. Within a short time Sun Lau and I used the same technique to record His bundle activity in patients undergoing right heart catheterization.

"It took approximately two years for the technique established in the experimental laboratory to reach fruition as a clinical procedure. Electrocardiography at this time had become the purview of fewer and fewer academicians. With the development of techniques to record transmembrane potentials from cardiac muscle cells, cardiac electrophysiology tended to polarize into basic and clinical compartments. The popularization of the His bundle recording technique became the basis for a new field called clinical electrophysiology which quickly attracted many young investigators. The insights gained from intracardiac recordings made in the cardiac catheterization laboratory served to bridge the gap between experimental studies done on the whole animal and in isolated tissues and clinical electrocardiography."

1. **Hoffman B F, Cranefield P F, Stuckey J H & Bagdonas A A.** Electrical activity during the P-R interval. *Circ. Res.* **8**:1200-11, 1960.
2. **Hoffman B F, Amer N S, Stuckey J H, Cappelletti A & Domingo R T.** Activation of the interventricular septal myocardium studied during cardiopulmonary bypass. *Amer. Heart J.* **59**:224-37, 1960.
3. **Scherlag B J, Helfant R H & Damato A N.** A catheterization technique for His bundle stimulation and recording in the intact dog. *J. Appl. Physiol.* **25**:425-8, 1968.

This Week's Citation Classic

CC/NUMBER 16
APRIL 18, 1983

Coumel P & Attuel P. Reciprocating tachycardia in overt and latent preexcitation: influence of functional bundle branch block on the rate of the tachycardia. *Eur. J. Cardiol.* **1**:423-36, 1974.
[Hôpital Lariboisière, Paris, France]

This paper deals with two original ways for diagnosing latent preexcitation in patients with paroxysmal junctional reciprocating tachycardias: the phenomenon of paradoxically premature atrial capture by ventricular stimulation, and the influence of functional bundle branch block on the tachycardia rate. [The *SCI*® indicates that this paper has been cited in over 115 publications since 1974, making it the most-cited paper ever published in this journal.]

Philippe Coumel
Department of Cardiology
Hôpital Lariboisière
75015 Paris
France

February 15, 1983

"My interest in preexcitation syndromes dates from the early days of clinical electrophysiology; this discipline started in the late-1960s. Several groups realized that stimulating the heart chambers was a fantastic tool for exploring the arrhythmias. The atrioventricular (AV) junction was the most fruitful area for verifying the long proposed concept of reentry, but attention was focused on proving the reciprocating mechanism rather than locating it. It was supposed to be extranodal every time a preexcitation pattern was present, and the reverse was taken for granted.

"Mendez and Moe[1] were the first to demonstrate experimentally the reality of reentry in the AV node, and actually it was only after reading their publication that we understood what we had done in our first explored patient.[2] Again, Moe and his group called attention, in 1971, to the probability of accessory pathways conducting only retrogradely.[3] Precisely at that time it was also our impression, after having manipulated many junctional tachycardias, that they reacted identically whether or not the evidence of preexcitation was present. Progressively, just initiating and terminating tachycardias became less attractive than influencing their course: the yes or no question was replaced by the how and why. Instead of measuring RR or P'P' intervals, we started measuring the stimulation-P': shortening the cardiac cycle by more than the stimulus prematurity defined the paradoxically premature capture, which is sufficient to prove the existence of an extranodal circuit.

"The influence of the bundle branch block on the tachycardia rate is just an extension of this mode of reasoning. The time relationships between P' and R during reciprocating tachycardias were irrelevant in the classical conception of upper, middle, and lower nodal rhythms with initial and final common pathways, so that people working in this field were not paying enough attention to their variations. Measuring the retrograde conduction times during the capture phenomenon helped us to realize how meaningful the principles of goniometry were; and when these conduction times were disturbed in coincidence with the presence or absence of a bundle branch block, we were forced to realize that the only possible explanation was the route of the impulse. Once the principle was known, it could be extended to the other phenomena, most recently to the coupling interval of ventricular premature beats.[4]

"I think that this paper has been cited frequently because it is the first which deals directly with the problem of latent accessory pathways and proposes a diagnostic approach. Having a paper frequently or not frequently cited is a matter of chance, and language, rather than value: we published a more documented paper on this subject one year later,[5] and it was almost completely ignored. Since that time, many studies have been devoted to the same problem. They mainly use the technique of atrial capture and its time and space relationships with the ventricular activation and ventriculo-atrial conduction, in addition to the atrial mapping.[6,7] These different approaches to the geometry of the pathways have permitted extension of the notion of accessory routes not only to partial atrio-His or His-ventricle bundles, but also to accessory nodal formations, particularly in the permanent form of reciprocating tachycardia."[2,8]

1. **Mendez C & Moe G K.** Demonstration of a dual AV nodal conduction in the isolated rabbit heart. *Circ. Res.* **19**:378-93, 1966.
2. **Coumel P, Cabrol C, Fabiato A, Gourgon R & Slama R.** Tachycardie permanente par rythme réciproque. I. Preuves du diagnostic par stimulation auriculaire et ventriculaire. *Arch. Mal. Coeur Vaisseaux* **60**:1830-49, 1967.
3. **De La Fuente D, Sasyniuk B & Moe G K.** Conduction through a narrow isthmus in isolated canine atrial tissue: a model of the W.P.W. syndrome. *Circulation* **44**:803-9, 1971.
4. **Billak S A & Denes P.** The effect of intermittent bundle branch block on the coupling interval of ventricular premature depolarizations. *Circulation* **66**:1120-3, 1982.
5. **Coumel P, Attuel P, Motté G, Slama R & Bouvrain Y.** Les tachycardies jonctionnelles paroxystiques. Évaluation du point de jonction inférieur du circuit de rentrée. Démembrement des "rythmes réciproques intra-nodaux." *Arch. Mal. Coeur Vaisseaux* **68**:1255-68, 1975.
[The *SCI* indicates that this paper has been cited in over 25 publications since 1975.]
6. **Sellers T D, Jr., Gallagher J J, Cope G D, Tonkin A M & Wallace A G.** Retrograde atrial preexcitation following ventricular premature beats during reciprocating tachycardia in the Wolff-Parkinson-White syndrome. *Eur. J. Cardiol.* **4**:283-94, 1976.
7. **Gallagher J J, Pritchett E L C, Benditt D G, Tonkin A M, Campbell R W F, Dugan F A, Bashore T M, Tower A & Wallace A G.** New catheter techniques for analysis of the sequence of retrograde atrial activation in man. *Eur. J. Cardiol.* **6**:1-14, 1977.
8. **Gallagher J J & Sealy W C.** The permanent form of junctional reciprocating tachycardia: further elucidation of the underlying mechanism. *Eur. J. Cardiol.* **8**:413-30, 1978.

This Week's Citation Classic

CC/NUMBER 9
MARCH 3, 1980

Severinghaus J W. Blood gas calculator. *J. Appl. Physiol.* **21**:1108-16, 1966. [Dept. Anesthesia and Cardiovascular Res. Inst., Univ. California Med. Sch., San Francisco, CA]

The paper describes a slide rule for calculating human blood O_2 saturation from Po_2, pH, temperature and base excess, blood gas temperature corrections, the Henderson-Hasselbalch equation for blood and CSF, base excess, and BTPS *vs.* STPD factors. However, its primary use by physiologists is the standard O_2 dissociation curve I prepared from 11 publications and new measurements, with a graph of the fall of the temperature coefficient, $\Delta \log Po_2/\Delta T$, at high saturation. [The *SCI*® indicates that this paper has been cited over 645 times since 1966.]

John W. Severinghaus
Department of Anesthesia
and the Cardiovascular Research Institute
School of Medicine
University of California
San Francisco, CA 94143

December 27, 1979

"The idea of devising a slide rule for O_2 dissociation occurred to me while on sabbatical in Copenhagen in 1964. It resulted from talks with Poul Astrup about his proposed, formidable nomogram for calculating O_2 saturation, with four full sets of rectangular and bi-diagonal logarithmic grids. A slide rule multiplies numbers by adding logarithms, and this is needed to correct Po_2 for pH, temperature, BE, and P50. That evening, I constructed the first cardboard rule, adding other scales to it over succeeding weeks by using all the experts around town. Siggaard-Andersen helped with the base excess grid, the most complex calculation. Asmussen and I usually had lunch together, and he helped with the gas factors. I was able to join Naeraa's group in Aarhus to finish their studies of the separate roles of pH and Pco_2 on the Bohr coefficient[1] and, with help from Astrup and Xenia Brun, fill in the missing top and bottom of the O_2 dissociation curve. F.J.W. Roughton invited me to Cambridge for final discussions on details, from which grew our subsequent yearly summer dissociation curve studies in San Francisco until his death in 1972.[2] Scale drafting and design required frequent stops at Radiometer Co., halfway from home to work. The coincidence of so many important factors near Copenhagen was the more remarkable since I had chosen my sabbatical there to work on blood brain barrier transport with H.H. Ussing and P. Kruhøffer and on cerebral circulation with Niels Lassen. Also, I helped teach the WHO 11-month postgraduate course for anesthesiologists from underdeveloped countries. Each of these collaborations and contacts were to continue for many years, and led, on June 1, 1979, to my promotion to Doctor Medicine Honoris Causa on the occasion of the 500th anniversary of the University of Copenhagen (Hafnensis in Latin).

"The article has been widely used as the standard oxygen dissociation curve, and the standard for temperature correction and for calculation of the effects of pH, Pco_2, and base excess on oxygen tension, thus accounting for its frequent citation.

"It is less than 20 years since commercial blood gas analyzers became available. We are still seeing rapid growth in their use. As automated blood gas analyzers, computers, and pocket and desk calculators replace the slide rule, using the equations in this paper, the need for a simple accurate equation for the O_2 dissociation curve has become acute. The Adair and other equations are both complex and not very accurate. I recently modified Hill's too-simple equation enough to compute O_2 saturation from 0-100% to within $\pm 0.5\%$, and added other simple equations expressing the variations of the temperature and Bohr coefficients with saturation, and an iterative computation of O_2 content from either Po_2 or saturation, thus updating the 1966 papers."[3]

1. **Naeraa N, Strange-Petersen E, Boye E & Severinghaus J W.** pH and molecular components of the Bohr effect in human blood. *Scand. J. Clin. Lab. Invest.* **18**:96-102, 1966.
2. **Roughton F J W & Severinghaus J W.** O_2 dissociation curve analysis above 98% saturation for human blood. *J. Appl. Physiol.* **35**:861-9, 1973.
3. **Severinghaus J W.** Simple accurate equations for human blood O_2 dissociation computations. *J. Appl. Physiol.* **46**:599-602, 1979.

This Week's Citation Classic

de la Lande I S & Rand M J. A simple isolated nerve-blood vessel preparation. *Aust. J. Exp. Biol. Med. Sci.* **43**:639-56, 1965.
[Dept. Human Physiol. and Pharmacol., Univ. Adelaide, Adelaide, South Australia]

The isolated perfused rabbit ear artery responded by vasoconstriction to noradrenaline and to periarterial stimulation of intramural sympathetic nerves. Acetylcholine caused dilatation, but only when the tone was raised by sympathetic nerve stimulation; 5-hydroxytryptamine had only weak vasoconstrictor activity, but markedly potentiated the effects of noradrenaline. [The *SCI*® indicates that this paper has been cited over 145 times since 1965.]

I.S. de la Lande
Department of Clinical
and Experimental Pharmacology
University of Adelaide
Adelaide, South Australia 5001
Australia

April 11, 1980

"The paper described the pharmacology of an isolated perfused artery which responded rapidly and reproducibly to sympathetic nerve stimulation. As a result, the preparation has come into widespread use for the study of adrenergic transmission in arteries and of the modification of transmission by drugs, in particular nowadays, drugs acting via pre-synaptic receptors.

"The preparation was essentially a 'spin-off' from a collaborative study on sympathetic neurotransmitter release in the perfused rabbit ear carried out in 1963 while I was on 12 months' study leave from the department of human physiology and pharmacology, University of Adelaide, in W.D.M. Paton's laboratory at Oxford. Bill Paton, Barbara Waud, and I spent much of the year being baffled by the tiny amounts of transmitter released during seemingly massive vasoconstrictor responses to periarterial sympathetic nerve stimulation. We finally investigated the possibility that much of the response may have been localized to the region of the artery immediately distal to the site of stimulation. Small segments of the artery when perfused in identical fashion to the whole ear did indeed prove to be highly responsive. As my leave had expired, we concluded the study at that stage, but I arranged to explore further the potential of the isolated segment preparation on my return to Adelaide.

"Progress in 1964 was slow and went little beyond defining the optimal conditions for perfusing the vessel; however, the situation changed dramatically when Michael Rand, a former colleague from PhD student days, spent a short period in our department towards the end of 1964. His extensive experience in the area of adrenergic pharmacology was just what was needed to get the pharmacological characterization of the isolated rabbit ear artery 'off the ground,' and there followed several weeks of intensive activity during which most of the basic pharmacology described in the paper was defined. Indeed, my recollection is that the only 'recreation' Michael enjoyed during that time in Adelaide was to assist in the removal of a large orange tree from my garden in near-century heat! Predictably, in addition to providing a simple model for studying established vascular phenomena, the study gave us tantalizing glimpses of hitherto unsuspected phenomena. The mechanism of one of these—cholinergic inhibition of the response to sympathetic transmission—subsequently has been explained in terms of pre-synaptic receptors; however, another (serotonin-induced sensitization of other vasoactive agents) still awaits explanation after 15 years!

"I believe that two messages emerge from the history of the research which led to this publication. One is that it is yet another reminder of the way a new and useful technique can emerge as an unexpected bonus from a purely basic research project, in this instance, the study at Oxford. The other is that it illustrates the importance of collaboration between individuals who can bring quite different points of view and expertise into the solution of a problem of common interest, as was the case with Rand and myself."

CC/NUMBER 41
OCTOBER 12, 1981

This Week's Citation Classic

Strandness D E, Jr., Schultz R D, Sumner D S & Rushmer R F. Ultrasonic flow detection: a useful technic in the evaluation of peripheral vascular disease. *Amer. J. Surg.* **113**:311-20, 1967.
[Depts. Surgery and Physiol. and Biophys., Univ. Washington Sch. Med., and Third Univ. Surgical Serv., Veterans Admin. Hosp., Seattle, WA]

This paper describes the use of the ultrasonic velocity detector in the evaluation of patients with a wide variety of vascular disorders. The great appeal of this method is that it is safe, noninvasive, and can be applied to study arterial and venous disease involving all segments of the upper and lower extremities. [The *SCI*® indicates that this paper has been cited over 155 times since 1967.]

D.E. Strandness, Jr.
Department of Surgery
School of Medicine
University of Washington
Seattle, WA 98195

August 11, 1981

"This paper was the end result of a fortuitous happening which occurs so often in the lives of many of us. As a young surgeon, I was convinced there had to be better objective methods of evaluating patients with peripheral vascular disease. The traditional, time-tested approaches were clearly inadequate in describing the pathophysiology of vascular disease and monitoring the effects of therapy.

"Because of my training in surgery, I was ill-prepared to launch myself into more quantitatively oriented disciplines such as physiology and engineering which would provide me with the necessary background. Fortunately, R.F. Rushmer had an intensive summer course in electronics, physics, and bioengineering which introduced me to a whole new field and most importantly changed my outlook and approach to applied research.

"It was during this time that I was first exposed to ultrasonic techniques as available for both experimental and early clinical application.[1,2] I immediately recognized that ultrasound could and would with time become one of the most useful modalities available to those interested in studying peripheral vascular function, both in the normal state and as affected by disease. For the first time, we had access to arteries and veins at all levels of the limbs and could safely and repetitively study patients with a wide variety of diseases.

"Initially, and even to some extent today, these methods were considered unnecessary by those favoring more traditional approaches. However, with time and improvements in the technology, ultrasound has come to occupy a very important place in the evaluation of patients with peripheral vascular disease. Advances in the field are continuing to occur at a very rapid pace.[3]

"This publication has been so widely cited because it was possibly the first to describe in some detail the potential application of ultrasonic methods to evaluate vascular disease. It presented an entirely new approach which with time has become commonplace to those persons interested in this important area. Fortunately, most of the conclusions reached at the time it was published remain true today."

1. **Franklin D L, Schlegel W A & Rushmer R F.** Blood flow measured by Doppler frequency shift of backscattered ultrasound. *Science* **134**:564-5, 1961.
2. **Rushmer R F, Baker D W & Stegall H F.** Transcutaneous Doppler flow detection as a nondestructive technique. *J. Appl. Physiol.* **21**:554-66, 1966.
3. **Strandness D E, Jr.** The use of ultrasound in the evaluation of peripheral vascular disease. *Progr. Cardiovasc. Dis.* **20**:403-22, 1978.

CC/NUMBER 40
OCTOBER 6, 1980

This Week's Citation Classic

Mason D T. Usefulness and limitations of the rate of rise of intraventricular pressure (dp/dt) in the evaluation of myocardial contractility in man.
Amer. J. Cardiol. **23**:516-27, 1969.
[Sect. Cardiopulmonary Med., Depts. Med. and Physiol., Univ. California Sch. Med., Davis, CA]

Clinical determination of ventricular pressure rate of rise (dp/dt) constitutes an important new advancement for evaluating myocardial contractility of the intact human heart in health and disease. This paper delineates the proper use, interpretation, and rationale of the dp/dt approaches obtained by cardiac catheterization: peak dp/dt, dp/dt corrected for mechanical factors, and contractile element shortening velocity in intra and interpatient studies. [The *SCI*® indicates that this paper has been cited over 295 times since 1969.]

Dean T. Mason
Section of Cardiovascular Medicine
University of California
School of Medicine
Davis, CA 95616

August 21, 1980

"It is indeed gratifying to learn that my 1969 article has been so frequently cited, and to recognize the progress in cardiac function research since then. This was the first paper presenting the sequence of developments in ventricular dp/dt methodology and its value in examining contractility, which consisted of principal accomplishments of my series of studies in assessing ventricular performance in patients.[1] Thus the article served both as a continuation of my first investigations on the concept's validity and a springboard for my later publications extending this knowledge to myocardial force-velocity properties in quantifying contractility in intact human hearts.[2]

"The publication occurred fortuitously at an important time in my early academic career. The 1968 American College of Cardiology's Scientific Program Committee asked me to formulate and chair a ventricular function symposium. This paper represents the publication of my presentation at that annual meeting. Furthermore, the timing is noteworthy, since I was negotiating my present position: professor of medicine and physiology and chief of cardiovascular medicine at the University of California School of Medicine at Davis. The previous seven years, I was assistant section chief of cardiovascular diagnosis in the cardiology branch of the National Heart Institute in Bethesda (1961-1968), having completed my internal medicine residency on the Johns Hopkins Hospital's Osler Service (1958-1961) upon graduating from Duke University Medical School.

"In 1968, at age 35, I had authored 100 original articles on cardiovascular science and clinical cardiology. Subsequently, in the past 12 years here at UC Davis, academic activities have gone well for me as evidenced by 800 such articles and 12 books, and service on 20 scientific journals' editorial boards, American Board of Internal Medicine Cardiovascular Diseases member, past president of the Western Society of Clinical Research, past president of the American College of Cardiology, and currently editor-in-chief of the *American Heart Journal*. In addition, this landmark paper has been largely responsible for over 500 visiting professorships and more than 70 professional honors, including the ASPET Experimental Therapeutics Award, the ATS Research Award, and the Distinguished Duke University Alumnus Award.

"In my opinion, from scientific and practical standpoints, the reason why this paper has been highly cited and is considered a hallmark contribution to progress in ventricular function is that fundamental techniques and explanations were provided for credibility of ventricular dp/dt equations as readily available indices of contractile state for pharmacologic and physiologic investigations which now enjoy widespread, standard application in clinical research and patient care. I consider it insight that dynamic (dp/dt), rather than static, measures of performance emerged from my youthful experiences in professional baseball. Moreover, the paper established the launching pad leading to the impetus for expanding the concept to more complex force-velocity contractility indices of ventricular function clinically by us and other investigators."[3]

1. **Mason D T & Braunwald E.** Effects of ouabain on the nonfailing human heart. *J. Clin. Invest.* **42**:1105-14, 1963.
2. **Mason D T, Spann J F & Zelis R.** Quantification of the contractile state of the intact human heart. *Amer. J. Cardiol.* **26**:248-57, 1970.
3. **Mason D T.** *Congestive heart failure.* New York: Dun-Donnelley, 1976. 448 p.

CC/NUMBER 36
SEPTEMBER 5, 1983

This Week's Citation Classic

DeBakey M E & Simeone F A. Battle injuries of the arteries in World War II. An analysis of 2,471 cases. *Ann. Surg.* **123**:534-79, 1946.
[Office of the Surgeon General, Washington, DC]

An effort was made in this report to present information on 2,471 acute arterial injuries in American forces during World War II, with respect to incidence, types, location, and morbidity. For the results of this study, which are too lengthy to abstract, the reader is referred to the original article. [The *SCI*® indicates that this paper has been cited in over 215 publications since 1961.]

Michael E. DeBakey
Texas Medical Center
Baylor College of Medicine
Houston, TX 77030

July 25, 1983

"As a member of the Surgical Consultants' Division of the Office of the Surgeon General during World War II, I became interested in diseases and injuries of the circulation, owing to my interests and research activities in this field of endeavor before entering the service. Accordingly, I began an exhaustive review of the publications on this subject for all previous wars. It soon became apparent from this review that there was considerable confusion concerning the incidence, site of occurrence, treatment, and results of treatment of battle injuries of the arteries in previous wars. Even the official histories of World War I, including the American, British, German, and French, provided inadequate reports for proper evaluation of incidence and results of treatment. Moreover, during the first two years of World War II, reports received in the Surgeon General's office from various theaters of operations provided inadequate data for proper evaluation and basis for development of good concepts of treatment. It thus became clearly evident that special efforts were needed to study this problem and to collect data that would permit a more reliable analysis and more useful information from which proper concepts of treatment could be developed.

"For this purpose, I obtained the cooperation of our surgical consultants in various theaters of operations and asked them to collect data on this subject in accordance with certain guidelines I provided them. Moreover, I personally visited three of the armies (Third, Fifth, and Seventh) in the European theater of operations on a temporary duty basis. During these visits, I made a special effort to obtain firsthand information and collect data from the surgeons working in the field hospitals. During my visit to the Fifth Army, I met Fiorindo A. Simeone, who showed a particular interest in this problem and had already collected a considerable amount of data from the battle experience in that army. We agreed to collaborate on this subject, and this resulted in the preparation of the manuscript that is the subject of this commentary.

"The primary significance of this article lies in the fact that it was the first comprehensive review of battle injuries of the arteries that included World War II and previous wars and provided extensive statistical data on incidence, location of the injury, complications, methods of treatment, and results of treatment. It also indicated the need for better methods of treatment in both military and civilian arterial injuries. I believe that it provided a stimulus for efforts in this direction which have been fruitful, as evidenced by subsequent published reports showing great improvement in the methods of treatment and results of treatment by the application of vascular surgical methods of repair and restoration of circulation both in military and civilian wounds."[1-8]

1. **DeBakey M E.** Acute vascular injuries. (Cole W H, ed.) *Operative technic in specialty surgery.* New York: Appleton-Century-Crofts, 1956. p. 1-9.
2. **Beall A C, Jr., Diethrich E B, Morris G C, Jr. & DeBakey M E.** Surgical management of vascular trauma. *Surg. Clin. N. Amer.* **46**:1001-11, 1966.
3. **Beall A C, Jr., Diethrich E B, Crawford H W, Cooley D A & DeBakey M E.** Surgical management of penetrating cardiac injuries. *Amer. J. Surg.* **112**:686-92, 1966.
4. **Beall A C, Jr., Diethrich E B, Cooley D A & DeBakey M E.** Surgical management of penetrating cardiovascular trauma. *Southern Med. J.* **60**:698-704, 1967.
5. **Beall A C, Jr. & DeBakey M E.** Cardiovascular injuries. (Cooper P, ed.) *The craft of surgery.* London: Churchill, 1971. Vol. I. p. 716-25.
6. **Pickard L R, Mattox K L, Espada R, Beall A C, Jr. & DeBakey M E.** Transection of the descending thoracic aorta secondary to blunt trauma. *J. Trauma* **17**:749-53, 1977.
7. **Graham J M, Feliciano D V, Mattox K L, Beall A C, Jr. & DeBakey M E.** Management of subclavian vascular injuries. *J. Trauma* **20**:537-44, 1980.
8. **Brown M F, Graham J M, Feliciano D V, Mattox K L, Beall A C, Jr. & DeBakey M E.** Carotid artery injuries. *Amer. J. Surg.* **144**:748-53, 1982.

Chapter

7

Endocrinology and Metabolic Disease

Among the phenomena that have contributed to the development of endocrinology within departments of medicine, surely the development of sensitive and specific radioimmunoassays (RIAs) can be considered as one. The seven Citation Classics based on RIAs in this chapter equal the number in Chapter 3 on Immunology and Rheumatology. The basis for this segregation is that the Classics in Chapter 3 relate primarily to the development of the procedure rather than its application.

Studies of pancreas function are recorded in the first five Classics in this chapter, of which the first two interrelate with lipids. Bierman's "This Week's Citation Classic" (TWCC) describes the result of analyses that demonstrated for the first time that insulin deficiency led to elevated blood levels of nonesterified fatty acids and that these acids might be precursors of the keto acids that circulate during diabetic ketosis. Karam and his co-investigators discovered that insulin levels of obese patients were much more elevated after a glucose load than was the case with normal controls. This was a useful indicator of early maturity onset of diabetes. Fortunately, Karam eventually found the right sweetbreads for his bovine insulin after proving that bovine thymus was insulin-free.

Examination of alpha cell function is the basis for the next two Classics, which share many of the same authors. In the first, glucagon secretion was evaluated in subjects fed high-protein or high-carbohydrate diets. Müller and Unger's description of the meals the subjects were obliged to eat would discourage many volunteers. In Unger's second TWCC is the comment that 259 rabbits were immunized in order to identify one glucagon-specific antiserum. Somehow this reduces the agony of screening dozens of the hybridomas that are now preferred as the source of specific monoclonal antisera to important biomolecules. The article by Kahn et al. is of interest inasmuch as their research identified an insulin receptor deficiency as a cause of insulin resistance. Receptor studies are now widespread, extending to hormone receptors, light receptors, neurotransmitter receptors, antigen receptors, and others of topical interest.

The difficulties in proving that prolactin existed as a human hormone with a function exactly parallel to its proven role in lower animals were burdensome until RIA was applied. It was then possible to demonstrate that thyrotropin-releasing hormone (p. 235) and the multiple hormonal changes associated with pregnancy (p. 236) stimulated prolactin secretion. Prolactin secretion can be specifically inhibited by bromocriptine (p. 237), thus assisting in the therapy of hypogonadism and galactorrhea.

Morris in 1953 discovered congenital, sex-linked testicular feminization, a condition dependent upon a loss of androgen receptors. Later, Haddad and Wilkins reviewed the congenital abnormalities in Turner's syndrome or gonadal aplasia. Both diseases have pronounced psychological effects in their victims, and Turner's syndrome has ocular abnormalities as part of its pathology. Haddad's TWCC eulogizes his co-author Wilkins as the instrument that shaped his career.

Again, the role of RIA in endocrine-hormone relations appears in the TWCC by Neill on the levels of luteinizing hormone and progesterone during the menstrual cycle. Another Citation Classic based exclusively on a study of female subjects is that of Sartwell on the positive relationship of thromboembolic disease and the use of oral contraceptives. This article was overshadowed by the earlier publication on the same topic by an expert committee (p. 241), but the paper by Sartwell et al. is remarkable for its clear proof of the stated relationship and the careful manner in which their data were collected. The RIA contribution is continued in the next two TWCCs, one on the synthesis of steroid hormones (p. 243) and the other on the production of growth hormone during the early, deep phase of sleep (p. 244).

The next four TWCCs continue the trend of the earlier reports by describing the release of a hormone under a specific stimulus, a receptor for a hormone, or the influence of a hormone in a disease process. The fourth described the novel role of hormones in gene control in metamorphosing insects.

The metabolic pathway chart so often seen posted in biochemistry laboratories has been both blessed and damned by students. The blessings derive from the utility of this chart, which ably condenses and unifies in graphic form the multitude of chemical reactions that are essential to the living creature. The damnations arise because of the ever increasing number of these reactions and interactions that are the substance of the chart. Fortunately this chapter does not demand a total recall of this monstrous map since only a few of its highways are considered. A scant half dozen plus two of the following TWCCs on metabolic disease relate to genetic road blocks that interrupt these highways and create metabolic disease. The last two TWCCs describe an instance of DNA repair failure and a successful text on inherited disease. Other TWCCs that pertain to the subjects of specific chapters—e.g., Hematology or Immunology and Rheumatology—have been placed in the appropriate chapters.

The first TWCC in this series on metabolic disorders describes the early application of creatine kinase assays in the diagnosis of muscular dystrophy. In the Duchenne type of muscular dystrophy, the two normal intracellular enzymes, creatine kinase and aldolase, are both elevated in the blood. Since muscular dystrophy is transmitted as a sex-linked, congenital disease, the detection of female carriers is of obvious importance, and the creatine kinase test designed by Dreyfus et al. proved sufficient for this purpose. Assays for this enzyme are also useful in evaluating myocardial infarction.

Homocystinuria is a genetic disorder that exists in three variations, all of which result in the urinary excretion of homocystine. In the form of this disorder described by Carson in her TWCC, the missing enzyme is cystathionine β synthase, an enzyme that links homocysteine with serine to produce cystathionine. A genetic deficiency of this enzyme is more common in Ireland (1 in 40,000 births), where Carson and Neill studied this condition, than in other countries. As indicated in the TWCC, mental retardation is one of the serious complications of the disease. In Carson's last paragraph, the positive response of patients to vitamin B_6 refers to the requirement of the synthase for a pyridoxal coenzyme. Clearly a dietary deficiency of this vitamin would contribute to homocystinuria even if the enzyme were fully available in an active form.

Methylmalonic aciduria is closely related to maple syrup urine disease since both are related to the metabolism of the branched-chain amino acids valine, leucine, and isoleucine. Removal of the amino group from these three molecules produces the corresponding keto acids. Under normal conditions, these keto acids are decarboxylated to form methylmalonic acid. When the decarboxylase is missing, maple syrup urine disease results (p. 251). However, if the methylmalonic acid is not converted to succinic acid, then the result is methylmalonic aciduria (p. 252). Oberholzer and his co-investigators discovered the latter condition, a defect that has the highest frequency of the organic acidurias. An unexpected honor from this was the opportunity to tour the English Queen through the new and spacious biochemistry laboratories.

Lesch has written an interesting TWCC on how, as a freshman medical student, he entered into a research program that later enabled the identification of a familial hyperuricemia that bore his name. The Lesch-Nyhan syndrome is due to the loss of a transferase that would normally metabolize the purines through a salvage pathway that minimizes uric acid formation.

Fabry's disease is classified as a lipidosis based on an inherited defect in the enzyme ceramide trihexosidase. It should not be confused with Farber's disease, a distinct genetic disease also involving lipid metabolism. Fabry's disease is a sex-linked illness associated with an excessive deposition of lipid in the tissues, ocular opacities, vascular complications, and eventually renal failure. The defective enzyme normally removes the terminal (third) saccharide from ceramide glucosylgalactosylgalactoside. Fabry's disease is one of the more common of the sphingolipid storage diseases. The discovery of the enzymatic basis of this disease resulted from the use of a tritiated terminal galactose in the enzyme substrate. This galactose was labeled by exposing the molecule to radioactive hydrogen gas in a sealed chamber!

The impact of genetics on human medicine was foreseen by McKusick in the early 1950s, and the first edition of his book *Heritable Disorders of Connective Tissue* was published in 1961. Prior to March 1979, this important volume was cited more than 1,085 times. McKusick has provided an interesting description of how the book was conceived, the difference between diseases *in* and *of* connective tissue, and several other features, including the erroneous citation of his book as *Veritable Disorders of Connective Tissue.*

The reviews listed below continue the theme of the TWCCs in this chapter on insulin, prolactin, thyroid hormones, oral contraception, and inborn errors of metabolism. The widespread interest in these subjects is manifest by the distribution of these 17 references through 13 different journal sources.

Bartlett K. Vitamin-responsive inborn errors of metabolism. *Adv. Clin. Chem.* **23:**141–98, 1983.

Ben-Jonathan N. Dopamine: a prolactin-inhibiting hormone. *Endocrinol. Rev.* **6:**564–89, 1985.

Blackwell R E. Diagnosis and treatment of hyperprolactinemic syndromes. *Obstet. Gynecol. Annu.* **14:**310–27, 1985.

Chaudhuri G. Physiologic aspects of prostaglandins and leukotrienes. *Semin. Reprod. Endocrinol.* **3:**219–30, 1985.

Cheng K & Larner J. Intracellular mediators of insulin action. *Annu. Rev. Physiol.* **47:**405–24, 1985.

Edwards N L & Fox I H. Disorders associated with purine and pyrimidine metabolism. *Spec. Top. Endocrinol. Metab.* **6:**95–140, 1984.

Evans W S & Thorner M O. Mechanisms for hypogonadism in hyperprolactinemia. *Semin. Reprod. Endocrinol.* **2:**9–22, 1984.

Fotherby K. Oral contraceptives, lipids and cardiovascular disease. *Contraception* **31:**367–94, 1985.

Glew R H, Basu A, Prence E M & Remaley A T. Lysosomal storage diseases. *Lab. Invest.* **53:**250–69, 1985.

Hindmarsh J T. Clinical disorders of prophyrin metabolism. *Clin. Biochem.* **16:**209–19, 1983.

Kahn C R. The molecular mechanism of insulin action. *Annu. Rev. Med.* **36:**429–51, 1985.

Lenzer S & Bailey C J. Thyroid hormones, gonadal and adrenocortical steroids and the function of the islets of Langerhans. *Endocrinol. Rev.* **5:**411–34, 1984.

Lewis U J. Variants of growth hormone and prolactin and their posttranslational modifications. *Annu. Rev. Physiol.* **46:**33–42, 1984.

Murphy B D & Rajkumar K. Prolactin as a luteotrophin. *Can J. Physiol. Pharmacol.* **63:**257–64, 1985.

Ray R A, Howanitz P J & Howanitz J H. Controversies in thyroid function testing. *Clin. Lab. Med.* **4:**671–82, 1984.

Seltzer W K, Firminger H, Klein J, Pike A, Fennessey P & McCabe E R B. Adrenal dysfunction in glycerol kinase deficiency. *Biochem. Med.* **33:**189–99, 1985.

Walters M R. Steroid hormone receptors and the nucleus. *Endocrinol. Rev.* **6:**512–43, 1985.

CC/NUMBER 51
DECEMBER 17, 1984

This Week's Citation Classic™

Bierman E L, Dole V P & Roberts T N. An abnormality of nonesterified fatty acid metabolism in diabetes mellitus. *Diabetes* **6**:475-9, 1957.
[Hospital of the Rockefeller Institute and New York Hospital, New York, NY]

This paper demonstrated for the first time that insulin deficiency causes elevated levels of nonesterified fatty acids (NEFA), reversible with insulin treatment. In patients with ketoacidosis, injection of insulin caused a dramatic drop of NEFA levels paralleling the fall in blood glucose and preceding by several hours the elimination of ketone bodies. It was also demonstrated that diabetics tend to have elevated fasting NEFA levels and abnormally delayed responses to hyperglycemia induced by oral glucose or injection of glucagon. [The *SCI*® indicates that this paper has been cited in over 330 publications since 1957.]

Edwin L. Bierman
Department of Medicine
Division of Metabolism and Endocrinology
University of Washington
Seattle, WA 98195

September 20, 1984

"This work represents one of my earliest major research papers, emerging from the first year of my research apprenticeship in the laboratory of Vincent P. Dole at the Rockefeller Institute for Medical Research (now Rockefeller University). I was offered the position there toward the end of my internship across the street at New York Hospital. Dole had just worked out a simple method for measuring the tiny concentration of nonesterified fatty acids (NEFA) in plasma,[1] and he theorized that NEFA was indeed the long sought-after high-energy fuel released from fat tissue. A single preliminary study suggested that NEFA levels were elevated in a patient with uncontrolled diabetes and that NEFA might be the precursor of ketone acids (and hence involved in the pathogenesis of diabetic ketoacidosis).

"Because of my interest in diabetes and metabolism, a research career, and temporary postponement of military service, and despite my appalling prior lack of knowledge about fat metabolism, I accepted the challenge of defining abnormalities of NEFA metabolism in diabetes. My first task was to follow the course of NEFA levels before and during treatment of patients with diabetic ketoacidosis entering the emergency room. I did the analyses myself at any hour of the day or night that the blood became available. This included laborious analyses of plasma bicarbonate levels performed on one of the early hand-operated mercury machines, developed and built by Donald D. Van Slyke and left over in the lab as part of his legacy.

"The excitement of following the decline of NEFA levels coincident with insulin treatment, and preceding the fall in blood glucose, can only be imagined. These results led directly to our animal studies demonstrating that insulin inhibits fatty acid release from fat tissue stores. The additional finding that the fall in NEFA levels after a glucose or glucagon-induced hyperglycemic challenge is impaired in diabetics not in ketoacidosis is a major topic of the cited paper. An abstract of this work was presented at the plenary session of the American Society for Clinical Investigation, and the paper generated much interest.[2]

"I think that this publication is so frequently cited because it was the first documentation that insulin deficiency causes fatty acid mobilization and elevated NEFA levels, reversible with insulin treatment. It also raised the level of awareness that the abnormal metabolic state of the diabetic patient reflected in the circulation consists of more than hyperglycemia and, in fact, suggested that abnormal regulation of fat mobilization plays an important role. These results have been amply confirmed and have stood the test of time. Furthermore, they opened up a new area of research focus in diabetes in many laboratories, and led directly to the discovery of insulin regulation of a new enzyme, hormone-sensitive lipase, in adipose tissue.[3] The fact that NEFA mobilization is an early step in the pathogenesis of ketoacidosis is now well established."[4,5]

1. **Dole V P.** A relation between non-esterified fatty acids in plasma and the metabolism of glucose. *J. Clin. Invest.* **35**:150-4, 1956. (Cited 3,710 times since 1956.)
2. **Dole V P, Bierman E L & Roberts T N.** Plasma NEFA as an index of carbohydrate utilization. (Abstract.) *J. Clin. Invest.* **36**:884, 1957. (Cited 35 times since 1957.)
3. **Rizack M A.** An epinephrine-sensitive lipolytic activity in adipose tissue. *J. Biol. Chem.* **236**:657-62, 1961. (Cited 260 times.)
4. **Kreisberg R A.** Diabetic ketoacidosis: new concepts and treatment. *Ann. Intern. Med.* **88**:681-95, 1978.
5. **Foster D W & McGarry J D.** The metabolic derangements and treatment of diabetic ketoacidosis. *N. Engl. J. Med.* **309**:159-69, 1983.

NUMBER 14
APRIL 2, 1979

This Week's Citation Classic

Karam J H, Grodsky G M & Forsham P H. Excessive insulin response to glucose in obese subjects as measured by immunochemical assay. *Diabetes* **12**:197-204, 1963.

This paper shows that obese, non-diabetic subjects had levels of serum immunoreactive insulin three to four times higher than those of non-obese, normal subjects after identical rapid intravenous glucose loads. These findings established the relevance of obesity in interpreting the excessive insulin responses to glucose in early maturity-onset diabetics. [The *SCI*® indicates that this paper has been cited over 335 times since 1963.]

John H. Karam
Metabolic Research Unit
University of California
San Francisco, CA 94143

January 25, 1978

"In late 1960, after a year of laboratory research at Hammersmith Hospital in London, I began an endocrinology fellowship in Peter H. Forsham's Metabolic Research Unit at the University of California in San Francisco, where a new modification of the radioimmunoassay of insulin had just been developed by Gerold M. Grodsky.[1] My interest in the clinical potential of this method derived from two earlier years spent as a resident physician at the Bronx VA Hospital, where Berson and Yalow had initiated the exciting technology of radioimmunoassay and had reported that early maturity-onset diabetics had a greater insulin-secretory response to oral glucose than normal subjects.[2]

"I was fortunate to be assigned to Jerry Grodsky's lab and was advised to learn the insulin immunoassay by obtaining from a local meatpacking plant some fresh beef pancreas, from which insulin might be extracted and assayed. However, my first harrowing venture into a slaughterhouse so dulled my discriminatory sense that I passively accepted abattoir terminology of 'sweetbreads' for my requested 'pancreas.' My initial attempts to estimate insulin repeatedly failed. Eventual histological evidence that the frozen tissue was not pancreas at all but thymus ('neck sweetbreads'), and subsequent recovery of insulin from true pancreas ('abdominal sweetbreads'), salvaged my research career, confirmed the specificity of the Grodsky-Forsham insulin assay, and, to no one's concern at the time, suggested a lack of immunoreactive insulin in beef thymus gland.

"As my primary interest was in clinical research, I submitted a protocol to compare the effects of intravenous glucose versus galactose in stimulating insulin secretion in humans. To verify that my technical skills were adequate to measure circulating insulin in serum, I administered glucose intravenously to a maturity-onset mild diabetic, and, as reported by Yalow and Berson, confirmed that the insulin response was considerably higher than after a similar dose of glucose given to a normal subject.[2] In discussing this result with Jerry Grodsky and Peter Forsham, I commented that my diabetic subject was markedly obese, weighing 370 lb. Since his extreme obesity far surpassed his mild hyperglycemic disorder, it raised the question of whether obesity itself contributed to the excessive insulin response to glucose seen in our patient as well as in Yalow and Berson's early diabetics, whose weights were not reported but in whom obesity is known to have a high frequency.

"Subsequent findings in 9 of 10 non-diabetic, obese subjects demonstrated that obesity itself was clearly associated with a supra-normal insulin response to glucose. This led to the conclusion that the presence of obesity should be 'weighed' carefully whenever evaluating insulin levels in either the diabetic or the non-diabetic.

"That this finding has achieved the distinction of being one of the most cited papers in its field is most satisfying to the three of us, who have continued close collaboration in a research unit that emphasizes a balanced relationship between basic and clinical research."

Reference

1. **Grodsky G M & Forsham P H.** An immunochemical assay of total extractable insulin in man. *J. Clin. Invest.* **39**:1070-9, 1960.
2. **Yalow R S & Berson S A.** Plasma insulin concentrations in non-diabetic and early diabetic subjects: determinations by a new sensitive immunoassay technic. *Diabetes* **9**:254-60, 1960.

CC/NUMBER 32
AUGUST 8, 1983

This Week's Citation Classic

Müller W A, Faloona G R, Aguilar-Parada E & Unger R H. Abnormal alpha-cell function in diabetes. Response to carbohydrate and protein ingestion. *N. Engl. J. Med.* **283**:109-15, 1970.
[Dept. Internal Medicine, Univ. Texas Southwestern Med. Sch., and Veterans Admin. Hosp., Dallas, TX]

Carbohydrate ingestion reduced glucagon secretion in nondiabetics, but not in diabetics. Protein meals doubled plasma glucagon in both. Induced hyperglycemia abolished the glucagon response to protein ingestion in nondiabetics, but had no effect in diabetics. This inappropriate hyperglucagonemia appears to be a hallmark of diabetes mellitus and worsens its metabolic state. [The *SCI*® indicates that this paper has been cited in over 260 publications since 1970.]

Walter A. Müller
rue du Musée 9
2000 Neuchâtel
Switzerland
and
Roger H. Unger
Department of Internal Medicine
University of Texas Health Science Center
Dallas, TX 75235

June 2, 1983

"In 1960, Rosalyn S. Yalow and Solomon A. Berson reported on the first radioimmunoassay used to measure insulin.[1] During the same time period, Roger H. Unger and Anne M. Eisentraut in Dallas started to produce antisera against glucagon with the goal of measuring it in plasma by a similar assay. In contrast to the rapidly working insulin immunoassay, the glucagon immunoassay required another decade to become of equal quality. The common efforts of Unger and his co-workers Eisentraut and Virginia Harris made this possible.

"Müller was fortunate to join the team at the Veterans Administration Research Center in Dallas in 1969, shortly after the first antiserum, generously produced by the rabbit G-58, was capable of measuring true glucagon in peripheral blood from animals and humans. Eugenio Aguilar-Parada introduced Müller to the human studies, teaching him how to perform arginine infusions and feeding strange meals to the laboratory staff and the diabetic US veterans.

"The first two papers appeared in 1969 and in April 1970[2,3] describing in humans the inhibition of glucagon secretion by glucose and its stimulation by arginine infusions. Diabetics exhibited higher plasma glucagon concentrations. We then tested physiologic situations of feeding carbohydrate and protein. Patients and controls were asked to rapidly eat dry steaks kept warm in the oven used otherwise for drying glassware. Despite the even more unpalatable carbohydrate meals consisting of bread, spaghetti, rice, potatoes, and corn, our patients did not reject the food.

"It appears to us that there are two reasons why this paper has been cited so often. First, it was the first publication reporting reliable measurements of plasma glucagon in a physiological situation, namely, in response to ingested food, an important facet of human physiology and nutrition. Second, it revealed a new aspect of the pathophysiology of diabetes mellitus: diabetics exhibit higher glucagon concentrations and abnormal alpha-cell function, a possible pathogenetic feature of this disease. Indeed, we found it in all forms of diabetes that we studied.[4]

"The results were presented to the Southern Society for Clinical Investigation in New Orleans and to the American Society for Clinical Investigation in Atlantic City in 1970. With minor revisions, the manuscript was accepted for publication by the *New England Journal of Medicine*. We were proud that Unger was subsequently honored by receiving the Banting and Claude Bernard Medals. Unger has since made numerous contributions to the understanding of islet cell physiology and pathophysiology, particularly with respect to the interaction of the different islet cell hormones,[5] whereas Müller was lately involved in studying the role of glucagon in protein metabolism."[6]

1. **Yalow R S & Berson S A.** Immunoassay of endogenous plasma insulin in man. *J. Clin. Invest.* **39**:1157-75, 1960. [Citation Classic. *Current Contents* (14):9, 4 April 1977.]
2. **Aguilar-Parada E, Eisentraut A M & Unger R H.** Pancreatic glucagon secretion in normal and diabetic subjects. *Amer. J. Med. Sci.* **257**:415-19, 1969.
3. **Unger R H, Aguilar-Parada E, Müller W A & Eisentraut A M.** Studies of pancreatic alpha cell function in normal and diabetic subjects. *J. Clin. Invest.* **49**:837-48, 1970. [Citation Classic. *Current Contents/Clinical Practice* **8**(2):10, 14 January 1980.]
4. **Müller W A, Faloona G R & Unger R H.** The effect of experimental insulin deficiency on glucagon secretion. *J. Clin. Invest.* **50**:1992-9, 1971.
5. **Unger R H & Orci L.** Glucagon and the A cell. Physiology and pathophysiology. *N. Engl. J. Med.* **304**:1518-24; 1575-80, 1981.
6. **Müller W A, Cüppers H J, Zimmermann-Telschow H, Micheli H, Wyss T, Renold A E & Berger M.** Amino acids and lipoproteins in plasma of duodenopancreatectomized patients: effects of glucagon in physiological amounts. *Eur. J. Clin. Invest.* **13**:141-9, 1983.

CC/NUMBER 2
JANUARY 14, 1980

This Week's Citation Classic

Unger R H, Aguilar-Parada E, Müller W A & Eisentraut A M. Studies of pancreatic alpha cell function in normal and diabetic subjects. *J. Clin. Invest.* **49**:837-48, 1970. [Dept. Int. Med., Univ. Texas, Southwestern Med. Sch., Dallas; and VA Hospital, Dallas, TX]

A-cell function was characterized in non-diabetics and juvenile-type and adult-type diabetics. In normals glucagon rose during arginine infusion and declined during hyperglycemia. In diabetics glucagon was high relative to glucose and overresponded to arginine. Diabetic A-cell dysfunction may contribute pathogenetically to the metabolic abnormalities of diabetes. [The *SCI*® indicates that this paper has been cited over 390 times since 1970.]

Roger H. Unger
Department of Internal Medicine
University of Texas Health Science Center
at Dallas
Southwestern Medical School
Dallas, TX 75235

October 22, 1979

"This paper is widely cited because it is the first valid study of human A-cell function. It provided the first evidence that glucagon was a hormone in man, characterized normal human A-cell function, and showed that A-cell function was abnormal in diabetics. For Anna M. Eisentraut and me, it marked the end of a nine-year effort to develop an immunoassay for glucagon in human plasma. In 1959, helped by advice from Berson and Yalow, we had developed a glucagon radioimmunoassay.[1] But valid measurements of glucagon in human plasma were impeded by inadequate sensitivity of our antisera against glucagon, nonspecificity of most of these antisera, and damage to the labeled glucagon when incubated in human plasma. For these reasons, between 1959 and 1968 we confined our work to dogs, in which the foregoing problems could be circumvented; incubation damage of the glucagon tracer in canine plasma was relatively slight, and by selective catheterization of the pancreatic and mesenteric veins and the inferior vena cava, the need for a highly sensitive assay was reduced and discrimination between immunoreactivity of pancreatic and intestinal origin made possible.

"Although the dog work strongly suggested that glucagon was a true hormone, at least in that species, efforts to establish this in man were largely frustrated until 1968 when two fortunate unrelated events occurred. First, Anne Eisentraut, Nancy Whissen, and I observed that aprotinin (Trasylol) prevented incubation damage. Second, Anne Eisentraut discovered that the antiserum from one of 259 rabbits then undergoing immunization, rabbit G58, was remarkably different from that of the others. Not only was it highly sensitive, but it did not react appreciably with extrapancreatic sources of glucagon-like immunoreactivity, i.e., it was almost 'specific' for pancreatic glucagon. A valid assay for human glucagon was quickly developed and used for explorations of A-cell function reported in this and subsequent papers.

"Briefly, we found that in normal subjects glucagon was suppressed by hyperglycemia and stimulated by starvation, hypoglycemia, protein meals, and arginine infusion, suggesting that pancreatic glucagon behaved as a true hormone of 'glucose need' in normal man. This ended a controversy that had begun with the discovery of glucagon by Kimball and Merlin in 1923.[2] We also found that in diabetics the fasting levels of glucagon were high relative to the ambient blood glucose level, could not be suppressed by hyperglycemia, and were hyperresponsive to arginine infusion. This demonstration of abnormal A-cell function in diabetics has led to the 'bihormonal abnormality' concept of diabetes. This holds that certain of its metabolic abnormalities are the consequence, not of the insulin lack alone, but of insulin lack *plus* excessive glucagon secretion.[3] Glucagon suppression can reduce both the marked endogenous hyperglycemia and hyperketonemia of diabetes, a fact which may have therapeutic implications for this disease."

1. **Unger R H, Eisentraut A M, McCall M S, Keller S, Lanz H C & Madison L L.** Glucagon antibodies and their use for immunoassay for glucagon. *Proc. Soc. Exp. Biol. Med.* **102**:621-3, 1959.
2. **Unger R H.** Diabetes and the alpha cell (Banting Memorial Lecture). *Diabetes* **25**:136-51, 1976.
3. **Raskin P & Unger R H.** Hyperglucagonemia and its suppression: importance in the metabolic control of diabetes. *N. Engl. J. Med.* **299**:433-6, 1978.

CC/NUMBER 50
DECEMBER 10, 1984

This Week's Citation Classic™

Kahn C R, Flier J S, Bar R S, Archer J A, Gorden P, Martin M M & Roth J. The syndromes of insulin resistance and acanthosis nigricans. Insulin-receptor disorders in man. *N. Engl. J. Med.* **294**:739-45, 1976.
[Diabetes Branch, Natl. Inst. Arthritis, Metabolism, and Digestive Dis., NIH, Bethesda, MD and Dept. Pediatrics, Georgetown Univ. Sch. Med., Washington, DC]

Six patients are described representing two syndromes of insulin resistance associated with acanthosis nigricans. The Type A patients are young females with virilization and have insulin resistance due to a decrease in the number of insulin receptors on cells. The Type B patients have an autoimmune syndrome with autoantibodies to the insulin receptor. [The *SCI*® indicates that this paper has been cited in over 345 publications since 1976.]

C. Ronald Kahn
Research Division
Joslin Diabetes Center
One Joslin Place
Boston, MA 02215

August 15, 1984

"Although the concept of specific cellular receptors for hormones and drugs dates back to the turn of the century, direct measurement of the receptor for peptide hormones did not become possible until 1969. When I arrived as a clinical associate at the National Institutes of Health in July 1970, most of the effort of what was then a small section on diabetes, under the direction of Jesse Roth and Phil Gorden, was devoted to defining these receptors. A colleague and I were actually assigned to work on the problem of ACTH receptors, but this proved impossible to master, moving my interest into the area of insulin receptors and driving my colleague into dermatology!

"As soon as it became apparent that insulin receptors could be defined by direct binding studies, we turned our attention to possible abnormalities in disease states. We were able to demonstrate defects in insulin binding to liver membranes from obese mice. But for human studies we were restricted to the study of circulating blood cells, and the significance of insulin receptors on these cells was uncertain.

"As the medical community recognized our interest in diseases associated with defects in insulin action, we were gradually referred several patients with syndromes of extreme insulin resistance—some requiring thousands of units of insulin per day. These were clinically challenging cases, but even more interesting in that they provided a way to test the importance of the insulin receptor. As we had hoped, when insulin binding to its receptor was measured using circulating monocytes from these patients, there was a marked decrease. Jeffrey Flier recognized the importance of the immune features in some of these patients and developed an assay to directly measure anti-receptor antibodies.

"Although the syndromes of insulin resistance and acanthosis nigricans are quite rare (about 12 cases of the Type A and 30 cases of the Type B syndrome have been identified), they are now well recognized as discrete forms of diabetes. They have also provided important insights into insulin action. The Type A patients have been shown to have a series of genetic defects in the insulin receptor molecule or its biosynthesis. The Type B patients have provided a source of anti-receptor antibodies that have been valuable probes of receptor structure and function. Thus, this is another example in which studies of a rare disease have shed light on both normal physiology and the physiology of many disease states.

"As a result of this and related studies of insulin receptors, the diabetes section grew into a large branch, and many of the fellows involved in these studies now head independent diabetes clinical and research groups at several university hospitals. This body of work has also been recognized by a number of awards given to the investigators involved, and the field of insulin receptors has grown to a size large enough for several international meetings and many written reviews."[1-3]

1. **Kahn C R.** The insulin receptor and insulin. The lock and key to diabetes. *Clin. Res.* **31**:326-35, 1983.
2. **Bar R S, Harrison L C, Muggeo M, Gorden P, Kahn C R & Roth J.** Regulation of insulin receptors in normal and abnormal physiology in humans. *Advan. Internal Med.* **24**:23-46, 1979.
3. **Olefsky J M & Kolterman O G.** Mechanisms of insulin resistance in obesity and noninsulin-dependent (Type II) diabetes. *Amer. J. Med.* **70**:151-68, 1981.

CC/NUMBER 5
FEBRUARY 2, 1981

This Week's Citation Classic

Jacobs L S, Snyder P J, Wilber J F, Utiger R D & Daughaday W H. Increased serum prolactin after administration of synthetic thyrotropin releasing hormone (TRH) in man. *J. Clin. Endocrinol. Metab.* **33**:996-8, 1971. [Endocrine Divs., Depts. Med., Washington Univ. Sch. Med., St. Louis, MO, Northwestern Univ. Sch. Med., Evanston, IL, and Univ. Pennsylvania Sch. Med., Philadelphia, PA]

Intravenous thyrotropin-releasing hormone (TRH) caused a prompt rise in serum prolactin in normal subjects, and slight fasting hyperprolactinemia was shown to occur in primary hypothyroidism. TRH or a structurally similar molecule was suggested as the mediator of hypothalamic stimulation of prolactin secretion. [The *SCI*® indicates that this paper has been cited over 295 times since 1971.]

Laurence S. Jacobs
Clinical Research Center
University of Rochester
Medical Center
Rochester, NY 14642

January 16, 1981

"Many investigators were convinced, by 1970, that human prolactin must exist despite the inability to isolate it biochemically at that time. A series of elegant biosynthetic and immunologic experiments then underway led to the development of a radioimmunoassay for human prolactin in Friesen's laboratory.[1] At that time, I was a postdoctoral fellow in Daughaday's lab; he had been working at the prolactin problem using a rodent mammary bioassay. I decided to attempt the measurement of human prolactin with combinations of animal prolactins and their antisera, and was lucky to obtain a satisfactory result with one of the early experiments. The cited paper grew out of a convergence of this work with the early clinical experiments with TRH, the first of the hypothalamic peptides to be isolated and tested in man. TRH has been shown to release only TSH in normal subjects, and total specificity of action was assumed. When we and Friesen became able to measure human prolactin by radioimmunoassay, roughly simultaneously, one of the first questions we asked related to possible effects of TRH on prolactin. Tashjian's lab[2] had shown that TRH stimulated prolactin synthesis by cultured rat pituitary tumor cells. Our paper, demonstrating the potent prolactin releasing effect of TRH, was published essentially simultaneously with one from Friesen's laboratory showing similar results, in late 1971.[3] The full description of our heterologous assay system was not published until six months later.[4]

"Peter Snyder, Jack Wilber, and Bob Utiger, with whom we collaborated, had saved every possible scrap of serum from their TRH-TSH study. This laudable pack-rat behavior, so common in clinical investigation, made possible the 'freezer' study we then performed. Wilber and Utiger, who also had served as fellows in Daughaday's lab, have gone on to head endocrine-metabolism units of their own, and all of us have remained actively engaged in both clinical and bench research in neuroendocrinology.

"A number of factors undoubtedly contribute to the frequent citation of our paper, including the explosive growth of the neurosciences and especially clinical neuroendocrinology during the past decade. In addition, prolactin pathophysiology has touched upon many areas; pituitary tumors, dopaminergic neuro-regulation of the pituitary, thyroid disease, hypogonadism and reproductive endocrinology, hormonal control of breast function, and biochemical effects of neuroleptics are some of these areas. The extent and intensity of fundamental bench and clinical investigations on prolactin which were rapidly undertaken can be appreciated by noting that three major international symposia devoted to prolactin had already taken place by the summer of 1973. It was a red-hot area then, and remains quite warm today."

1. **Hwang P, Guyda H & Friesen H.** *Proc. Nat. Acad. Sci. US* **68**:1902-6, 1971.
2. **Tashjian A H, Barowsky J & Jensen D K.** *Biochem. Biophys. Res. Commun.* **43**:516-23, 1971.
3. **Bowers C Y, Friesen H G, Hwang P, Guyda H J & Folkers K.** *Biochem. Biophys. Res. Commun.* **45**:1033-41, 1971.
4. **Jacobs L S, Mariz I K & Daughaday W H.** *J. Clin. Endocrinol. Metab.* **34**:484-90, 1972.

CC/NUMBER 33
AUGUST 15, 1983

This Week's Citation Classic

Tyson J E, Hwang P, Guyda H & Friesen H G. Studies of prolactin secretion in human pregnancy. *Amer. J. Obstet. Gynecol.* **113**:14-20, 1972.
[Dept. Gynecology and Obstetrics, Johns Hopkins Univ. Sch. Med., Baltimore, MD and McGill Univ. Clinic, Royal Victoria Hosp., Montreal, Quebec, Canada]

This paper reported the rise in prolactin concentrations throughout human gestation and in the puerperium in response to suckling. Very high amniotic fluid prolactin levels compared to maternal and fetal blood levels suggested there was an extrapituitary source of prolactin production during pregnancy. [The *SCI*® indicates that this paper has been cited in over 245 publications since 1972.]

John E. Tyson
Department of Obstetrics, Gynecology, and Reproductive Sciences
University of Manitoba
Winnipeg, Manitoba R3E 0W3
Canada

June 23, 1983

"In 1966, while a fellow in gynecology and obstetrics at Johns Hopkins Hospital, I participated in an investigation of pregnant women suffering from isolated growth hormone deficiency.[1] These women were known to experience postpartum lactation presumably in the absence of either pituitary growth hormone or prolactin. When Frantz and Kleinberg described prolactin-like activity in human serum using a mouse mammary gland bioassay,[2] Henry Friesen called me from McGill University asking if I could fly to Montreal with any blood samples left over from my lactating dwarf study. Like most November days, it was cold and damp when I arrived in Montreal. Peter Hwang, then a research fellow in Friesen's lab, was wrestling with the immunoassay for prolactin while Harvey Guyda, who had recently returned from the US, was perfecting techniques for affinity chromatography. Over the next six days we extracted my samples and assayed them for this ubiquitous pituitary polypeptide. By the weekend we were ecstatic to have found high prolactin-like activity in each and every sample.

"By late January 1971, I had completed the first large study of the dynamics of prolactin secretion in pregnant and puerperal women. Friesen and I drafted an abstract from these results in time for the annual meeting of the Endocrine Society. The results, which formed the body of our paper, included the normal range for prolactin values for pregnancy, the suckling-induced prolactin response to nipple stimulation, and the levels of prolactin in amniotic fluid. I was later to describe along with others that a suckling-induced increment in prolactin is present beyond the 90th postpartum day.[3] What had happened in our original study was an error in sampling which did not take into account the frequency and intensity of the suckling stimulus.

"There are several reasons for the high citation of this paper. Our original paper was replete with observational data, and the discussion included a number of personal hypotheses. These had been drawn up by Friesen and me as we sat in a small French restaurant during the November visit. Fantasizing over a glass of white wine, we arbitrarily divided up future research possibilities. Friesen was to expand his work on pituitary physiology and the role of prolactin in the etiology of mammary carcinoma. I was more interested in female reproduction. Our original article was the first to suggest that prolactin might be produced in extraglandular sites during pregnancy. Since then, my lab has confirmed that amniotic fluid prolactin is synthesized by human decidua.[4] Other studies have shown a definite effect of prolactin on fetoplacental osmoregulation.[5-7]

"The field of prolactin research has expanded exponentially during the last 12 years, yet the personal satisfaction which I obtained from those early 'lean years' in clinical research is inestimable. Unfortunately, in spite of nearly 13 years of basic and applied research, prolactin remains principally a marker of other disease processes especially in the area of the hypothalamus."

1. **Tyson J E, Barnes A C, Merimee T J & McKusick V A.** Isolated growth hormone deficiency: studies in pregnancy. *J. Clin. Endocrinol. Metab.* **31**:147-52, 1970.
2. **Frantz A G & Kleinberg D L.** Prolactin: evidence that it is separate from growth hormone in human blood. *Science* **170**:745-7, 1970.
3. **Tyson J E.** Nursing and prolactin secretion: principal determinants in the mediation of puerperal infertility. (Crosignani P G & Robyn C, eds.) *Prolactin and human reproduction.* London: Academic Press, 1977. p. 97-108.
4. ------------. Role of the human decidua in the elaboration of polypeptide hormones. (Choate J W, Dolan T E & Thiede H A, eds.) *Transcript of the Seventh Rochester Trophoblast Conference. October, 1977.* Rochester, NY: University of Rochester School of Medicine & Dentistry, 1977. p. 18-24.
5. **Leontic E A & Tyson J E.** Prolactin and fetal osmoregulation: water transport across isolated human amnion. *Amer. J. Physiol.* **232**:R124-7, 1977.
6. **Leontic E A, Schruefer J J, Andreassen B, Pinto H & Tyson J E.** Further evidence for the role of prolactin on human fetoplacental osmoregulation. *Amer. J. Obstet. Gynecol.* **133**:435-8, 1979.
7. **Tomita K, McCoshen J A, Fernandez C S & Tyson J E.** Immunologic and biologic characteristics of human decidual prolactin. *Amer. J. Obstet. Gynecol.* **142**:420-6, 1982.

This Week's Citation Classic

CC/NUMBER 35
AUGUST 30, 1982

Thorner M O, McNeilly A S, Hagan C & Besser G M. Long-term treatment of galactorrhoea and hypogonadism with bromocriptine.
Brit. Med. J. **2**:419-22, 1974.
[Medical Professorial Unit and Dept. Chemical Pathology, St. Bartholomew's Hospital, London, England]

Seventeen women and four men with galactorrhea and associated hypogonadism were treated with bromocriptine for two to 28 months. Serum prolactin levels were elevated in 12 of 17 patients. Bromocriptine therapy led to cessation of galactorrhea, lowered prolactin levels to normal, and restored gonadal function. [The *SCI*® indicates that this paper has been cited in over 330 publications since 1974.]

Michael O. Thorner
Department of Internal Medicine
University of Virginia
School of Medicine
Charlottesville, VA 22908

June 28, 1982

"Prolactin is secreted by the anterior pituitary gland. Until 1971 many eminent physiologists did not accept that prolactin existed as a distinct and separate hormone from growth hormone in the human. The pioneering work of Friesen[1] finally led to the extraction of prolactin from the human pituitary. This prolactin was then used to raise antibodies to prolactin for the development of a radioimmunoassay for human prolactin. The radioimmunoassay was immediately used to measure prolactin levels in various physiological and pathological conditions. It became rapidly apparent that elevated circulating prolactin levels were often found in patients with galactorrhea and hypogonadism. At the same time, Flückiger[2] (working at Sandoz, Basel) had developed bromocriptine, an ergot drug, with specific prolactin lowering properties which acted directly at the pituitary to lower the prolactin levels.

"Some of the first clinical studies with bromocriptine in hyperprolactinemic patients were performed at St. Bartholomew's Hospital in London by G. Michael Besser.[3] The study which became this *Citation Classic* was the follow-up of that study; a larger group of patients was carefully studied before, during, and after withdrawal of treatment. Twenty-one patients were treated for up to 28 months. Included in this group were nine patients with pituitary tumors and their prolactin levels also fell to normal and gonadal function was restored.

"This paper demonstrated several important points: (1) hyperprolactinemia, irrespective of the presence of a demonstrable pituitary tumor, can be effectively treated by bromocriptine; (2) gonadal function, which is disordered in hyperprolactinemic states, is restored to normal in the majority of patients when prolactin levels are restored to normal; (3) gonadotropin secretion in hyperprolactinemia may be disordered due to a hypothalamic defect. Although at that time we believed that prolactin might induce hypogonadism by acting at the gonadal level, we now believe that it causes hypogonadism predominantly by interfering with gonadotropin-releasing hormone secretion at the hypothalamic level.

"The year 1974 was a crossroads for the understanding of hyperprolactinemia and the mechanism of action of bromocriptine at the pituitary level. MacLeod[4] had shown in 1969 that catecholamines could inhibit prolactin secretion *in vitro* at the pituitary level. The explanation for the widely observed direct inhibition of prolactin secretion by ergot drugs, including bromocriptine, only appeared after 1974 when the following observations were made: (1) bromocriptine inhibited dopamine turnover in the brain; (2) the inhibition of prolactin secretion by ergots could be blocked with neuroleptic drugs; and (3) dopamine receptors were identified in the pituitary and bromocriptine and other ergots had high affinity for these receptors.

"I believe the reason our paper is a *Citation Classic* is that it showed, for the first time, in a large group of patients, that medical therapy of hyperprolactinemia is effective in the long term. In recent years it has become clear that this therapy is also effective in reducing the size of these tumors and is becoming the treatment of choice for large prolactin secreting tumors. For a more recent review, see *Bromocriptine: A Clinical and Pharmacological Review*."[5]

1. **Hwang P, Guyda H & Friesen H.** A radioimmunoassay for human prolactin. *Proc. Nat. Acad. Sci. US* **68**:1902-6, 1971.
2. **Flückiger E & Wagner H.** 2-Br-α-ergokryptin: beeinflussung von fertilität und laktation bei der ratte. *Experientia* **24**:1130-1, 1968.
3. **Besser G M, Parkes L, Edwards C R W, Forsyth I A & McNeilly A S.** Galactorrhoea: successful treatment with reduction of plasma prolactin levels by brom-ergocryptine. *Brit. Med. J.* **3**:669-72, 1972.
4. **MacLeod R M.** Influence of norepinephrine and catecholamine-depleting agents on the synthesis and release of prolactin and growth hormone. *Endocrinology* **85**:816-923, 1969.
5. **Thorner M O, Flückiger E & Calne D B.** *Bromocriptine: a clinical and pharmacological review.* New York: Raven Press, 1980. 181 p.

CC/NUMBER 35
AUGUST 29, 1983

This Week's Citation Classic

Morris J M. The syndrome of testicular feminization in male pseudohermaphrodites. *Amer. J. Obstet. Gynecol.* **65**:1192-211, 1953.
[Department of Obstetrics and Gynecology, Yale University School of Medicine, New Haven, CT]

Testicular feminization was the name given to a syndrome found in individuals with female external genitalia and breast development, absent pubic and axillary hair, absent uterus, and intra-abdominal or inguinal testes. It is an X-linked recessive disorder related to an absence of androgen receptors. [The *SCI*® indicates that this paper has been cited in over 245 publications since 1961.]

John McLean Morris
Department of Obstetrics and Gynecology
School of Medicine
Yale University
New Haven, CT 06510

June 24, 1983

"I was working with the late Hans Kottmeier at the Radiumhemmet in Stockholm on an American Cancer Society fellowship when he asked me to see a patient who had been treated for a dysgerminoma of the ovary. The fact that she had no uterus, no axillary or pubic hair, but otherwise appeared to be a normal female, reminded me of a similar case I had encountered while working as assistant to J.V. Meigs at the Massachusetts General Hospital in Boston. Meigs's case was thought to be a true hermaphrodite. I had reviewed the slides on that patient and found tubules and ovarian-like stroma but no follicular elements. Review of the slides in Stockholm showed rudimentary testicular tubules scattered through the dysgerminoma (seminoma).

"By spending long hours in the library, I was able to unearth 80 similar cases in the literature going back to 1817. Some were reported as a special form of pseudohermaphroditism, but others because of their completely feminine appearance were incorrectly assumed to have ovaries, often with germinomas, arrhenoblastomas, or other tumors. If men as distinguished as Meigs and Kottmeier did not recognize that their patients had this disorder, it seemed worth calling attention to as an entity.

"The selection of a name for the syndrome was a problem. Karyotypes, Barr bodies, hormone receptors, and radioimmunoassays were unknown at that time. Because patients who were castrated prior to puberty did not get significant breast development, and therefore the testes appeared to be producing estrogens, 'testicular feminization' seemed an acceptable term. The suggestion made subsequently by Lawson Wilkins[1] that the syndrome might be due to androgen insensitivity did not in my mind explain the breast development, until a former Yale resident, O.J. Miller, asked me one day, 'How do you know that you would not have female breasts if they were not suppressed by your testosterone?' My initial negative response was altered when I recalled an untreated case of congenital adrenal hyperplasia who had no breast development in spite of the presence of ovaries because of suppression by her adrenal androgens.

"Further studies carried out with Mahesh,[2] Kase,[3] VandeWiele, Dorfman,[4] and Lubs[5] showed normal male androgen production and XY karyotypes. Ultimately, lack of androgen receptors was found to be the etiology of the disorder. Griffin and Wilson[6] have recently summarized the work to date on various androgen resistant syndromes. Other reviews have also appeared.[7,8]

"While this syndrome should therefore be called familial congenital androgen receptor deficiency, we all have our egos. Mine was bolstered when I heard of *Tfm* mice—and even more when my secretary showed me my name in *Stedman's Medical Dictionary* with the word syndrome attached to it.

"Sexual differentiation is a provocative subject. The original article called attention to a generally unrecognized entity. Although there was an unwillingness on the part of some gynecologists to accept the fact that such completely feminine appearing individuals were XY with testes, the syndrome accounts for seven to ten percent of cases of primary amenorrhea."

1. **Wilkins L.** *The diagnosis and treatment of endocrine disorders in childhood and adolescence.* Springfield, IL: Charles C. Thomas, 1957. p. 276.
2. **Morris J M & Mahesh V B.** Further observations on the syndrome, "testicular feminization." *Amer. J. Obstet. Gynecol.* **87**:731-45, 1963.
3. **Kase N & Morris J M.** Steroid synthesis in the cryptorchid testes of three cases of the "testicular feminization" syndrome. *Amer. J. Obstet. Gynecol.* **91**:102-5, 1965.
4. **Southren A L, Ross H, Sharma D C, Gordon G, Weingold A B & Dorfman R I.** Plasma concentration and biosynthesis of testosterone in the syndrome of feminizing testes. *J. Clin. Endocrinol. Metab.* **25**:518-25, 1965.
5. **Lubs H A, Jr., Vilar O & Bergenstal D M.** Familial male pseudohermaphroditism with labial testes and partial feminization: endocrine studies and genetic aspects. *J. Clin. Endocrinol. Metab.* **19**:1110-20, 1959.
6. **Griffin J E & Wilson J D.** The syndromes of androgen resistance. *N. Engl. J. Med.* **302**:198-209, 1980.
7. **Morris J M.** Gonadal anomalies and dysgenesis. (Behrman S J & Kistner R W, eds.) *Progress in gynecology.* Boston: Little, Brown, 1975. p. 265-79.
8. **Simmer H H, Pion R J & Dignam W J.** *Testicular feminization.* Springfield, IL: Charles C. Thomas, 1965. 108 p.

This Week's Citation Classic

NUMBER 9
FEBRUARY 26, 1979

Haddad H M & Wilkins L. Congenital anomalies associated with gonadal aplasia. *Pediatrics* **23**: 885-902, 1959.

The paper reviews congenital anomalies in 55 cases with gonadal aplasia (Turner's syndrome). In addition to the characteristic stigmata of the disease, which each patient displayed, there were congenital anomalies, particularly ocular, which were quite prevalent in these patients. [The *SCI*® indicates that this paper has been cited 150 times since 1961.]

Haskel M. Haddad
Clinical Profesor of Ophthalmology
New York Medical College
New York, NY

January 4, 1978

"It is gratifying to learn that this article, which I wrote in collaboratiaon with the late Dr. Lawson Wilkins, is one of the most cited papers in the field. The reason for this, in my opinion, is that this paper is the only comprehensive review of the largest number ever published of gonadal aplasia patients.

"When Wilkins was preparing to rewrite his book *The Diagnosis and Treatment of Endocrine Diseases in Childhood and Adolescence,* he asked me to review the cases with gonadal aplasia which we had seen in the Pediatric Endocrinology Clinic at Johns Hopkins Hospital. The review proved to be revealing in the abundance of congenital anomalies which these patients displayed. It was thus decided to increase the scope of the review to actual statistical analysis of the anomalies displayed for a separate publication.

"The obstacles encountered were those that one usually encounters in any review article, especially when thoroughness is not always achieved. Even though almost all the patients had ophthalmological evaluations, not all patients had complete ophthalmological examinations including color vision, etc. Thus, the ocular manifestations might not be as accurate as other manifestations reported in the paper.

"The other difficulty was the writing of the paper. This manuscript was written and rewritten over twenty times, until it came into shape and form that was suitable for publication. To give a review article on such a subject would have been lengthy. However, we had to make it short and suitable for quick review of the congenital anomalies in gonadal aplasia, and thus it required considerable rewriting and editing. Also, the review of the literature had to be comprehensive and one could not always follow up the reported cases in the literature, especially in the Spanish and other foreign languages. This created tremendous hardship, because many of the publications which are cited in the references of the paper were not available in the Cumulative Index Medicus.

"All in all, the experience in writing this paper was very gratifying. It was a great learning experience for me personally, especially considering the fact that the late Lawson Wilkins was a great teacher with vivid ability for critique and editing. Without his help, the manuscript would not have come to light.

"May I add that the experience with the late Lawson Wilkins encouraged me in my path to develop the field of metabolic ophthalmology with subsequent formation of the International Society on Metabolic Eye Disease and its official publication, *Metabolic Ophthalmology*. The Society has introduced three international symposia with one book published called *Metabolic Eye Disease*. I consider this all a tribute to the late Lawson Wilkins."

This Week's Citation Classic

CC/NUMBER 34
AUGUST 25, 1980

Neill J D, Johansson E D B, Datta J K & Knobil E. Relationship between the plasma levels of luteinizing hormone and progesterone during the normal menstrual cycle. *J. Clin. Endocrinol. Metab.* **27**:1167-73, 1967.
[Dept. Physiol., Univ. Pittsburgh Sch. Med., Pittsburgh, PA]

A rapid and relatively simple competitive protein binding assay for the steroid hormone, progesterone, was developed and applied to the measurement of plasma progesterone levels daily throughout the human menstrual cycle. [The *SCI*® indicates that this paper has been cited over 365 times since 1967.]

Jimmy D. Neill
Department of Physiology
and Biophysics
University of Alabama
Birmingham, AL 35294

June 23, 1980

"I joined the laboratory of Ernst Knobil, department of physiology, University of Pittsburgh, as a postdoctoral fellow in the Fall of 1965 to study the hormonal control of the menstrual cycle in the rhesus monkey. These studies required measurement of circulating hormone levels so I visited A. Rees Midgley, department of pathology, University of Michigan, to learn the radioimmunoassay for human luteinizing hormone (LH) that he had recently developed[1] (in fact, when I visited, his method had been published only in abstract form). Next we turned to the measurement of progesterone. All of the available methods were extremely laborious, lacked sensitivity, and required the expertise of an organic chemist. Fortunately for us, Beverly Murphy published an abstract in the Spring of 1966 describing a simple and highly sensitive assay for a related steroid hormone, cortisol, based on the 'competition' between radioactive and non-radioactive cortisol for binding to a plasma protein, corticosteroid binding globulin (CBG or transcortin).[2] Our initial plan was to enzymatically convert progesterone, isolated from plasma, to cortisol and then use her method for quantification. However, when we phoned her to get additional details about the method, she told us that progesterone itself also bound to CBG and could be measured directly without the conversion step. I added a thin-layer chromatographic step to her method so that it would be specific for progesterone, and on July 4, 1966, obtained the first convincing evidence that the method could be applied to measurement of progesterone in plasma.

"Because the human LH radioimmunoassay turned out to be unsuitable for measuring monkey LH, we studied the human menstrual cycle by collecting daily blood samples from four women for simultaneous measurements of progesterone and LH (of the group of co-authors, only Johansson was a physician). Ours and Murphy's manuscripts were submitted simultaneously for publication with instructions to the editor that our paper should appear one month after Murphy's, and it did.

"This paper was cited frequently for several reasons. First, it ushered-in an era of relatively rapid and simple measurements of plasma steroid hormone levels; indeed, many people visited our laboratory to learn the method long before it was published. Second, and of more lasting significance, it established unequivocally and for the first time the relationship between the secretion of progesterone and LH. At that time, progesterone was believed to be the ovarian stimulus for the increased LH secretion that results in ovulation. Our paper showed that progesterone secretion increased only after the increase in plasma LH and hence was not the ovarian signal. It also established that the regression of the corpus luteum—as signified by a decrease in plasma progesterone levels—was not associated with changes in the secretion of its luteotrophic hormone, LH."

1. **Midgley A R, Jr.** Radioimmunoassay: a method for human chorionic gonadotropin and human luteinizing hormone. *Endocrinology* **79**:10-18, 1966.
2. **Murphy B E P.** Some studies of the protein-binding of steroids and their application to the routine micro and ultramicro measurements of various steroids in body fluids by competitive protein binding radioassay. *J. Clin. Endocrinol. Metab.* **27**:973-90, 1967.

CC/NUMBER 44
NOVEMBER 3, 1980

This Week's Citation Classic

Inman W H W & Vessey M P. Investigation of deaths from pulmonary, coronary, and cerebral thrombosis and embolism in women of child-bearing age. *Brit. Med. J.* **2**:193-9, 1968.
[Committee on Safety of Drugs, Queen Anne's Mansions, and Med. Res. Council, Stat. Res. Unit, Univ. Coll. Hosp. Med. Sch., London, England]

A study in which women who died from various types of thromboembolism in the United Kingdom during 1966 were practice-matched with healthy women revealed a significant excess of oral contraceptive use among those dying from cerebral thrombosis or pulmonary embolism. [The *SCI*® indicates that this paper has been cited over 315 times since 1968.]

W. H. W. Inman
Drug Surveillance Research Unit
University of Southampton
Southampton SO2 3FL
England

October 20, 1980

"Shortly after my appointment as senior medical officer in charge of monitoring the adverse drug reactions reported to the Committee on Safety of Drugs (CSD), small numbers of suspected associations between oral contraceptive use and thromboembolic disease began to appear on the Committee's yellow cards. In the 12 months ending August 1965, the total of 16 reported deaths was very close to the 13 that would have been expected among the 400,000 women believed to have been using the pill at that time. If all deaths had been reported, use of the pill would appear to present no hazards, but lack of confidence in the completeness of the reporting led me to conduct, with the encouragement of the CSD, what proved to be the earliest study to show a significant relationship.

"During 1965 I had recruited a team of about 35 medically-qualified part-time fieldworkers and their first major assignment was to investigate deaths from thromboembolism of women aged between 20 and 44 occurring in the United Kingdom in 1966, identified by means of certificates provided by the Registrar General. At each interview with a general practitioner they obtained details about use of oral contraceptives by the dead woman and by healthy controls in the same practice. By the end of August it became apparent that there was significantly greater use of the pill by the dead women.

"Because of the alarm that might have been caused by premature publicity, the CSD waited for the results of two further studies by the College of General Practitioners, commenced in July 1966, and by the Medical Research Council, commenced in December 1966. A meeting was arranged at the request of the Committee in January 1967 at which the results of the three studies were reviewed and in April a preliminary communication was prepared by a working group.[1] This was the start of my long association with Martin Vessey and other workers in Oxford. By mid-1967 most of the fieldwork in the CSD was complete and Vessey accepted my invitation to become the coauthor and give expert epidemiological help in the preparation of the final report.

"After studying 385 deaths, we estimated the excess risk from pulmonary embolism and cerebral thrombosis attributable to use of the pill to be 1.3 deaths per 100,000 women aged 20 to 34, and 3.4 per 100,000 women aged 35 to 44, roughly a sevenfold risk among pill users. The risk of fatal myocardial infarction was not quite statistically significant, but if added to the above estimates brought the totals to 2.3 and 4.5 per 100,000 respectively.

"While studying voluntary reports to the CSD in 1966, I suspected that the preparations containing mastranol might carry a greater risk than those containing ethinyloesteradiol; later it became apparent that the total dose of estrogen determined the risk and this hypothesis was developed in a further publication with Vessey and colleagues from Scandinavia in 1970.[2] I have reviewed the history of these early pill studies elsewhere."[3]

1. **Medical Research Council.** Risk of thromboembolic disease in women taking oral contraceptives. A preliminary communication to the Medical Research Council by a sub-committee. *Brit. Med. J.* **2**:355-9, 1967.
2. **Inman W H W, Vessey M P, Westerholm B & Engelund A.** Thromboembolic disease and the steroidal content of oral contraceptives. *Brit. Med. J.* **2**:203-9, 1970.
3. **Inman W H W.** Role of drug-reaction monitoring in the investigation of thrombosis and "The Pill." *Brit. Med. Bull.* **26**:3, 248-56, 1970.

CC/NUMBER 42
OCTOBER 20, 1980

This Week's Citation Classic

Sartwell P E, Masi A T, Arthes F G, Greene G R & Smith H E. Thromboembolism and oral contraceptives: an epidemiologic case-control study.
Amer. J. Epidemiol. **90**:365-80, 1969.
[Dept. Epidemiol., Sch. Hygiene and Pub. Health, Johns Hopkins Univ., Baltimore, MD]

We made a case-control study of 175 women aged 15-44, hospitalized with idiopathic thromboembolism, and 175 matched hospital patients as controls. By interview, the relative risk of thrombosis for users of oral contraceptives within the month preceding onset was found to be 4.4. [The *SCI*® indicates that this paper has been cited over 170 times since 1969.]

Philip E. Sartwell
38 Cloutman Lane
Marblehead, MA 01945

October 1, 1980

"This study can be traced to an innocent remark over cocktails that the problems of the Food and Drug Administration (FDA) in detecting and evaluating adverse drug reactions were epidemiological. This led to an appointment in 1965 to the FDA's Advisory Committee on Obstetrics and Gynecology, whereupon I learned that the most serious question then before the Committee was whether use of oral contraceptives was a cause of thrombophlebitis, pulmonary embolism, and other intravascular clotting. Although several erudite committees had already debated this question, there were no answers because no one had begun to collect really useful data to test the hypothesis.

"I outlined a proposal for a case-control (retrospective) study, whereupon the representatives of the drug industry who attended the meeting drafted a commentary explaining why it wouldn't work. Despite this opposition, the agency supported the study wholeheartedly.

"Alfonse Masi, who doubled as epidemiologist and internist, and I recruited a field team, including Federico Arthes, internist, and Helen Smith, project supervisor. Later, Gerald Greene joined us on loan from CDC. Others, named in the paper, provided invaluable assistance.

"We determined to include only women with no apparent reason to develop intravascular clotting, and spent considerable time polling authorities as to what conditions should be considered cause for rejection of a case. We found it necessary to reject the great majority of patients for this and other reasons. This selectivity necessitated the collaboration of 43 hospitals in five large eastern cities. After we had begun work we learned that W.H.W. Inman, R. Doll, M.P. Vessey, and others had similar studies under way in the UK.[1,2] They were able to complete and publish their investigations well before we did.

"Subjects (women aged 15-44 meeting the study requirements) were interviewed at home by employees of a survey research company using a pretested structured questionnaire. We devised special methods to obtain complete medical and reproductive histories, and to have the subjects identify the drugs taken, and over what period. There were 350 subjects (175 cases, 175 controls).

"The study yielded an overall 'relative risk' of 4.4 (idiopathic thrombosis 4½ times more frequent in users of OCs than nonusers). For deep thrombosis, pulmonary embolism alone, and intracranial lesions, the risk ratio was significantly increased. A subsequent paper[3] provided further information as to our methods and results.

"Why so many citations? Certainly because of the importance of this finding to many millions of women and their physicians and because this was the first study of its kind done in the US. The study has been vigorously challenged, but enough work has been done by others to consider the hypothesis established."

1. **Inman W H W & Vessey M P.** Investigation of deaths from pulmonary, coronary and cerebral thrombosis and embolism in women of child-bearing age. *Brit. Med. J.* **2**:193-9, 1968.
2. **Vessey M P & Doll R.** Investigation of relation between use of oral contraceptives and thromboembolic disease. A further report. *Brit. Med. J.* **2**:651-7, 1969.
3. **Sartwell P E.** Oral contraceptives and thromboembolism: a further report. *Amer. J. Epidemiol.* **94**:192-201, 1971.

CC/NUMBER 24
JUNE 15, 1981

This Week's Citation Classic

Tait J F. Review: the use of isotopic steroids for the measurement of production rates *in vivo. J. Clin. Endocrinol. Metab.* **23**:1285-97, 1963.
[Worcester Foundation for Experimental Biology, Shrewsbury, MA]

Theoretical considerations and experimental procedures involved in the measurement of metabolic clearance rate (MCR) and blood production rate were compared and described, e.g., single injection and continuous infusion methods. Emphasis was placed on applications in endocrinology and particularly for steroid hormones. [The *SCI*® indicates that this paper has been cited over 275 times since 1963.]

James F. Tait
Department of Physics as
Applied to Medicine
Middlesex Hospital
Medical School
London W1P 6DB
England

May 6, 1981

"Applications in endocrinology of the experimental procedures and theoretical considerations for the estimation of metabolic clearance rate, largely originating from the work of Hamilton and co-workers,[1] were a feature of this review. The concept of blood production rate was also introduced.

"This concept arose because the labelled reagent methods for the estimation of nanomole amounts or less of biologically important substances in blood had become generally applicable. These originated in Bethesda with the radioactive pipsyl method and had been applied there and elsewhere to the estimation of steroid hormones using labelled pipsyl, acetic anhydride, and thiosemicarbazide reagents. These methods have now been supplanted by immunoassay procedures, but were the first practical methods in blood for important steroids such as aldosterone, androstenedione, and testosterone. Although laborious they were quite accurate and indeed it is doubtful whether some of the estimates of secretion rates for blood production rates then made could have been achieved with the present accuracy of routine immunoassays.

"The blood production rate is the metabolic clearance rate multiplied by the blood concentration of hormone and represents its secretion rate plus the amount irreversibly converted to it from precursors. These concepts originated mainly from the general theoretical ideas of E. Gurpide and co-workers.[2] The blood concepts, which proved to be more generally valid than those involving measurement of urinary metabolites, were largely evolved from the experimental work by myself and colleagues[3] on aldosterone metabolism which presented a starting point for consideration of more complicated situations such as when steroids were converted peripherally. Their development also followed extensive discussions with J. Coghlan of the Florey Institute of Experimental Biology and Medicine, Melbourne, Australia, and S. Burstein, who worked, as did I then, at the Worcester Foundation for Experimental Biology, US. The S^{35} thiosemicarbazide method, which was probably both the most difficult and sophisticated labelled reagent method ever developed, was vital for the critical estimation of androstenedione which first showed that concentrations of this prehormone in female and male plasma were similar. The use of this reagent was developed with the chemical advice of Marcel Gut at Worcester.

"If the review has been highly cited and has had some influence it is because it was timely and the concepts, although not completely original in general physiology, had not been appreciated generally in endocrinology. Appropriate experimental methods had also just become available.

"Later work at the Worcester Foundation followed this review when experimental collaborative studies with R. Horton, C. Longcope, and D. Baird[4] exploited these concepts culminating in a presentation at the Laurentian Hormone Conference."

1. **Hamilton W F & Remington J W.** Comparison of the time concentration curves in arterial blood of diffusible and non-diffusible substances when injected at a constant rate and when injected instantaneously. *Amer. J. Physiol.* **148**:35-9, 1947.
2. **Gurpide E, Mann J, VandeWiele R L & Lieberman S.** A discussion of the isotope dilution method for estimating secretory rates from urinary metabolites. *Acta Endocrinol.* **39**:213-22, 1962.
3. **Tait J F, Little B, Tait S A S & Flood C.** The metabolic clearance rate of aldosterone in pregnant and nonpregnant subjects estimated by both single-injection and constant-infusion methods. *J. Clin. Invest.* **41**:2093-100, 1962.
4. **Baird D T, Horton R, Longcope C & Tait J F.** Steroid dynamics under steady-state conditions. *Recent Progr. Hormone Res.* **25**:611-64, 1969.

CC/NUMBER 6
FEBRUARY 11, 1980

This Week's Citation Classic

Takahashi Y, Kipnis D M & Daughaday W H. Growth hormone secretion during sleep. *J. Clin. Invest.* **47**:2079-90, 1968.
[Washington Univ. Sch. Med., Dept. Med., Metabolism Div., St. Louis, MO]

In young adults a remarkable peak of GH secretion occurs about one hour after the onset of deep sleep. This GH secretion is clearly entrained with the onset of deeper levels of sleep and not with discernible metabolic stimuli. [The *SCI*® indicates that this paper has been cited over 285 times since 1968.]

William H. Daughaday
Metabolism Division
Department of Internal Medicine
School of Medicine
Washington University
St. Louis, MO 63110

December 19, 1979

"In September 1966, Yasuro Takahashi came to the metabolism division of the department of medicine of Washington University as a research fellow for only one year to learn immunoassay procedures and endocrine physiology. He arrived with a sound background in neurophysiology, particularly in the area of sleep physiology, which he had obtained at the Neuropsychiatric Research Institute in Tokyo. He was intrigued with earlier preliminary reports suggesting increased GH secretion during the night and wished to correlate GH secretion with the stages of sleep. Our division provided radioimmunoassay resources, an excellent Clinical Research Center equipped with a small but adequate sleep study room, and an active research program of study of growth hormone and insulin secretion. Within a very short period Takahashi initiated this study by recruiting the subjects, personally monitoring their sleep by EEG and EMG, and conducting many of the assays. Truly this was a remarkable performance of varied technical skills and Japanese industry.

"The results of this study were clear. The early period of deep sleep in young adults is associated with a major peak of growth hormone secretion unassociated with detectable changes in plasma glucose, fatty acid, insulin, or cortisol concentrations. GH secretion was clearly entrained with sleep as shown by sleep delay and sleep interruption studies. Administration of five CNS active drugs did not inhibit GH secretion with the possible exception of imipramine which did block GH secretion in two of the four subjects.

"We concluded that the GH secretion of early sleep was regulated by primary hypothalamic mechanisms unrelated to metabolic clues.

"As in many clinical investigations, this study brought together ideas and techniques from a number of disciplines which characterized an important human neuroendocrine function. The results of our study were rapidly confirmed and extended in other laboratories. The findings still have important implications in the study of human growth because for most subjects the sleep related GH peak represents the most active period of GH secretion for the entire 24 hours.

"This paper attracted much reader interest and stimulated others to undertake physiologic, neuropharmacologic, and clinical projects because of the direct linkage of growth hormone secretion with a specific neural mechanism—the sleep process. This, I think, accounts for the frequent citation of this paper."

CC/NUMBER 33
AUGUST 16, 1982

This Week's Citation Classic

Boyd A E, Lebovitz H E & Pfeiffer J B. Stimulation of human-growth-hormone secretion by L-dopa. *N. Engl. J. Med.* **283**:1425-9, 1970.
[Divs. Endocrinology and Neurology, Dept. Medicine, Duke Univ. Medical Ctr., Durham, NC]

This paper showed clearly that the administration of L-dopa, a precursor of central nervous system catecholamines, stimulated the release of growth hormone in man. The data indicated that a dopaminergic mechanism in the median eminence or norepinephrine sensitive site in the hypothalamus was involved in human growth hormone regulation. [The ***SCI®*** **indicates that this paper has been cited in over 360 publications since 1970.]**

A.E. Boyd
Departments of Medicine and Cell Biology
Baylor College of Medicine
Houston, TX 77030

June 7, 1982

"In 1969, I started an endocrine fellowship working with Harold Lebovitz at Duke University in Durham, North Carolina. I had just completed three years of training in medicine at Boston City Hospital and Duke after graduating from medical school at Washington University in St. Louis. Like many ideas in clinical medicine, the genesis of our studies on L-dopa was at the bedside. I saw a patient of John Pfeiffer who was taking a new experimental therapy, L-dopa, for Parkinson's disease. The patient was a mild diabetic and we worried about the effect of the new medication on his diabetes. We thought that this precursor of catecholamines might inhibit the release of the patient's endogenous insulin and result in deterioration of the diabetes. We set up a clinical study of Pfeiffer's patients to investigate the effect of L-dopa on glucose metabolism. When I reviewed the literature it also became obvious that this amino acid would cross the blood-brain barrier, increasing turnover of dopamine and norepinephrine in the hypothalamus, and could be used as a probe to study control of the pituitary by catecholamines. On the basis of the animal data in which amines had been injected directly into the ventricles or hypothalamus, I thought that L-dopa might stimulate the release of the gonadotropins. To our surprise, instead, L-dopa stimulated a dramatic rise in growth hormone levels in the patients we studied, and it did not alter the pituitary hormones which control the adrenal, thyroid, or gonadal axis. The L-dopa-induced rise in growth hormone could not be blocked by either oral or intravenous glucose. This latter information was obtained serendipitously from the studies in which we had administered the drug prior to glucose, and subsequently measured insulin secretion. Since L-dopa was a precursor of both dopamine and norepinephrine, growth secretion appeared linked to dopamine pathways in the median eminence or norepinephrine in the hypothalamus. Subsequent studies by a number of investigators have indicated that both dopaminergic and noradrenergic pathways control the release of growth hormone by increasing the secretion of a putative growth hormone-releasing factor.

"In 1970 it was not clear that prolactin was a distinct human hormone, but in 1971 it became possible to measure serum prolactin levels in man,[1] and L-dopa was shown to have a potent inhibitory effect on prolactin secretion.[2] After our studies in parkinsonian patients, I enthusiastically recruited all of the endocrine fellows at Duke to come to Lebovitz's home on Sunday mornings to take the drug. L-dopa is a powerful emetic and my bloodletting was frequently interrupted by the rush of my friends to the bathroom. These studies were soon interrupted more definitely by my entering the Army after one year of fellowship.

"This publication is frequently cited because it was the first study to directly test the monoaminergic control of pituitary function in man. In addition, the L-dopa test has become a standard clinical means of evaluating growth hormone secretion. In acromegaly, a pituitary disorder with excess growth hormone secretion, L-dopa and dopamine agonists have a paradoxical effect lowering the elevated growth hormone levels and are now used to treat this disease. Similar success is seen in the therapy of disorders of excess prolactin secretion."

1. **Martin J B.** Neural regulation of growth hormone secretion. Medical progress report. *N. Engl. J. Med.* **288**:1384-93, 1973.
2. **Malarkey W B, Jacobs L S & Daughaday W H.** Levodopa suppression of prolactin in non-puerperal galactorrhea. *N. Engl. J. Med.* **285**:1160-3, 1971.

CC/NUMBER 46
NOVEMBER 17, 1980

This Week's Citation Classic

Hamolsky M W, Stein M & Freedberg A S. The thyroid hormone-plasma protein complex in man. II. A new *in vitro* method for study of "uptake" of labelled hormonal components by human erythrocytes.
J. Clin. Endocrinol. Metab. **17**:33-44, 1957.
[Dept. Med., Harvard Med. Sch.; Med. Res. Dept., Yamins Res. Lab.; and Med. Serv., Beth Israel Hosp., Boston, MA]

A new *in vitro* method is presented, based on the 'uptake' of I-131 T-3 by red blood cells from whole blood. The simple test accurately differentiates hyper-, hypo-, and euthyroidism, is unaffected by iodine exposure, avoids administration of radioactivity to patients, and indicates several epiphenomena of wide biologic and clinical interest. [The *SCI*® indicates that this paper has been cited over 320 times since 1961.]

Milton W. Hamolsky
Department of Medicine
Brown University
Rhode Island Hospital
Providence, RI 02902

October 30, 1980

"Our studies were based on a) the fact that thyroxin (T-4) and triiodothyronine (T-3) molecules are both hydrophilic and lipophilic, and b) the notion that their hormonal action might therefore involve alignment at, and alteration of, the aqueous plasma-lipid membrane interface.

"We found: I-131 T-4 or I-131 T-3 passed *in vitro* from buffers to olive or mineral oil, lipid extracts of tissue or cell components, to the rat diaphragm, to foreskin of seven-day old males. Attempts to isolate human white blood cells to study uptakes were premature in 1952, so we turned to human red blood cells—then considered 'simple' sacs of hemoglobin. The addition of increasing amounts of plasma to the buffer solution progressively decreased transfer of T-4 or T-3 to the lipid extracts or tissues; the decrease in transfer was always greater for T-4 than T-3. These studies antedated notions of specific plasma protein binders (TBG or TBPA) of thyroid hormones. We thought we were studying 'active' lipid or tissue 'uptake' of T-4 or T-3.

"The next step was study of 'uptakes' from whole plasma. With hyper-, eu-, and hypothyroid plasmas, the rat diaphragm, foreskin, or red blood cell nicely 'diagnosed' the thyroid status of the plasma donor—'uptakes' were greater from hyper- than from euthyroid plasmas and less from hypo- than from euthyroid plasmas. The standard clinical test involved addition of I-131 T-3 to a 3 ml. aliquot of whole blood, incubation at 37° for two hours, determination of percent incorporation of T-3 by the washed red cell mass, corrected for hematocrit. 'Crisscross' studies (euthyroid cells in hyperthyroid plasmas, etc.) revealed that 'uptakes' were determined by the thyroid status of the *plasma* donor. This served as the basis for widespread use of resins, coated charcoal, clay, etc., in place of the red cell as the competitive binder of I-131 T-3 from plasma or serum.

"We offered then the *in vitro* T-3 uptake test which was simple, rapid, reproducible, avoiding administration of radioactivity to the patient, with a differential diagnostic accuracy equal or superior to then available methods, accurate in following therapy of hyper- or hypothyroidism. The test was modified—for pediatrics—to use only 0.5 ml. whole blood. Results were not affected by prior exposure to iodine containing compounds or X-ray dyes which vitiated the then current PBI or I-131 thyroid uptake tests.

"In continuing series (3,900 tests[1]), we found uptakes were decreased by estrogen and pregnancy (failure of lowered uptake in pregnancy presaged miscarriage) and in families with excess TBG, increased in nephrosis, acidoses, anticoagulant therapy, Dilantin—phenomena which led to studies in many laboratories around the world. For, in addition to the above advantages, citation of our article may be attributed to its introduction at a time of explosive ferment of biological and clinical studies of the thyroid gland.

"In 1977, I was selected by the Mallinckrodt Company as a 'Founder of Nuclear Medicine' for the development of 'the first T-3 *in vitro* diagnostic test.' "

1. **Hamolsky M W, Golodetz A & Freedberg A S.** The plasma protein-thyroid hormone complex in man. III. Further studies on the use of the *in vitro* red blood cell uptake of I-131-l-triiodothyronine as a diagnostic test of thyroid function. *J. Clin. Endocrinol. Metab.* **19**:103-16, 1959.

CC/NUMBER 21
MAY 21, 1984

This Week's Citation Classic™

Bywaters E G L, Dixon A S J & Scott J T. Joint lesions of hyperparathyroidism. *Ann. Rheum. Dis.* **22**:171-87, 1963.
[Postgraduate Medical School, London, and MRC Rheumatism Research Unit, Taplow, Berkshire, England]

Patients with hyperparathyroidism and less commonly those with osteomalacia may suffer crush lesions of juxta-articular bone with a traumatic type of synovitis manifest by effusions and disability. Later, osteoarthrosis occurs. Some of these cases may mimic clinically and radiologically cases of rheumatoid arthritis. However, calcification in the synovial membrane and cartilage, common in these cases, is never seen in rheumatoid arthritis. It is important to recognize such presentations and to proceed to appropriate treatment. [The *SCI*® indicates that this paper has been cited in over 155 publications since 1963.]

Eric G.L. Bywaters
Rheumatology Division
Royal Postgraduate Medical School
Hammersmith Hospital
London W12 0HS
England

February 29, 1984

"'Accident' is how we describe the way things start. The background of our paper on the joint lesions of hyperparathyroidism was a result of a long-term interest in rheumatoid arthritis starting for me in 1936. By 1939, I was responsible for rheumatology at the British Postgraduate Medical School at Hammersmith Hospital, London, and, over the course of years, had many talented and later famous colleagues training in that fabulous environment of medical advancement headed by Jack McMichael. But in those early days, we had no support in rheumatology from the pathologists and little from radiologists (until Robert Steiner came in the late 1950s). We had to do our own pathological and radiological interpretations.

"Against this background, we were referred, more or less by accident from the orthopaedic surgeon, a woman aged 66 with 'rheumatoid arthritis.' Although polyarticular, the surgeon contemplated doing knee arthrodeses on the grounds of incapacity. She had been unable to walk beyond the house for two years. Examination showed multiple joint swellings with pain. At our regular weekly session with the radiologists, we reviewed the knee X rays and initially concurred in the diagnosis of 'erosive rheumatoid arthritis' and indeed there were multiple severe erosions as well as other rather bizarre lesions. The hand X rays, however, showed not only carpal wrist and styloid erosions but also characteristic sawtooth subperiosteal erosions of the phalanges. Despite removal of the parathyroid adenoma, the patient died of renal failure 16 months later, vaguely aware to the last that she had been a patient of more than usual interest, although perhaps not appreciating her precise role in the advancement of clinical knowledge.

"We studied in detail the bone pathology of this and another case, as well as the X rays of 17 other cases and ten with osteomalacia. We were in a very fortunate position because Russell Fraser, chief of endocrinology, and his renowned team had a special interest in metabolic bone disease. Calcific deposits in cartilage were likened to the chondrocalcinosis described by Zitnan and Sitaj in 1963,[1] although they had not yet been characterized as due to calcium pyrophosphate dihydrate.

"The mimicry of rheumatoid arthritis (despite normal sedimentation rate and absence of rheumatoid factor) was, we thought from the pathological studies, due to bone collapse and the development of a 'traumatic' synovitis. This was important to recognise early because progress could be halted with appropriate treatment.

"In addition, urate metabolism was studied in this group of patients.[2] Hyperuricaemia was found to be common, attributable only partly to general renal failure: it was suggested that there was a certain type of renal lesion associated with calcium deposition in those parts of the tubule concerned with uric acid secretion.

"The frequent citation of this paper is due probably to previous neglect of such combined clinical, pathological, and radiological studies in the field of skeletal disorders. More recent studies in metabolic joint disease from this pathological viewpoint include accounts of haemachromatosis,[3] acromegaly,[4] and ochronosis[5] reviewed in Sokoloff."[6]

1. **Zitnan D & Sitaj S.** Chondrocalcinosis articularis. 1. Clinical and radiological study. *Ann. Rheum. Dis.* **22**:142-52, 1963. (Cited 125 times.)
2. **Scott J T, Dixon A S J & Bywaters E G L.** Association of hyperuricaemia and gout with hyperparathyroidism. *Brit. Med. J.* **1**:1070-3, 1964. (Cited 60 times.)
3. **Bywaters E G L, Hamilton E B D & Williams R.** The spine in idiopathic haemachromatosis. *Ann. Rheum. Dis.* **30**:453-65, 1971.
4. **Bluestone R, Bywaters E G L, Hartog M, Holt P J L & Hyde S.** Acromegalic arthropathy. *Ann. Rheum. Dis.* **30**:243-58, 1971.
5. **Bywaters E G L, Dorling J & Sutor J.** Ochronotic densification. *Ann. Rheum. Dis.* **29**:563, 1970.
6. **Bywaters E G L.** The pathology of the spine. (Sokoloff L, ed.) *The joints and synovial fluid.* New York: Academic Press, 1980. Vol. 2. p. 427-47.

NUMBER 37
SEPTEMBER 10, 1979

This Week's Citation Classic

Karlson P. New concepts on the mode of action of hormones.
Perspect. Biol. Med. **6**:203-14, 1963.
[Department of Physiological Chemistry, University of Munich, Germany]

The paper presents the concept that hormones control gene activity. This was based on an experiment, i.e., puff induction in giant chromosomes by the insect hormone ecdysone. In biochemical terms, stimulation of transcription and translation, i.e., enzyme induction, was postulated as primary mechanism of action of hormones. [The *SCI*® indicates that this paper has been cited over 140 times since 1963.]

P. Karlson
University of Marburg
Institute of Physiological Chemistry 1
D-3550 Marburg
Federal Republic of Germany

May 29, 1979

"The paper is essentially a theoretical interpretation of a series of experiments carried out in 1959 together with Ulrich Clever on the control of puffing patterns in salivary gland chromosomes in *Chironomus tentans.* Clever had been studying puffing patterns in giant chromosomes; I was interested in the biochemical and physiological effects of the moulting hormone ecdysone, an insect steroid hormone.

"In the course of a discussion, it became clear that the change of puffing pattern observed by Clever which occurred shortly before pupation might be the action of the moulting hormone. To test this idea, I worked for a week in Clever's laboratory in October 1959. Two months later the essential result became clear: ecdysone induces puffs in giant chromosomes. The experimental results were published in the summer of 1960.[1]

"During our discussions, we were well aware of the implication of our experimental results. Ecdysone seemed to be a timing device for the control of gene activity, turning on certain genes. This was quite a new concept on the mechanism of hormone action; earlier investigators had always looked for a direct influence of steroids on the activity of certain enzymes.

"My review, laying emphasis on the induction of enzyme synthesis by hormones, appeared at about the same time as the well-known paper by Jacob and Monod on the nature of enzyme induction in *E. coli,* i.e., the repressor concept.[2] Both theories fit together quite easily. That might have been one of the reasons why my review article became so widely known and is so often cited.

"It may be pointed out that my 'Citation Classic' had a forerunner.[3] But this review was written in German and published in a medical journal; therefore, it did not reach the international scientific audience.

"The new ideas presented above resulted in a new line of research for our laboratory (possibly also for other laboratories). We dropped many of the research projects in which we were engaged previously, and I interested most of my co-workers to follow up, in various biochemical systems, the mode of action of hormones. We selected steroid hormones, mainly corticosteroids, for our investigations since it was already known that corticosteroids induce enzyme synthesis. This was fortunate; it is nowadays generally accepted that this mechanism of action is restricted to steroid hormones."

1. **Clever U & Karlson P.** Induktion von Puffveränderungen in den Speicheldrüsenchromosomen von *Chironomus tentans* durch Ecdyson. *Exp. Cell. Res.* **20**:623-6, 1960.
2. **Jacob F & Monod J.** Genetic regulatory mechanisms in the synthesis of proteins. *J. Mol. Biol.* **3**:318-56, 1961.
3. **Karlson P.** Biochemische Wirkungsweise der Hormone. *Deut. Med. Wochenschr.* **86**:668-74. 1961.

CC/NUMBER 47
NOVEMBER 23, 1981

This Week's Citation Classic

Dreyfus J C, Schapira G, Demos J & Alexandre Y. Étude de la créatine-kinase sérique chez les myopathes et leurs familles.
Rev. Fr. Étud. Clin. Biol. 5:384-6, 1960.
[Laboratoire de Recherches de Biochimie Médicale, Hôpital des Enfants-Malades, Paris, France]

A new technique for serum creatine-kinase activity determination made it possible for the first time to detect with a sufficient degree of confidence the carrier state for progressive muscular dystrophy. It was the starting point for the carrier detection method which is still in use today. [The ***SCI®*** **indicates that this paper has been cited over 110 times since 1961.]**

Jean-Claude Dreyfus
and Georges Schapira
Institut de Pathologie Moléculaire
24, rue du Faubourg St. Jacques
75674 Paris
France

August 7, 1981

"The cited paper was part of a continuous effort to understand mechanisms of progressive muscular dystrophy, undertaken with Fanny Schapira. In 1953, we described an increase in serum aldolase activity, which was the first enzymatic test for the disease.[1] Other enzymatic methods were described by our group; this type of research culminated with the creatine-kinase test discovered by Japanese researchers.[2] The technique was relatively crude, and improvements were necessary to test the hypothesis that healthy carriers, mothers or sisters of patients, could be detected by creatine-kinase determination. While patients display a very large increase, much smaller elevations were expected in heterozygous carriers. A more precise colorimetric method was then devised that allowed recognition of a number of high values in definite carriers. A combination of aldolase and the creatine-kinase determination test permitted the detection of about half of the carriers.[3] Our results met with general incredulity, which changed into general agreement when the technique was improved to include reducing agents. Three years later,[4] the creatine-kinase test detected 75 percent of carriers, and it is somewhat sad that after 20 years no generally accepted improvement has been made in this field.

"It may be worth mentioning that a companion paper[5] contained the first description of serum creatine-kinase increase in myocardial infarction. It might perhaps deserve to become a *Citation Classic*, in view of the overflow of papers on creatine-kinase and its isozymes in this disease.

"The quoted paper was published in French in a French journal, which has since changed its name to *Biomedicine*. This was indeed a handicap, but perhaps not as big as it would be nowadays. We must say that we were not aware that it was so widely quoted. The reason may be that it was the first paper convincing enough in the field of carrier detection for any disease, in which a rapid expansion took place in the next few years. After a decline for at least ten years, many new attempts have been made lately to find other tests for carrier or antenatal detection of progressive muscular dystrophy, especially on membrane abnormalities, which were already suspected by us 20 years ago on grounds of enzyme efflux from muscle into plasma.

"One of us (J.C. Dreyfus) was awarded the International Gallanti Prize for Clinical Enzymology in 1979, partly for our enzymological work in muscle diseases."[6]

1. **Schapira G, Dreyfus J C & Schapira F.** L'élévation du taux de l'aldolase sérique, test biochimique des myopathies. *Sem. Hôp. Paris* **29**:1917-20, 1953.
2. **Ebashi S, Toyokura Y, Momoi H & Sugita H.** High creatine phosphokinase activity of sera of progressive muscular dystrophy. *J. Biochem. Tokyo* **46**:103-4, 1959.
3. **Schapira F, Dreyfus J C, Schapira G & Demos J.** Étude de l'aldolase et de la créatine kinase du sérum chez les mères de myopathes. *Rev. Fr. Étud. Clin. Biol.* **5**:990-4, 1960.
4. **Dreyfus J C, Schapira F, Demos J, Rosa J & Schapira G.** The value of serum enzyme determination in the identification of dystrophic carriers. *Ann. NY Acad. Sci.* **138**:304-14, 1966.
5. **Dreyfus J C, Schapira G, Resnais J & Scebat L.** La créatine-kinase sérique dans le diagnostic de l'infarctus myocardique. *Rev. Fr. Étud. Clin. Biol.* **5**:386-7, 1960.
[The *SCI* indicates that this paper has been cited over 85 times since 1961.]
6. **Dreyfus J C.** Some problems in clinical and molecular enzymology. (Burlina A & Galzigna L, eds.) *Clinical enzymology symposia 2.* Padua, Italy: Piccin Medical Books, 1979. p. 13-26.

CC/NUMBER 30
JULY 23, 1984

This Week's Citation Classic™

Carson N A J & Neill D W. Metabolic abnormalities detected in a survey of mentally backward individuals in Northern Ireland.
Arch. Dis. Child. **37**:505-13, 1962.
[Royal Belfast Hosp. for Sick Children, and Royal Victoria Hosp., Belfast, Northern Ireland]

During screening of mentally retarded persons in Northern Ireland for metabolic disorders using simple qualitative tests and two-way paper chromatography, two sisters were discovered to be excreting homocystine, a previously unrecognised metabolic error. [The *Science Citation Index* (*SCI*®) and the *Social Sciences Citation Index*® (*SSCI*®) indicate that this paper has been cited in over 195 publications since 1962.]

Nina A.J. Carson
Department of Child Health
The Queens University
Belfast
Northern Ireland

June 28, 1984

"In the 1950s, while working in a children's hospital laboratory, I became interested in developing paper chromatographic techniques to screen patients with suspected amino acid disorders. In 1959, I was given a research grant to extend this work and screen the mentally retarded population of Northern Ireland for metabolic errors. During this research, two sisters were discovered who appeared to be excreting cystine in their urine. I had the opportunity to examine the children and was impressed by the similarity and unusual nature of their symptoms, i.e., mental retardation, fits, ectopia lentis, and skeletal abnormalities (they both later died as a result of thrombotic episodes).

"Chromatographic examination of urine specimens which had shown a normal amino acid pattern when fresh, after two weeks' storage, revealed large spots in the cysteic acid position. The urine was also found to give a positive nitroprusside/cyanide test, suggesting the presence of a sulphur-containing amino acid. It is known that the phenol solvent which we used is detrimental to thiol groups but not to the oxidised product. This would explain the presence of the normal amino acid pattern on the fresh specimen of urine. As it is unusual to find a specific cystinuria without the presence of the basic amino acids lysine, orithine, and arginine (all three were absent in these children), and as I did not possess an amino acid analyser, the specimens were sent to Dent at University College, London. In the meantime, the children were given a cystine load. On examination of the postload urines using large size chromatography paper and oxidising with hydrogen peroxide, two spots were evident, one of which co-chromatographed with cysteic acid. Dent, while first confirming our finding of cysteic acid, telegraphed excitedly a few days later that what we had was homocysteic and not cysteic acid.

"This experience highlights the fact that no one person is responsible for any new discovery. The children were referred to me by Claude Field, paediatrician, because he suspected the presence of an inherited metabolic disorder. My colleague and mentor D.W. Neill, senior biochemist, encouraged me to pursue the investigation, and Dent and his co-workers with their expertise in amino acids were responsible for the undoubted identification of homocystine. Other patients were discovered in Northern Ireland and a typical clinical picture emerged.

"In 1964, Mudd *et al.*[1] reported that homocystinuria was due to inactivity of cystathionine synthase (CS), an enzyme on the trans-sulphuration pathway which converts homocystine to cystathionine. Since then, three genetically determined enzyme defects are now known in the remethylation pathway from homocystine to methionine. (For a review of homocystinurias, see reference 2.)

"Treatment initially was by giving a low methionine diet, then Barber and Spaeth[3] in 1967 reported three patients on a normal diet who responded biochemically to pharmacological doses of B_6, thus establishing the original form of homocystinuria as an early example of a vitamin dependent inborn error. About 40 percent of our patients are B_6 responsive. The reason for this often quoted reference is therefore because we were the first group to discover CS homocystinuria. Later in 1962, Gerritsen, Vaughn, and Waisman[4] described the first North American patient."

1. **Mudd S H, Finkelstein J D, Irreverre F & Laster L.** Homocystinuria: an enzymatic defect. *Science* **143**:1443-5, 1964. (Cited 215 times.)
2. **Carson N A J.** Homocystinuria—clinical and biochemical heterogeneity. (Cockburn F & Gitzelmann R, eds.) *Inborn errors of metabolism in humans.* New York: Liss, 1982. p. 53-67.
3. **Barber G W & Spaeth G L.** Pyridoxine therapy in homocystinuria. *Lancet* **1**:337, 1967. (Cited 85 times.)
4. **Gerritsen T, Vaughn J G & Waisman H A.** The identification of homocystine in the urine. *Biochem. Biophys. Res. Commun.* **9**:493-6, 1962. (Cited 125 times.)

This Week's Citation Classic

CC/NUMBER 20
MAY 14, 1979

Menkes J H, Hurst P L & Craig J M. A new syndrome: progressive familial infantile cerebral dysfunction associated with an unusual urinary substance. *Pediatrics* **14**:462-6, 1954.

The paper describes the clinical course of what the authors later termed 'Maple Syrup Disease,' a syndrome involving a rapidly progressive cerebral dysfunction commencing during the first week of life, and marked by the excretion of urine having a characteristic 'maple syrup' odor. [The *SCI*® indicates that this paper has been cited over 140 times since 1961.]

John H. Menkes
9615 Brighton Way
Beverly Hills, CA 90210

January 9, 1978

"In 1952, I had just begun my internship at Boston Children's Hospital. Peter Hurst was junior resident, and John Craig was the pathologist. The only disorder of amino acid metabolism recognized at that time was phenylketonuria, and although the methodology for paper chromatography had been described some 18 years before, it was used at only one laboratory at the Children's Hospital, that of the late David Hsia.

"The patient was brought in to our medical center because two of three earlier born siblings had succumbed to a disease that was thought to be an atypical form of kernicterus. William Pfeffer had been selected as attending physician, since he had been interested in erythroblastosis.

"In obtaining the infant's history I was told that the mother had noted that the infants who died had an unusual odor, while the girl who was well did not.

"Our baby did indeed develop an unusual odor and shortly thereafter began to have neurologic symptoms. We began to collect urine, and wondered what the odor was. I am sure I must have asked nearly everyone in the hospital, but could get no better reply other than that it smelled like maple syrup. After all, we were in New England.

"One rainy Saturday afternoon Hurst and I went to see Louis Fieser, then Professor of Organic Chemistry at Harvard, and author of the textbook from which I had studied the subject. He was not of much more help, but allowed us to roam through his stock room. Urine bottles in hand, we began to sniff our way through the chemicals. I started at the A's, Peter Hurst at the Z's. Not too much later I had what I then thought was the answer: 'Acid Malic.'

"We were dealing with a disorder of the Krebs Cycle, and an enzyme deficiency which, in analogy to phenylketonuria, caused malic acid to accumulate, and was responsible for the neurologic symptoms.

"Titration of the urine did indeed indicate the presence of an organic acid, but at that point I could go no further. A sample was sent to David Hsia for amino acid chromatography, but not having established norms for newborns, he was unable to help us.

"The infant died, and we used up the last bit of urine for a variety of tests, none of which brought us any closer to the answer. A few months later I did learn from an industrial firm that artifical maple syrup contained a cyclic ketone, and in 1957, when I was given urine from another patient with this disease, I was able to use this information to demonstrate the presence of the branched-chain keto acids[1] and to identify the 'Maple Syrup' odor.[2] By then I was a trainee in Pediatric Neurology and had a research budget—$35.

"I view the importance of this paper as lying not in that it was the first description of a rare disease, but rather in that it emphasizes that the combination of clinical skills (in this instance, obtaining a thorough history) and a good basic science background (in this instance, chemistry) are important ingredients for advancing medical knowledge."

REFERENCES

1. **Menkes J H.** Maple syrup disease, investigations into the metabolic defect. *Neurology* **9**:826-35, 1959.
2. **Menkes J H.** Maple syrup disease, isolation and identification of organic acids in the urine. *Pediatrics* **23**:348-53, 1959.

This Week's Citation Classic™

CC/NUMBER 12
MARCH 19, 1984

Oberholzer V G, Levin B, Burgess E A & Young W F. Methylmalonic aciduria. *Arch. Dis. Child.* **42**:492-504, 1967.
[Queen Elizabeth Hospital for Children, London, UK]

Large amounts of methylmalonic acid were detected in the urine of a child with persistent metabolic acidosis. Two cases are described and evidence presented indicating a new syndrome resulting from a block in the conversion of methylmalonyl coenzyme A to succinyl CoA. [The *SCI*® indicates that this paper has been cited in over 180 publications since 1967.]

Victor G. Oberholzer
Department of Clinical Biochemistry
Queen Elizabeth Hospital for Children
London E2 8PS
UK

January 17, 1984

"Following World War II, the Queen Elizabeth Hospital servicing the children in the East End of London became a centre for paediatric teaching of undergraduates. Among the number of gifted members on the staff, the consultant pathologist Barnett Levin (now retired) was responsible for creating and developing the clinical biochemistry section. As part of the general pathology department, this was housed in a series of basement rooms partly below ground. Despite the overcrowded conditions, important contributions to inherited disorders of metabolism were made. In 1962, we reported the first cases of ornithine transcarbamylase deficiency, an inherited disorder of urea synthesis.[1]

"One of the patients at this time was a girl believed to have a form of renal tubular acidosis. She had been successfully managed since birth through many severe acidotic episodes and is now 24 years old and physically and mentally well. During one of her hospital admissions at the end of 1965, the resident medical officer, M.N. Buchanan, who must be given credit for first challenging the diagnosis, asked me to explain why this child under controlled treatment with alkalies was producing an acid urine. Somewhat puzzled, I said I'd see what I could find in the urine. Screening for organic acids was not then a routine procedure. My initial guess from chemical and chromatographic evidence as to the identity of the organic acid found in the urine fortunately was soon confirmed by an adaptation of a newly described colour reaction for the measurement of methylmalonic acid in pernicious anaemia.[2] The appearance of the specific emerald green colour was the high point of my investigation. In methylmalonic aciduria, the term we used for this condition, apart from ketone bodies, large amounts of only one organic acid are excreted. This undoubtedly made it easier to identify. The survival of our patient allowed us to study her disorder in detail.

"Winifred Young had remembered a previous patient with a similar history of recurrent acidosis and ketosis who had died in 1959. Luckily, a small amount of this child's plasma had been kept. The discovery that it contained a high level of methylmalonic acid was another exciting moment.

"A reward for all the research work done by the hospital has been the new Research Building, following the launch of our research appeal at the end of 1965. It was officially honored by the Queen in 1972, and I was given the honour of showing Her Majesty around the spacious biochemistry department.

"The frequent citation of this paper is most likely due to its being a first report of a new disorder and one that has been found to have the highest frequency of occurrence among the organic acidurias.

"More recent studies in the synthesis of the vitamin B12 cofactor, 5′ deoxyadenosyl cobalamin, necessary for the conversion of methylmalonyl CoA to succinyl CoA, widened the field of interest and has led to a better understanding of the biochemical heterogeneity of the inherited defects in methylmalonic acid metabolism. An excellent review has recently been published."[3]

1. **Russell A, Levin B, Oberholzer V G & Sinclair L.** Hyperammonaemia: a new instance of an inborn enzymatic defect of the biosynthesis of urea. *Lancet* **2**:699-700, 1962. (Cited 120 times.)
2. **Giorgio A J & Plaut G W E.** A method for the colorimetric determination of urinary methylmalonic acid in pernicious anemia. *J. Lab. Clin. Med.* **66**:667-76, 1965. (Cited 100 times.)
3. **Matsui S M, Mahoney M J & Rosenberg L E.** The natural history of the inherited methylmalonic acidemias. *N. Engl. J. Med.* **308**:857-61, 1983.

This Week's Citation Classic

Lesch M & Nyhan W L. A familial disorder of uric acid metabolism and central nervous system function. *Amer. J. Med.* **36**:561-70, 1964.
[Dept. Pediat., Johns Hopkins Univ. Sch. Med., Baltimore, MD and Univ. Miami Sch. Med., Miami, FL]

A syndrome consisting of hyperuricemia, choreoathetosis, self-destructive behavior, and mental retardation is described. Marked abnormalities, quantitatively greater than any previously reported, of urate synthetic rates are described. [The *SCI*® indicates that this paper has been cited over 460 times since 1964.]

Michael Lesch
Department of Medicine
Northwestern University
Medical School
Northwestern Memorial Hospital
Chicago, IL 60611

July 23, 1981

"As a freshman medical student I applied for a student research position too late to work in the biochemistry department. The dean suggested I speak to a young assistant professor of pediatrics whose research interests were in biochemistry. I made the appointment with Bill Nyhan and on arrival, found that he barely had any area that could be called an office. Moreover, my interview began by talking to a pair of feet, the rest of Nyhan's body being submerged in the 'innards' of an early model Beckman amino acid analyzer.

"When he crawled out of the machine, I met a man to whom I took an instant liking and, as I recall, I was immediately hired. That summer I worked for Nyhan trying to separate various nucleoproteins isolated from the nuclei of an experimental tumor. The summer passed rapidly; I accomplished little other than to ruin some glassware but Nyhan and I became close friends. He entered me into a Hopkins program that allowed me to spend an entire year between my sophomore and junior years in his laboratory but still graduate with my class. The following summer I reported to his lab ready to isolate those 'damn' proteins once and for all.

"Work on this project progressed slowly. Part of our laboratory effort was related to Nyhan's interests in disorders of amino acid metabolism and, as such, the laboratory provided a 'service' function to the pediatrics department and frequently performed routine blood and urine amino acid analyses. One such specimen was sent to the laboratory labeled 'cystinuria' but we could find no cystine in the specimen. Nyhan, who trusted his Beckman more than he did the clinical judgment of a pediatrics house officer, insisted on seeing the patient. In a short time he recognized the crystals in the urine to be urate. The rarity of gout in the pediatric age group, coupled with the child's obvious bizarre neurologic deficit, suggested something of significance to Nyhan. This suspicion was heightened when the mother said, 'You think this kid is something, you should see the other one I have at home.'

"My work on nucleoproteins was immediately halted and Nyhan asked me to read up on methods of studying urate metabolism. At that time, such studies included determination of pool size and turnover time, and injection of labeled glycine to determine incorporation rates of glycine into urate. The two brothers were admitted, appropriate control subjects were identified, and I became a urate chemist for six months. The work progressed smoothly as we were utilizing previously published methods.[1,2] It took me almost two months to write and rewrite the manuscript, which was accepted without change.

"In retrospect, my contribution to the discovery of the Lesch-Nyhan syndrome was marginal. I simply was fortunate to be in the right place at the right time and to be working for a senior investigator who was gracious enough to allow a medical student to be first author on a manuscript.

"The publication laid the groundwork for the subsequent discovery[3] in J. Seegmiller's laboratory of the absence of hypoxanthine-guanine phosphoribosyl transferase in these children which in turn opened new concepts as to the regulation of purine metabolism. For this reason and the obvious features of a 'new' genetic disease, this paper has been oft quoted. See *The Metabolic Basis of Inherited Disease* for more recent work in the field."[4]

1. **Benedict J D, Forsham P H & Stetten D, Jr.** The metabolism of uric acid in the normal and gouty human studied with the aid of isotopic uric acid. *J. Biol. Chem.* **181**:183-93, 1949.
2. **Benedict J D, Roche M, Yü T F, Bien E J, Gutman A B & Stetten D, Jr.** Incorporation of glycine nitrogen into uric acid in normal and gouty man. *Metabolism* **1**:3-12, 1952.
3. **Seegmiller J R, Rosenbloom F M & Kelley W N.** An enzyme defect associated with a sex linked human neurological disorder and excessive purine synthesis. *Science* **155**:1682-4, 1967.
4. **Kelley W N & Wyngaarden J B.** The Lesch-Nyhan syndrome. (Stanbury J B, Wyngaarden J B & Fredrickson D S, eds.) *The metabolic basis of inherited disease.* New York: McGraw Hill, 1978. p. 1011-36.

CC/NUMBER 39
SEPTEMBER 24, 1984

This Week's Citation Classic™

Brady R O, Gal A E, Bradley R M, Martensson E, Warshaw A L & Laster L.
Enzymatic defect in Fabry's disease: ceramidetrihexosidase deficiency.
N. Engl. J. Med. **276**:1163-7, 1967.
[Lab. Neurochem., Natl. Inst. Neurological Dis. and Blindness, and Sect. Gastroenterol., Metabolic Dis. Branch, Natl. Inst. Arthritis and Metabolic Dis., NIH, Bethesda, MD]

Fabry's disease is an inherited metabolic disorder in which a lipid called ceramidetrihexoside accumulates throughout the body. The condition was shown to be due to a deficiency of the enzyme that catalyzes the hydrolytic cleavage of the terminal molecule of galactose of ceramidetrihexoside. [The *SCI*® indicates that this paper has been cited in over 290 publications since 1967.]

Roscoe O. Brady
Developmental and Metabolic
Neurology Branch
National Institute of Neurological
and Communicative Disorders and Stroke
National Institutes of Health
Bethesda, MD 20205

July 5, 1984

"Fabry's disease is transmitted as an X-chromosome-linked recessive disorder. Hemizygous males frequently have a reddish-purple maculopapular rash on their skin. They experience acroparesthesias in the hands and feet that get worse with exercise and hot weather. The clinical picture is further characterized by corneal opacities, tortuosity of retinal vessels, generalized atherosclerosis, propensity to premature myocardial infarction and stroke, and eventual renal shutdown. Heterozygotes usually have much milder manifestations although severe signs may be apparent in occasional individuals.

"Original descriptions of this condition were published by dermatologists W. Anderson[1] and J. Fabry[2] in 1898. Eventually, it became apparent that there was a generalized accumulation of lipid in the tissue of these patients. In 1963, Charles C. Sweeley and Bernard Klionsky reported that ceramidetrihexoside [galactosylgalactosylglucosylceramide, (CTH)] was the major accumulating material in Fabry's disease.[3] Much of this lipid appears to be derived from glycolipids in the stroma of senescent erythrocytes.

"In 1965 and 1966, David Shapiro, Julian N. Kanfer, and I synthesized several sphingolipids labeled with ^{14}C with which the metabolic defects in Gaucher's disease and Niemann-Pick disease were established. Based on these findings, I anticipated that Fabry's disease was caused by a deficiency of an enzyme that cleaves the terminal molecule of galactose from CTH.[4] However, in 1966, it was not possible to synthesize CTH chemically with a radioactive tracer in the critical terminal molecule of galactose. Andrew E. Gal joined my group and succeeded in labeling ceramidetrihexoside throughout the molecule by exposing it to radioactive hydrogen gas in a sealed vessel (the Wilzbach procedure). Since the terminal galactose contained radioactive 3H, we were able to trace the fate of this moiety. We discovered that mammalian tissues contain an enzyme that catalyzes the hydrolytic cleavage of this galactose and that intestinal mucosa had the highest activity in this regard.[5] Optimal conditions for measuring the activity of this enzyme were determined and lactosylceramide was identified as the product of the reaction. When this information became available, Andrew L. Warshaw and Leonard Laster obtained biopsy specimens of human small intestinal mucosa from 12 controls, from men with Fabry's disease, and from the mother of one of the patients. Ceramidetrihexosidase activity was readily demonstrated in the specimens from the controls, whereas no activity was detected in the biopsies from the men with Fabry's disease. The activity of the enzyme in the sample from the female carrier was 25 percent of the mean of the controls, a value considerably less than might have been expected for a heterozygote, but compatible with the Lyon hypothesis for X-chromosome inactivation. Furthermore, this level of enzyme activity was consistent with her clinical presentation.

"I believe the paper is frequently cited because Fabry's disease is one of the more common sphingolipid storage disorders. Numerous investigations on the pathogenesis of the clinical manifestations in this condition and approaches to the control[6] and therapy[7] of this disorder have been reported. A review of historical aspects and summary of recent studies on Fabry's disease is available."[8]

1. **Anderson W.** A case of angiokeratoma. *Brit. J. Dermatol.* **10**:113-17, 1898. (Cited 70 times since 1955.)
2. **Fabry J.** Ein Beitrag zur Kenntnis der Purpura haemorrhagica nodularis (Purpura papulosa haemorrhagica Hebrae). *Arch. Dermatol. Syphilis* **43**:187-200, 1898. (Cited 105 times since 1955.)
3. **Sweeley C C & Klionsky B.** Fabry's disease: classification as a sphingolipidosis and partial characterization of a novel glycolipid. *J. Biol. Chem.* **238**:PC3148-50, 1963. (Cited 230 times.)
4. **Brady R O.** Sphingolipidoses. *N. Engl. J. Med.* **275**:312-18, 1966. (Cited 110 times.)
5. **Brady R O, Gal A E, Bradley R M & Martensson E.** The metabolism of ceramide trihexosides. I. Purification and properties of an enzyme that cleaves the terminal galactose molecule of galactosylgalactosylglucosylceramide. *J. Biol. Chem.* **242**:1021-6, 1967. (Cited 75 times.)
6. **Brady R O, Uhlendorf B W & Jacobson C B.** Fabry's disease: antenatal diagnosis. *Science* **172**:174-5, 1971. (Cited 90 times.)
7. **Brady R O, Tallman J F, Johnson W G, Gal A E, Leahy W E, Quirk J M & Dekaban A S.** Replacement therapy for inherited enzyme deficiency: use of purified ceramidetrihexosidase in Fabry's disease. *N. Engl. J. Med.* **289**:9-14, 1973. (Cited 120 times.)
8. **Brady R O.** Fabry's disease. (Dyck P J, Thomas P K, Lambert E H & Bunge R, eds.) *Peripheral neuropathy*. Philadelphia: Saunders, 1984. p. 1717-27.

This Week's Citation Classic

NUMBER 13
MARCH 26, 1979

McKusick V A. *Heritable disorders of connective tissue.* St. Louis: C. V. Mosby Company, 1972 (4th ed.). 878 p. [The Johns Hopkins Hospital, Baltimore, MD 21205]

The monograph presents a synthesis of information from the literature and the author's clinical experience, delineating mendelian disorders of collagens, elastins or mucopolysaccharides and presents a precis of normal biology of connective tissue and of clinical genetics as background. [The *SCI*® indicates that this book has been cited over 1085 times since 1961.]

Victor A. McKusick
The Johns Hopkins University
School of Medicine and
The Johns Hopkins Hospital
Baltimore, MD 21205

December 19, 1977

"The work on which this monograph was based began in 1950 when I saw a patient with the Marfan syndrome and severe aortic complications. I was then a resident. I became fascinated with the disorder, probably because it combined areas in which I had already worked: hereditary disorders (e.g., Peutz-Jeghers syndrome) and cardiology (e.g., electrokymography and constrictive pericarditis).

"When the book was published in June of 1956, the publisher produced, I am told, only 1,000 copies, on the advice that it would have limited interest, mainly to geneticists. What was not appreciated was that the wide distribution of connective tissue in the body is paralleled by a wide range of specialties that are concerned with these disorders. The first edition was sold out before the end of 1956!

"*Heritable disorders of connective tissue* has been almost as successful a title as Garrod's *Inborn errors of metabolism.* I selected 'heritable' as the adjective because it indicates that the disorders are capable of being transmitted genetically, although in the individual case the disorder (those that are dominant, at least) may have arisen by new mutation.

"Rheumatologists are wont to refer to some of the conditions they treat as connective tissue diseases, e.g., SLE, scleroderma, even rheumatoid arthritis. I like to chide them, saying that 'their' diseases are, yes, diseases *in* connective tissue, but not diseases *of* connective tissue; battle is fought in connective tissue and the connective tissue elements, as innocent bystanders, are injured, but 'mine' are the true diseases *of* connective tissue. Consequently, imagine my satisfied amusement when, in the list of references of an article published in the 1960s, I saw my monograph referred to as *Veritable disorders of connective tissue.* A one-letter change, although resulting in an inaccuracy, conveyed a profound truth.

"The monograph (which had subsequent editions in 1960, 1966, and 1972, with a 5th edition presently in the mill, probably for 1979 publication) grew with the field—and the field grew with the book.

"My research, presented in the monograph, can be labelled genetic nosology, which I define as the delineation of genetic diseases. I have been lucky in my colleagues in many branches of clinical medicine, in genetics, and in biochemistry. I was fortunate in working in a large general hospital that gave me access to patients in the pediatric, ophthalmologic, cardiologic, orthopedic, and other areas where patients with these protean diseases may first present. Bentley Glass, long Professor of Biology at Hopkins, encouraged and guided me in my self-education in general genetics.

"Collaborators with special expertise joined me in the study of these groups of patients: S. Harvey Mudd of the NIH (homocystinuria), David Kaplan of Downstate Medical Center (the specific mucopolysaccharidurias), Elizabeth F. Neufeld of the NIH (the metabolic and enzymatic characteristics of cells from patients with mucopolysaccharidoses) and George R. Martin of the NIH (biochemial abnormalities of collagen in the Ehlers-Danlos syndromes and osteogenesis imperfecta). Through the years I have also been helped in all this by a large group of the able junior associates. The nosology of these diseases illustrates the catalytic and mutually potentiating interaction between clinical, genetic, and biochemical study."

Chapter

8

Gastroenterology and Liver Disease

The 19 Citation Classics on the digestive system include two reviews and two pairs of TWCCs by the same authors. Gordon was the sole author of one Classic and contributed to another, whereas Davenport was the sole author of both of his Classics. One of the review articles was written in two parts (p. 262), so this, being a chapter of pairs, has been organized to emphasize gastrointestinal and liver disease.

Among the many curses of alcoholism is cirrhosis. Less well known among the lay public is the development of fatty livers and jaundice. Credit for discovering the triad of jaundice, hyperlipemia, and hemolytic anemia in alcoholic patients is given to Zieve, who implies that a question about "the so-called Zieve's syndrome" on the Board Examination in Internal Medicine may have established the popularity of his report. Unfortunately even Citation Classic status was insufficient to maintain Zieve's syndrome as a standard textbook term. Theoretically, this condition is easily treated since rapid improvement follows the withdrawal of alcohol. Alcohol oxidation in the liver by liver alcohol dehydrogenase generates NADH which then influences other enzyme systems. This "direct" NADH toxic effect of alcoholism as opposed to indirect effects of malnutrition was determined by examining the metabolism of alcohol by liver slices *in vitro*. To accomplish this Lieber had to travel through the streets of Boston from his laboratory to the only available scintillation counter at New England Nuclear. Another untoward effect of excess NADH is the inhibition of the conversion of galactose to glucose by the UDP galactose-4-epimerase. Discussions of this and other direct toxic effects of ethanol were described by Isselbacher and Greenberger in their review for the *New England Journal of Medicine.*

The tedious labor of examining 1,000 patients by scintillation scanning of the liver has been done not once but twice (p. 263). The application of technetium as the label has improved the sensitivity of this procedure, and the use of target-specific carriers for the isotope may enable even further improvements. In any event, the ponderous equipment once a hazard to patients has now been replaced. The purpose of these tracer studies was to define the configuration of the liver and to locate abnormalities.

Hans Popper serves as the spokesman for that group of hepatologists known as the "Gnomes of Zurich" because of their first meeting site. His "This Week's Citation Classic" (TWCC) is based on this group's since amended classification scheme for chronic hepatitis originally published in 1976.

Gallstone dissolution by dietary changes has been suggested on numerous occasions, and altering the composition of bile can induce it to carry more cholesterol. A dietary supplement of chenodeoxycholic acid thus aids the dissolution of gallstones that are largely cholesterol in nature. The detergent nature of this compound causes diarrhea, however (p. 265). The hectic pace by which the manuscript was produced in 48 hours attests to the writing skills of the authors. The small Chiba or Okuda needle minimized the hazard associated with the earlier use of larger needles for percutaneous cholangiography (p. 266).

Hypoproteinemia was a partially understood condition until studies in the late 1950s began to identify possible etiologies (other than hypercatabolism) and remove it from its grouping with other idiopathic conditions. Gordon demonstrated a genuine loss of protein from tissues into the lumen of the intestinal tract as a cause of hypoproteinemia. The appearance of ^{131}I polyvinyl pyrrolidone in the intestine tract after intravenous injection was an important confirmatory experiment. Waldmann and his co-workers, among them Gordon, showed that much of the protein loss was from the lymphatic system. In the condition they termed intestinal lymphangiectasia, the intestinal lymphatics become dilated or display a disordered channeling that permits the protein loss.

Chemical alteration of the gastric mucosa by aspirin leads to ulceration and thus to bleeding. Davenport's study of this came, as he mentions in his TWCC, as an afterthought to his work with eugenol. The mechanism for this is the passage of H^+ from the lumen into the tissue and the balanced diffusion of Na^+ from tissue into the lumen. Hydrogen protons are the source of the mucosal injury. These events in the small intestine can also be produced by detergents and urea, as described by Davenport in his second TWCC. Bile salts, because of their detergent property, are able to interrupt the integrity of cell membranes. Cells of the gastric mucosa are as sensitive to this as cells from other tissues. Because of this excess bile, the mucosal barrier is destroyed. This property of bile has been extensively reviewed (p. 271). Stress, of course, is considered an important cause of gastric ulcers and is also dependent upon H^+ diffusion (p. 272).

Lower bowel disease is represented by two TWCCs, the first demonstrating that colonic infarcts are an important cause of ischemic colitis. Marston's analysis of the original paper 17 years after its publication is what many scientists must feel—that the work was important even if some things were stated which could not be totally agreed upon today. Crohn's disease is the subject of the other TWCC, the message being that it is a clearly different illness than ulcerative colitis (p. 274).

Lactosuria is accompanied by a chronic diarrhea resulting from an osmotic imbalance in the intestinal tract and the flux of water into the bowel. Durand uses I^2 to indicate his agreement with others who believe that the absence of a lactose disaccharidase and transport system are the more common causes of the disease. Rarer forms include the delayed adult lactase deficiency syndrome and those secondary to other intestinal diseases. In a further paper on lactose malabsorption, the veterinary use of lactose as a laxative for domestic animals depends upon the disappearance of lactase from the gut of the young animal after nursing ceases (p. 276). Partial loss of human intestinal lactose as a basis for intestinal malabsorption is thus an interesting parallel. Malabsorption is also a component of celiac disease. The patient group examined by Rubin had profound abnormalities in the structure of the villi that enabled him to illustrate his paper in a convincing fashion. The author of the last TWCC states that an incident "following an evening of mild intemperance" was a key stimulant to his research endeavor on the aspiration of stomach acid into the lungs, an event that can be lethal.

Clinics in Gastroenterology and *Seminars in Liver Diseases* are the most visible sources of review articles related to the title of this chapter. Infrequent reviews appear in the *American Journal of Gastroenterology,* and summaries titled as progress articles are an occasional feature of *Gastroenterology.* Since major review journals are limited in this field, other review journals in medicine, physiology, allergy, etc., must be consulted.

The TWCCs in this chapter considered several important problems, among them alcoholic cirrhosis and fatty livers, erosion of the mucosal surface by bile and acid, lactosuria, malabsorption, and Crohn's disease. Several of these subjects have continued to capture the interest of gastroenterologists, as the listing that follows confirms.

Ackroyd F W & Hedberg S E. Colonic polyps. *Annu. Rev. Med.* **36:**619–25, 1985.

Baillie J & Soltis R D. Systemic complications of inflammatory bowel disease. *Geriatrics* **40:**53–60, 1984.

Dobbins W O III. Dysplasia and malignancy in inflammatory bowel disease. *Annu. Rev. Med.* **35:**33–48, 1984.

Ferguson A, Ziegler K & Strobel S. Gluten intolerance (coeliac disease). *Ann. Allergy* **53:**637–42, 1984.

Frank D. Alcohol-induced liver disease. *Alcoholism (NY)* **9:**66–82, 1985.

Hofmann A F & Roda A. Physiochemical properties of bile acids and their relationship to biological properties: an overview of the problem. *J. Lipid Res.* **25:**1477–89, 1984.

Lieber C S. Alcohol and the liver: 1984 update. *Hepatology* **4:**1243–60, 1984.

Malinkowska D H & Sachs G. Cellular mechanisms of acid secretion. *Clin. Gastroenterol.* **13:**309–26, 1984.

Marston A. Ischaemia. *Clin. Gastroenterol.* **14:**847–62, 1985.

Rossi E & Lentze M J. Clinical significance of enzymatic deficiencies in the gastrointestinal tract with particular reference to lactose deficiency. *Ann. Allergy* **53:**649–56, 1984.

Shorter R G. Intestinal cancer in Crohn's disease. *Bull. N.Y. Acad. Med.* **60:**980–6, 1984.

CC/NUMBER 39
SEPTEMBER 26, 1983

This Week's Citation Classic

Zieve L. Jaundice, hyperlipemia and hemolytic anemia: a heretofore unrecognized syndrome associated with alcoholic fatty liver and cirrhosis.
Ann. Intern. Med. **48**:471-96, 1958.
[Dept. Med. and Radioisotope Serv., Veterans Admin. Hosp., and Univ. Minnesota, Minneapolis, MN]

Twenty alcoholic patients were described with jaundice, hyperlipemia, and hemolytic anemia. The illness and chemical abnormalities improved rapidly once drinking stopped. Hemolysis was slight and short in duration. The liver biopsy showed fatty infiltration and minimal to moderate cirrhosis. [The *SCI*® indicates that this paper has been cited in over 260 publications since 1961.]

Leslie Zieve
Department of Medicine
Hennepin County Medical Center
University of Minnesota
Minneapolis, MN 55415

July 26, 1983

"As a resident in internal medicine I observed a few jaundiced alcoholic patients who were sent to surgery for obstructive jaundice, but were found to have fatty livers instead. These patients had hyperlipemia, usually only documented as an elevated blood cholesterol concentration. I looked carefully at the hospital records of a series of such patients with lipemia and noted a pattern of abnormalities not previously recognized. The jaundiced patients had lipemia or at least hypercholesterolemia and evidence of hemolysis. Both the lipemia and hemolysis were usually of short duration. On liver biopsy all of the patients had fatty infiltration and some had mild to moderate cirrhosis. None ever had severe cirrhosis. The occurrence of lipemia in alcoholics was fairly well known; however, the simultaneous occurrence of hemolysis had not previously been recognized. One of the confusing factors was the rapid improvement that occurred in these alcoholics once they stopped drinking upon becoming sick. The lipemia and the hemolysis improved spontaneously, often within a week, and only partial evidence of what had occurred remained. This did not fit into a known pattern, and the findings were usually ignored as the patient improved without treatment. The cases with persistence of elevated serum cholesterol and alkaline phosphatase for more than a week were suspected of having obstructive jaundice, and some were operated on for gallstone obstruction of the common bile duct, which wasn't found at surgery.

"To me, understanding that the coexistence of jaundice, hyperlipemia, and hemolysis in an alcoholic patient was an entity with a predictable rapid recovery rate was important because one could eliminate from consideration the possibilities of more serious and prolonged liver diseases, and one did not confuse these cases with those of extrahepatic common duct obstruction and thus avoided surgical exploration. I therefore assembled data on 20 patients and presented a paper at an American College of Physicians meeting.

"The response to my paper by hepatologists was one of indifference for about two years. However, I heard from residents in training and from recent graduates of specialty training programs who wanted to discuss similar cases. Four years after my paper, a report of six similar cases introduced the term 'Zieve's syndrome' and discussed my paper in great detail.[1] This seemed to generate some interest in the subject, and prompted somebody to ask a question on the American Board Examination in Internal Medicine about the entity. Widespread interest in this area developed promptly among trainees in internal medicine across the country. Case reports describing similar patients appeared in many parts of the world over the next decade. In 1966, I contrasted the two types of hemolysis occurring in liver diseases.[2] A few skeptics are unconvinced there is anything to the syndrome, and they speak of the 'so-called Zieve's syndrome.' Others have studied possible etiologic mechanisms and have added to our understanding of possible pathogenesis, though the final answer is not in.[3-5]

"This paper has been cited whenever the differential diagnosis of alcoholic liver disease or the occurrence of lipemia or hemolysis in liver disease is discussed."

1. **Kessel L.** Acute transient hyperlipemia due to hepatopancreatic damage in chronic alcoholics (Zieve's syndrome). *Amer. J. Med.* **32**:747-57, 1962.
[The *SCI* indicates that this paper has been cited in over 50 publications since 1962.]
2. **Zieve L.** Hemolytic anemia in liver disease. *Medicine* **45**:497-505, 1966.
3. **Balcerzak S P, Westerman M P & Heinle E W.** Mechanism of anemia in Zieve's syndrome. *Amer. J. Med. Sci.* **255**:277-87, 1968.
4. **Kunz F & Stummvoll L W.** The significance of plasma phospholipids in Zieve syndrome. *Blut* **21**:210-26, 1970.
5. **Goebel K M, Goebel F D, Schubotz R & Schneider J.** Hemolytic implications of alcoholism in liver disease. *J. Lab. Clin. Med.* **94**:123-32, 1979.

This Week's Citation Classic

Lieber C S & Schmid R. The effect of ethanol on fatty acid metabolism; stimulation of hepatic fatty acid synthesis *in vitro*. *J. Clin. Invest.* **40**:394-9, 1961. [Thorndike Mem. Lab. and Second and Fourth (Harvard) Med. Services, Boston City Hosp., and Dept. Med., Harvard Med. Sch., Boston, MA]

Liver slices incubated with ethanol had a significant increase in total fatty acids. The incorporation of acetate-C^{14} into fatty acids was stimulated and $C^{14}O_2$ production from palmitate-1-C^{14} depressed. Another NADH generating system reproduced this effect, while a hydrogen receptor reversed it. [The *SCI*® indicates that this paper has been cited over 210 times since 1961.]

Charles S. Lieber
Alcoholism Research and Treatment Center
VA Medical Center
Bronx, NY 10468
and
Mount Sinai Medical Center
New York, NY 10029

December 1, 1979

"This investigation was carried out at the Thorndike Memorial Laboratory of the Harvard Medical School, where I had joined Charlie Davidson in 1958 to study alcoholic liver disease. The accepted dogma at the time was that liver disease of the alcoholic was not due to alcohol itself, but merely to the malnutrition commonly associated with alcoholism, a view most clearly enunciated by the Nobel laureate Charles Best, who wrote in 1949 that 'there is no more evidence of a specific toxic effect of pure ethyl alcohol upon liver cells than there is for one due to sugar.'[1] However, since it was known that alcohol is oxidized almost exclusively in the liver, I was fascinated by the possibility that it might cause disease through some interference with liver metabolism. A direct way to test this hypothesis was to add alcohol to liver tissue *in vitro* to ascertain whether any change could be observed. Liver slices were therefore incubated in the presence of labeled substrates with or without ethanol. Rudi Schmid, who had joined the unit a year before, taught me the *in vitro* techniques. For tracing of the labels, a liquid scintillation counter was needed. The only instrument then available in Boston was located in the New England Nuclear plant. We rented it on a 'minute' basis; I regularly rushed through the snowy streets to count a few vials. The results were worth the effort: alcohol was found to exert striking effects on the metabolism of the liver, including promotion of lipogenesis and inhibition of lipid oxidation. Since oxidation of ethanol is associated with reduction of NAD to NADH, I hypothesized that the redox shift may be responsible. Indeed, effects of ethanol were mimicked by another NADH generating system (sorbitol) and prevented by a hydrogen acceptor (methylene blue).

"This paper is often quoted because it documented two new fundamental concepts: (1) Ethanol exerts direct effects on the liver which might play a role in the development of liver disease. (2) Some of these effects on the liver could be traced to the metabolism of ethanol. The hepatotoxicity was subsequently established *in vivo*: with the development of a new alcohol feeding technique as part of a nutritionally adequate, totally liquid diet, rats were shown to develop a fatty liver, the first stage of alcoholic liver disease, in the absence of dietary deficiencies. This was later confirmed in man.[2] Eventually, the final and irreversible stage of liver disease, namely cirrhosis, was produced in the baboon despite adequate diets.[3] The second key idea, namely the link between ethanol effects and its metabolism, led to the demonstration by us and others that alcoholic hyperuricemia, ketosis, hypoglycemia, and various other metabolic complications can be ultimately attributed to such a mechanism. Extension of this concept prompted studies concerning the hepatotoxicity of acetaldehyde. Further investigation of the metabolism of ethanol resulted in the discovery of an alternate pathway in the microsomes associated with activation and inactivation of drugs, hepatotoxic agents, carcinogens, and endogenous steroids."[4]

1. **Best C H, Hartroft W S, Lucas C C & Ridout J H.** Liver damage produced by feeding alcohol or sugar and its prevention by choline. *Brit. Med. J.* **2**:1001-6, 1949.
2. **Lieber C S, Jones D P & DeCarli L M.** Effect of prolonged ethanol intake: production of fatty liver despite adequate diets. *J. Clin. Invest.* **44**:1009-21, 1965.
3. **Lieber C S, DeCarli L M & Rubin E.** Sequential production of fatty liver, hepatitis and cirrhosis in sub-human primates fed ethanol with adequate diets. *Proc. Nat. Acad. Sci. US* **72**:437-41, 1975.
4. **Lieber C S.** Liver adaptation and injury in alcoholism. *N. Eng. J. Med.* **288**:356-62, 1973.

CC/NUMBER 23
JUNE 9, 1980

This Week's Citation Classic

Isselbacher K J & Greenberger N J. Metabolic effects of alcohol on the liver. *N. Engl. J. Med.* **270**:351-6, 402-10, 1964.
[Dept. Med., Harvard Med. Sch., and Med. Serv., Gastrointestinal Unit, Mass. Gen. Hosp., Boston, MA]

Alcohol has many effects on hepatic, carbohydrate, protein, and lipid metabolism. Many of the actions of alcohol on the liver cell are of a direct or toxic nature. Other effects are indirect and the result of changes in the redox state of the hepatocyte secondary to ethanol oxidation. Our knowledge of the metabolic actions of alcohol has provided insight into the mechanism of alcohol-induced hyperlipidemia, hyperuricemia, and hypoglycemia. [The *SCI*® indicates that these papers have been cited over 350 times since 1964.]

Kurt J. Isselbacher
Gastrointestinal Unit
Departments of Medicine
Massachusetts General Hospital and
Harvard Medical School
Boston, MA 02114

November 1, 1979

"My interest in alcohol and alcohol metabolism, which served as a basis of this article, had a somewhat unique origin. In 1955-56, while an investigator at the NIH and working in association with Herman Kalckar, we were fortunate to discover the mechanism of the genetic defect causing the hereditary disorder galactosemia.[1] The fundamental defect in galactosemia was shown to involve a deficiency in the enzyme, galactose-1-PO_4 uridyl transferase. In the course of studying the reactions involved in the normal interconversion of galactose to glucose, it became evident to us that in addition to uridyl transferase, there was also the step involving the isomerase reaction whereby UDP-galactose is converted to UDP-glucose. This isomerization is catalyzed enzymatically by UDP-galactose-4-epimerase, which requires and is stimulated by NAD but is inhibited by NADH.

"I was aware of numerous older clinical studies showing that alcohol ingestion results in impairment of galactose metabolism by the liver, an observation which in fact had served as the basis of the (now abandoned) galactose tolerance test to assess liver disease and alcohol-induced liver injury. Combining this observation with the then recently described reactions involving the uridine nucleotides in the metabolism of galactose and glucose, it seemed reasonable to postulate that alcohol might be interfering with hepatic galactose metabolism at one of these enzymatic steps. From my studies with Kalckar, I knew that the UDP-galactose-4-epimerase enzyme was extremely sensitive to inhibition by NADH. Since the oxidation of alcohol by the liver involved the reduction of NAD to NADH, it appeared to me therefore the most likely step to be inhibited by alcohol was the one involving the interconversion of UDP-galactose and UDP-glucose. I then was able to confirm this postulate[2] with my colleague, Stephen M. Krane (now well recognized for his work in collagen metabolism in rheumatoid arthritis) who at the time was measuring changes in NAD/NADH levels under various experimental conditions. It was thus shown by us, and amply confirmed later by others, that alcohol metabolism by the liver affects the redox level in the liver cell, and that the resultant increased NADH concentration inhibits the hepatic oxidation of alcohol at the epimerase step.

"Numerous alcohol-related studies followed. I temporarily abandoned further studies on galactosemia and examined the effects of alcohol on hepatic metabolism. These metabolic effects proved to be legion—the major ones involving interference in carbohydrate, protein (including lipoprotein), and lipid metabolism. It was our research in this area that led the then editor of the *New England Journal of Medicine* (Joseph Garland) to invite me to review this area for a broad medical audience. This resulted in this highly cited article which I prepared with one of my most able research fellows, Norton J. Greenberger, now chairman and professor of medicine at the University of Kansas Medical Center.

"Although from 1964 to the present my research has taken me to other areas (esp. studies of intestinal and malignant cell surface structure and function), I have attempted to continue my studies of alcohol metabolism. Our studies have resulted in further observations on the role and possible mechanism of alcohol in the inhibition of intestinal nutrient transport, interference with liver cell regeneration, and potentiation of hepatic viral injury. An update of our many investigations in this area led to the publication of a more recent review dealing with alcohol and its metabolic effects."[3]

1. **Isselbacher K J, Anderson E P, Kurshashi K & Kalckar H M.** *Science* **123**:635-6, 1957.
2. **Isselbacher K J & Krane S M.** *J. Biol. Chem.* **236**:2394-8, 1962.
3. **Isselbacher K J.** *N. Engl. J. Med.* **296**:612-6, 1977.

CC/NUMBER 35
AUGUST 27, 1984

This Week's Citation Classic™

McAfee J G, Ause R G & Wagner H N, Jr. Diagnostic value of scintillation scanning of the liver: follow-up of 1,000 studies.
Arch. Intern. Med. **116**:95-110, 1965.
[Depts. Radiology and Radiological Science, Johns Hopkins Schools of Medicine and Hygiene and Public Health, Baltimore, MD]

One thousand diagnostic studies of the liver were performed by rectilinear scintillation scanning using colloidal Au-198, or I-131 rose bengal, or colloidal albumin, and correlated with clinical, laboratory, and pathological findings. Normal variations in hepatic configuration, and scanning abnormalities in diffuse and focal hepatic lesions, were described. [The *SCI*® indicates that this paper has been cited in over 225 publications since 1965.]

John G. McAfee
Department of Radiology
Division of Radiological Sciences
State University of New York
Upstate Medical Center
Syracuse, NY 13210

July 6, 1984

"These studies were done because internists had trouble in differentiating focal hepatic lesions, such as metastases, from diffuse diseases, such as cirrhosis. The earlier studies were performed with a primitive rectilinear scanner jury-rigged from commercial and homemade parts put together by an engineer, James Mozley, in a small 12′ × 13′ room in the radiology department of Johns Hopkins Hospital. My associate, Henry Wagner, performed many of these studies alone at night, while he was chief resident in medicine. Only one near-catastrophe happened—one day, while scanning a patient, the scintillation detector came loose from its moorings with its 75-pound shield and fell, fortunately to the floor and not on the patient. Robert Ause, a resident in radiology at the time, painstakingly accumulated the clinical laboratory and pathological data on these patients.

"It is surprising that this paper has been highly cited. At that time, many other centers had similar equipment for rectilinear scanning, and the radioactive agents we used were not new. We had already published a paper on the same subject in the same journal four years previously,[1] and about 50 related papers had appeared since 1957. One equally large series of 1,000 hepatic scans had been reported previously.[2] Perhaps this paper appeared at the right time, when nuclear imaging by rectilinear scanning was just becoming popular, and when no other methods for hepatic imaging were available. We did show that rectilinear scanning usually could distinguish between focal and diffuse hepatic lesions. The paper documented many normal variations in hepatic configuration and size, and systematically analyzed the abnormalities encountered in congenital and acquired lesions. Prior to this paper, it was probably not appreciated that such a wide variety of lesions could produce focal photopenic defects in liver images, and that adjacent extrinsic masses could markedly deform this organ.

"The methods described in our paper are now totally obsolete. In the intervening years, the rectilinear scanner has become a historical relic, replaced by the more efficient Anger scintillation scanner. The older radioactive agents have been superseded by Tc-99m sulfur or microaggregated albumin colloids. Although these technical advances improved the spatial resolution of radionuclide images, the objective findings in various hepatic lesions have not changed markedly. Despite the advent of competing noninvasive modalities (ultrasonography, computed tomography, and magnetic resonance imaging), radionuclide imaging still has maintained a role in the investigation of liver disease.[3]

"Wagner has received numerous awards including the George von Hevesy Medal from the Gesellschaft für Nuklearmedizin, the Hevesy Nuclear Pioneer Award from the Society of Nuclear Medicine, and the Francis E. Schwentker Award of Johns Hopkins Hospital. I have received a Gold Medal Award and the Paul C. Aebersold Award from the Society of Nuclear Medicine and a Designated Scholar Award from the State University of New York. We both have received the Hermann L. Blumgart Award of the New England Chapter, Society of Nuclear Medicine. We suspect that these awards were not granted on the basis of this particular paper."

1. **Wagner H N, Jr., McAfee J G & Mozley J M.** Diagnosis of liver disease by radioisotope scanning. *Arch. Intern. Med.* 107:324-8, 1961. (Cited 95 times.)
2. **Nagler W, Bender M A & Blau M.** Radioisotope photoscanning of liver. *Gastroenterology* **44**:36-43, 1963. (Cited 140 times.)
3. **McAfee J G, Grossman Z D, Winstow B W, Bryan P J & Cohen W N.** Relative merits (computed tomography, ultrasonography and nuclear medicine in disease of the liver and biliary tract). (Margulis A R & Burhenne H J, eds.) *Alimentary tract radiology. Volume III. Abdominal imaging.* St. Louis: Mosby, 1979. p. 226-47.

This Week's Citation Classic

CC/NUMBER 11
MARCH 17, 1980

De Groote J, Desmet V J, Gedigk P, Korb G, Popper H, Poulsen H, Scheuer P J, Schmid M, Thaler H, Uehlinger E & Wepler W. A classification of chronic hepatitis. *Lancet* **2**:626-8, 1968.

Since 'chronic hepatitis' covers various conditions of differing clinical significance and pathologic appearance, chronic persistent hepatitis was histologically distinguished from chronic aggressive hepatitis and subdivided into moderate (A) and severe (B) varieties. [The *SCI*® indicates that this paper has been cited over 330 times since 1968.]

Hans Popper
Mount Sinai School of Medicine
City University of New York
New York, NY 10029

January 30, 1980

"Until the 1960s, 'chronic hepatitis' was an ill-defined term and the emphasis was on cirrhosis as chronic liver disease. Several factors increased interest in chronic hepatitis. The wide use of liver biopsy, facilitated by the new Menghini needle, revealed histologic features which could not be easily classified and correlated with clinical manifestations. Moreover, the spreading determinations of the transaminases detected milder chronic liver disease, associated often with clinical symptoms previously not related to the liver. The confusion in terminology and interpretation was even more disturbing if immunosuppressive therapy with its adverse side effects was to be instituted.

"To meet this challenge, a group consisting mostly of pathologists, but also some clinicians, constituted itself at a meeting of the European Association for the Study of the Liver in 1967. This group is often designated as the 'Gnomes of Zurich' because of the site of its first organized meeting. The small, loosely organized and, in a way, self-annointed fraternity has held yearly meetings ever since, in different cities, to discuss histologic slides circulated before and reviewed together. The group has only slightly been enlarged and the yearly meetings have created a bond of understanding and friendship. Besides problems of chronic hepatitis, others were discussed, and, when a consensus was reached, a statement was published.[1]

"The original distinction of chronic persistent from chronic aggressive hepatitis turned out to be the first step in a prognostic separation of forms of chronic hepatitis. Since chronic persistent hepatitis implied a nonprogressive disease, in contrast to the aggressive variety, only the latter appeared to be a candidate for immunosuppressive therapy. This nomenclature spread unexpectedly through the international medical community. Soon, several flaws in this simplistic terminology appeared and stimulated the search for better information.

"The original group published two modifying statements.[2,3] Since chronic hepatitis was subsequently defined as an hepatic disorder lasting longer than six months and, thus, encompassing prolonged manifestations of acute viral hepatitis, a third group, chronic lobular hepatitis, was introduced. Moreover, the histologic criteria for potential progression to cirrhosis were better defined and emphasis was placed on the etiology, when serum and tissue markers became available for forms of hepatitis. However, improvement of histologic identification correlated with the evolution of the disease is still required.

"The frequent citation of the original, now 12-year-old statement appears explained by the seminal value of a group consensus in introducing a first step in a therapeutic differential diagnosis. It indeed provided a stimulus (1) to establish the natural history of the various types of chronic hepatitis, (2) to study their pathogenesis, and (3) to confirm therapeutic indications in clinical trials, in part underway and in part accomplished."

1. **Bianchi L, De Groote J, Desmet V J, Gedigk P, Korb G, Popper H, Poulsen H, Scheuer P J, Schmid M, Thaler H & Wepler W.** Guidelines for diagnosis of therapeutic drug-induced liver injury in liver biopsies. *Lancet* **1**:854-7, 1974.
2. ---. Morphological criteria in viral hepatitis. *Lancet* **1**:333-7, 1971.
3. ---. Acute and chronic hepatitis revisited. *Lancet* **2**:914-9, 1977.

CC/NUMBER 29
JULY 19, 1982

This Week's Citation Classic

Danzinger R G, Hofmann A F, Schoenfield L J & Thistle J L. Dissolution of cholesterol gallstones by chenodeoxycholic acid. *N. Engl. J. Med.* **286**:1-8, 1972. [Gastroenterology Unit, Mayo Clinic and Mayo Foundation, Rochester, MN]

This paper demonstrated that the ingestion of a pure, naturally occurring human bile acid, chenodeoxycholic acid (CDC), produced gradual dissolution of radiolucent (cholesterol) gallstones in four of seven women. Dissolution took from six to 22 months with the only notable side effect of dose-related diarrhea. This work, therefore, opened a whole new vista for the management of a common human disease. [The *SCI®* indicates that this paper has been cited in over 355 publications since 1972. It more than fulfilled Ingelfinger's expectations.]

Rudy G. Danzinger
Department of Surgery
University of Manitoba
St. Boniface General Hospital
Winnipeg, Manitoba R2H 2A6
Canada

April 26, 1982

"In 1969, as the only Canadian and surgeon among a group of internationally recognized gastroenterologists, I learned that Les Schoenfield and John Thistle had demonstrated that the ingestion of pure chenodeoxycholic acid (CDC) (which Alan Hofmann had obtained in small quantity from Weddel Pharmaceuticals in England) by patients with gallstones greatly improved the solvent capacity of their bile for cholesterol. A fellow was required to see if such altered bile would induce dissolution of cholesterol gallstones. I leaped at the opportunity!

"Our initial problem was to obtain an adequate supply of encapsulated pure CDC. Then we proceeded to convince physicians in the Mayo Clinic to allow us to 'shanghai' patients who had come for surgical treatment of their gallstones. Simultaneously, we faced the problem of obtaining precise radiographs for accurate follow-up measurements of stone size, i.e., the gallbladder is mobile and its contained movable stones are seldom spheres. Complete dissolution presented a lesser problem, but that, too, had hazards since tiny stones could easily hide in the contrast material. Definitions were made and limitations for accepting change in size were reluctantly accepted.

"Nothing is ever new! Rewbridge had reported the disappearance of gallstones after the ingestion of bile salts in 1937,[1] but was unable to repeat his initial results with subsequent supplies. Although he had not analyzed his original batch of bile salts, we guessed that his initial supply must have been extremely rich in CDC.

"We presented our initial results to an NIH-sponsored symposium in Phoenix in October 1971, where Franz Ingelfinger, then editor of the *New England Journal of Medicine*, was present. Intrigued by our presentation, he proposed, over cocktails, that if he had the manuscript when he left in 48 hours, it might be the lead article for 1972. You can imagine our enthusiasm and resolve. We rented a typewriter, each of us took a segment, and we began to write furiously. Without figures and photographs (which we promised would follow within ten days), the manuscript was completed at 6:00 a.m., whereupon I hailed a taxi to the Phoenix airport where I placed it in Ingelfinger's hand just before his flight left for Boston. We made it!

"The best recent review is that of the NIH-supported National Cooperative Gallstone Study.[2] Perhaps 20 percent of all patients with gallstones could benefit from this form of therapy. Recurrence rate after dissolution has not been resolved. Stone recurrence could necessitate several episodes of therapy during a patient's life or continued small daily doses after dissolution. CDC and its 7-beta, hydroxy epimer—ursodeoxycholic acid—are available for routine therapy in Japan and many European countries. We are presently attempting to supply knowledge gained from these compounds to manipulate bile composition more efficiently and to prepare more potent pharmaceutical agents."

1. **Rewbridge A G.** The disappearance of gallstone shadows following the prolonged administration of bile salts. *Surgery* 1:395-400, 1937.
2. **Schoenfield L J, Lachin J M, the Steering Committee (Baum R A, Habig R L, Hanson R F, Hersh T, Hightower N C, Jr., Hofmann A F, Lasser E C, Marks J W, Mekhjian H, Okun R, Schaefer R A, Shaw L, Soloway R D, Thistle J L, Thomas F B, Tyor M P) & the National Cooperative Gallstone Study Group.** Chenodiol (chenodeoxycholic acid) for dissolution of gallstones: the National Cooperative Gallstone Study. *Ann. Intern. Med.* **95**:257-82, 1981.

CC/NUMBER 29
JULY 18, 1983

This Week's Citation Classic

Okuda K, Tanikawa K, Emura T, Kuratomi S, Jinnouchi S, Urabe K, Sumikoshi T, Kanda Y, Fukuyama Y, Musha H, Mori H, Shimokawa Y, Yakushiji F & Matsuura Y. Nonsurgical, percutaneous transhepatic cholangiography—diagnostic significance in medical problems of the liver. *Amer. J. Digest. Dis. New Ser.* **19**:21-36, 1974.

[1st Dept. Med. and Dept. Radiol., Chiba Univ. Sch. Med.; 2nd Dept. Med., Kurume Univ. Sch. Med.; Med. Serv., Kimitsu Gen. Hosp.; and Med. Serv., Yame Public Hosp., Japan]

Percutaneous transhepatic cholangiography was carried out from the right flank on 314 patients using a very thin needle. Intrahepatic bile ducts were visualized in 67.5 percent of those who had no to minimal dilation. Practically no complication was encountered in patients with medical problems of the liver. [The *SCI*® indicates that this paper has been cited in over 285 publications since 1974.]

Kunio Okuda
First Department of Medicine
Chiba University School of Medicine
Chiba 280
Japan

May 20, 1983

"Percutaneous transhepatic cholangiography had been carried out for the diagnosis of obstructive jaundice by surgeons who could immediately open the abdomen of the patient for control of bile leak which was inevitable because of the size of the needle used.[1,2] In those days, direct cholangiography could not be thought of as a medical procedure. One group of surgeons at Chiba University Hospital began puncturing intrahepatic bile ducts around 1966.[3] Various factors determined success or failure in entering intrahepatic bile ducts for diagnostic cholangiograms. Our group at the first department of medicine at the same hospital improved their technique further by selecting the midaxillary line for entry and applying a positive pressure on the syringe containing contrast medium instead of suctioning bile in search of an intrahepatic bile duct.[4] The needle should be as thin as possible without losing its aiming capability. These simple ideas proved very successful, and changed percutaneous cholangiography to a nonsurgical technique. With the help of my previous students at affiliated hospitals, I could gather data on more than 300 patients within a short period of time. Although this technique had already spread throughout Japan at the time I wrote the paper, I thought that the technique was worth describing in an English-language journal. While preparing the manuscript, I felt that the thin needle with our specification should be called the 'Chiba needle' because a number of people at Chiba University Hospital had been involved in its development.

"The reaction was overwhelming and requests poured in for sample needles. I sent out several hundred needles, two for each request. Within a year or two, reports began appearing at various meetings throughout the world, some of them calling the needle 'Okuda's needle.' Reprint requests also poured in. I understand that the needles are now available in a disposable form in the US. Reynolds and his group at Los Angeles used the same needle for measuring intrahepatic portal vein pressure.[5] Since this technique was so widely used in the US, with some people starting without experience and with a loose selection of patients, complications became frequent. Mary Jean Kreek had to conduct a national survey on the frequency of complications. In due time, endoscopic cholangiography became popular, and the percutaneous approach has yielded considerably to the former in the indication and selection of patients.

"The reason for this paper being cited very often is that many radiologists and gastroenterologists began using this needle and technique, and reported their experiences in the past eight years or so. They had to quote our paper in their publications, and many of them acknowledged my supply of the needles to them.

"Perhaps because of this paper, I became known in gastroenterology and hepatology throughout the world. I was sometimes compared to Menghini, from Italy, who invented a one-second biopsy needle.[6] It may have contributed indirectly to my current position as vice president of the Organisation Mondiale de Gastro-Enterologie (OMGE), and my past presidency of the International Association for the Study of the Liver (IASL)."

1. **Nurick A W, Patey D H & Whiteside D G.** Percutaneous transhepatic cholangiography in the diagnosis of obstructive jaundice. *Brit. J. Surg.* **41**:27-30, 1953.
2. **Kidd H A.** Percutaneous transhepatic cholangiography. *Arch. Surg.* **72**:262-8, 1956.
3. **Ueno K.** Systematic investigation of puncture for percutaneous cholecystocholangiography. *Jpn. J. Gastroenterol.* **63**:520-37, 1966. (In Japanese.)
4. **Okuda K.** Thin needle percutaneous transhepatic cholangiography—historical review. (Editorial.) *Endoscopy* **12**:2-7, 1980.
5. **Boyer T D, Triger D R, Horisawa M, Redeker A G & Reynolds T B.** Direct transhepatic measurement of portal vein pressure using a thin needle. Comparison with wedged hepatic vein pressure. *Gastroenterology* **72**:584-9, 1977.
6. **Menghini G.** One-second biopsy of the liver—problems of its clinical application. *N. Engl. J. Med.* **283**:582-5, 1970.

CC/NUMBER 13
MARCH 30, 1981

This Week's Citation Classic

Gordon R S, Jr. Exudative enteropathy: abnormal permeability of the gastrointestinal tract demonstrable with labelled polyvinylpyrrolidone. *Lancet* **1**:325-6, 1959.
[Lab. Cellular Physiology and Metabolism, National Heart Institute, US Public Health Service, Bethesda, MD]

PVP labeled with ^{131}I was shown to be a practical diagnostic test for the recognition of hypoproteinemia due to loss into the digestive tract. [The *SCI*® indicates that this paper has been cited over 280 times since 1961.]

Robert S. Gordon, Jr.
Office of the Director
National Institutes of Health
Bethesda, MD 20205

February 13, 1981

"This investigation exemplifies the virtues of serendipity, and the merits of having a large and varied scientific and clinical research endeavor under one roof at the National Institutes of Health. F. Bartter admitted a patient with 'hypercatabolic hypoproteinemia' for studies of nitrogen balance. I saw her with the intention of measuring her levels of free fatty acids (my research interest at that time), and guessed that her 'hypercatabolism' might really be due to loss of plasma proteins into the gut, followed by digestion and absorption of amino acids. With the help of J. Davidson (who was set up for duodenal intubations) and E. Middleton (who had prepared rabbit antiserum to human albumin for a study of chylomicrons), I tested her duodenal juice for albumin and got a strongly positive result. This observation was the beginning of a collaborative effort to study conditions associated with gastrointestinal protein loss.

"It was not difficult to postulate that an injectable, recognizable, nonbiodegradable macromolecule such as radioactive PVP would be a good diagnostic agent. It was difficult to make one; in fact, the commercial manufacturer of PVP said it could not be done. It could be, but only with the continued help of another colleague, H. Fales, a knowledgeable and well-equipped organic chemist. After almost a year, I was ready to test the same patient, whose continued participation was also essential to the project, with ^{131}I-PVP. It worked. Whereas normals excreted only traces of an injected dose in their stools, hers were highly radioactive.

"I then began preparing labeled PVP on a regular monthly schedule. The assistance of W. Briner, pharmacist, was invaluable in sterilizing, safety-testing, and calibrating the product. With his facilities, we could scale up the monthly production, and offer experimental quantities of the material to investigators all over the world who had reported patients who appeared to have a similar condition. Wide distribution of the diagnostic agent led to other studies which showed how many diseases could result in the same pathophysiology.[1] This is the main reason for the frequent citation of my initial small study. I believe that the paper is also cited because of my mention of our use of disposable paint cans for collecting and handling feces for laboratory examination, avoiding most of the unpleasantness of transferring, homogenizing, and disposing of samples.

"^{131}I-PVP has since been supplanted by other diagnostic agents, usually human albumin labeled with ^{51}Cr. The condition has come to be known as protein-losing gastroenteropathy, and knowledge of its many etiologies is still expanding. It was all initiated by a chance observation on an unusual patient in an unusually diversified research environment—a study which could never have been planned.

"Recently, T.A. Waldmann prepared a chapter on this subject in the book *Gastroenterology*."[2]

1. **Waldmann T A, Steinfeld J L, Dutcher T F, Davidson J D & Gordon R S, Jr.** The role of the gastrointestinal system in "idiopathic hypoproteinemia." *Gastroenterology* **41**:197-207, 1961. [Citation Classic. *Current Contents/Clinical Practice* (15):16, 14 April 1980.]
2. **Waldmann T A.** Protein-losing enteropathies. (Bockus H L, ed.) *Gastroenterology*. Philadelphia: W.B. Saunders, 1975. Vol. II. p. 361-85.

Waldmann T A, Steinfeld J L, Dutcher T F, Davidson, J D & Gordon R S, Jr. The role of the gastrointestinal system in "idiopathic hypoproteinemia." *Gastroenterology* **41**:197-207, 1961. (Metab. Serv. and Pathological Anat. Br., Nat. Cancer Inst., and Lab. Cell. Physiol. and Metab., Nat. Heart Inst., Bethesda, MD)

A new syndrome we termed 'intestinal lymphangiectasia' was described in patients previously diagnosed as 'idiopathic hypoproteinemia.' Intestinal lymphangiectasia is characterized by a generalized disorder of lymphatic channels including dilated small intestinal lymphatics that leads to excessive gastrointestinal protein loss and to hypoproteinemia and edema. [The *SCI*® indicates that this paper has been cited over 215 times since 1961.]

Thomas A. Waldmann
Metabolism Branch
National Cancer Institute
National Institutes of Health
Bethesda, MD 20205

February 22, 1980

"Shortly after the NIH Clinical Center opened, investigators from different institutes joined in a study of patients with 'idiopathic hypoproteinemia.' Frederic Bartter followed the fate of IV human albumin in these patients by metabolic balance techniques and found several cases with increased catabolism. Jesse Steinfeld using radioiodinated proteins then showed that hypoproteinemia in many patients was due to shortened protein survival rather than decreased synthesis.[1] Citrin at SUNY Upstate Medical Center using IV ^{131}I-albumin demonstrated loss of albumin into the gastric secretions in a patient with Menetrier's disease.[2] However, no practical test for protein loss was available until Robert S. Gordon, Jr.'s development of radioiodinated polyvinylpyrolidone (PVP),[3] a macromolecule that is unaffected by mammalian enzymes and is not absorbed from the intestine. The hypoproteinemic patients excreted excessive quantities of IV PVP into their feces demonstrating that their hypoproteinemia was due to excessive gastrointestinal loss. We then joined in a study of 18 patients to define the cause of the protein losing enteropathy demonstrated in patients who did not have a previously described gastrointestinal disease.

"Three new syndromes defined in these patients formed the basis for the cited publication. One patient had transient protein loss, two protein loss secondary to constrictive pericarditis, and 15 a previously undescribed disease we termed 'intestinal lymphangiectasia.' A generalized disorder of lymphatic channel development was suggested by chylous effusions and asymmetrical edema observed in many of these patients. The suspected disorders of small intestinal lymphatics were demonstrated on peroral biopsies. The disorder of intestinal lymphatics leads to excessive protein loss, hypoproteinemia, edema, and chylous effusions.

"This description of a new syndrome and pathophysiologic mechanism led to the numerous citations and to the reproduction of this paper in the silver anniversary issue of *Gastroenterology*.[4] We subsequently developed new macromolecules, including ^{51}Cr albumin, to quantitate gastrointestinal protein loss.[5] In addition, we demonstrated a new immunodeficiency state characterized by hypogammaglobulinemia, lymphocytopenia, skin anergy, and impaired homograft rejection in patients with intestinal lymphangiectasia.[6] These defects were due to excessive gastrointestinal loss of immunoglobulins and lymphocytes through the disordered lymphatic channels.

"Thus, studies of patients with the ill defined disorder 'idiopathic hypoproteinemia' led to the discovery of a new common cause of hypoproteinemia, protein losing enteropathy, to the identification of a new disease, intestinal lymphangiectasia, and to the definition of an associated immunodeficiency with a previously unrecognized pathogenic mechanism leading to disordered immunity."

1. **Bartter F C, Steinfeld J L, Waldmann T A & Delea C S.** Metabolism of infused serum albumin in hypoproteinemia of gastrointestinal protein loss and in analbuminemia. *Trans. Assoc. Amer. Phys.* **44**:180-94, 1961.
2. **Citrin Y, Sterling K & Halsted J A.** Mechanisms of hypoproteinemia associated with giant hypertrophy of gastric mucosa. *N. Eng. J. Med.* **257**:906-12, 1957.
3. **Gordon R S, Jr.** Exudative enteropathy: abnormal permeability of the gastrointestinal tract demonstrable with labelled polyvinylpyrolidone. *Lancet* **1**:325-6, 1959.
4. **Waldmann T A, Steinfeld J L, Dutcher T F, Davidson J D & Gordon R S, Jr.** The role of the gastrointestinal system in "idiopathic hypoproteinemia." *Gastroenterology* **54**:794-6, 1968.
5. **Waldmann T A.** Gastrointestinal protein loss demonstrated by ^{51}Cr-labelled albumin. *Lancet* **2**:121-3, 1961.
6. **Strober W, Wochner R D, Carbone P P & Waldmann T A.** Intestinal lymphangiectasia: a protein losing enteropathy with hypogammaglobulinemia, lymphocytopenia and impaired homograft rejection. *J. Clin. Invest.* **46**:1643-56, 1967.

CC/NUMBER 7
FEBRUARY 16, 1981

This Week's Citation Classic

Davenport H W. Gastric mucosal injury by fatty and acetylsalicylic acids. *Gastroenterology* **46**:245-53, 1964.
[Section of Physiology, Mayo Clinic and Mayo Foundation, Rochester, MN]

This paper demonstrated that short chain fatty acids and acetylsalicylic acid (aspirin) break the gastric mucosal barrier when they diffuse into the gastric mucosa in fat soluble form. Once the barrier is broken, H^+ in the lumen diffuses into the mucosa, and Na^+ in mucosal interstitial fluid diffuses into the lumen. The consequences of back-diffusion of H^+ into the mucosa include cell destruction, copious output of fluid into the lumen, shedding of plasma proteins, and frank bleeding. These consequences can be prevented or ameliorated by neutralizing the contents of the stomach. [The *SCI*® indicates that this paper has been cited over 275 times since 1964.]

Horace W. Davenport
Department of Physiology
University of Michigan
Ann Arbor, MI 48109

January 27, 1981

"That this paper should be frequently cited is something of a joke. In 1962, being exhausted by my duties at the University of Michigan and at a dead end in my research, I went on sabbatical leave to the section of physiology at the Mayo Clinic to work under Charles F. Code. I told Code to treat me like a postdoctoral fellow, and he assigned me the problem of explaining why the gastric mucosa, previously irrigated with eugenol, secretes fluid low in H^+ and high in Na^+. I proposed that eugenol breaks the gastric mucosal barrier, allowing secreted H^+ to disappear by back diffusion and Na^+ to leak into the lumen. Code and I demonstrated that my proposal was correct, and he wrote up the results in what turned out to be, if I may be truthful as well as immodest, a classic paper.[1]

"In the few weeks remaining to me at the Clinic, I tackled the obvious problems: What is the nature of the gastric mucosal barrier, and what happens when it is broken? I studied the effects of fatty acids and their salts for the reason that I knew the barrier must behave like a lipid membrane. Halfway through that work it dawned on me that aspirin should behave the same way.[2] I thought of aspirin for three reasons. 1. At that time the clinical world was having one of its recurrent spasms about gastric bleeding induced by aspirin, but there were no sensible explanations of the reason. 2. My wife had been junior author of a notorious paper[3] demonstrating gastric damage induced by massive parenteral doses of aspirin. 3. Any scientifically sound work on the gastric effects of aspirin would be sure to stir up the animals. I did the work very quickly and wrote up the paper immediately upon my return to Michigan. It was published before the much more important paper,[1] for the reason that it took some time for Code to write the better one and to see it through the Clinic's section of publications.

"As the *Science Citation Index*® shows, the aspirin paper did stir up the animals. The work started at the Mayo Clinic occupied me for 16 years and has resulted in a substantial body of new knowledge, provided by many others as well as by myself. That knowledge has, as Morton Grossman predicted, revolutionized the physiology of the stomach, and it has made a considerable contribution to patient care. I am pleased to have participated in that revolution, and I am equally pleased that my work has earned me the William Beaumont Professorship, election to the National Academy of Sciences, and the American Gastroenterological Association's Friedenwald Medal."

1. **Davenport H W, Warner H A & Code C F.** Functional significance of gastric mucosal barrier to sodium. *Gastroenterology* **47**:142-52, 1964.
[The *SCI*® indicates that this paper has been cited over 180 times since 1964.]
2. **Hogben C A M, Schanker L S, Tocco D J & Brodie B B.** Absorption of drugs from the stomach. II. The human. *J. Pharmacol. Exp. Ther.* **120**:540-5, 1957.
3. **Barbour H G & Dickerson V C.** Gastric ulceration produced in rats by oral and subcutaneous aspirin. *Arch. Int. Pharmacodyn. Ther.* **58**:78-87, 1938.

CC/NUMBER 14
APRIL 4, 1983

This Week's Citation Classic

Davenport H W. Destruction of the gastric mucosal barrier by detergents and urea. *Gastroenterology* **54**:175-81, 1968.
[Department of Physiology, University of Michigan, Ann Arbor, MI]

This paper demonstrates that bile salts (10, 20, and 40 mM in neutral solution, 40 mM in a liquid meal, and 10 mM in acid solution), decyl sulfate (10 or 20 mM in neutral solution), and urea (1, 2, and 4 M in neutral solution) all break the dog's gastric mucosal barrier and permit back-diffusion of acid into the mucosa. [The *SCI*® indicates that this paper has been cited in over 335 publications since 1968.]

Horace W. Davenport
Department of Physiology
University of Michigan
Ann Arbor, MI 48109

January 20, 1983

"This is my second paper to achieve the notoriety of becoming a *Citation Classic*. The first was on aspirin damage to the gastric mucosa,[1] and when I wrote it I knew that anything making sense about aspirin in the stomach was sure to stir up the animals. This second paper contained a beast-goad in the form of bile salts I did not recognize at the time.

"The gastric mucosal barrier is the property of the stomach that allows it to contain the acid it secretes. If the barrier is broken, as by aspirin in acid solution, acid diffuses back into the mucosa, causing all sorts of damage extending to fatal exsanguinating hemorrhage.[2] For many years after I had shown that aspirin in acid solution breaks the barrier, I tried to discover the nature of the barrier by some simpleminded experiments in which I attempted to reinforce it or to destroy it. I never published the reinforcing experiments, for they accomplished nothing. To partition the barrier I used urea just as I used acetylcysteine later.[3] Lipids of the cell membrane must be part of the barrier, and I dispersed the lipids with some decyl sulfate given me by the DuPont Company years before. Both broke the barrier.

"Eventually it dawned on me that bile had been acting at oil-water interfaces long before DuPont synthesized decyl sulfate. I got bile from dogs in the student laboratory, and I demonstrated that it broke the barrier and permitted back-diffusion of acid. At the time, I was totally ignorant of the clinical supposition that regurgitated bile is a cause of gastric ulceration, and I did the experiments solely in pursuit of information about the structure of the barrier. I knew I should repeat the experiments with a pure conjugated bile salt. In those days, bile salts were just becoming fashionable, and the conjugated ones were not in supply-house catalogs. I asked Alan Hofmann for advice, and he told me about a magician-chemist who was conjugating bile acids in King Mark's court in Cornwall. I got 100 grams of sodium taurocholate from Tintagel. After I had established that a pure bile salt behaves like bile in breaking the barrier, I knew there were many more experiments to be done. I should run up and down the pH and concentration scales and so on. However, I thought: 'I have done enough. Let some clinician do the rest.'

"It seems that I had done enough. Clinicians immediately took up the problem of the significance of bile regurgitation in breaking the barrier, permitting acid back-diffusion and causing gastric hemorrhage. Until they had papers of their own to cite, they liberally cited mine."

1. **Davenport H W.** Gastric mucosal injury by fatty and acetylsalicylic acids. *Gastroenterology* **46**:245-53, 1964. [Citation Classic. *Current Contents/Clinical Practice* **9**(7):16, 16 February 1981.]
2. --------------------. The gastric mucosal barrier; past, present, and future. *Proc. Mayo Clin.* **50**:507-14, 1975.
3. --------------------. Protein-losing gastropathy produced by sulfhydryl reagents. *Gastroenterology* **60**:870-9, 1971.

This Week's Citation Classic

CC/NUMBER 35
SEPTEMBER 1, 1980

Hofmann A F & Small D M. Detergent properties of bile salts: correlation with physiological function. *Annu. Rev. Med.* **18**:333-76, 1967.
[Gastroenterol. Unit, Mayo Clinic and Foundation, Rochester, MN; and Dept. Med., Boston Univ. Sch. Med., Boston, MA]

This interpretative review summarized the behavior of amphipathic molecules in water and then considered the physical chemistry of bile acid solutions and the behavior of physiologically relevant additives. It discussed the composition of bile, gallstone formation, and fat digestion in physicochemical terms. [The *SCI*® indicates that this paper has been cited over 280 times since 1967.]

A.F. Hofmann
Division of Gastroenterology
Department of Medicine
University of California
San Diego, CA 92103

June 24, 1980

"This review was a labor of love written by Donald Small, who is now director of the division of biophysics in the department of medicine at Boston University, and myself, when I was a member of the department of medicine of the Mayo Clinic.

"The review had two aims. The first was to describe the detergent properties of bile acids using the language and principles of colloid chemistry. The second was to correlate the distinctive detergent properties with their physiological role of lipid transport, in particular, the transport of cholesterol in bile and of triglyceride digestion products in the intestinal lumen. The review has been popular, I think, because it was among the first discussions of micelle formation in the medical literature and because it attempted to relate human physiology and disease to colloid chemistry.

"Both Small and I had been trained in internal medicine. I had spent three years in the department of physiological chemistry at the University of Lund, Sweden, working with Bengt Borgström. Here I had shown that bile acids readily solubilize fatty acids and monoglycerides to form mixed micelles and then had isolated a micellar phase by ultracentrifugation of intestinal content obtained during the digestion of a meal in man. Small had worked at the Institut Pasteur in Paris with the great biophysicist, Dervichian, defining the phase equilibria of simulated bile, as well as the surface properties of bile acids.

"There are some novel ideas in the review. We reversed the McBain phase diagram for the soap-water system, putting the aqueous side on the left; we drew structures of molecular organization of the mesomorphic phases; and we proposed the term 'critical micellar temperature' to replace the older term 'Krafft point.' We used the term 'swelling amphipath' and stressed the importance of transition temperatures for liquid crystalline states.

"Since then I have continued as a clinical investigator, studying the metabolism of bile acids in health and disease; more recently, I have worked on the medical dissolution of cholesterol gallstones with certain bile acids. Small has focused on the structure and function of lipoproteins and has become a world authority on cholesterol metabolism. Interest in bile acids has expanded enormously (even though they are not yet an ASCA® topic). Small and I have each received the Distinguished Achievement Award of the American Gastroenterological Association, and we shared (together with Jan Sjövall) the Eppinger Prize.

"We like to think that our review helped to make certain biological processes comprehensible to colloid chemists and showed that understanding of simple concepts of colloid chemistry aids in understanding the pathogenesis of digestive disease. The physical chemistry of bile acids as it relates to bile and gallstone formation has subsequently been characterized in greater detail,[1] and micelles and liquid crystalline phases have moved from the detergent literature into the exploding areas of membranology.[2,3] Finally, research on the biological effects of bile acids has also expanded greatly; bile acid researchers gather biennially for an international conference sponsored by the Falk Foundation."[4]

1. **Carey M C & Small D M.** The physical chemistry of cholesterol solubility in bile. Relationship to gallstone formation and dissolution in man. *J. Clin. Invest.* **61**:998-1026, 1978.
2. **Hellenius A & Simons K.** Solubilization of membranes by detergents. *Biochem. Biophys. Acta* **415**:29-79, 1975.
3. **Mazer N A, Carey M C & Benedek G B.** Quasielastic light scattering studies of aqueous bilary lipid systems. Mixed micelle formation in bile salt-lecithin solutions. *Biochemistry* **19**:601-15, 1980.
4. **Paumgartner G, Stiehl A & Gerok W,** eds. *Biological effects of bile acids. Proceedings of the 26th Falk Symposium, 5th Bile Acid Meeting, Freiburg im Breisgau, West Germany, June, 1978.* Lancaster, UK: MTP Press, 1979. 318 p.

This Week's Citation Classic™

CC/NUMBER 20
MAY 14, 1984

Skillman J J, Gould S A, Chung R S K & Silen W. The gastric mucosal barrier: clinical and experimental studies in critically ill and normal man, and in the rabbit. *Ann. Surg.* **172**:564-84, 1970.

[Department of Surgery, Harvard Medical School and Beth Israel Hospital, Boston, MA]

Permeability of the gastric mucosa to instilled hydrochloric acid and acid secretion was studied in 26 seriously ill patients, in normal human subjects, and in rabbits. Half of the seriously ill patients (in whom use of steroids, hypotension, renal failure, jaundice, and a lethal outcome was more common) had strikingly increased back-diffusion of H^+ ions in comparison to the less seriously ill patients and to normal subjects. The rabbit experiments showed that a short period of hemorrhagic shock also had a disruptive effect on the gastric mucosal barrier to H^+. The data suggested that disruption of the stomach's normal functional barrier to secreted acid might be a clue to the pathogenesis of acute stress ulceration. [The *SCI*® indicates that this paper has been cited in over 155 publications since 1970.]

John J. Skillman
Department of Surgery
Beth Israel Hospital
Harvard Medical School
Boston, MA 02215

February 10, 1984

"Our work on the gastric mucosal barrier was stimulated by the experiments of the eminent physiologist from Michigan, Horace Davenport, whose work on this subject, which was started in 1962 at the Mayo Clinic during a sabbatical year with Charles Code,[1] revived an even older concept of the regulation of the acidity in the stomach proposed by the Swedish medical chemist Torsten Teorell. Teorell proposed, in 1939, that there was a continuous diffusion of hydrochloric acid from the gastric lumen into mucosa, which he called 'back-diffusion,' and a simultaneous diffusion of sodium chloride from mucosa to lumen that accounted for the reduction in acidity in the stomach.[2] Based on his experiments with agents which produced damage to the gastric mucosa,[3,4] Davenport suggested the possibility in 1965 that the apparent low rates of acid secretion in patients with chronic gastric ulcer disease might be caused by increased back-diffusion of acid across a damaged mucosa.[5]

"In 1969, we found that eight of the first 150 patients admitted to our newly opened respiratory-surgical intensive care unit had massive hemorrhage from acute, multiple, gastric ulcers, almost all of which were located in the fundus of the stomach.[6] Seven of these eight patients died. The presence of respiratory failure, hypotension, sepsis, jaundice, and renal failure suggested a clinical syndrome which set the stage for the development of acute stress ulceration.

"Investigations in our seriously ill patients were stimulated by the unsolved clinical problem (stress ulceration) and the concepts on the damage to the gastric mucosa suggested by Davenport's timely work. Our own study showed that the gastric mucosa of seriously ill patients (especially those with multiple complications) had strikingly abnormal permeability to instilled acid. The status of the gastric mucosal integrity could not be predicted from standard tests of gastric secretion (basal acid output and augmented histamine tests). We suggested that abnormal permeability of the stomach to acid in the presence of poor mucosal perfusion might be related to the subsequent development of acute gastric ulceration and hemorrhage. Subsequent experiments in animals by Kivilaakso, working in William Silen's laboratory, showed that impairment of buffering capacity in the gastric mucosa, rather than tissue anoxia, is the key factor leading to ulceration during hemorrhagic shock.[7]

"There may be two reasons why this paper has been cited frequently. First, it was one of the first human studies of the barrier function of the stomach in critically ill patients. The work attempted to dissect a clinical problem in intensive care units which was often fatal and which was occurring with an alarming frequency. Second, the paper provided a rational basis for a regimen of prevention of stress ulceration with antacid based on the experiments of hemorrhagic hypotension in rabbits. The experiments in rabbits, which were conducted by Raphael Chung in Silen's laboratory, showed that buffering of gastric acid with sodium lactate significantly reduced the amount of back-diffusion of acid and prevented gastric ulceration.

"Titration of gastric juice to a pH > 3.5 by the hourly instillation of antacid in seriously ill patients has become the mainstay of stress ulceration prophylaxis in most intensive care units.[8] This regimen has eliminated almost completely the clinical problem of acute stress ulceration of the stomach. A recent review of stress ulceration can be found in an entire issue of the *World Journal of Surgery*."[9]

1. **Davenport H W, Warner H A & Code C F.** Functional significance of gastric mucosal barrier to sodium. *Gastroenterology* **47**:142-52, 1964. (Cited 220 times.)
2. **Teorell T.** On the permeability of the stomach mucosa for acids and some other substances. *J. Gen. Physiol.* **23**:263-74, 1939. (Cited 90 times since 1955.)
3. **Davenport H W.** Gastric mucosal injury by fatty and acetylsalicylic acids. *Gastroenterology* **46**:245-53, 1964.
4. --------------------. Citation Classic. Commentary on *Gastroenterology* **46**:245-53, 1964. *Current Contents/Clinical Practice* **9**(7):16, 16 February 1981.
5. --------------------. Is the apparent hyposecretion of acid by patients with gastric ulcer a consequence of a broken barrier to diffusion of hydrogen ions into the gastric mucosa. *Gut* **6**:513, 1965. (Cited 90 times.)
6. **Skillman J J, Bushnell L S, Goldman H & Silen W.** Respiratory failure, hypotension, sepsis and jaundice—a clinical syndrome associated with lethal hemorrhage from acute stress ulceration of the stomach. *Amer. J. Surg.* **117**:523-30, 1969. (Cited 95 times.)
7. **Kivilaakso E & Silen W.** Pathogenesis of experimental gastric-mucosal injury. *N. Engl. J. Med.* **30**:364-9, 1979.
8. **Priebe H J & Skillman J J.** Methods of prophylaxis in stress ulcer disease. *World J. Surgery* **5**:223-33, 1981.
9. **Ritchie W P, Jr.**, ed. Stress ulcer and erosive gastritis. (Whole issue.) *World J. Surgery* **5**(2), 1981. 162 p.

CC/NUMBER 44
OCTOBER 31, 1983

This Week's Citation Classic

Marston A, Pheils M T, Thomas M L & Morson B C. Ischaemic colitis. *Gut* 7:1-15, 1966.
[Dept. Surgical Studies, Middlesex Hosp., London; Dept. Surgery, St. Peter's Hosp., Chertsey; Dept. Radiology, St. Thomas's Hosp.; and Dept. Pathology and Research Dept., St. Mark's Hosp., London, England]

This paper brings a conceptual unity to the clinical problems of ischaemia attacking the gut and describes the three syndromes which may occur. On the basis of postclinical and experimental work, a classification of ischaemic colitis into gangrenous, stricturing, and transient forms is proposed. It is suggested that ischaemia of the colon, occurring in the same age group and from the same causes as myocardial infarction, accounts for certain cases of 'segmental' colitis, particularly those involving the splenic flexure. [The *SCI*® indicates that this paper has been cited in over 285 publications since 1966.]

Adrian Marston
Middlesex and Royal Northern Hospitals
University of London
London W1N 8AA
England

July 26, 1983

"In 1951, when I was an 'intern' in a small hospital on the periphery of London, I admitted a middle-aged woman with acute abdominal pain, who died two days later, in spite of surgery, from a mesenteric embolus. What puzzled me at that time was that although this was an accepted cause of death, I could not see precisely why she had died, because at autopsy her intestine was perfectly viable. It occurred to me that some physiological process must be at work, other than simple necrosis and peritonitis. This idea nestled in my mind for a number of years, when I encountered another case of intestinal ischaemia, but this time of a different nature. The patient was a 47-year-old man who presented with what I thought was a peridiverticular abscess. When I (by now a senior resident) operated upon him, I found a long length of inflamed colon which was not obviously necrotic, and I constructed a proximal colostomy. A few weeks later, barium studies showed that the lumen of the intervening bowel had completely disappeared. Obviously no closure was possible, so I resected the abnormal area and joined up the two ends. The pathologist reported that this was an infarction of the colon, with a thrombosed mesenteric artery.

"On the basis of these two cases and my study of the literature, I became convinced that there must be abnormalities in the intestinal circulation which could result in degrees of infarction similar to those seen in the brain, myocardium, and kidneys.

"In the early 1960s, an opportunity presented itself to study this problem at Harvard Medical School, with such famed figures as Francis Moore and Richard Warren. The year in Boston was spent in an experimental study of the ischaemic small bowel which was published in two papers in the *Annals of Surgery*.[1,2] My interest in the colon persisted, however, and it was borne in upon me that my case of spontaneous colonic ischaemia was similar, both clinically and radiologically, to those seen following cardiac and vascular surgery and that many patients with obscure colonic disease in fact had infarcts, similar to those appearing in other circulatory territories. This prompted a critical review of our experience in London, at St. Thomas's Hospital and St. Mark's Hospital, with the cooperation of Basil Morson, director of pathology at St. Mark's. From this was born the concept of 'ischaemic colitis,' which was a new category of colonic disease, clinically and pathologically distinct from other forms of inflammatory bowel disease such as ulcerative colitis and Crohn's disease. The paper was published in *Gut* in 1966.

"The study was based on 16 patients, but our experience is now of nearly two hundred, and the original classification, and suggested management of the condition, have changed. In particular, the concepts of 'transient' and 'stricturing' disease are misleading, and it is better to think of colonic gangrene on the one hand (often with no vascular occlusion) and (nongangrenous) ischaemic colitis on the other. Subsequent authors have confirmed this.[3-5]

"This paper has been highly cited because it was the first attempt to categorize and describe graduated colonic infarction and related the fields of vascular and intestinal surgery in an original way. Like all 'classical' papers, it has been frequently misquoted and misapplied and rereading it now, I would disagree with much that it says. Nonetheless, it remains true that in 1966 the concept of ischaemic disease of the colon was new, and one which caused people to reexamine accepted models, and I am pleased to think that the work should still be quoted."

1. **Marston A.** Causes of death in mesenteric arterial occlusion. I. Local and general effects of devascularization of the bowel. *Ann. Surg.* **158**:952-9, 1963.
2. --------------. Causes of death in mesenteric arterial occlusion. II. Observations on revascularization of the ischemic bowel. *Ann. Surg.* **158**:960-70, 1963.
3. **De Dombal F T, Fletcher D M & Harris R S.** Early diagnosis of ischaemic colitis. *Gut* **10**:131-4, 1969.
4. **Boley S J, Schwartz S S & Williams L F, Jr.,** eds. *Vascular disorders of the intestine.* New York: Appleton-Century-Crofts, 1971. 657 p.
5. **Wittenberg J, Athanasoulis C A, Williams L F, Jr., Paredes S, O'Sullivan P & Brown B.** Ischemic colitis: radiology and pathophysiology. *Amer. J. Roentgenol.* **123**:287-99, 1975.

CC/NUMBER 7
FEBRUARY 18, 1980

This Week's Citation Classic

Lockhart-Mummery H E & Morson B C. Crohn's disease of the large intestine. *Gut* 5:493-509, 1964.
[St. Mark's Hospital, London, England]

This paper sets out clearly the clinical and pathological features of Crohn's disease of the large intestine as seen in a series of 75 patients. This combined clinical and pathological study makes it clear that Crohn's disease is a different disease from ulcerative colitis and that the two do not occur together in the same patient. [The *SCI*® indicates that this paper has been cited over 230 times since 1964.]

H.E. Lockhart-Mummery
149 Harley Street
London, W1N 2DE
England

December 27, 1979

"Following my appointment to the consultant staff of St. Mark's Hospital in the early 1950s, I had the opportunity of working with Cuthbert Dukes in his laboratory there. At that time, colectomy for inflammatory bowel disease was beginning to be practised more frequently and many colon specimens from patients with 'colitis' were coming to the laboratory for pathological examination. The pathological changes in the large bowel produced by ulcerative colitis had never been properly studied, and there were no good accounts in the literature, except some on postmortem material.[1,2] Although a surgeon, I thought this would be a useful field for further study and, encouraged by Dr. Dukes, examined the macroscopic and microscopic appearances of every case of inflammatory bowel disease that came into the laboratory for some years. The findings of these studies formed the basis of an MD thesis.

"At that time, most patients with inflammatory bowel disease were regarded as having ulcerative colitis and it was thought that Crohn's disease did not affect the colon. However, from the now fairly large series of cases studied, it was apparent that some of the cases did not conform to the usual macroscopic and microscopic pattern of ulcerative colitis. Basil Morson had by then succeeded Dukes as head of the department of pathology at St. Mark's Hospital and I asked him to reexamine all the unusual specimens. He suggested that these might all be cases of Crohn's disease of the colon, a concept which opposed previously accepted teaching. We then decided to reexamine in detail the clinical and radiological features of these cases. From then on the research became more exciting as it gradually became apparent that there were in many cases clinical and radiological features as well as pathological ones that were different from those of ulcerative colitis. We first published the tentative findings in 1959 and 1960,[3,4] but by 1963 we had a sufficiently large series, adequately studied and documented, to be certain that these were in fact cases of Crohn's disease and to publish the paper.

"Although there had been other papers suggesting that Crohn's disease could in fact affect the large bowel,[5,6] we think that ours has been frequently cited because it was the first to present in detail the whole clinical, radiological, and pathological picture of Crohn's disease as it affects the large bowel. Therefore, this was a step forward in clarifying and classifying the several diseases which had for too long been lumped together as 'colitis.'

"It is of interest to recall that the concept of Crohn's disease of the colon and rectum and its separation from ulcerative colitis met with considerable resistance from surgeons, gastroenterologists, and pathologists for a good many years after this paper, but that it is now firmly established."

1. **Wilks S & Moxon W.** *Lectures on pathological anatomy.* London: Churchill, 1875. 672 p.
2. **Hawkins H P.** An address on the natural history of ulcerative colitis and its bearing on treatment. *Brit. Med. J.* **1**:765-70, 1909.
3. **Morson B & Lockhart-Mummery H E.** Crohn's disease of the colon. *Gastroenterologia (Basel)* **92**:168-73, 1959.
4. **Lockhart-Mummery H E & Morson B.** Crohn's disease (regional enteritis) of the large intestine and its distinction from ulcerative colitis. *Gut* **1**:87-105, 1960.
5. **Brooke B N.** Granulomatous diseases of the intestine. *Lancet* **2**:745-9, 1959.
6. **Wells C.** Ulcerative colitis and Crohn's disease. *Ann. Roy. Coll. Surg.* **11**:105-20, 1952.

CC/NUMBER 31
AUGUST 2, 1982

This Week's Citation Classic

Durand P. Lattosuria idiopatica in una paziente con diarrea cronica ed acidosi. (Idiopathic lactosuria in a patient with chronic diarrhea and acidosis.) *Minerva Pediat.* **10**:706-11, 1958.
[G. Gaslini Institute, Genova-Quarto, Italy]

This paper provides support for the suggestion that a lactose intolerance might be a cause of chronic diarrhoea and failure to thrive in infancy. The interest stimulated by this suggestion has resulted in the accumulation of a considerable amount of knowledge on intestinal disaccharide absorption and malabsorption. [The *SCI*® indicates that this paper has been cited in over 120 publications since 1961, making it the most-cited paper published in this journal, 1961-80.]

Paolo Durand
Third Department of Pediatrics
G. Gaslini Institute
16148 Genova-Quarto
Italy

May 4, 1982

"Twenty-four years ago, when this paper was published, it was not clear whether the tempo would justify the publication. In the intervening years, it has become apparent that the rate of accumulation of new knowledge on the absorption and malabsorption of carbohydrates and its relevance to man has exceeded all my expectations.

"The paper reported the case of a 13-month-old girl, daughter of consanguineous and unaffected parents, who was weak and malnourished, and suffered from chronic diarrhoea, abdominal pain, dehydration, and symptoms of vomiting. She showed severe lactosuria, renal acidosis, and intermittent proteinuria. A galactose tolerance test showed normal results and a lactose tolerance test showed a low rise in blood sugar with an increase of lactosuria. On a lactose-free diet she improved temporarily, but died at 15 months. Postmortem examination revealed atrophic enteritis as well as hepatic and adrenal atrophy and renal tubular degeneration. I suggested that the patient was affected by a congenital deficiency of intestinal lactase.

"It seemed to me that the diarrhoea developed because the lactose failed to undergo hydrolysis, remained in the lumen, and, by its osmotic effect, moved water into the lumen from the absorptive cells. Lactose passing through an abnormally permeable enteric mucosa led to lactosuria. The clinical syndrome lacked a biochemical demonstration of lactase deficiency but at that time the methods were not available for obtaining and assaying peroral biopsies of the small intestine.[1] However, a reason for the slow development of these methods was a general acceptance of the erroneous concept that digestive enzymes are excreted from the intestinal wall into the lumen.

"Since 1958 some additional cases having similar clinical manifestations have been reported and the number of papers on lactose intolerance has been increasing logarithmically.

"The contributors and I[2] came to the conclusion that there are two categories of carbohydrate intolerance: the first, rare, of congenital absence of a disaccharidase or of the transport mechanism, and the second, frequent, of one or more disaccharidases and of transport mechanism, secondary to many intestinal diseases. My first patient was probably affected by lactose intolerance without lactase deficiency; the etiology is unknown but a gastrogenic origin of the disorder is likely.[3] Other types of lactose intolerance are the very rare lactase deficiency in infants and young children; the lactase deficiency in adults, especially in black Americans, Asians, African Bantus, and Indians; and the frequent secondary and transient lactase deficiency in a variety of diseases in which the small intestine is or is not directly involved.

"There was a polite polemic about the priority of discovery of lactose intolerance by myself (1958) and by Holzel *et al.*[4] Certainly these first studies contributed to the creation of the chapter on intestinal disaccharidase deficiencies and to development of pediatric gastroenterology with many clinical, laboratory, and commercial implications.

"These factors contribute to the unexpected frequency of citation of my paper. Finally, this experience convinced me to publish in English the successive papers that I and my friends and colleagues judged of some interest."

1. **Dahlqvist A.** Method for assay of intestinal disaccharidases. *Anal. Biochem.* **7**:18-25, 1964.
2. **Durand P.** *Disorders due to intestinal defective carbohydrate digestion and absorption.* Rome: Il Pensiero Scientifico, 1964. 190 p.
3. **Berg N O, Dahlqvist A & Lindberg T.** A boy with severe infantile gastrogen lactose intolerance and acquired lactase deficiency. *Acta Paediat. Scand.* **68**:751-8, 1979.
4. **Holzel A, Schwarz V & Sutcliffe K W.** Defective lactose absorption causing malnutrition in infancy. *Lancet* **1**:1126-8, 1959.

This Week's Citation Classic™

CC/NUMBER 52
DECEMBER 26, 1983

Haemmerli U P, Kistler H, Ammann R, Marthaler T, Semenza G, Auricchio S & Prader A. Acquired milk intolerance in the adult caused by lactose malabsorption due to a selective deficiency of intestinal lactase activity. *Amer. J. Med.* **38**:7-30, 1965. [Depts. Med. and Medical Out-Patient Dept., Kantonsspital, and Dept. Biochem. and Children's Hosp., Univ. Zürich, Switzerland]

Acquired selective intestinal lactase deficiency with lactose malabsorption was demonstrated in nine patients with a history of intolerance to the ingestion of milk by means of carbohydrate tolerance tests with lactose, maltose, and a combination of glucose and galactose, as well as by measurements of the intestinal disaccharidases lactase, maltase, isomaltase, and sucrase in peroral jejunal biopsies. Results were compared with 12 normals and three patients with celiac sprue. [The *SCI*® indicates that this paper has been cited in over 190 publications since 1965.]

Urs Peter Haemmerli
Department of Medicine
Stadtspital Triemli
CH-8063 Zürich
Switzerland

October 27, 1983

"During my training as assistant resident in medicine at Mount Sinai Hospital in New York (1957-1959), the Sippy regimen was still used for ulcer patients. Not infrequently, we observed that individuals receiving milk every two hours developed colicky abdominal pains and diarrhea. The symptoms disappeared when milk was replaced by a normal diet. In 1959, I heard the Dutch pediatricians Weijers and van de Kamer talk on their recent discovery of a syndrome of congenital lactose intolerance in infants, which was published a year later.[1] The description was based on a selective malabsorption of one disaccharide among many tested. Intestinal enzymes could not be determined at that time.

"I suddenly wondered whether our ulcer patients on a Sippy regimen did not have a similar, but acquired, lactase deficiency. During 1960-1962, Dahlqvist, at the department of physiological chemistry in Lund, Sweden, developed a method to determine human intestinal disaccharidases in intestinal mucosa.[2] In 1962, he started to work at the department of pediatrics at the University of Zürich and taught his method to biochemists Auricchio and Semenza. Meanwhile, I had returned from New York to the department of medicine at the University of Zürich, bringing along the method of peroral jejunal biopsy which pediatricians there were not yet using.

"Combining the different facilities, Kistler and I started examining patients recruited from the outpatient department of medicine at Kantonsspital with intolerance to the ingestion of milk. Among many cranks and neurotics (which were really the hardest part of the study!), we discovered nine patients with the expected syndrome: we could demonstrate an isolated intestinal lactase deficiency combined with a flat blood glucose curve after lactose ingestion. The other disaccharides tested were absorbed normally. We postulated an acquired syndrome, because we knew that in the congenital variety observed in infancy the symptoms disappear as the patients grow older. Intolerance to milk was also present in the three sprue patients examined, but of course all intestinal disaccharidases were deficient.

"Meanwhile, Dahlqvist had gone to the VA Hospital in Hines near Chicago with his method, and Armand Littman's group published the same syndrome in a preliminary report of three patients in 1963,[2] a few months after we had reported our first four patients in Bern before the Swiss Society for Internal Medicine on May 12, 1963.

"The nearly simultaneous discovery of the syndrome in Switzerland and the US produced an avalanche of papers in the literature. The entity is now contained in every standard textbook of medicine, and has recently been treated in a monograph.[3] Our own paper has been cited widely because it was the first description in detail of a new, but quite common, clinical syndrome.

"However, nothing is new in science. Among veterinarians, lactose had long been used as a laxative, as all mammals lose their intestinal lactase after the suckling period, and of course fowls never have any lactase in their gut. The California sea lion became a favorite object of study because it has no lactose in its milk.

"The first patient with documented lactase deficiency may well have been the German physician M. Traube, who in 1881 reported the successful treatment of his own chronic constipation with lactose.[4]

"Our paper was awarded the Biennial Prize of the Swiss Society for Gastroenterology. It later led us to create our own 'artificial' disaccharide malabsorption syndrome: in 1966 we introduced successfully the synthetic disaccharide lactulose for the treatment of chronic hepatic coma.[5] Man has no intestinal enzyme to digest lactulose. Lactulose is—as unabsorbed lactose—fermented by bacteria in the colon to organic acids. Acidification of fecal contents prevents ammonia formation and lowers elevated blood ammonia levels in hepatic coma."

1. **Weijers H A, van de Kamer J H, Mossel D A A & Dicke W K.** Diarrhoea caused by deficiency of sugar-splitting enzymes. *Lancet* **2**:296-7, 1960. (Cited 75 times.)
2. **Dahlqvist A, Hammond J B, Crane R K, Dumphy J V & Littman A.** Intestinal lactase deficiency and lactose intolerance in adults. Preliminary report. *Gastroenterology* **45**:488-91, 1963. (Cited 120 times.)
3. **Paige D M & Bayless T M,** eds. *Lactose digestion: clinical and nutritional implications.* Baltimore, MD: Johns Hopkins University Press, 1981. 280 p.
4. **Traube M.** Ueber den Milchzucker als Medikament. *Deut. Med. Wochenschr.* **7**:113-14, 1881.
5. **Bircher J, Mueller J, Guggenheim P & Haemmerli U P.** Treatment of chronic portal-systematic encephalopathy with lactulose. *Lancet* **1**:890-3, 1966.

CC/NUMBER 23
JUNE 4, 1979

This Week's Citation Classic

Rubin C E, Brandborg L L, Phelps P C & Taylor H C. Studies of celiac disease, 1. The apparent identical and specific nature of the duodenal and proximal jejunal lesion in celiac disease and idiopathic sprue. *Gastroenterology* **38**:28-49, 1960. [Univ. Washington Sch. Med., Seattle, WA]

From infancy to old age abnormalities of villous architecture were found in duodenojejunal biopsies from all patients with celiac disease or idiopathic sprue. Such abnormalities were not seen in normals or in patients with a wide variety of other types of malabsorption. Ileal mucosal morphology was normal in two celiac sprue patients with abnormal duodenojejunal mucosa. [The *SCI*® indicates that this paper has been cited over 320 times since 1961.]

Cyrus E. Rubin
Department of Medicine RG-20
University of Washington
Seattle, WA 98195

February 8, 1978

"Our research on celiac sprue began accidentally when we were studying the gastric mucosa of some of Dr. Louis Diamond's patients with juvenile pernicious anemia. Before that time we'd never performed a small bowel biopsy, but we wanted to see whether the intestinal mucosa was normal in these patients, because a duodenal abnormality had just been reported in one type of malabsorption—celiac disease. With Dr. Harry Schwachman's encouragement and help, we not only biopsied our study patients but also several of his celiacs. The findings were so fascinating that completion of our studies of juvenile pernicious anemia had to wait eight years while we pursued celiac sprue.

"The research reported in this paper probably made the Plenary Session of the 'Young Turks' because it contained quantitative data to prove a histologic difference between normal controls and celiac sprue that was *visually obvious*. The presentation was almost entirely morphologic and so distractingly beautiful that the auidence failed to notice the paucity of precise measurements.

"This study raised several questions: Was the lack of correlation between the severity of malabsorption and the severity of the duodenal and proximal jejunal mucosal abnormality somehow explained by the normal ileal mucosa? Actually it was: our subsequent studies of the whole length of the small bowel of patients with celiac sprue showed that the severity of malabsorption correlated with the length of bowel lined by abnormal mucosa, i.e., if the ileum and distal jejunum were normal, malabsorption was milder than if they were involved. If we had hypothesized correctly that the mucosal lesion of celiac sprue was pathognomonic, why was the lesion indistinguishable from that seen in tropical sprue? We now know that our hypothesis was wrong because several other rare illnesses cause the same lesion, although only celiac sprue responds to a gluten-free diet. The presence of the identical proximal intestinal lesion in children with celiac disease, and in adults with idiopathic sprue, suggested that they were the same disease and that is why we call the illness celiac sprue; a hypothesis that is now generally accepted.

"In retrospect the main contribution of this paper was to make morphologic research a respectable scientific pursuit for gastroenterologists; this was accomplished by demonstrating the validity of blind review for testing subjective histologic criteria, by emphasizing the need for orientating biopsies precisely before fixation and by sectioning them serially to obtain maximal information."

CC/NUMBER 27
JULY 4, 1983

This Week's Citation Classic

Mendelson C L. The aspiration of stomach contents into the lungs during obstetric anesthesia. *Amer. J. Obstet. Gynecol.* **52**:191-205, 1946.
[Dept. Obstetrics and Gynecology, Cornell Univ. Medical Coll., and New York Hosp., NY]

This study described a new type of adult respiratory distress syndrome due to aspiration of gastric hydrochloric acid. The pertinent etiologic, pathologic, clinical, diagnostic, therapeutic, and prophylactic features were presented. [The *SCI®* indicates that this paper has been cited in over 270 publications since 1961—the 5th most-cited paper published in that journal.]

Curtis L. Mendelson
5427 Alta Way
Lake Worth, FL 33463

May 5, 1983

"While serving as obstetric consultant to the New York City Health Department I observed high maternal mortality locally, throughout the country, and abroad due to aspiration complicating general anesthesia. Personal experiences demonstrated the common occurrence of gastric retention during labor with copious fluid being vomited at the time of delivery.

"I attended a case having massive liquid aspiration with clinical findings resembling those of an acute asthmatic attack. The cardiopulmonary status deteriorated rapidly and pulmonary edema ensued. X rays revealed fluffy densities throughout the lungs, and normal mediastinal position. This differed significantly from the classic syndrome of solids aspiration, namely, either suffocation due to complete obstruction; or atelectasis, segmental consolidation, and mediastinal shift due to incomplete obstruction.

"The clue to etiology of the liquid aspiration syndrome was apparent when I inadvertently inhaled gastric fluid following an evening of relative intemperance. Accordingly, I presented an investigative protocol to the Cornell University Medical College—and rabbits, funds, and facilities were soon forthcoming. In the animal experiments, hydrochloric acid produced bronchiolar spasm, peribronchiolar exudation, and congestion which frequently culminated in pulmonary edema.

"I stressed that gastric retention during labor subjects ALL PARTURIENTS to the PREVENTABLE HAZARD of aspiration. Getting this message across was—and still is—a serious problem. Prophylactic recommendations included: withholding all oral feeding during labor; wider use of conduction anesthesia; gastric alkalinization; and emptying the stomach prior to general anesthesia. Treatment of aspiration was directed toward alleviating bronchiolar spasm, maintaining oxygenation and cardiopulmonary function, and preventing secondary bacterial infection: pneumonia and lung abscess.

"Other investigators[1-6] have confirmed the findings and have made important additional observations and recommendations. Prophylactic measures emphasize avoiding oversedation and hypotension, administering antacids during labor, and practicing refined techniques of general anesthesia: rapid smooth induction; universal intubation with an inflatable endotracheal cuff; cricoid pressure to seal off the esophagus during the interval between loss of consciousness and successful intubation; and extubation after the patient is completely responsive. Raising gastric pH above 2.5 reduces intensity of aspiration pneumonitis although particulate antacid in the aspirate is also irritating.

"The goal of therapy is maintenance of adequate oxygenation through careful and continued monitoring of blood gases, preferably in an intensive care environment. There are conflicting reports concerning therapeutic effects of tracheostomy, steroids, and lyophilized urea.

"I am honored by creation of the term 'Mendelson's syndrome' but hasten to note the dubious distinction of being identified with a vomiting tableau. I believe my study is cited frequently because aspiration is so common and so lethal. The prevalence is undoubtedly related to the rising incidence of cesarean section and the mortality associated with aspiration is 70 percent and higher. Surgeons, anesthesiologists, dentists, and veterinarians have also come to more fully relate the syndrome to their respective specialties. If all these facts and figures serve to spread the word, perhaps there is hope for greater safety in childbearing and in surgery."

1. **Nicholl R M, Holland E L & Brown S S.** Mendelson's syndrome: its treatment by tracheostomy and hydrocortisone. *Brit. Med. J.* **2**:745-6, 1967.
2. **Chapman R L, Jr.** Treatment of aspiration pneumonitis. *Int. Anesthesiol. Clin.* **15**:85-96, 1977.
3. **Dines D E, Baker W G & Scantland W A.** Aspiration pneumonitis—Mendelson's syndrome. *J. Amer. Med. Assn.* **176**:229-31, 1961.
4. **Johnson H.** Pulmonary aspiration of gastric acid: Mendelson's syndrome. Successful treatment with lyophilized urea and 10% invert sugar. *J. Amer. Med. Assn.* **179**:900-2, 1962.
5. **Roberts R B.** Aspiration and its prevention in obstetrical patients. *Int. Anesthesiol. Clin.* **15**:49-70, 1977.
6. **Wynne J W, Reynolds J C, Hood C I, Auerbach D & Ondrasick J.** Steroid therapy for pneumonitis induced in rabbits by aspiration of foodstuff. *Anesthesiology* **51**:11-19, 1979.

Chapter 9

Nephrology

In this brief chapter that contains but 10 "This Week's Citation Classic" (TWCC) commentaries, four stem from review articles.

The 54-page review by Wrong and Davies on acid excretion during renal disease opens the chapter. At the time their research project was conceived, both were junior scientists at Manchester Medical School. By ammonium chloride loading of patients with various forms of kidney disease, they were able, in 4 years, to plot the acid excretion pattern for most renal diseases. Their job was so thorough (in part because of the extra workload they assumed on Sundays) that their chairman prophetically stated, "Of course, it will be a classic." A second review on the excretion of organic acids and bases also achieved Citation Classic status. In this instance (p. 283) the paper was invited by the editor of the *American Journal of Medicine.* A major contribution of this report was the emphasis on reabsorption rather than secretion alone. The third review also resulted from an invitation, in this instance to participate in a conference whose proceedings were to be published. The article by Ullrich et al. became a Citation Classic. The principal concept described in the review was how the urine becomes more concentrated in the kidney medulla. Delicate measurements of the tubular osmolarity and of blood indicated that a countercurrent movement of numerous electrolytes, urea, amino acids, and creatinine was responsible for this concentration along the tubule. The last review focuses on calcification in the soft tissues as a result of uremia. Calcium salts deposit in the arteries, skin, viscera, and eyes as a result of hyperphosphatemia. This review too was written at the invitation of a symposium organizer, and the author made good use of *Current Contents* during his illness. The papers from this conference were published in a series of four issues, and of those several articles, only this one became a Citation Classic (p. 285).

Brown's TWCC clearly explains the technique he and Wickham used to measure urethral pressure at different points along its length. Brown admits his embarrassment at the simplicity of the method but is now able to take the remark of a fellow Ph.D. student that other people in the department "make discoveries of that magnitude every day" with only a tinge of bitterness.

The phenomenon of encephalopathy as a terminal illness in uremic patients was a painful experience for attending physicians who had high expectations for dialysis therapy. The condition renders the victim mute, helpless, and moribund often within a period of 6 to 9 months. A search for toxic elements in tissue collected at autopsy failed, but the neurotoxicity of aluminum was known to the authors, who soon identified it in the dialysis fluid. Thereafter the elimination of dialysis encephalopathy was a simple matter (p. 287).

Dialysis of patients with kidney disease is expensive, and proponents of kidney transplantation as a substitute for dialysis have always anticipated that a more economic relief of uremic patients would come from their specialty. The obvious problems were the availability of kidneys and the difficulty in maintaining them in a viable condition during transport. The UCLA transplant team found that perfusion with fluids high in K^+ and Mg^{2+} followed by packing in ice would retain tissue viability for 30 hours. The article was first rejected by *Lancet,* but a knowledgeable British transplant surgeon interceded successfully.

The renal toxicity of the anesthetic methoxyflurane was found to be due to its release of free fluorine (p. 289). An *in vivo* animal model in rats and *in vitro* data clearly supported this conclusion.

The final two TWCCs describe unrelated studies. The first is on vitamin B_{12} excretion in patients with pernicious anemia. The feeding of a large dose of unlabeled vitamin (the cold carrier) after a smaller dose of radioactive vitamins caused sufficient B_{12} to appear that an assessment of B_{12} absorption in these patients was possible. The final TWCC is built around a familiar scene in medical school toilet facilities—the collection of large volumes of urine in buckets, carboys, flasks, or other large vessels. In this instance the Aussie investigators wished to isolate a colony growth stimulating factor from urine. Their only disappointment was that visits to a nearby pub did not increase the recovery of the growth factor. Otherwise, it would have made construction of the grant budget a true pleasure.

If one were to list the half dozen most visible areas of study in kidney physiology and kidney disease, it is a certainty that renal transplantation, the immunologic basis of kidney disease, hormonal influences (renin-angiotensin-aldosterone) on kidney function, and kidney dialysis, including continuous ambulatory peritoneal dialysis, would all be good candidates for this list. Yet of the 10 TWCCs in this chapter only one, on kidney preservation, would fall into this listing. Significant attention is accorded problems in kidney transplantation by the journals *Transplantation Proceedings* and *Transplantation,* the latter in the form of occasional review articles. The former is more inclined to whole issues or issue supplements centering on a specific aspect of transplantation. Four issues of *Transplantation Proceedings* published as part of volume 17 in 1985 were of this nature. These were titled New Trends in Transplantation, Cyclosporine-associated Renal Injury, Relevant Immunologic Factors in Clinical Kidney Transplantation, and Organs for Transplantations. In 1983, the journal *Kidney* included a 93-page supplement (supplement 14) to its volume 23 titled Advances in Renal Transplantation. The entire November issue (vol. 6, no. 5, 1985) of the *American Journal of Kidney Diseases* deals with aluminum toxicity.

True review-style journals in nephrology and urology are limited to *Advances in Nephrology* and *Contributions to Nephrology. The Kidney* publishes only mini-reviews, often of only four pages. Persons seeking review articles on the current status of kidney disease may need to consult other review journals in medicine, physiology, etc., depending upon the logical cross-referencing of the disease in question.

Anagnostopoulos T, Edelman A, Teulon J & Planelles G. Mechanisms of proximal tubular reabsorption: contribution of electrophysiologic techniques. *Adv. Nephrol.* **12:**63–84, 1983.

Antonovych T T. Drug-induced nephropathies. *Pathol. Annu.* **19:**165–96, 1984.

Friedman E A. Critical appraisal of continuous ambulatory peritoneal dialysis. *Annu. Rev. Med.* **34:**233–48, 1984.

Halperin B D & Feeley T W. The effect of anesthesia and surgery on renal function. *Int. Anesthesiol. Clin.* **22:**157–68, 1984.

Kassirer J P. Life-threatening acid-base disorders. *Adv. Nephrol.* **14:**67–85, 1985.

Kon V & Ichikawa I. Hormonal regulation of glomerular filtration. *Annu. Rev. Med.* **36:**515–31, 1985.

Simon P, Allain P, Ang K S, Cam G & Mauras Y. Prevention and treatment of aluminum intoxication in chronic renal failure. *Adv. Nephrol.* **14:**439–78.

This Week's Citation Classic

CC/NUMBER 50
DECEMBER 10, 1979

Wrong O & Davies H E F. The excretion of acid in renal disease. *Quart. J. Med.* **28**:259-313, 1959.
[Univ. Dept. Med., Manchester Royal Infirmary and Medical Unit, Cardiff Royal Infirmary, UK]

The paper describes the urinary response to an acid load, taken as a single oral dose of ammonium chloride. Study of normal subjects and patients with different forms of kidney disease distinguished the factors influencing urinary acidification and ammonium excretion. [The ***SCI***® **indicates that this paper has been cited over 475 times since 1961.]**

Oliver Wrong
Department of Medicine
University College Hospital
Medical School
Medical Unit
London WC1E 6JJ
England

January 30, 1978

"This work was conceived in 1954 at the Manchester Medical School, where I was a junior teacher in the department of medicine of Robert Platt, then the doyen of British renal physicians. I was single, with military service, medical residencies, and exams behind me, and had just returned from Boston anxious to put the lessons learnt from Fuller Albright and Alex Leaf into effect. The University provided a pittance of £640 a year as salary, lodging in the nearby student residence, laboratory facilities, and modest clinical and teaching responsibilities. The seniors in the department, Douglas Black and Bill Stanbury, were liberal with ideas and expertise, but did not try to enroll me in their research, so I teamed up with Howard Davies, then a Medical Research Council research fellow, to study renal tubular function in hyperparathyroidism—a topic combining two of the main departmental interests.

"We naively proposed to study *all* tubular functions, concentrating on the distal tubule as being more important clinically. Water conservation had been fairly well worked out, so we turned to acid excretion, meaning to later tackle the more difficult problems of sodium and potassium conservation. It was easy to establish an acid load test which was completed in a working day (and so did not require hospital admission). In fact, we never changed our initial protocol as this test caused excretion of a maximally acid urine within two hours of the acid load.

"We were fortunate that one of our first patients without parathyroid disease had renal calcification (nephrocalcinosis) and turned out to have a marked defect in urinary acidification without acidosis, which we named 'the incomplete syndrome of renal tubular acidosis.' Inevitably we extended our interests to other forms of renal disease. Manchester colleagues referred us many patients of interest, and Charles Dent in London generously collected patients whom I drove down to study on Sundays, spending the small hours of the morning running urine analyses and getting to know the hospital where I now work. Within four years, 68 subjects had been studied and we had a mammoth manuscript which Robert Platt thought too indigestible to stand much chance of publication, though he was kind (or prescient) enough to remark, 'Of course, it will be a classic.'

"I suspect the paper has been quoted mainly by those following our test procedure, though some of our other findings were of greater theoretic interest, particularly the low urinary PCO_2 in tubular disease and the direct relationship of stimulated ammonium excretion to glomerular filtration rate in all forms of renal disease. In retrospect we attached too much importance to potassium depletion as a cause of acidification defect, but the paper's chief omission was our failure to recognise proximal ('Type II') renal tubular acidosis, then undescribed, and so rare that we didn't encounter a case.

"Looking back to my years in Manchester, I realise what an excellent education they provided by giving me time to tackle my own problems under a benign yet critical supervision. Because of earlier marriage, and the rigidity of our postgraduate medical training programme, few of our present graduates feel able to afford such self-indulgence."

CC/NUMBER 27
JULY 6, 1981

This Week's Citation Classic

Weiner I M & Mudge G H. Renal tubular mechanisms for excretion of organic acids and bases. *Amer. J. Med.* **36**:743-62, 1964.
[Dept. Pharmacology and Exp. Therapeutics, Johns Hopkins Univ., Sch. Med., Baltimore, MD and Dept. Pharmacology and Toxicology, Dartmouth Med. Sch., Hanover, NH]

The review covered renal excretory patterns of various organic electrolytes including uric acid. Special emphasis was placed on the recently discovered phenomenon of bidirectional transport of drugs: active tubular secretion and passive reabsorption by nonionic diffusion. [The *SCI*® indicates that this paper has been cited over 215 times since 1964.]

I.M. Weiner
Department of Pharmacology
State University of New York
Upstate Medical Center
Syracuse, NY 13210

May 20, 1981

"This paper was one of a series of short reviews in a symposium issue of the *American Journal of Medicine*. The guest editor, R.W. Berliner, had invited G.H. Mudge to prepare the review and the latter asked me to collaborate. Until two years earlier I had been one of Mudge's junior colleagues. To a considerable extent the review was based on material which followed from our 1959 paper.[1] The paper had been published in an institutional journal, the very vehicle used by E.K. Marshall, Jr., for his initial proof of tubular secretion in the mammalian kidney.[2] Mudge, who is about to retire from laboratory work, was and still is as fond of historical connections as he is of experiments yielding unexpected results.

"Our contributions in this area stemmed from a fortuitous event. We had been trying to understand why acidification of the urine enhanced and alkalinization diminished the renal response to organic mercurials, a class of diuretics which is now virtually obsolete. It was of interest to learn the sites of acidification within the nephron. Our plan was to do stop-flow experiments in animals treated with salicylate. Stop-flow experiments allow crude localizations of nephron functions and salicylate was thought to distribute across the tubular epithelium by nonionic diffusion, i.e., it was to serve as the pH indicator for the fluid in various nephron segments. Our initial results with salicylate made no sense in this context and further work demonstrated that salicylate is subjected to active tubular secretion as well as reabsorption by nonionic diffusion. This complex excretory pattern had been entertained as a possibility for antimalarial drugs years earlier by Jailer, Rosenfeld, and Shannon[3] but the idea seems to have been treated with total, perhaps benign, neglect. We, and others, were unaware of the suggestion at the time of our initial work. As indicated in our review and by much subsequent work, this excretory pattern for organic electrolytes is quite common, but not universal. Recent reviews of this subject are cited in the article by Barbara Rennick.[4]

"It is difficult to pinpoint the reason or reasons why a review is cited frequently. Several ideas come to mind. First, most of the more recent reviews of this subject have appeared in books. Books may be too expensive for many individuals or libraries. Second, an area of research may not progress rapidly and an older review may retain its usefulness. Third, a review sometimes contains the most explicit exposition of an idea. Finally, editors of reviews tend to be more generous than editors of scientific reports; this factor makes it easier for authors of reviews to cover interrelationships, some speculative, that might be excluded from a regular paper."

1. **Weiner I M, Washington J A, II & Mudge G H.** Studies on the renal excretion of salicylate in the dog. *Bull. Johns Hopkins Hosp.* **105**:284-97, 1959.
2. **Marshall E K, Jr. & Vickers J L.** The mechanism of the elimination of phenolsulphonephthalein by the kidney—a proof of secretion by the convoluted tubules. *Bull. Johns Hopkins Hosp.* **34**:1-7, 1923.
3. **Jailer J W, Rosenfeld M & Shannon J A.** The influence of orally administered alkali and acid on the renal excretion of quinacrine, chloroquine and santoquine. *J. Clin. Invest.* **26**:1168-72, 1947.
4. **Rennick B R.** Renal tubular transport of organic cations. *Amer. J. Physiol.* **240**:F83-9, 1981.

CC/NUMBER 4
JANUARY 25, 1982

This Week's Citation Classic

Ullrich K J, Kramer K & Boylan J W. Present knowledge of the counter-current system in the mammalian kidney. *Progr. Cardiovasc. Dis.* **3**:395-431, 1961.

Counter-current systems achieve considerable final effects by multiplying small, single effects along a distance. Kuhn and Wirz proposed that such a system constitutes the basis for urine concentration in renal medulla.[1] The cited article reviewed the experimental evidence for this hypothesis. [The *SCI*® indicates that this paper has been cited over 195 times since 1961.]

K.J. Ullrich
Max-Planck-Institut für Biophysik
6000 Frankfurt am Main 70
Federal Republic of Germany

November 11, 1981

"My studies since 1954 have been concerned with verification of the counter-current theory by Kuhn and Wirz.[1] After my data, published in German,[2,3] became known in the US, I was asked by C. Friedberg 'to join a group of outstanding investigators in a symposium on heart, kidney, and electrolytes.' The symposium was published in *Progress in Cardiovascular Diseases*, my contribution to which has now become a *Citation Classic*. In 1960 I felt that a review on the renal counter-current system was overdue because the then available experimental data seemed not only to readily answer all critical questions of the Kuhn-Wirz theory, but also to provide unequivocal evidence for it. I was lucky to have as coauthors my teachers Kurt Kramer, an expert on oxymetry applied to renal circulation, and John Boylan, at that time a visiting professor at the Physiologisches Institut in Göttingen.

"As the citations in our review show, the situation in that field of research in 1961 was as follows: the Kuhn-Wirz theory of urine concentration by the medullary counter-current system in its main formulation of 1951 postulates that the osmolarity in the structures of the kidney medulla rises from the base to the tip and is not very different in horizontally adjacent structures. This was supported in 1951 by Wirz, Hargitay, and Kuhn applying direct cryoscopy to papillary slices;[1] in 1953 by Wirz's determination of the osmolarity of urine taken from the tip of Henle's loop and of blood from adjacent vasa recta; in 1955-1956 by our measurements of osmolality as well as the profile of Na^+, K^+, Ca^{2+}, Mg^{2+}, Cl^-, P_i, urea, amino acids, and creatinin in the papilla;[2] in 1956 by Wirz showing that the fluid leaving Henle's loop into the distal tubule is hypotonic; in 1958 by our microcatheter studies of the reabsorption of water, Na^+, Cl^-, and urea from the collecting duct as well as our measurement of the Na^+-stimulated respiration of slices from the outer medulla;[3] in 1959 by Gottschalk's confirmation of Wirz's micropuncture data of 1953 and 1956.

"In joint experiments at Chapel Hill during 1959-1960, Gottschalk, B. Schmidt-Nielsen, and I elucidated the urea recirculation in kidney medulla. In 1960-1961, Kramer together with Thurau and Deetjen evaluated the mutual influence of vascular and tubular counter-currents, while my group determined the skimming and shrinking behavior of erythrocytes in the papillary vessels during formation of hypertonic urine. Other important data, obtained during that year, were the degree of oxygen saturation of red cell hemoglobin during passage through the renal papilla, measured by Kramer's group, as well as the rate of anaerobic and aerobic glycolysis of papillary tissue, measured by my research group.

"I think that our review has been so highly cited because: a) it compiled the early experimental proof for the theory that concentrated urine is formed in the renal medulla by a counter-current system, and b) the data available at that time were published in German and, furthermore, in European journals and therefore were not easily accessible to the majority of American scientists. This holds even today, 20 years later, as shown by a citation in a recent publication on this topic.[4]

"For my work on the counter-current system in the renal medulla I received, in 1961, the British-German Feldberg prize in experimental medicine."

1. **Wirz H, Hargitay B & Kuhn W.** Lokalisation des Konzentrierungsprozesses in der Niere durch direkte Kryoskopie. *Helv. Physiol. Pharmacol. Acta* **91**:196-207, 1951.
2. **Ullrich K J & Jarausch K H.** Untersuchungen zum Problem der Harnkonzentrierung und -verdünnung. *Pflügers Arch. Ges. Physiol.* **262**:537-50, 1956.
3. **Hilger H H, Klümper J D & Ullrich K J.** Wasserruckresorption und Ionentransport durch die Sammelrohrzellen der Säugetierniere. *Pflügers Arch. Ges. Physiol.* **267**:218-37, 1958.
4. **Hogg R J & Kokko J P.** Renal counter-current multiplication system. *Rev. Physiol. Biochem. Pharmacol.* **86**:95-135, 1979.

CC/NUMBER 32
AUGUST 6, 1984

This Week's Citation Classic™

Parfitt A M. Soft tissue calcification in uremia.
Arch. Intern. Med. **124**:544-56, 1969.
[Depts. Med., Cedars-Sinai Med. Ctr., Los Angeles, CA, and Univ. Queensland, Brisbane, Australia]

In chronic renal failure, calcium salts can be deposited in the tunica media of large and small arteries, in the cornea and conjunctiva, as nodular or tumoral masses around joints, in the skin and subcutaneous tissues, and in viscera such as lungs, kidney, stomach, and heart, with a wide spectrum of clinical effects. Pathogenesis depends on chronic hyperphosphatemia and on alterations in connective tissue proteins from a variety of causes to form a calcifiable matrix that binds calcium and phosphate ions. [The *SCI*® indicates that this paper has been cited in over 170 publications since 1969.]

A. Michael Parfitt
Bone and Mineral Research Laboratory
Henry Ford Hospital
Detroit, MI 48202

July 2, 1984

"In August 1968, I began a sabbatical leave in Los Angeles at the invitation of Charles R. (Chuck) Kleeman, who was busy organizing the third National Institutes of Health supported conference on chronic renal failure and dialysis, to be held in November at the Miramar Hotel, Santa Barbara. He had asked me to cover the subject of soft tissue calcification and I had reluctantly agreed, in the spirit that in the country of the blind the one-eyed man was king! My presentation was based on extensive clinical experience, both of renal osteodystrophy and its geographic variation in three continents, and of mineral metabolism generally, which I now had the opportunity to reflect upon and to codify. I also made a detailed but selective analysis of the experimental literature from a clinical perspective, a task made easier by the superb medical library at the University of California in Los Angeles.

"After the conference, Chuck was disappointed that I did not begin some experimental work on the subject, but my research interests were shifting away from the kidney and systemic mineral metabolism toward the bone. Completion of the manuscript was interrupted by my falling ill with hepatitis, but with my wife, Elaine, as courier, and my first systematic use of *Current Contents*®, I was able to get all the material needed and to keep abreast of recent developments. The conference proceedings were published in four consecutive issues of *Archives of Internal Medicine*, later collected into a single symposium volume entitled *Divalent Ion Metabolism and Osteodystrophy in Chronic Renal Failure*[1] with Chuck as guest editor. For several years this was an indispensable reference source, marred only by some excessively pedantic subediting.

"I believe the paper has been frequently cited for three main reasons. First, it was the earliest review of the subject during the modern era of treatment for chronic renal failure; hemodialysis and renal transplantation had only recently been widely applied, with a manifold increase in the number of patients at risk. Second, I was able to put what had been an area of great confusion into some sort of order. The clinical classification I proposed is still in use, with minor modifications,[2] and each clinical type was compared with a counterpart occurring in the absence of uremia. I clarified the relationships between several different syndromes of articular and periarticular calcification, so that the article was useful to rheumatologists and orthopedists as well as to nephrologists. Concerning pathogenesis, I emphasized the interplay of both local factors leading to so-called dystrophic calcification, and systemic factors leading to so-called metastatic calcification. Third, substantial improvement in the control of hyperphosphatemia and secondary hyperparathyroidism in renal patients has greatly reduced the incidence of all forms of soft tissue calcification, so that the subject has since received comparatively little investigative attention. The most important subsequent advances[2,3] have been the identification of different calcium salts, such as oxalate[3] and a magnesium-containing compound resembling Whitlockite,[4] the increasing recognition of cardiopulmonary complications of calcium deposition[3,5] and their detection with variable success by scintigraphy,[6] and the likely role of abnormal pyrophosphate metabolism in pathogenesis."[7]

1. **Kleeman C R,** ed. *Divalent ion metabolism and osteodystrophy in chronic renal failure.* Chicago: American Medical Association, 1969. 54 p.
2. **Coburn J W & Slatopolsky E.** Vitamin D, parathyroid hormone and renal osteodystrophy. (Brenner B M & Rector F C, eds.) *The kidney.* Philadelphia: Saunders, 1981. Vol. II. p. 2213-305.
3. **Parfitt A M.** Soft tissue calcification in uremia. *Dialysis Transplant.* **5**:17-24, 1976.
4. **LeGeros R Z, Contiguglia S R & Alfrey A C.** Pathological calcifications associated with uremia. Two types of calcium phosphate deposits. *Calcified Tissue Res.* **13**:173-85, 1973.
5. **Conger J D, Hammond W S, Alfrey A C, Contiguglia S R, Stanford R E & Huffer W E.** Pulmonary calcification in chronic dialysis patients. *Ann. Intern. Med.* **83**:330-6, 1975. (Cited 70 times.)
6. **De Graaf P, Schicht I M, Pauwels E K J, Souverijn J H M & de Graeff J.** Bone scintigraphy in uremic pulmonary calcification. *J. Nucl. Med.* **20**:201-6, 1979.
7. **Alfrey A C, Solomons C C, Ciricillo J & Miller N L.** Extraosseous calcification. Evidence for abnormal pyrophosphate metabolism in uremia. *J. Clin. Invest.* **57**:692-9, 1976.

CC/NUMBER 9
FEBRUARY 28, 1983

This Week's Citation Classic

Brown M & Wickham J E A. The urethral pressure profile.
Brit. J. Urol. **41**:211-17, 1969.
[Depts. Urology and Medical Electronics, St. Bartholomew's Hosp., London, England]

A method was developed for measuring the urethral closure pressure and presenting this as a plot of pressure against distance along the urethra. The method, though very simple and easy to perform with commonly available apparatus, was shown to be accurate and difficult to misuse. [The *SCI*® indicates that this paper has been cited in over 190 publications since 1969.]

Malcolm C. Brown
Bioengineering & Medical Physics Unit
Royal Liverpool Hospital
Liverpool L7 8XP
England

December 9, 1982

"From 1967 to 1971, I was a PhD student in medical electronics, working with a urological surgeon (John Wickham) at St. Bartholomew's Hospital, London. We were conducting a trial of the performance of implantable electrical stimulators for the treatment of urinary incontinence, and required a measurement to assess the effect of the stimulation on the inside of the urethra, which could be used for finding the correct siting for electrodes and for assessing the performance of the stimulator once implanted.

"The method we devised used a plain plastic catheter with side holes opening against the urethral wall through which water was forced at a very slow rate. The pressure inside the catheter was recorded remotely and we were able to show by theoretical and practical methods that the recorded pressure was equal to the urethral wall pressure, plus a small known error due to the infusion. By drawing the catheter along the urethra, a complete profile of urethral pressure was drawn in just a few seconds and this could be repeated after a change in the electrical stimulation level.

"After my PhD, I moved to Liverpool to work on other aspects of biomedical engineering. I visited the US in 1977 and was surprised to find the method in widespread use, though it was interesting to find from the *Science Citation Index*® that there were few citations before 1974 (five years after publication). It had been used in studies of urethral physiology, neuromuscular behaviour of the urethra, and in pharmacological studies. Alternative methods (membrane catheters, or miniature transducers in the urethra) were generally more costly, and required greater attention during experiments. A large number of citations came from work which attempted to classify urethral disorders from the urethral pressure profile parameters. This was rather unsuccessful since the individual variations are large. However, sequential profiles on the same cases do appear to be useful.

"The key to the success of the method must be its simplicity. Indeed, it was so simple I was embarrassed at first. A fellow PhD student at St. Bartholomew's Hospital told me the idea was 'trivial' and that other people in the department 'make discoveries of that magnitude every day.' I often wonder if his contribution to medical research has ever been recognized.

"The discovery of the interest in such simple methods of measurement has led me to associate with a research group in Liverpool working on urinary incontinence in women. We have recently developed two new measurement techniques, one to demonstrate the severity of urinary incontinence,[1] and another to show incompetence at the bladder neck.[2,3] Both of these new measurements use the most simple apparatus, provide readily comprehensible information, and cannot easily be misused. Based on experience with the 1969 paper, we expect it to be some years before we can properly assess their impact."

1. **Sutherst J, Brown M & Shawer M.** Assessing the severity of urinary incontinence in women by weighing perineal pads. *Lancet* **1**:1128-30, 1981.
2. **Brown M C & Sutherst J.** A test for bladder neck competence: the fluid bridge test. *Urol. Int.* **34**:403-7, 1979.
3. **Shawer M, Brown M & Sutherst J.** Diagnosis of bladder neck incompetence without use of capital equipment. *Brit. Med. J.* **283**:760-1, 1981.

CC/NUMBER 7
FEBRUARY 14, 1983

This Week's Citation Classic

Alfrey A C, LeGendre G R & Kaehny W D. The dialysis encephalopathy syndrome: possible aluminum intoxication. *N. Engl. J. Med.* **294**:184-8, 1976. [Renal Sect., Denver Veterans Admin. Hosp., and Div. Renal Medicine, Univ. Colorado Medical Ctr., Denver, CO]

This report documented that brain aluminum levels were higher in dialyzed uremic patients dying of dialysis encephalopathy than in dialysis patients dying of other causes. It was the first hint that aluminum intoxication was responsible for this disease. [The *SCI*® indicates that this paper has been cited in over 320 publications since 1976.]

Allen C. Alfrey
Veterans Administration
Medical Center
1055 Clermont Street
Denver, CO 80220

December 28, 1982

"Upon my return to the University of Colorado Medical Center in late-1970, my staff and I began observing a unique neurological syndrome (dialysis encephalopathy) in uremic patients on chronic maintenance hemodialysis. This disease had distinctive features with all the patients presenting with speech disturbances. Death occurred some seven months later at which time patients were totally mute and unable to perform any purposeful movements. This illness was responsible for 50 percent of the deaths on our dialysis program and prevented any patient from living longer than six years.

"To watch our patients dying from such a devastating disease had a profound effect on the morale of our staff, as well as on the surviving patients and their families. We resolved to find its cause. When we first reported this syndrome, others felt it was unique to the Denver area, and one publication called it the 'Denver disease.' It soon became apparent, however, that it was occurring worldwide but with marked variations in frequency. For instance, it would occur in epidemic proportions in some units but was rarely, if ever, seen in other units. This, in association with the lack of anatomical changes in the brains of patients who had died of this disease, suggested that some environmental toxin, such as a trace element, might be responsible for the illness. Using an X-ray fluorescence method which measures all elements between the atomic numbers of 19 and 92, we could find no consistent differences in trace elements in brains of patients who had died of the disease. Because aluminum was known to be a neurotoxin, yet was too light to measure with this technique, we decided to develop a method to determine aluminum levels in biological samples. Over a period of three years, after attempting a variety of unsuccessful techniques, we finally developed a satisfactory flameless atomic absorption procedure to measure aluminum. When we applied this method to the brains of patients who had died of this neurological syndrome—as well as to the brains of dialysis patients who had died of other causes—it became immediately apparent that although brain aluminum was increased in all the patients studied, it was consistently higher in patients who had suffered from this neurological ailment. This finding was subsequently confirmed by other investigators.[1,2] In addition, large epidemiological studies showed that all units having frequent cases of this disease also had aluminum-contaminated dialysate, whereas units without this disease had dialysate free of aluminum. It was then found that the disease could virtually be eliminated from all involved units by dialyzing patients with aluminum-free dialysate.

"I believe this article is frequently cited because it documented the etiology of the first new disease described in dialysis patients and was instrumental in establishing water standards for the preparation of dialysate, making it possible to eradicate a disease which had been responsible for major mortality. Moreover, it opened up a new area of research into the role aluminum plays in the pathogenesis of a disabling bone disease of dialysis patients."[3]

1. **Cartier F, Allain P, Gary J, Chatel M, Menault F & Pecker S.** Encéphalopathie myoclonique progressive des dialysés. Rôle de l'eau utilisée pour l'hémodialyse. *Nouv. Presse Méd.* 7:97-102, 1978.
2. **McDermott J R, Smith A I, Ward M K, Parkinson I S & Kerr D N S.** Brain-aluminum concentration in dialysis encephalopathy. *Lancet* 1:901-3, 1978.
3. **Hodsman A B, Sherrard D J, Alfrey A C, Ott S, Brickman A S, Miller N L, Maloney N A & Coburn J W.** Bone aluminum and histomorphometric features of renal osteodystrophy. *J. Clin. Endocrinol. Metab.* 54:539-46, 1982.

CC/NUMBER 32
AUGUST 11, 1980

This Week's Citation Classic

Collins G M, Bravo-Shugarman M & Terasaki P I. Kidney preservation for transportation. Initial perfusion and 30 hours' ice storage. *Lancet* **2**:1219-22, 1969. [Dept. Surgery, Center for Health Sci., Univ. Calif., Los Angeles, CA]

This article described a method for kidney preservation by which the organ could be stored in ice for up to 30 hours with minimal damage. The main departure from previously used methods was in the composition of the flush solution, which was formulated to resemble the intracellular rather than the extracellular ionic content. [The *SCI*® indicates that this paper has been cited over 340 times since 1969.]

Geoffrey M. Collins
Veterans Administration Hospital
3350 La Jolla Village Drive
San Diego, CA 92161

June 10, 1980

"My work in organ preservation began in 1968 in Paul Terasaki's laboratory at UCLA. The advantage conferred by histocompatibility matching for living donor kidney transplants was becoming evident, and it was believed that these benefits could be extended to cadaveric kidney transplantation if only there were a suitable method for preservation and transportation to a selected recipient. It was anticipated that it would frequently be necessary to send the preserved kidney to a recipient in another city by air transport. At that time the only preservation technique which had been shown to be capable of keeping kidneys in good condition for more than eight hours required a bulky perfusion machine and therefore did not seem practicable for transportation by air. The alternative method, used in the majority of transplant centers which did not possess a perfusion machine, was to immerse the organ in iced saline and flush out the vascular compartment with an electrolyte solution of the type used for intravenous infusions. My reading on the subject led me to doubt whether such an approach conferred any benefit by comparison with ice immersion alone. In fact, on many occasions, the results seemed worse with the former method. The explanation for this appeared to lie in a report by Keeler *et al.*,[1] which described a rapid loss of intracellular ions, principally potassium and magnesium, when kidneys were perfused with cold electrolyte solutions of extracellular type. It seemed logical to try flushing the kidney with a solution formulated to resemble the intracellular, i.e., high in potassium and magnesium, rather than the extracellular ionic content. Compared with our previous findings, the results using an intracellular type flush solution were surprisingly good. Dog kidneys could be preserved in excellent condition for more than 24 hours by a single flush with a few milliliters of an intracellular type solution followed by immersion in ice. This appeared to be the technique we were looking for, and we were therefore more than a little surprised when the manuscript was turned down by *Lancet*. Fortunately, Grant Williams, a British transplant surgeon, interceded on our behalf with the editor who then agreed to publish the manuscript. Williams was particularly well placed to present our case since he was very familiar with the work, having preceded me in the same laboratory on a kidney preservation project.

"A scientific argument continues as to the precise mode of action of an 'intracellular' flush solution and which of cold storage or perfusion is the better method for clinical use. Perhaps this controversy is one of the reasons for the article's frequent citation. Nevertheless, our ability to preserve kidneys for a day or so has greatly altered the logistics of clinical kidney transplantation during the past ten years."

1. **Keeler R, Swinney J, Taylor R M R & Uldall P R.** The problem of renal preservation. *Brit. J. Urol.* **38**:653-6, 1966.

CC/NUMBER 24
JUNE 11, 1984

This Week's Citation Classic™

Mazze R I, Trudell J R & Cousins M J. Methoxyflurane metabolism and renal dysfunction: clinical correlation in man. *Anesthesiology* **35**:247-52, 1971.
[Dept. Anesthesia, Stanford Univ. Sch. Med., and Vet. Admin. Hosp., Palo Alto, CA]

This was the first controlled study to demonstrate that postoperative nephrotoxicity in surgical patients anesthetized with methoxyflurane was due to biodegradation of the anesthetic to inorganic fluoride. Metabolic pathways were proposed to support the hypothesis, since confirmed, that inorganic fluoride caused methoxyflurane nephrotoxicity. [The *SCI*® indicates that this paper has been cited in over 190 publications since 1971.]

Richard I. Mazze
Department of Anesthesia
Stanford University School of Medicine
and
Anesthesiology Service
Veterans Administration Medical Center
Palo Alto, CA 94304

March 8, 1984

"In 1966, Crandell[1,2] reported that methoxyflurane caused high-output renal insufficiency in surgical patients. However, because of numerous errors in study design and lack of confirmatory studies, most anesthesiologists, myself included, did not accept Crandell's conclusion and methoxyflurane usage actually increased during the next five years to a rate of approximately two million administrations per year. To set aside what I believed was an unfair indictment, I designed a prospective, randomized, controlled clinical study[3] which would overcome the flaws in Crandell's work. To my surprise, all 12 patients administered methoxyflurane showed signs of renal dysfunction. Just prior to publication of this study, Taves[4] reported the case of a patient anesthetized with methoxyflurane who had an elevated plasma fluoride level and clinical nephrotoxicity. Michael Cousins, James Trudell, and I (the cited article) then measured inorganic fluoride and oxalic acid levels in the stored serum of patients from my earlier study.[3] We showed a correlation between the degree of nephrotoxicity and the extent of methoxyflurane biotransformation to these metabolites and suggested that inorganic fluoride was the principal nephrotoxin. For the first time, a clear cause-and-effect relationship had been established between methoxyflurane administration, its biotransformation to inorganic fluoride, and the clinical syndrome of postanesthetic high-output renal insufficiency.

"Subsequently, Cousins and I developed an animal model for methoxyflurane nephrotoxicity in Fischer 344 rats in which we could demonstrate dose-related biochemical and renal morphological lesions similar to those seen in humans.[5] In my opinion, this is one of the best animal models of a clinical disease entity available to date. We followed this study with several other animal studies in which we demonstrated that: induction of hepatic microsomal enzymes increased the extent of the renal lesion; there was toxic interaction between nephrotoxic antibiotics, such as gentamicin, and methoxyflurane; and oxalic acid was not of primary importance in the methoxyflurane renal lesion. In later clinical studies, we were able to precisely establish the dose-related nature of the methoxyflurane renal lesion and to demonstrate that the threshold level of inorganic fluoride necessary to produce nephrotoxicity was approximately 40-50 μM.[6] In addition to *in vivo* human and animal studies, we performed *in vitro* studies with hepatic microsomal preparations in which we compared the defluorination and nephrotoxic potential of methoxyflurane with that of the other clinically available fluorinated inhalation anesthetics—halothane, enflurane, and isoflurane—and with several experimental agents.

"Since 1971, my laboratory has published more than 50 scientific articles relating to the defluorination and renal effects of anesthetic agents. The cited article established the basis for these studies and those of other investigators studying anesthetic nephrotoxicity. As a result, methoxyflurane has all but dropped from clinical usage and most hospital pharmacies do not even have a bottle on their shelves. In the early 1970s, there was a great deal of interest in our studies and pressure from the manufacturers of methoxyflurane regarding our work, so there was a constant air of excitement in the laboratory. The atmosphere is less charged today, but we have a sense of satisfaction knowing that our research helped to shape clinical practice and, no doubt, to decrease anesthetic morbidity and mortality. The subject has recently been reviewed."[7]

1. **Crandell W B, Pappas S G & Macdonald A.** Nephrotoxicity associated with methoxyflurane anesthesia. *Anesthesiology* **27**:591-607, 1966.
2. **Crandell W B.** Citation Classic. Commentary on *Anesthesiology* **27**:591-607, 1966. *Current Contents/Life Sciences* **22**(30):10, 23 July 1979.
3. **Mazze R I, Shue G L & Jackson S H.** Renal dysfunction associated with methoxyflurane anesthesia: a randomized, prospective clinical evaluation. *J. Amer. Med. Assn.* **216**:278-88, 1971. (Cited 135 times.)
4. **Taves D R, Fry B W, Freeman R B & Gillies A J.** Toxicity following methoxyflurane anesthesia. II. Fluoride concentrations in nephrotoxicity. *J. Amer. Med. Assn.* **214**:91-5, 1970. (Cited 160 times.)
5. **Mazze R I, Cousins M J & Kosek J C.** Dose-related methoxyflurane nephrotoxicity in rats: a biochemical and pathological correlation. *Anesthesiology* **36**:571-87, 1972. (Cited 115 times.)
6. **Cousins M J & Mazze R I.** Methoxyflurane nephrotoxicity: a study of dose-response in man. *J. Amer. Med. Assn.* **225**:1611-16, 1973. (Cited 120 times.)
7. **Mazze R I.** Nephrotoxicity of fluorinated anaesthetic agents. (Mazze R I, ed.) *Inhalation anaesthesia.* London: Saunders, 1983. p. 469-84.

CC/NUMBER 38
SEPTEMBER 17, 1984

This Week's Citation Classic™

Schilling R F. Intrinsic factor studies. II. The effect of gastric juice on the urinary excretion of radioactivity after the oral administration of radioactive vitamin B_{12}. *J. Lab. Clin. Med.* **42**:860-6, 1953.
[Dept. Medicine, Univ. Wisconsin Medical School, Madison, WI]

This paper describes a urinary excretion test for estimating a patient's ability to absorb vitamin B_{12}. The most common cause of failure to absorb vitamin B_{12} is pernicious anemia, but several other conditions also cause B_{12} malabsorption and can be diagnosed or suspected on the basis of studies of vitamin B_{12} absorption. [The *SCI*® indicates that this paper has been cited in over 740 publications since 1955.]

Robert F. Schilling
Department of Medicine
University of Wisconsin
Madison, WI 53792

May 22, 1984

"After spending two thoroughly stimulating years in Harvard's Thorndike Laboratory at the Boston City Hospital, I returned to the University of Wisconsin in 1951 and was given time and space to pursue my research interest in nutritional anemia. The use of radioisotopes as tracers in the study of biology, including human physiology, was relatively new but obviously capable of answering many questions. Rosenblum and Woodbury[1] had recently prepared radioactive vitamin B_{12} by providing ^{60}Co in the biosynthetic process. Heinle and his colleagues[2] had shown that the absorption of vitamin B_{12}, estimated by measuring fecal radioactivity for seven days, was greatly below normal in patients with pernicious anemia.

"I was attempting to measure absorption of the vitamin by determining radioactivity in plasma or urine in normal subjects, but no radioactivity was detected with the relatively insensitive apparatus available to me. I had been reading about cold carrier techniques in a radiochemistry text and decided to use what might be called an *in vivo* cold carrier technique: I injected a large amount of nonradioactive B_{12} after having drunk a physiologic quantity of radioactive B_{12}. The urine collected over the next 24 hours contained easily detectable and quantifiable radioactivity indicating that the orally ingested material had been absorbed. A trial of the technique on a patient known to have pernicious anemia produced no detectable urine radioactivity.

"The urine radioactivity test has been widely used as a test for vitamin B_{12} absorption because of its simplicity and utility. It has been carefully compared with fecal excretion and whole body counting methods, and the correlation of results is good. Vitamin B_{12} absorption tests have enabled studies which have significantly increased our understanding of gastrointestinal physiology.

"Physicians and patients are always hopeful that the patient's symptoms are due to a curable disorder. This urine radioactivity test is useful in sorting out the mechanisms of conditions leading to vitamin B_{12} deficiency, an ideally treatable or even preventable illness. For a recent review, see reference 3."

1. **Rosenblum C & Woodbury D T.** Cobalt 60 labeled vitamin B_{12} of high specific activity. *Science* **113**:215, 1951.
2. **Heinle R W, Welch A D, Scharf V, Meacham G C & Prusoff W H.** Studies of excretion (and absorption) of Co^{60}-labeled vitamin B_{12} in pernicious anemia. *Trans. Assn. Am. Physician.* **65**:214-22, 1952. (Cited 235 times since 1955.)
3. **Chanarin I.** *The megaloblastic anaemias.* Oxford: Blackwell Scientific, 1979. 800 p.

CC/NUMBER 20
MAY 18, 1981

Stanley E R & Metcalf D. Partial purification and some properties of the factor in normal and leukaemic human urine stimulating mouse bone marrow colony growth *in vitro*. *Aust. J. Exp. Biol. Med. Sci.* **47**:467-83, 1969. [Cancer Res. Unit, Walter and Eliza Hall Inst., Royal Melbourne Hosp., Victoria, Australia]

The growth factor in human urine which stimulates the formation of macrophage clones from murine bone marrow cells in agar culture was purified 200-fold. This colony stimulating factor (CSF) was active at concentrations of less than 100 ng/ml and appeared to be an acidic glycoprotein. [The *SCI*® indicates that this paper has been cited over 150 times since 1969.]

E. Richard Stanley
Department of Microbiology
and Immunology
Albert Einstein College of Medicine
Yeshiva University
Bronx, NY 10461

April 22, 1981

"The work reported in this paper was initiated in late 1967 during the first year of my PhD with Don Metcalf at the Walter and Eliza Hall Institute in Melbourne. Don was away on sabbatical for my first nine months there. During this time, Bill Robinson, Gordon Ada, and I, with the help of Ray Bradley (the originator of the agar culture method for bone marrow colony formation), had concluded, on the basis of studies with mouse serum, that CSF was not a transforming virus, as some had thought, but probably a protein or glycoprotein. Following our discovery of CSF in human urine[1] and Don's subsequent return from sabbatical, we set about purifying it from this potentially abundant source.

"From preliminary studies with 2.0 l. batches of urine, it became clear that we were dealing with a minor urinary component and that considerable volumes of urine would be required. The resources of the entire male staff of the Institute were mobilized and urine was collected in white buckets placed by the urinals. These buckets, with their accompanying poster requesting contributions (and subsequent graffiti), became an Institute conversation piece. On Fridays, many Institute members would spend an hour or two at the local 'pub' but loyally returned to the Institute afterwards to donate. Collections on these days were almost overflowing but, to our subsequent dismay, contained subnormal CSF concentrations!

"The handling of 20-100 l. quantities of urine presented several new occupational hazards. I recall opening the door of the lab early one morning to step into three inches of water—the result of a failure in the 'automatic' system I had set up for the dialysis of large volumes.

"The division of labor was such that I was able to concentrate on the biochemistry. However, the *in vitro* agar culture assay for CSF, although sensitive, takes seven days. Progress seemed slow to me and even slower to Don. Nevertheless, during this study, we became convinced that because of its specificity, occurrence, and action at very low concentrations, we were studying a potent growth factor and that the key to understanding its role was its complete purification and radiolabeling. Despite considerable difficulties, complete purification and radiolabeling of this type of CSF was achieved.[2] We now know that human urinary CSF is a macrophage growth factor and only one subclass of the CSFs that stimulate granulocyte and/or macrophage production.[3]

"I think this publication has been highly cited because it was the first detailed description of the characteristics of a white blood cell growth factor. It indicated that complete purification was feasible and emphasized its possible physiological role as a humoral regulator of hemopoiesis.

"I am pleased to see a thoroughly Australian paper become a *Citation Classic*. I hope this can continue in spite of the low priority given to the funding of basic research by the Australian government."

1. **Robinson W A, Stanley E R & Metcalf D.** Stimulation of bone marrow colony growth *in vitro* by human urine. *Blood* **33**:396-9, 1969.
2. **Stanley E R & Heard P M.** Factors regulating macrophage production and growth. Purification and some properties of the colony stimulating factor from medium conditioned by mouse L cells. *J. Biol. Chem.* **252**:4305-12, 1977.
3. **Stanley E R.** Colony stimulating factor (CSF) radioimmunoassay: detection of a CSF subclass stimulating macrophage production. *Proc. Nat. Acad. Sci. US* **76**:2969-73, 1979.

Chapter

10

Perinatology

A modest number of 12 Citation Classics are listed here, but among these few are several important as well as popular articles. The first, by Noyes, was published as the lead article in the first issue of *Fertility and Sterility.* This 22-page article was heavily illustrated to document histologic changes in the endometrium following ovulation until menses. Noyes' co-authors are responsible for his name as first author although Hertig received the editor's request for the article. Another important report published in the early 1950s is that by Thiersch on the abortifacient and teratogenic property of a folic acid antagonist. This was an advance and tragically unheeded warning that some compounds would have dramatic and disastrous effects on the developing fetus with little outward influence on the metabolism of the mother. A decade later, the mandatory study of the teratogenic potential of drugs for women was enacted into U.S. law. The unexplained phenomenon that operating room nurses have a miscarriage rate nearly four times higher than general duty nurses is matched by an equal discrepancy among anesthesiologists versus physicians in other specialties (p. 297). Anesthetic gases were the unproved cause, but this concept is indirectly supported by similar data from dental technologists who use nitrous oxide.

Shelley became the "glycogen girl" in her laboratory while studying pregnancy toxemia in sheep and was able to associate glycogen stores in fetal animals with their ability to survive in anaerobic environments. Shelley cites a publication by Robert Boyle in 1670 as an original investigation in this field and states that Claude Bernard also noted the presence of glycogen in fetal tissues. Of course, Shelley's data do not mean that fetal or newborn pO_2 is unimportant, and blood drawn from blood vessels of the fetal scalp is the earliest way to secure this information (p. 299). This research has been cited as a part of the origin of fetal medicine, along with amniocentesis and fetal transfusion, even though the first application for funds to support this project was denied.

Surviving newborn infants undersize for their term have been grouped as "preemies," but the "This Week's Citation Classic" (TWCC) by Warkany et al. notes that this is an error. Since the growth rate varies between individuals and growth begins at the earliest moment of intrauterine life, variations in growth rate will produce infants of different sizes at equivalent ages. As a consequence, such infants are not preemies; they are only "small for date."

That thermal regulation by newborn infants is as fully developed as that in adults will be a surprise to many (p. 301). The reason that 33 to 34°C is the optimal air temperature and thus used in the newborn nursery as opposed to 27°C for adults is the result of differences in body size, blood flow, sweat secretion, body fat, and other variables.

High oxygen tension was normally therapeutic for infantile respiratory distress syndrome (RDS) even though many patients did poorly under this treatment. Northway evaluated medical records and X-rays, and concluded that 13 of the 32 infants he had studied had a hitherto undescribed syndrome which was termed bronchopulmonary dysplasia. The etiologic agent was the high tension of oxygen used in the respirator (see also TWCC in Chapter 11 on Respiratory Disease).

The RDS, a combination of vascular and respiratory complications that may affect adults as well as children, was found 25 years ago to involve failure of the heart's left ventricle and patency of the ductus arteriosus in newborn infants. Rudolph mentions that this study might not be possible under the present conditions of institutional review. Lack of pulmonary surfactant and the consequent restraint of lung expansion is another associate of RDS. Amniocentesis is an avenue to the prediagnosis of hyaline membrane disease, and a high lecithin-sphingomyelin ratio foretells inadequate lung development in utero. A slight modification of the published method is virtually 100 percent accurate in predicting lung maturity.

The fourth article on RDS recommended that steroids be administered in utero if a risk for incomplete lung development exists. *Lancet* rejected what was later to become a Citation Classic. The original idea was derived from studies of prematurely born lambs that had been given ACTH. Though these lambs were preemies, their lungs were mature, air-filled organs. From this the therapy for human preemies followed.

Kawasaki has written a revealing TWCC that explains how his self-confidence was shaken when he saw atypical patients with the disease that now bears his name. He feared that he may have erred is describing the limits of the new syndrome. A discussion about the true diagnosis of some difficult cases at the Tokyo Pediatric Association meeting established his priority in describing this novel lymph node syndrome. The first publication on Kawasaki disease appeared in a journal of allergology although the cause of the disease is still unknown.

Perinatology is itself too young to have spawned much in the way of review literature. The review journals *Seminars in Perinatology* and *Clinics in Perinatology* are still pre-pubescent, not yet having reached their ninth and twelfth birthdays. Nevertheless, readers interested in the subjects of the Citation Classics described in this chapter will be pleased to learn that the entire 1984 volume of *Seminars in Perinatology* was devoted to intrauterine growth retardation (17 articles), fetal and neonatal oxygenation (9 articles), and hyaline membrane disease (7 articles). These three subjects obviously continue to be of interest to perinatologists.

Occasionally, *Current Problems in Pediatrics* devotes an issue to some aspect of neonatology, as do *Clinics in Obstetrics and Gynaecology* and *Clinical Obstetrics and Gynecology.* Articles in recent issues include:

Campbell S, editor. Ultrasound in obstetrics and gynaecology: recent advances. *Clin. Obstet. Gynaecol.* **10:**369–643, 1983 (a collection of 13 articles).

Cowett R M. Pathophysiology, diagnosis and management of glucose homeostasis in the neonate. *Curr. Prob. Pediatr* **15:**(3), March 1985.

Cruikshank D P, editor. Antepartum fetal surveillance. *Clin. Obstet. Gynecol.* **25:**633–807, 1982 (a collection of 10 articles).

Donn S M, Faix R G & Gates M R. Neonatal transport. *Curr. Prob. Pediatr.* **15:**(4), April 1985.

Glaze D G & Zion T E. Infantile spasms. *Curr. Prob. Pediatr* **15:**(11), November 1985.

Merkatz I R, editor. Preterm birth. *Clin. Obstet. Gynecol.* **27:**537–694, 1984 (a collection of 11 articles).

Platt L D, editor. Obstetric ultrasound. *Clin. Obstet. Gynecol.* **27:**267–427, 1984 (a collection of 12 articles).

Other recent review articles in perinatology include:

Lin C C. Intrauterine growth retardation. *Obstet. Gynecol. Annu.* **14:**127–221, 1985.

Robinson A & Henry G P. Prenatal diagnosis by amniocentesis. *Annu. Rev. Med.* **36:**13–26, 1985.

Seeds J W. Impaired fetal growth: definition and clinical diagnosis. *Obstet. Gynecol.* **64:**303–10, 1984.

Varma T R. Low birth weight babies. The small for gestational age. A review of current management. *Obstet. Gynecol. Surv.* **39:**616–24, 1984.

This Week's Citation Classic

CC/NUMBER 14
APRIL 7, 1980

Noyes R W, Hertig A T & Rock J. Dating the endometrial biopsy. *Fert. Steril.* **1**:3-25, 1950.
[Free Hosp. Women, Brookline, MA and Dept. Gynecology, Harvard Med. Sch., Cambridge, MA]

Rapid changes in endometrial histologic patterns following ovulation permit assignment of 'dates' which correlate well with other timing measures of ovulation in the study of human fertility. This methodology paper includes a graph of histologic changes during the menstrual cycle, a series of representative photomicrographs, and clinical correlations among 300 patients. [The *SCI*® indicates that this paper has been cited over 330 times since 1961.]

Robert W. Noyes
334 Tennessee Lane
Palo Alto, CA 94306

February 1, 1980

"John Rock, pioneer fertologist now living in Temple, New Hampshire, and M. K. Bartlett first published on endometrial dating in 1937.[1] Arthur Hertig, eminent embryologist and gynecologic pathologist now at the New England Primate Center, improved the method[2] and used it extensively in his famous research with John Rock on early human ova.

"I first encountered endometrial dating in 1948 when I was a volunteer fellow in pathology at the Free Hospital for Women, Brookline, Massachusetts, where Hertig was chief pathologist. I learned much from an unpublished graph contributed by J. P. F. LaTour, currently professor of gynecologic oncology at the McGill University School of Medicine. Some of the younger clinicians, such as myself, were still wondering whether or not endometrial responsiveness could be accurately dated. Sensing this, Hertig suggested that I undertake, as a special project, a 'blind' comparison of endometrial dates with clinical endpoints such as basal body temperature and onset of succeeding menses.

"Just at this time, Pendleton Tompkins, editor of the future journal *Fertility and Sterility,* requested Hertig to submit a lead manuscript for volume 1. I readily agreed to add my clinical correlation results to this worthwhile cause, and to get some representative photomicrographs taken. But I was completely unprepared to find my name as first author on the published paper. Such is the generosity of truly great people like Arthur Hertig and John Rock. The photomicrographs were made by Leo Goodman at the Boston City Hospital, and I drafted the captions.

"The original interest in the 1950 paper may have been sustained by follow-up studies such as my report with J. O. Haman on 1,007 biopsies from infertile women,[3] my papers on the uniformity of secretory endometrium[4] and on the underdeveloped secretory endometrium,[5] plus chapters in books by Greenblatt,[6] Joel,[7] and Norris, Hertig, and Abell.[8] Endometrial dating has been found to correlate well with the ovulatory peak of luteotrophic hormone, and with electron microscopic and biochemical measures of endometrial responsiveness—all the work of many others. I am naturally pleased that this paper has been so widely cited, and I attribute this to a continuing need for an objective secretory phase time scale until someone discovers a way to pinpoint the moment of ovulation."

1. **Rock J & Bartlett M K.** Biopsy studies of human endometrium. *J. Amer. Med. Ass.* **108**:2022-8, 1937.
2. **Hertig A T.** Diagnosing the endometrial biopsy. (Engle E T, ed.) *Proceedings: conference on diagnosis in sterility.* Springfield, IL: Charles C. Thomas, 1946. p. 93-128.
3. **Noyes R W & Haman J O.** Accuracy of endometrial dating. *Fert. Steril.* **4**:504-17, 1953.
4. **Noyes R W.** Uniformity of secretory endometrium, multiple sections removed from 100 uteri. *Fert. Steril.* 7:103-8, 1956.
5. --------------. The underdeveloped secretory endometrium. *Amer. J. Obstet. Gynecol.* 77:929-45, 1959.
6. --------------. Endometrial dating for the detection of ovulation. (Greenblatt R, ed.) *Ovulation, stimulation, suppression, detection.* Philadelphia: J.B. Lippincott, 1966. p. 319-28.
7. --------------. Endometrial biopsy. (Joel C A, ed.) *Fertility disturbances in men and women.* Basel: S. Karger, 1971. p. 399-412.
8. --------------. Normal phases of the endometrium. (Norris H J, Hertig A T & Abell M R, eds.) *The uterus.* Baltimore: Williams and Wilkins, 1973. p. 110-35.

CC/NUMBER 7
FEBRUARY 13, 1984

This Week's Citation Classic™

Thiersch J B. Therapeutic abortions with a folic acid antagonist, 4-aminopteroylglutamic acid (4-amino P.G.A.) administered by the oral route. *Amer. J. Obstet. Gynecol.* **63**:1298-304, 1952.
[Dept. Pathology, Univ. Washington Medical School, Seattle, WA]

4-Aminopteroylglutamic acid (4-amino PGA) given in nontoxic doses to pregnant women induced malformation and death in the fetuses. With that, an entire new field was opened mandating investigation of all drugs given to pregnant women for their teratogenic effect on the fetus. A second specific effect was noted on the reduction of production of chorionic gonadotropins. [The *SCI*® indicates that this paper has been cited in over 205 publications since 1955.]

John B. Thiersch
7552 34th Street Northwest
Seattle, WA 98107

December 29, 1983

"It all started in 1948 at the Sloan-Kettering Institute in New York, while I was studying the toxicity of folic acid antagonists. A bitch, treated with a nontoxic dose of 4-aminopteroylglutamic acid (4-amino PGA), bled vaginally and aborted. The animal was not supposed to have been pregnant. I took this single observation seriously and followed it up with a number of experiments in mice, rats, and dogs studying the effects of folic acid antagonists in pregnant animals and fetuses. From this evolved the fact of a differential toxicity of drugs between mother and fetus with a teratogenic effect of the drugs in different stages of pregnancy. In the course of the study, it soon became evident that the idea to control reproduction of the pregnant female with antimetabolites was accompanied with the danger of malformation in surviving fetuses. The whole approach was therefore abandoned. However, the fact remains that the compounds given to human mothers might induce malformation in the offspring. This was demonstrated ten years later when, with thalidomide, the human experiments preceded the animal work and large numbers of malformations were induced in the human fetus.

"Subsequently, the teratogenic effects of drugs on the fetus led to legislation in the US in 1962 demanding careful evaluation of drug effects on the fetus before a compound is recommended for use in pregnant women. The striking inhibitory effects on the production of chorionic gonadotropins led to the introduction of folic acid antagonists into the therapy of chorionic carcinoma.

"The effect of 4-amino PGA in pregnant women and its teratogenic action on the human fetus was the forerunner of many other compounds coming out of the field of chemotherapy of cancer.[1,2]

"I believe this publication is so highly cited because it opened up a new field—the effect of drugs on the fetus *in utero.*"

1. **Thiersch J B.** Control of reproduction in rats with the aid of antimetabolites and early experiences with antimetabolites as abortifacient agents in man. *Acta Endocrinol.* (Suppl. 28):37-45, 1956.
2. ----------------. Effects of antimetabolites on the fetus and litter of the rat *in utero* (second review). *International Conference on Planned Parenthood, 6th, India, 1959. Report of the proceedings: family planning: motivations and methods.* London: International Planned Parenthood Federation, 1959. p. 154-64.

This Week's Citation Classic

Cohen E N, Bellville J W & Brown B W, Jr. Anesthesia, pregnancy, and miscarriage: a study of operating room nurses and anesthetists. *Anesthesiology* **35**:343-7, 1971.
[Departments of Anesthesia, and Community and Preventive Medicine, Stanford University School of Medicine, CA]

Retrospective surveys of 67 operating room nurses and 92 general duty nurses indicate that during the years 1966-1970, 29.7 percent of pregnancies in operating room nurses ended in spontaneous miscarriage compared with only 8.8 percent in the control group. A similar pattern was observed in a second study of 50 anesthetists and 81 physicians practicing in specialties other than anesthesia. During the period 1965-1970, the physician anesthetists evidenced a 37.8 percent spontaneous miscarriage rate compared with 10.3 percent in the control group. [The *SCI*® indicates that this paper has been cited in over 190 publications since 1971, making this the 3rd most-cited paper published in this journal.]

Ellis N. Cohen
Department of Anesthesia
Stanford University Medical Center
Stanford, CA 94305

June 16, 1983

"While attending the Third European Anesthesiology Conference in Prague in 1970, I heard with significant concern reports presented by Askrog[1] of Denmark and Lencz[2] of Rumania suggesting an association between work in the operating room and a high incidence of spontaneous abortion in female anesthetists. These investigators had, in turn, been stimulated by an earlier survey of female anesthetists in Russia reported by Vaisman[3] in 1967. Unfortunately, each of these three studies was technically defective, lacking adequate statistical control. Although epidemiology was far removed from my major interests in drug metabolism, I felt the need to initiate a well-controlled study to evaluate the problem and confirm or deny its existence.

"Accordingly, two retrospective surveys were planned and conducted. Each included an operating room-exposed and an unexposed control group. The first study comprised 159 married operating room and general duty nurses. The second study involved 131 anesthetists and physicians practicing in specialties other than anesthesia. Every effort was made to conduct the study so as to avoid bias. The first study of nurses was conducted by means of a long, detailed questionnaire. All questions were asked in fixed format by two trained observers. The second study in physicians was completed by mailed questionnaires. Only after completion of the questionnaire were the respondents instructed to open a second sealed envelope which explained the purpose of the study. Results of both studies were confirmatory and indicated large statistically significant differences between the experimental and control groups in the incidence of spontaneous abortion. We thus concluded the presence of a fetal lethality associated with work in the operating room, possibly due to the anesthetic gases, although we could not incriminate the anesthetic agents in a cause-effect relationship.

"Subsequent to publication of the above report, some 20 epidemiologic studies have been conducted in the US and abroad which largely confirm the presence of similar occupational hazards. Individuals at risk include physicians, nurses, technicians, dentists, and chairside assistants. In the US alone, this number exceeds some 214,000 individuals. The most recent survey conducted in 1980 among dentists and dental assistants establishes the additional presence of a serious neurological dysfunction among those anesthetically exposed and strongly suggests a causative role for nitrous oxide.[4]

"Frequent citation of our paper lies primarily in its broad public health concern. As a result of this small, carefully controlled study, the operating room environment was recognized as a new source of potential health hazard. Wide interest in this problem rapidly developed among occupationally exposed doctors, dentists, and nurses and from governmental agencies concerned with the control of health hazards in the workplace. These interests and concerns led to expanded studies serving to define the seriousness and extent of the problem."

1. **Askrog V F.** Teratogenic effects of inhalational anesthetics. (Abstract.) (Hoder J, Jedlička R & Pokorný J, eds.) *Advances in anaesthesiology and resuscitation: proceedings of the third European Congress of Anaesthesiology held in Prague 31.8.-4.9.1970.* Prague: Avicenum—Czechoslovak Medical Press, 1972. Vol. I. p. 383.
2. **Lencz L, Nemes C & Berta L.** Psychische Belastungen und Morbidität der Anaesthesisten. (Abstract.) (Hoder J, Jedlička R & Pokorný J, eds.) *Advances in anaesthesiology and resuscitation: proceedings of the third European Congress of Anaesthesiology held in Prague 31.8.-4.9.1970.* Prague: Avicenum—Czechoslovak Medical Press, 1972. Vol. II. p. 1581.
3. **Vaisman A I.** Working conditions in surgery and their effect on the health of anesthesiologists. *Eksp. Khir. Anest.* **3**:44-9, 1967.
4. **Cohen E N, Brown B W, Wu M L, Whitcher C E, Brodsky J B, Gift H C, Greenfield W, Jones T W & Driscoll E J.** Occupational disease in dentistry and chronic exposure to trace anesthetic gases. *J. Amer. Dent. Assn.* **101**:21-31, 1980.

This Week's Citation Classic

Shelley H J. Glycogen reserves and their changes at birth and in anoxia.
Brit. Med. Bull. **17**:137-43, 1961.
[Nuffield Inst. Medical Res., Univ. Oxford, Oxford, England]

This paper describes the changes in tissue glycogen concentration which occur during fetal life and the first few days after birth. Large amounts accumulate in the liver and skeletal muscles of many species as a store for use after birth. The high concentration in the heart enables the fetus to survive for long periods without oxygen. [The *SCI*® indicates that this paper has been cited over 265 times since 1961.]

Heather J. Shelley
University of Oxford
Nuffield Institute for Medical Research
Headington, Oxford OX3 9DS
England

February 1, 1980

"This was a review paper and one reason it has been cited so often is that reviews make convenient references. Another is that the timing was right. It was becoming clear that not only the survival but also the quality of the newborn child could be affected by events occurring before and immediately after birth. Evidence was accumulating that lack of oxygen or glucose during the perinatal period could cause permanent brain damage and clinicians were anxious to prevent this.

"The article summarized data showing that the fetus accumulates glycogen during the latter part of gestation and suggested that if these reserves were deficient, the newborn's chances of normal survival would be jeopardized. This suggestion was followed by a great deal of more sophisticated research, aimed at discovering whether I was right, how carbohydrate metabolism was regulated in the fetus and newborn, and whether it could be modified to their advantage, a debate which is still in progress.

"I did not foresee my debut as 'the glycogen girl.' In 1956 I was a research assistant investigating the aetiology of pregnancy toxaemia in sheep. My attention was focused on the mother's glycogen reserves, but the Institute's director, G.S. Dawes, had become intrigued by the ability of fetal and newborn animals to survive for long periods without oxygen, an ability which was lost with increasing maturity. The phenomenon had been described by Robert Boyle,[1] but the mechanism was still obscure. Energy was obtained by anaerobic glycolysis and Claude Bernard had noted the presence of glycogen in fetal tissues. It seemed possible that the amount available to a vital organ could be a factor limiting survival. To our delight, we found a good correlation between anoxic survival and the glycogen content of the heart. We compared data from fetal lambs, rodents, and, thanks to the generosity of the National Institutes of Health, rhesus monkeys studied in Puerto Rico, one of the more glamorous places to pursue research. The monkey data were added to the graphs just before the paper went to press, the day we came back from San Juan.

"The next task was to see if the animal data were applicable to man. The review included values obtained at abortion, but babies near term could only be studied *post mortem*. Having no medical qualifications, and being pregnant myself by then, I was wholly dependent on the help of clinical colleagues in three large hospitals. Their generous collaboration enabled me to confirm its relevance, and the work was a good example of how clinical data can be interpreted in the light of animal experiments. I am still working in the field, investigating the response of the fetus to hypo- and hyperglycemia, in the hope that the treatment of pregnant women and their children can be improved still further. More recent reviews have been prepared by myself[2] and W.W. Hay, Jr."[3]

1. **Boyle R.** New pneumatical experiments about respiration. *Phil. Trans.* **5**:2011-31, 1670.
2. **Shelley H J, Bassett J M & Milner R D G.** Control of carbohydrate metabolism in the fetus and newborn. *Brit. Med. Bull.* **31**:37-43, 1975.
3. **Hay W W, Jr.** Fetal glucose metabolism. *Semin. Perinatol.* **3**:157-76, 1979.

CC/NUMBER 34
AUGUST 20, 1984

This Week's Citation Classic™

Saling E. Neues Vorgehen zur Untersuchung des Kindes unter der Geburt: Einführung, Technik und Grundlagen. (New procedures for examining the fetus during labor: introduction, technique and basics.) *Arch. Gynäkol.* **197**:108-22, 1962.
[Städtischen Frauenklinik und Hebammenlehranstalt Berlin-Neukölln, Fed. Rep. Germany]

The paper describes the first fetal scalp sampling during labor. Basic findings concerning intrauterine blood gas and acid-base balance under the aspect of fetal circulation as well as the technique of sampling are presented. [The *SCI*® includes over 145 cites to this paper, making it one of the two most-cited papers for this journal.]

Erich Saling
Institute of Perinatal Medicine
Free University of Berlin
and
Department of Obstetrics
Frauenklinik Berlin-Neukölln
D-1000 Berlin 44
Federal Republic of Germany

March 7, 1984

"Primarily, we were working on other scientific and clinical projects. At the end of the 1950s, we wanted to prove which of the methods then used was the most effective one for resuscitating asphyctic newborns in the delivery room of our department.

"The groundwork for these investigations was based on two achievements. One was the first successful catheterisation of the aorta of the human newborn through the umbilical arteries. Originally this was used for a new technique of blood exchange in newborns with erythroblastosis,[1,2] and for collecting blood samples for gas analysis from the newborn during resuscitation.[3] The second achievement was the development—in cooperation with the biochemist K. Damaschke—of the first method for quick measurement of O_2 saturation in blood samples.[4]

"In order to start the exchange transfusion in cases of severe erythroblastosis immediately after delivery, we took blood samples from the presenting part of the fetus hours before birth for the necessary serologic and hematologic investigations.

"The available micromethod for O_2 analysis and the experience that blood samples can easily be withdrawn from the fetus gave us the now fairly simple idea of performing blood gas analyses too. This was the birth of fetal blood analysis (FBA). What then followed seems rather curious today. The first applications for research grants were turned down: one expert thought it ethically inadmissible to break the taboo of the unborn infant and to withdraw blood samples from the fetus. Another expert, whose statement was not based on any research findings, believed that the caput succedaneum (which does not by far occur during all labors), would basically eliminate any conclusions because blood drawn from this part of the circulation is not a suitable indicator of the central fetal circulation.

"Nevertheless, fetal blood analyses have proved their relevance in many places, both from the clinical side and from the point of view of research. Their reliability has been confirmed by numerous examiners both in animal experiments and in clinical use. We published an up-to-date review in English in 1981.[5]

"I think that the reason the original publication has been so frequently cited lies in the fact that FBA—combined with cardiotocography—represents the most modern clinical supervision of the fetus during labor. FBA has also become a basic method for clinical research in the past 22 years. From the historical point of view, FBA is a method which enabled the first direct approach to the human fetus by blood analysis. In 1966, two English authors, Dobbs and Gairdner, described our activities—along with the development of amniocentesis by Bevis and fetal transfusion by Liley—as being 'the start of the science of foetal medicine.'"[6]

1. **Saling E.** Austauchtransfusion beim Neugeborenen über die Aorta abdominalis. *Geburtsh. Frauenheilk.* **19**:230-5, 1959.
2. ----------. Die Zwei-Katheter-Verfahren für den Blutaustausch beim Neugeborenen. *Deut. Med. Wochenschr.* **86**:294-8, 1961.
3. ----------. Über die Wirksamkeit von älteren und neuen Asphyxiebehandlungsmethoden. *Geburtsh. Frauenheilk.* **20**:325-39, 1960.
4. **Saling E & Damaschke K.** Neue Mikroschnellmethode zur Messung des Blutsauerstoffs auf elektrochemischen Wege. *Klin. Wochenschr.* **39**:305-6, 1961.
5. **Saling E.** Fetal scalp blood analysis. *J. Perinatal Med.* **9**:165-77, 1981.
6. **Dobbs R H & Gairdner D.** Foetal medicine—who is to practise it? *Arch. Dis. Child.* **41**:453, 1966.

CC/NUMBER 49
DECEMBER 3, 1979

Warkany J, Monroe B B & Sutherland B S. Intrauterine growth retardation.
Amer. J. Dis. Child. **102**:249-79, 1961.
[Children's Hosp. Res. Found. and Dept. Pediat., Univ. Cincinnati, Coll. Med., Cincinnati, OH]

The concept of intrauterine growth retardation aided in differentiation of premature and pseudopremature small neonates is presented. The article illustrates how a long known phenomenon of human pathology can be concealed by terminological policies and be rediscovered by mothers' statements and animal experiments. [The *SCI*® indicates that this paper has been cited over 140 times since 1961.]

Josef Warkany
Children's Hospital Medical Center
Elland & Bethesda Avenues
Cincinnati, OH 45229

July 18, 1979

"It has long been known that some children are born undersized and underweight for their gestational age. Obstetricians knew this and spoke of 'microsomia' or 'placental insufficiency,' but many physicians paid no attention to the condition because they had little confidence in mothers' memories and estimates of pregnancy, and so they called small newborn babies simply prematures. This terminology generally persisted and in 1919 A. Ylppö, a pioneer in the treatment of premature babies, suggested that all newborns weighing less than 2500g be considered prematures, irrespective of their gestational age, and be given the care required by infants born too early.[1] Owing to this intentional misnomer, no distinction was made subsequently between immature (pseudopremature) and truly premature infants. This probably benefited the immatures but impeded research on etiology of microsomia and on the postnatal outcome of the condition.

"My attention was drawn to this shortcoming by some mothers of handicapped children who stated that their children had been small at birth and were called prematures by their pediatricians although they had been carried 9 months. Repeatedly they stated that their pregnancies had been unusual since there was no increase in size of their abdomens, that fetal activity in utero was feeble, and that the afterbirths were small. At the same time, I was taught by teratologic animal experiments in which times of fertilization and birth weights were accurately determined that intrauterine growth could be markedly retarded by adverse gestational conditions. This made me believe the mothers rather than the physicians who labeled all underweight newborns 'prematures.' Subsequently, we reviewed 27 of our cases, which according to mothers' histories, had marked intrauterine growth retardation (IUGR) and searched the literature for information about incidence, etiology, family and pregnancy histories, patients' properties, associated anomalies, placentas and outcome of IUGR. The prognosis of the children seen by us was generally poor but we realized that this could be due to selection. We pointed out the need for intensive and longitudinal studies of unselected cases of IUGR to learn more about the causes of slow prenatal growth and postnatal fate. Our article appeared at a favorable time, when pediatricians recognized that differentiation of prematures and pseudoprematures could be valuable, and a WHO Expert Committee on Maternal and Child Health recommended reassessment of the international definition of prematurity.[2] This was followed by a flood of publications of exact and detailed measurements, chemical determinations, and statistics. New names were coined for children with IUGR such as 'small for date babies,' 'dysmatures,' etc.

"In retrospect it seems that our article has been frequently quoted because it appeared at a time when neonatologists began intensive work on babies with very low birth weights which necessitated differentiation between normal and retarded prenatal growth."

1. **Ylppö A.** Zur Physiologie, Klinik und zum Schicksal der Fruhgeborenen. *Z. Kinderheilkd.* **24**:1-110, 1919.
2. **World Health Organization.** Expert Committee on Maternal and Child Health. Technical Report Service, 1961. p. 217.

CC/NUMBER 37
SEPTEMBER 15, 1980

This Week's Citation Classic

Brück K. Temperature regulation of the newborn infant.
Biol. Neonate 3:65-119, 1961.
[Inst. of Phys., University of Marburg, Frankfort, Fed. Rep. of Germany]

The demonstration showed that, in the neonate, the actions of the thermoregulatory control elements are more or less adjusted to the heat loss conditions which are determined by factors related to body size. It disproved the widespread concept of a grossly undeveloped thermoregulatory system. It is not the unresponsiveness but the very sensitive thermoregulatory reactions which require the observation of special environmental conditions for the well being of the neonate. [The *SCI®* indicates that this paper has been cited over 200 times since 1961.]

Kurt Brück
Institute of Physiology
Justus-Liebig-University Giessen
Aulweg 129, D 6300 Giessen
Federal Republic of Germany

July 2, 1979

"This paper appeared after the pediatric wards had been provided with thermostatized cribs—'incubators'—which made it possible to rear the low-birth-weight neonate at any desired thermal condition. However, at this time nobody knew exactly which ambient thermal condition was to be considered optimal. Like other functional systems, the neonatal thermoregulatory system was thought to be characterized merely by deficiencies in comparison with the adult. The paper not only showed that, unlike a poicilithermic organism, the neonate (including low-birth-weight neonates) is able to activate all effector elements known from the adult thermoregulatory system—thermogenesis, peripheral blood flow, sweat secretion—but that the temperature thresholds for the actuation of these control actions are appropriately adjusted to the smaller body size. In particular, it was shown that the increased heat production, which compensates for the enlarged heat loss in a cool environment, is based on a 'non-shivering' mechanism, whereas in the adult this heat arises solely from shivering.

"In a series of subsequent studies in my laboratory and in others it was shown that the neonate possesses a special tissue—brown adipose tissue—in which the extra heat is generated under the condition of cold exposure.[1]

"It could be inferred from our studies that the optimal environmental temperature is that at which the least thermoregulatory effort is needed to maintain deep body temperature at the normal value. This temperature—thermal neutral temperature—is much higher in the neonate (33-34° C) than in the adult (ca. 27° C).

"The plan for the experimental studies developed while I was working in the department of pediatrics, University of Hamburg. There, no technical means for performing such studies were then available. So I went back to physiology (University of Marburg) where I was able to develop the required methods and to interest the department of obstetrics and gynecology in these studies which were then carried out with the help of my wife, Monika, and an obstetrician, Horst Lemtis, in the Women's Hospital.

"The most delicate problem was to convince the nurses and parents that our machines would not harm the newborn babies. Our daughter helped us a great deal here. She was born in this hospital right at the time our set-up was ready for the first examination. She became our first 'subject'—the ice was broken. The first results of these studies were published in *Pflügers Archive* in the German language.[2,3] The '*Citation Classic*' was the first publication in English and it was thought of as a review of the preceding German papers.

"The studies in human neonates were followed by animal studies when we became interested in the neuronal and biocybernetic aspects of the interlocked control of shivering and non-shivering thermogenesis and the mechanism of long term adaptation of functional systems. It was felt that this could improve the understanding of the peculiarities in the neonate which have a lot in common with the special modifications in functional systems found during adaptation."

1. **Brück K & Wünnenberg B.** Studies on the significance of the multilocular brown adipose tissue for the thermogenesis in the newborn guinea pig. *Pflügers Arch.* **283**:1-16, 1965.
2. **Brück K, Brück M & Lemtis H.** Skin blood flow and temperature regulation in newborn infants. *Pflügers Arch.* **265**:55-65, 1957.
3. --. Thermoregulatory changes on energy metabolism in mature neonates. *Pflügers Arch.* **267**:382-91, 1958.

This Week's Citation Classic

CC/NUMBER 25
JUNE 21, 1982

Northway W H, Jr., Rosan R C & Porter D Y. Pulmonary disease following respirator therapy of hyaline-membrane disease: bronchopulmonary dysplasia. *N. Engl. J. Med.* **276**:357-68, 1967.
[Depts. Radiol., Pediat., and Pathol., Stanford Univ. Sch. Med., Stanford, CA]

Clinical, radiologic, and pathologic data are reported from a series of 32 newborn infants with severe respiratory distress syndrome (RDS), who were treated for 24 hours or more with warm, humidified 80-100 percent oxygen via an intermittent positive pressure respirator. Examples of acute, subacute, and chronic pulmonary disease, not previously described, are documented, and an idealized picture of a new syndrome termed bronchopulmonary dysplasia (BPD) is presented. [The *SCI*® indicates that this paper has been cited over 380 times since 1967.]

William H. Northway, Jr.
Department of Radiology
Stanford University Medical Center
Stanford, CA 94305

April 8, 1982

"Shortly after arriving at Stanford University Medical Center in 1964, I was asked to review a series of chest radiographs of an infant with severe respiratory distress syndrome (RDS). This infant was being treated with a then new therapy of artificial ventilation and high concentrations of supplemental oxygen and was having a prolonged and difficult course in the hospital. These chest radiographs showed an unusual progression of changes in the lungs from the initial picture of RDS to one resembling chronic obstructive pulmonary disease after one month of age. This was unusual because prior to this time infants with RDS either died by three or four days of age or were well by seven days of age. In order to determine what was occurring to infants receiving this therapy, I reviewed their records, radiographs, and pathology.

"This review was laborious since many of these infants were hospitalized for months and the concentration and duration of supplemental oxygen and duration of artificial ventilation and endotracheal intubation had to be thoroughly documented. At the outset these three variables and the severity of the initial underlying lung disease seemed most likely to be the factors associated with the development of the chronic lung disease. With completion of the review, it was evident that 13 of the 32 infants treated had developed a lung disease which had not previously been described.

"The data in this study also indicated that the appearance of the disease was most strongly associated with the prolonged use of 80-100 percent oxygen. I was, therefore, tempted to call the entity 'pulmonary oxygen toxicity in the newborn,' but after discussions with Rosan, who had reviewed the lung pathology, we decided to name it 'bronchopulmonary dysplasia' (BPD). This name accurately described our interpretation of the pathology without attributing an etiology.

"The report of this study faced a mixed reception at first from neonatologists, probably for two reasons. The first was that no physician wants to believe that a therapy he is employing may produce a problem such as chronic lung disease. The second reason was related to the fact that the study had been done by a young pediatric radiologist and not an experienced neonatologist.

"I believe this publication has been highly cited because it was the first to describe a new syndrome of acute, subacute, and chronic lung disease in the newborn infant with severe RDS. This syndrome was rapidly recognized as occurring throughout the world when newborn infants with respiratory difficulty were artificially ventilated with supplemental oxygen. Following recognition and acceptance of the BPD syndrome and its iatrogenic etiology, significant improvements in the technique of artificial ventilation occurred as well as changes in the use of supplemental oxygen in the newborn infant. These changes have resulted in improved survival of infants with severe RDS, but the problem of the development of BPD in these infants persists. The most recent review of BPD is 'Workshop on Bronchopulmonary Dysplasia' published in *Journal of Pediatrics*."[1]

1. Workshop on bronchopulmonary dysplasia. *J. Pediatrics* **95**(5-Pt. 2):815-920, 1979.

CC/NUMBER 27
JULY 2, 1979

This Week's Citation Classic

Gluck L, Kulovich M V, Borer R C Jr., Brenner P H, Anderson G G & Spellacy W N.
Diagnosis of the respiratory distress syndrome by amniocentesis.
Amer. J. Obstet. Gynecol. **109**:440-45, 1971.
[Depts. Pediat. & Obstet.-Gynecol., Univ. Calif., San Diego Sch. Med., La Jolla, CA]

Amniotic fluid surfactant phospholipids reflect fetal lung development during gestation. Sharply rising lecithin, falling sphingomyelin—ratio of L/S greater than 2.0—beyond 35 weeks marks maturity, when delivered newborns are free of respiratory distress syndrome (RDS), or hyaline membrane disease. [The *SCI*® indicates that this paper has been cited over 410 times since 1971.]

Louis Gluck
Department of Pediatrics
University of California
La Jolla, CA 92093

April 3, 1978

"I long had been interested in biochemical development, correlating molecular, morphologic, and physiologic events during growth and maturation of embryos and fetuses. Our model organ, the lung, ideally encompasses all major facets of development. Its unique morphogenesis, easily studied, correlates with its biochemical and physiological maturation. Definable enzymes produce quantifiable surfactant phospholipids in the alveolar lining which lower surface tension and stabilize alveoli, without which life is not possible. There even is a major disease from lack of surfactant in premature humans, hyaline membrane disease (HMD), or respiratory distress syndrome.

"Early in our pioneering studies on biosynthesis of surfactant phospholipids in developing fetal lung my associate Marie V. Kulovich and I found that surfactant is deposited into amniotic fluid. Understanding the developmental biochemistry of lung surfactant allowed these data to fulfill probably the greatest need in management of pregnancy, assessment of fetal lung maturity. Serial amniotic fluids established biochemical maturity of lung at 35-36 weeks gestation in normal pregnancy by matching surfactant phospholipid patterns with clinical maturity. Thus arose lecithin/sphingomyelin or L/S ratios, utilizing these two phospholipid indicators on TLC as a *ratio* to compensate for daily and even hourly variations in amniotic fluid volumes.

"In 1966, we were able to measure maturity of fetal lung by this method. The work began at Yale at a difficult time for obtaining amniotic fluid; only fluids for Rh incompatibility studies during pregnancy were available. A short stay at the University of Miami (academic 1968-69) yielded many samples to verify our findings. In 1969, at the University of California, San Diego, together with Drs. Robert Borer and Roger Freeman we began clinical trials in San Diego and Los Angeles to establish reliability. Thus after three years of laboratory work plus one and a half years of clinical evaluation we felt ready to publish the test for fetal lung maturity, in February 1971. At this time leaders in surfactant studies doubted surfactant was a key factor in hyaline disease, following reports of surplus surfactant in prematures' lungs to stabilize alveoli. The ability to predict fetal lung maturity and thus prevent hyaline membrane disease 'renewed faith' in the central role of surfactant in this disease. The rapid worldwide acceptance of our work has been very gratifying, with daily applicability anywhere babies are delivered, and because it has spurred widespread research into lung development.

"We since have progressed to a more complex, more informative group of measurements, the Lung Profile, including the L/S ratio and percentages of disaturated lecithin, phosphatidyl inositol and phosphatidyl glycerol.[1,2] These last two acidic phospholipids appear necessary to stabilize lecithin in the alveolar layer. The accuracy of prediction of fetal lung maturity by Lung Profile appears as close to 100 percent as a biological test is ever likely to be."

1. **Kulovich MV, Hallman MV & Gluck L.** The Lung Profile. 1. Normal pregnancy. *Amer J. Obstet. Gynecol.* In press.
2. **Kulovich MV & Gluck L.** The Lung Profile. 2. Complicated pregnancy. *Amer J. Obstet. Gyneco.* In press.

CC/NUMBER 25
JUNE 18, 1979

This Week's Citation Classic

Rudolph A M, Drorbaugh J E, Auld P A M, Rudolph A J, Nadas A S, Smith C A & Hubbell J P. Studies on the circulation in the neonatal period. The circulation in the respiratory distress syndrome. *Pediatrics* **27**:551-66, 1961.
[Dept. Pediatrics, Harvard Med. Sch.; Boston Lying-In Hospital; Children's Medical Center, Boston, MA]

Cardiac catheterization studies in newborn infants demonstrated that the ductus arteriosus is usually closed functionally in normal gestationally mature babies within 15-20 hours. Premature infants with respiratory distress had a widely patent ductus arteriosus with a large shunt, predominantly left-to-right, within the first 20 hours after birth. [The *SCI*® indicates that this paper has been cited over 250 times since 1961.]

Abraham M. Rudolph
Departments of Pediatrics, Physiology, and Obstetrics, Gynecology & Reproductive Sciences
University of California
San Francisco, CA 94143.

February 13, 1978

"At the time this work was done, a large proportion of premature infants were dying as a result of hyaline membrane disease (idiopathic respiratory distress syndrome). I had observed that many of these infants had a cardiac murmur, and this, combined with reports of the presence of hyaline membranes in the alveoli of children dying of cardiac failure, led me to consider that the respiratory distress syndrome was due to left ventricular failure associated with persistent patency of the ductus arteriosus. I proposed a study to confirm this hypothesis by performing cardiac catheterization studies in a series of normal infants and infants with respiratory distress. Extensive discussions regarding the ethics of these studies followed for a period of about six months before it was agreed that the studies were justified. In view of the high incidence of morbidity and mortality in infants of diabetic mothers, these families were most cooperative in granting permission for the procedures.

"In reflecting on the changes in attitude regarding human research over the past 15 years, I doubt that I would have considered performing these studies, or that approval would have been granted by an institutional committee in the present era. The study was, however, extremely important in formulating our current concepts about the high incidence of persistent patency of the ductus arteriosus in premature infants, and the role of large left-to-right shunts through the ductus, either in causing cardiorespiratory difficulties or in aggravating symptoms in premature infants with hyaline membrane disease.

"It is also of interest that the information presented in this paper was neglected for some years because, soon after it was published, the role of immaturity of pulmonary surfactant in preventing adequate lung expansion and causing hyaline membrane disease, received most attention. It was suggested that inadequate ventilation would cause hypoxia and pulmonary vasoconstriction and, if the ductus arteriosus were patent, a right-to-left, rather than a left-to-right shunt, would result.

"Later, it became apparent that although lack of pulmonary surfactant accounted for inadequate lung expansion, large left-to-right shunts through the ductus arteriosus often complicated the course of premature infants with respiratory distress syndrome. This paper first clearly documented the importance of left-to-right shunts with resultant cardiac failure in contributing to respiratory distress in premature infants, and stimulated us, as well as others, to recommend ligation of the ductus arteriosus to treat these infants. This has proved to be very effective in selected cases. More recently, prostaglandin synthetase inhibitors have been used to close the ductus arteriosus by pharmacologic means."

CC/NUMBER 13
MARCH 29, 1982

This Week's Citation Classic

Liggins G C & Howie R N. A controlled trial of antepartum glucocorticoid treatment for prevention of the respiratory distress syndrome in premature infants. *Pediatrics* **50**:515-25, 1972.
[Postgrad. Sch. Obstet. and Gynaecol., Univ. Auckland, Auckland, New Zealand]

Immature human fetuses responded with accelerated lung maturation when exposed for 24 to 72 hours to a synthetic corticosteroid. At birth, the treated infants in this double-blind trial were less likely to develop respiratory distress syndrome (RDS) and more likely to survive. [The *SCI*® indicates that this paper has been cited over 565 times since 1972.]

G.C. Liggins
Postgraduate School of Obstetrics
and Gynaecology
University of Auckland
Auckland, New Zealand

February 4, 1982

"In 1967, while investigating the mechanism by which fetuses control the time of their birth, I noticed that lambs born very prematurely as a result of fetal infusions of ACTH or dexamethasone were able to breathe effectively. At autopsy, the lungs were found to be partly air-filled instead of having the liver-like appearance characteristic of immaturity. No sophisticated tests were needed to postulate a connection between adrenal activity and lung maturation. Because we were inexperienced at that time in pulmonary physiology and were preoccupied with parturitional physiology, it was decided to pass on this intriguing finding to better equipped colleagues elsewhere, particularly Mary Ellen Avery[1] in Montreal, and William Tooley and John Clements in San Francisco.[2] The preliminary observations were soon confirmed and greatly extended, encouraging us to plan a clinical trial to find out whether corticosteroid treatment would hasten pulmonary maturation in human fetuses about to be born prematurely. The medical staff and nurses of the National Women's Hospital, Auckland, New Zealand, cooperated enthusiastically in a double-blind trial which eventually included over 1,000 women. The study was organized with the help of my coauthor, Ross Howie, a neonatologist who has a gift that I lack for meticulous attention to detail. The first patient was enrolled in December 1969. A paper describing a reduction in the incidence of RDS and early neonatal death in infants treated *in utero* with corticosteroids was offered to *Lancet* in 1972 but was rejected on grounds of lack of general interest. Whereupon the spelling was Americanized and an otherwise unamended manuscript was submitted with greater success to *Pediatrics*.

"Interest in the paper has come not only from clinicians who have confirmed our findings but more particularly from physiologists and biochemists to whom the work seems to have acted as a stimulus to the study of lung development, perhaps partly because of its appeal to mission-oriented granting agencies. Inevitably there are those who wish to record their dislike of fetal exposure to drugs in any shape or form. Reports in press of the long-term follow-up of surviving children now up to 11 years old show no adverse effects of their corticosteroid treatment as fetuses.

"It is an interesting reflection on the way that science progresses in fits and starts that 12 years after I first reported the relationship of the fetal adrenal to lung maturation, the nature of the relationship remains unclear. It seemed so simple then—cortisol induces an enzyme in the biosynthetic pathway to surfactant. Today, there is no agreement on what, if any, enzyme is induced, whether changes in structure or surfactant are more important, and whether the action of cortisol is dependent on other hormones. Fortunately, therapeutic success often is not dependent on a detailed knowledge of pharmacological action. The reason the paper is highly cited may stem partly from novelty but mainly from the fact that an equally well-controlled study was not published until five years later."[3]

1. **DeLemos R A, Shermeta D W, Knelson J H, Kotas R & Avery M E.** Acceleration of appearance of pulmonary surfactant in the fetal lamb by administration of corticosteroids. *Amer. Rev. Resp. Dis.* **102**:459-61, 1970.
2. **Platzker A C G, Kitterman J A, Mescher E J, Clements J A & Tooley W H.** Surfactant in the lung and tracheal fluid of the fetal lamb and acceleration of its appearance by dexamethasone. *Pediatrics* **56**:554-61, 1975.
3. **Papageorgiou A N, Desgranges M F, Masson M, Colle E, Shatz R & Gelfand M M.** The antenatal use of betamethasone in the prevention of respiratory distress syndrome: a controlled double-blind study. *Pediatrics* **63**:73-9, 1979.

CC/NUMBER 15
APRIL 11, 1983

This Week's Citation Classic

Kawasaki T, Kosaki F, Okawa S, Shigematsu I & Yanagawa H. A new infantile acute febrile mucocutaneous lymph node syndrome prevailing in Japan. *Pediatrics* **54**:271-6, 1974.
[Dept. Pediatrics, Japanese Red Cross Med. Ctr., and Dept. Epidemiology, Inst. Public Health, Tokyo, Japan]

This paper was the first paper in English describing what was thought to be a new disease afflicting infants and young children in Japan since 1960. The paper was also unusual because it included color and not black-and-white photos which illustrated clinical features of the disease. [The *SCI®* indicates that this paper has been cited in over 235 publications since 1974.]

Tomisaku Kawasaki
Department of Pediatrics
Japanese Red Cross Medical Center
4-1-22, Hiroo, Shibuya-ku
Tokyo
Japan

February 2, 1983

"On January 5, 1961, I saw at our hospital a 4-year, 3-month-old boy with high fever, cervical adenopathy, conjunctival congestion, cracked lips, and rash. Looking back, I now know that this patient was a typical mucocutaneous lymph node syndrome (MCLS) patient. Today this syndrome is more commonly known as Kawasaki syndrome or Kawasaki disease. At that time, however, I was unable to make a correct diagnosis and discharged the patient with diagnosis unknown.

"The clinical features of this patient made a strong impression on me and I could not forget them. In 1961, this was the only case that I had experienced, but in March 1962, a case of suspected sepsis was brought to me by another doctor. When I saw this case, I realized at a glance that the appearance was very similar to the case which I had seen the previous year. Fortunately, I subsequently experienced very similar cases.

"In the process of trying to categorize the features of the syndrome, I did not always see typical patients. When I saw atypical patients, my confidence was shaken. My experiences led me to question my initial observations but gradually my experiences led me to believe that my initial conclusions had been correct.

"Finally in 1965, the pediatricians in my hospital agreed that it was a new syndrome. In January 1967, at a meeting of the Tokyo Pediatric Association, a doctor reported on 'three cases of Stevens-Johnson syndrome.' At that meeting, several doctors said that the diagnosis of Stevens-Johnson syndrome was not correct. One of the doctors said that it was acute juvenile rheumatoid arthritis and discussion centered around this diagnosis. No conclusion could be reached. However, one of the doctors had read the manuscript of the paper which I had submitted and which had already been accepted for publication. My manuscript described the new syndrome and the doctor pointed out that the three cases were the same as the new syndrome which I had described in my paper.

"In March, my paper in Japanese[1] was published in the *Japanese Journal of Allergology*, describing my clinical observations of 50 cases. As a result, some pediatricians sent me personal communications agreeing with me that I had described a new syndrome.

"In 1970, the Ministry of Health and Welfare established a research committee for Kawasaki disease, and Itsuzo Shigematsu, an epidemiologist, carried out the first nationwide survey. In 1972, there was the second nationwide survey. The information from both surveys was combined and included in the paper which appeared in *Pediatrics*.

"Recently, awareness among pediatricians that there is a new disease has increased. Some of the patients of this disease suffer sudden death from coronary thrombosis based on coronary artery aneurysm. An interesting point is that fatal MCLS is indistinguishable from already known infantile periarteritis nodosa with coronary artery involvement. Pediatricians must become aware of this new disease if they are to know one of the causes of sudden death among children.

"This paper has been highly cited for the following reason. The etiology is still unknown but the disease is known in America and in all parts of the world. Awareness among pediatricians of the importance of this so-called 'mysterious disease' has increased and in order to discover the etiology of this disease, more and more research is being done, leading to citation of the paper."

1. **Kawasaki T.** M.C.L.S.—clinical observation of 50 cases. [In Japanese.] *Jpn. J. Allergol.* **16**:178-222, 1967.

Chapter

11

Respiratory Disease

Diseases of the respiratory system, like those of most tissues, can be cross-listed with several other subjects—infectious disease, oncology, immunology, etc. The Citation Classics grouped here emphasize lung physiology although only the first was issued from a department of physiology and pharmacology. The others originated from divisions of cardiopulmonary disease, pulmonary disease, or the like. For these reasons they have been placed in this separate chapter.

The first "This Week's Citation Classic" (TWCC) describes, almost as well as the Citation Classic itself, how to measure airway resistance in the lung. It is only necessary to place the subject in a closed vessel and measure changes in the air pressure within the chamber as the person breathes. As simple as this seems today, DuBois mentions two essentials to his success—a hobby in amateur radio that allowed him to understand the basics of the cathode ray oscillograph and spare-time reading in physics so that he knew how to apply Boyle's law to airflow problems. The availability of his co-authors' plethysmograph was another essential, of course. The site and nature of airway blockade in patients was determined by Hogg, Macklem, and Thurlbeck, who submitted a manuscript containing their results to *Lancet.* The article was rejected and resubmitted to the journal in which it became a Citation Classic, but not until after revision. Since their technique of embedding a catheter through the pleural surface could not be used on living patients, it had no diagnostic application, but a subsequent Classic by McCarthy et al. addressed this problem. The approach to measuring airway obstruction came from observing his teacher exhale tobacco smoke in a dimly lit room. The concentration of the smoke was noted to increase at the end of the expiration. This increased flow at low lung pressure is due to airway closure, and the volume of expired air at which this occurred is the "closing volume." Persons with abnormal closing volumes are subject to chronic air-flow limitation in later life in the form of emphysema or chronic bronchitis.

The mechanics of respiration can be interpreted by the parameters pressure, volume, and airflow, as defined by Fry and Hyatt. This has been considered a useful analytical approach to evaluate lung physiology, but it also introduced a new and simple parameter for pulmonary function—the minimal expiratory flow-volume derived from a simultaneous measure of airflow and lung volume.

Gadgeteering appears to be a necessary requisite for achieving Classic status in respiratory physiology. Wright admits its essentiality in the construction of his flow meter, an instrument used to measure the maximum flow rate of air from the lung. Although his first model was broken by a hobbyist rower who clearly had a powerful set of lungs, later models were more sturdy. It might be entertaining to read some of his friends' derogatory comments about his manuscript, but enough is already available in this vein—long winded, bag of wind, blowhard, etc.—that our imaginations may be enough.

Acute respiratory distress following trauma, blood infusions, shock, or other stimuli was first recognized by Ashbaugh et al. as a syndrome with common features despite variations in etiology. The failure of the usual respirator treatment to save their first patient and the threat that the second patient would also die even with high oxygen treatment caused them to reevaluate the accepted treatment protocol. Because their respirator model had the option of expiratory pressure, they added it, with a dramatic recovery of their patient.

Excessive oxygen in respiratory therapy can be toxic and is another example that contradicts the statement, "If a little is good more is better." Oxygen toxicity can be expressed as respirator lung syndrome in which a decrease in oxygen transport through the alveoli develops because continuous exposure to high concentrations of oxygen reduces alveolar transport (p. 316). A TWCC on this subject is also found in the preceding chapter on Perinatology.

The last two TWCCs treat other aspects of lung disease rather than air exchange problems. Asbestos exposure—to a particular form of asbestos—in miners was determined to be the irritant responsible for lung cancer. This important discovery, first published in 1960, has only recently been appreciated by the American public. Today, many communities are removing the asbestos insulation from their schools because of the threat of mesotheliomas (p. 317). The final TWCC describes the path to the discovery that a surfactant (detergent) property of the lung lining is missing or decreased in immature infants dying of hyaline membrane disease. Viral pneumonia and paraquat poisoning are two other conditions that remove the surfactant and lead to secondary pulmonary disease.

The seven review articles listed below nearly equal the number of TWCCs contained in this brief chapter. The review articles emphasize specific medical aspects of respiratory physiology rather than respiratory physiology per se. Readers more interested in the latter should consult *Advances in Cardiopul-*

monary Diseases, Annual Review of Physiology, and *Clinics in Chest Medicine.* The journals *Clinical Physiology* and *Clinical Respiratory Physiology* also publish review articles, but on a random basis.

Bernard G R & Brigham K L. The adult respiratory distress syndrome. *Annu. Rev. Med.* **36**:195–205, 1985.

Chang H K & Harf A. High-frequency ventilation: a review. *Respir. Physiol.* **57**:135–52, 1984.

Davis J M. The pathology of asbestos related disease. *Thorax* **39**:801–8, 1984.

Gitlin J D, Parad R & Taeusch H W, Jr. Exogenous surfactant therapy in hyaline membrane disease. *Semin. Perinatol.* **8**:272–82, 1984.

Lee K P. Lung response to particulates with emphasis on asbestos and other fibrous dusts. *CRC Crit. Rev. Toxicol.* **14**:33–86, 1985.

Vallyathan V & Green F H Y. The role of analytical techniques in the diagnosis of asbestos-associated disease. *CRC Crit. Rev. Clin. Lab. Sci.* **22**:1–42, 1985.

Ward P A, Johnson K J & Till G O. Current concepts regarding adult respiratory distress syndrome. *Ann. Emerg. Med.* **14**:724–8, 1985.

CC/NUMBER 6
FEBRUARY 9, 1981

This Week's Citation Classic

DuBois A B, Botelho S Y & Comroe J H, Jr. A new method for measuring airway resistance in man using a body plethysmograph: values in normal subjects and in patients with respiratory disease. *J. Clin. Invest.* **35**:327-35, 1956.
[Department of Physiology and Pharmacology, Graduate School of Medicine, University of Pennsylvania, Philadelphia, PA]

This method provides a specific measurement of airway resistance (alveolar pressure/airflow) in man. The alveolar pressure can be measured by seating the person inside a closed chamber and recording pressure fluctuations of the air in the chamber during the breathing cycle. The box pressure change is converted to alveolar pressure change using Boyle's law and appropriate calibration constants. Normal airway resistance was 0.6 to 2.4, whereas in patients with obstructed airways it was as much as 10.8 cm H_2O/liter per sec. [The ***SCI***® **indicates that this paper has been cited over 730 times since 1961.]**

Arthur B. DuBois
John B. Pierce Foundation Laboratory
290 Congress Avenue
New Haven, CT 06519

January 23, 1981

"A physics text which I read while stationed at the US Naval Academy in 1948 said that if you know the length and diameter of a hollow tube, you can calculate its resistance to airflow. I reasoned that if one could measure human airway resistance, it would be possible to tell whether the airways were narrowed. Fenn allowed me to pursue this idea in his laboratory in the department of physiology, University of Rochester Medical School, where I began to display pressure against flow using the X and Y axes of a cathode ray oscillograph (CRO). And I explored higher breathing frequencies with an oscillating pump made from an aircraft piston and cylinder.

"Later, in Comroe's department at the University of Pennsylvania I turned to a problem which Comroe and Botelho had begun, but which had been set aside because of theoretical and technical difficulties. They had constructed an airtight chamber which was intended to allow the measurement of compressible gas volume (FRC) in the chest, using Boyle's law to calculate the volume from the degree of volume change resulting from a pressure change generated during the subject's effort to compress the alveolar gas. They also hoped to record volume changes of the alveolar gas due to its compression and decompression during breathing, and to calculate alveolar pressure changes from those volume changes. However, the obstacles were that alveolar air also changes its volume due to rapid warming and wetting of the air during inspiration, and due to CO_2 coming out of solution from the lung tissue during inspiratory airflow. The capacitance manometers were unstable radio-frequency bridges, and the method of recording and replotting data was cumbersome.

"I displayed box pressure against mouth pressure on a CRO, and at once found that the lung volume calculated from the slope of the line generated during voluntary straining equalled the FRC. Next day, I set up a flowmeter channel (Y axis) *vs.* box pressure (X axis) on the CRO, rebreathed through the flowmeter into a hot water bottle, and found an S-shaped line of alveolar pressure *vs.* airflow. Then, I discovered that with panting, the hot water bottle could be removed, simplifying the method.

"It took only one day to set up the plethysmographic FRC method, and another day for the airway resistance methods. But the outcome hinged on: a) an earlier hobby of amateur radio, b) a spare time reading of physics, c) the measurement of instantaneous gas exchange, and d) the exploration of lung mechanics at rapidly oscillating frequencies. All these had been necessary to prepare for those two successful days. Similarly, it had taken Comroe and Botelho years to conceive of[1] and build[2] the body plethysmograph which was then used to make the actual measurements.

"I consider it a tribute to Comroe's foresight and skill[3] that this manuscript was subsequently chosen for *Citation Classics*."

1. **Comroe J H, Jr.** Retrospectroscope: Man-Cans (conclusion). *Amer. Rev. Resp. Dis.* **116**:1091-9, 1977.
2. **Comroe J H, Jr., Botelho S Y & DuBois A B.** Design of a body plethysmograph for studying cardiopulmonary physiology. *J. Appl. Physiol.* **14**:439-44, 1959.
3. **DuBois A B.** Introduction. (DuBois A B & van de Woestijne K P, eds.) *Progress in respiration research, vol. 4: body plethysmography.* Basel: S. Karger, 1969. p. VII-XI.

CC/NUMBER 52
DECEMBER 27, 1982

This Week's Citation Classic

Hogg J C, Macklem P T & Thurlbeck W M. Site and nature of airway obstruction in chronic obstructive lung disease. *N. Engl. J. Med.* **278**:1355-60, 1968. [Dept. Pathology, McGill Univ., and Joint Cardio-Respiratory Service, Royal Victoria Hosp., Montreal, Canada]

A small catheter was wedged in 2 mm airways to measure central and peripheral airways resistance. We found that peripheral airways resistance accounted for 25 percent of total in normal lungs and that it was increased from four to 40 times in lungs with obstructive pulmonary disease. The fact that peripheral airways resistance is small in normal lungs and greatly increased in diseased lungs suggests that significant small airways disease may be present and undetected during the transition from healthy to diseased lungs. [The *SCI*® indicates that this paper has been cited in over 340 publications since 1968.]

James C. Hogg
Pulmonary Research Laboratory
St. Paul's Hospital
University of British Columbia
Vancouver, British Columbia V6Z 1Y6
Canada

October 29, 1982

"Our study was based on some fundamental observations made on airways resistance by Peter Macklem and Jerry Mead working at the Harvard School of Public Health in Boston. Macklem had been interested in measuring bronchial pressures for some time and had obtained some interesting data during bronchoscopy by using a small tube which he pushed down the bronchoscope. He tells me that while he was a fellow in Mead's laboratory, Mead got the idea for the retrograde catheter while they were discussing the problems of measuring pressure in the bronchial tree. The methodology is based on a somewhat similar technique used by Colin Caro[1] to measure pressure in the pulmonary vascular bed and involves introducing a catheter in a retrograde fashion. This simply means that a catheter is pushed down into the tracheobronchial tree as far as it can go and a thin piano wire is pushed through that catheter until it breaks through the pleural surface. The original catheter is then removed and a new catheter is fastened to the piano wire extending from the trachea and pulled down the tracheobronchial tree in a retrograde fashion until it comes through the pleural surface. This meant that the pressure drop along the airways could be partitioned accurately for the first time. Macklem and Mead exploited this new technique and published a classic physiological paper in 1967.[2]

"Macklem completed his fellowship in Mead's laboratory and returned to Montreal where I joined him as his postdoctoral fellow in 1966. I was actually an MRC postdoctoral research fellow in the department of pathology at McGill University, but, as Thurlbeck, who was my immediate supervisor, and Macklem were great friends, I had the opportunity to work on a joint project. As the Macklem and Mead technique is unsuitable for living patients, the obvious thing to do was to study postmortem lungs. I carried out a study in Macklem and Thurlbeck's laboratory from 1966 until 1968 where we used the technique to partition airways resistance in normal lungs and in the lungs from patients with chronic bronchitis and emphysema. The data showed that the distribution of airways resistance in the human lung was similar to that in the dog and showed that the major site of airways obstruction in the lungs of patients with chronic obstructive pulmonary disease was in the peripheral airways.

"When we wrote up our first paper, we submitted it to *Lancet* and it was rejected by return mail. We then submitted it to the *New England Journal of Medicine* where it was returned with a long letter from Ingelfinger, the then-editor. The paper was revised and resubmitted and was eventually published in 1968. The paper itself has taught me a great deal. First of all, it was a great experience to work with Macklem and Thurlbeck and the excitement of the project made me decide on a career in research. The rejection from *Lancet*, while devastating at that time, has become a less painful memory. The lesson for the young investigator in this situation is not to give up in the face of a rejected manuscript.

"The fact that the work has become highly cited is of course gratifying. However, the reason for this is primarily because it provided measurements of the distribution of resistance in both normal and diseased lungs. The concept that the peripheral airways are a major site of obstruction had been speculated about since the time of Laennec and our data simply provided important supporting evidence for this concept.

"A recent book in this field is *The Lung in the Transition between Health and Disease.*"[3]

1. **Caro C G & McDonald D A.** The relation between pulsatile pressure and flow in the pulmonary vascular bed. *J. Physiol.—London* **157**:426-53, 1961.
2. **Macklem P T & Mead J.** Resistance of central and peripheral airways measured by a retrograde catheter. *J. Appl. Physiol.* **22**:395-401, 1967.
3. **Macklem P T & Permutt S,** eds. *The lung in the transition between health and disease.* New York: Dekker, 1979. 435 p.

This Week's Citation Classic

CC/NUMBER 27
JULY 5, 1982

McCarthy D S, Spencer R, Greene R & Milic-Emili J. Measurement of "closing volume" as a simple and sensitive test for early detection of small airway disease. *Amer. J. Med.* **52**:747-53, 1972.
[Respiratory Div., Dept. Med., Royal Postgrad. Med. Sch., Hammersmith Hosp., London, England]

Chronic airflow limitation (chronic bronchitis and emphysema), which is largely a disease of cigarette smokers, is a major cause of morbidity and mortality. The closing volume test appears to identify abnormality of the lung function in smokers long before the disease becomes symptomatic or other more routine tests of lung function become abnormal. It is possible that subjects with abnormal closing volumes are destined to develop chronic airflow limitation as a clinical disease. [The *SCI*® indicates that this paper has been cited over 295 times since 1972.]

D.S. McCarthy
D.A. Stewart Respiratory Centre
Department of Medicine
University of Manitoba
Winnipeg, Manitoba R3E 0V8
Canada

May 13, 1982

"Ironic as it might seem, my inspiration came from a stream of tobacco smoke exhaled by a remarkable teacher. His name was J. Milic-Emili, a professor of physiology at McGill University who at the time was spending a sabbatical year at the Royal Postgraduate Medical School situated at Hammersmith Hospital, London, England. At that time he smoked cheroots, a habit he has since abandoned. I was a fellow assigned to him during his sabbatical year. Shortly after his arrival I was summoned to his office. A shaft of sunlight traversed the dimly lit room passing about one foot before his face. After some preliminary pleasantries, he remarked, 'Observe this closely.' He then breathed all the air out of his lungs, filled his mouth with tobacco smoke, and inhaled slowly to maximum lung capacity. He then exhaled slowly across the shaft of light. I noted the gray shades of smoke but as he approached minimal lung volume, the concentration of smoke increased remarkably. 'That is what I want you to investigate,' he said. The increase in tobacco smoke at low lung volumes was due to airway closure in the dependent lung regions. The lung volume at which airways closed was called the 'closing volume.'[1]

"The research reported was conceived because of the need for a simple and sensitive test of lung function to detect presymptomatic airflow limitation in smokers and other subjects at risk to develop lung disease. The alternative tests, at the time, required more subject cooperation, more complex equipment and analysis, and were usually limited to lung function laboratories. The closing volume test on the other hand was a simple test for the subject to perform, it required relatively unsophisticated equipment, and it was suitable for large-scale epidemiological studies. The vital question was and is whether abnormality of closing volume, which occurred frequently in smokers in contradistinction to nonsmokers, predicted the ultimate development of severe chronic airflow limitation in some of these subjects. Clearly this question will require longitudinal studies over many years to provide an answer. Such epidemiological studies have already been established.[2] If it turns out that closing volume does indeed predict the development of chronic airflow limitation, then a relatively simple test is available which will identify individuals who are at risk to develop significant clinical lung disease hopefully at a stage when the process is reversible.

"The paper was first submitted to *Lancet* in England, but was rejected because of little clinical interest."

1. **Dollfuss R E, Milic-Emili J & Bates D V.** Regional ventilation of the lung, studies with boluses of ^{133}xenon. *Resp. Physiol.* **2**:234-46, 1967.
2. **Buist A S, Ghezzo H, Anthonisen N R, Cherniack R M, Ducic S, Macklem P T, Manfreda J, Martin R R, McCarthy D & Ross B B.** Relationship between the single breath N_2 test and age, sex, and smoking habit in three North American cities. *Amer. Rev. Resp. Dis.* **120**:305-18, 1979.

CC/NUMBER 7
FEBRUARY 15, 1982

This Week's Citation Classic

Fry D L & Hyatt R E. Pulmonary mechanics: a unified analysis of the relationship between pressure, volume and gasflow in the lungs of normal and diseased human subjects. *Amer. J. Med.* **29**:672-89, 1960.
[Cardiodynamics Sect. Natl. Heart Inst., NIH, Bethesda, MD and Cardiopulmonary Lab., Beckley Memorial Hosp., Beckley, WV]

The mechanical behavior of the human lung may be described by three simultaneous variables, 'intrapleural' pressure (P), respiratory gas flow (F), and lung volume (V), which can be viewed in a three-dimensional diagram. This provided a unified picture of the interrelated mechanical events during breathing and led to the description of the 'expiratory flow-volume curve.' [The *SCI*® indicates that this paper has been cited over 255 times since 1961.]

Donald L. Fry
Laboratory of Experimental Atherosclerosis
College of Medicine
Ohio State University
Columbus, OH 43210

December 9, 1981

"Bob Hyatt and I are pleased that 'Pulmonary mechanics' has proved to be a useful reference in the field of pulmonary physiology and pathophysiology. This work allowed us to organize observations from many workers into a simpler, conceptually more easily assimilated, pattern of information.

"Earlier work had introduced the concept of pulmonary isovolume pressure-flow curves.[1] We extended this concept to show that the mechanical behavior of the lung could be described rather uniquely by three simultaneous variables, 'intrapleural' pressure (P), respiratory gas flow (F), and lung volume (V), which could be viewed in three-dimensional space as a PFV surface. All respiratory maneuvers could be represented as circuitous trajectories on this surface.

"We found various disease states to be associated with characteristic distortions of the shape of the PFV surface which suggested that early pathological changes should be associated with more subtle changes. We set about examining various ways of quantifying these changes with the goal of correlating these with various lesions in the lung. These efforts resulted in only modest progress toward the ultimate objective because of the enormous difficulty of making the necessary local mechanical measurements to correlate with the global behavior of the PFV surface.[2]

"In retrospect, the most useful result of these activities occurred at the outset when one day we were looking at the PFV diagram and noted an obvious and invariant feature of the diagram, namely, the shape of its silhouette projected onto the expiratory half of the flow-volume coordinate plane. We named the perimeter of this projection the 'maximum expiratory flow-volume' (MEFV) curve. This curve represents a plot of the flow maxima of the expiratory isovolume pressure-flow curves versus the corresponding volumes.[3] The MEFV curve is easily obtained from the simultaneous measurement of respiratory flow and lung volume. This measurement requires very little patient cooperation, does not require the measurement of the 'intrapleural' pressure, is invariant in a given subject, and, most importantly, is sensitive to changes inherent to the pulmonary system since the MEFV curve is determined solely by the aerodynamics, conduit geometry, and rheological properties of the intrathoracic pulmonary system.[2,3] It has become a valuable objective measurement of pulmonary mechanical function with a variety of diagnostic and investigative applications.[4]

"Thus there are probably two reasons for the frequent citing of this paper: first, it provided a useful unified analysis of pulmonary mechanical function which facilitated one's ability to conceptualize the interrelated set of mechanical events associated with breathing. Second, it directed attention to the significance of a simple but unique parameter of pulmonary function, the MEFV curve."

1. **Fry D L, Ebert R V, Stead W W & Brown C C.** The mechanics of pulmonary ventilation in normal subjects and in patients with emphysema. *Amer. J. Med.* **16**:70-97, 1954.
2. **Fry D L.** A preliminary lung model for simulating the aerodynamics of the bronchial tree. *Comput. Biomed. Res.* **2**:111-34, 1968.
3. **Hyatt R E, Schilder D P & Fry D L.** Relationship between maximum expiratory flow and degree of lung inflation. *J. Appl. Physiol.* **13**:331-6, 1958.
4. **Hyatt R E & Black L F.** The flow-volume curve. A current perspective. *Amer. Rev. Resp. Dis.* **107**:191-9, 1973.

CC/NUMBER 11
MARCH 16, 1981

This Week's Citation Classic

Wright B M & McKerrow C B. Maximum forced expiratory flow rate as a measure of ventilatory capacity—with a description of a new portable instrument for measuring it. *Brit. Med. J.* **2**:1041-7, 1959.
[Natl. Inst. Med. Res., Mill Hill, London, England and Pneumoconiosis Res. Unit (Cardiff), Llandough Hosp., Penarth, Glamorgan, Wales]

The advantages of the maximum forced expiratory flow rate as a measure of ventilatory capacity are considered and the history of the use of the measurement is reviewed. A new instrument, the peak flow meter, for making the measurement is described, and an account given of the method of calibration. [The *SCI*® indicates that this paper has been cited over 270 times since 1961.]

B.M. Wright
Department of Bioengineering
Clinical Research Centre
Harrow, Middlesex HA1 3UJ
England

February 19, 1981

"I developed the peak flow meter (PFM) while working as a pathologist at the MRC Pneumoconiosis Research Unit (PRU) in the Welsh coal fields, studying the effect of dust on the lungs of animals. Although officially a pathologist my real love was gadgeteering, and the PRU was ideal for it because the respiratory physiologists were all gadget-minded so the unit had a well equipped workshop.

"My experiments were long term so I had time on my hands and began to poke my nose into other people's business. One of the basic physiological problems was the measurement of ventilatory capacity for which the standard test, the Maximum Breathing Capacity, was exhausting for the subject and the apparatus so cumbersome that Colin McKerrow, who was working on it, when asked whether it would be suitable for field use, remarked, 'You'd be l-lucky to g-get it into a f-field!'

"Mike Kennedy[1] started the idea of peak flow measurement in 1949, using a spirometer which was still too clumsy and complicated for survey use. As Ian Higgins said, if someone opened the door to you, but you had to go back for your apparatus, when you returned the door would be shut. I therefore set out to design something simple and portable and the result was the PFM. Charles Fletcher, the unit director, who had rowed for Cambridge, broke the blade of my first model by blowing nearly 1000 1/min. Nevertheless he backed it enthusiastically, especially after he returned to clinical medicine and became a world expert on bronchitis.

"The physiologists were a bit sniffy about the PFM, holding that the proper way to measure flow is by volume and time, but Colin McKerrow and Margery McDermott kindly did a very thorough calibration study. I wrote the paper after I had left to become a full-time gadgeteer at the National Institute for Medical Research in London, and sent it back to the PRU for comments. I got many, some quite rude, but the result was a much improved paper which Colin decided he would quite like to have his name on after all.

"I think the paper has been cited so much because it describes a test and an instrument which are practical and useful. In those days there was also room to put in a decent historical review and quite a bit of discussion and useful detail. Some years ago I noticed that, although the PFM was mentioned, and was often the key to the whole work, there was no longer any reference to our paper. It was evidently assumed that the PFM had been created by God. I have never got any award or honour but the Minimeter,[2] a sort of paperback version, got a Design Award and is selling hundreds of thousands, because it can be used by patients at home. My reward is knowing that I have made a substantial and perhaps permanent contribution to clinical medicine."

1. **Kennedy M C S.** Practical measure of maximum ventilatory capacity in health and disease. *Thorax* **8**:73-83, 1953.
2. **Wright B M.** A miniature Wright peak flow meter. *Brit. Med. J.* **2**:1627-8, 1978.

NUMBER 44
OCTOBER 29, 1979

This Week's Citation Classic

Ashbaugh D G, Petty T L, Bigelow D B & Harris T M. Continuous positive-pressure breathing (CPPB) in adult respiratory distress syndrome. *J. Thorac. Cardiovas. Surg.* **57**:31-41, 1969. [Depts. Surg. and Med. & Respiratory Care Unit, Univ. Colorado Med. Ctr., Denver, CO]

The clinical syndrome of acute respiratory distress in the adult is defined both physiologically and pathologically. The use of CPPB in treatment of these patients has resulted in a dramatic improvement in morbidity and mortality. [The *SCI*® indicates that this paper has been cited over 205 times since 1969.]

David G. Ashbaugh
Cardiovascular &
Chest Surgical Associates, P.A.
125 E. Idaho
Boise, ID 83702

February 28, 1978

"This paper is one of a series of papers coauthored by myself and Thomas Petty, which dealt with the acute respiratory distress syndrome in older children and adults.[1] This was our first clinical paper in which the use of continuous positive pressure breathing (CPPB), or positive end expiratory pressure as it is now known, was stressed as an effective treatment modality.

"As is so often found in the understanding of clinical problems, our initial interest was stimulated by failure rather than success. Serendipitous observation eventually played a large role in identifying CPPB as a therapeutic tool that could be evaluated both clinically and in the laboratory. Recognizing the acute respiratory distress syndrome as a clinical entity was a major step forward in focusing attention on acute respiratory failure that arose following a variety of bodily insults.

"There had been, in the previous literature, a number of reports[2] describing isolated instances of progressive respiratory failure following trauma, fat embolism, excessive administration of blood, and shock. However, no one had seen or noticed the similarities in clinical presentation and course or had done much to investigate the physiologic consequences. Petty and I, having finished chief residencies in medicine and surgery respectively, at the University of Colorado, were both interested in providing better respiratory care for our patients and organized a joint medical and surgical respiratory care team. We had no designated space in the hospital and saw patients wherever they happened to be. By present-day standards our equipment was meager and mostly begged, borrowed, or stolen.

"The first patient in which we observed acute respiratory distress was a 29-year-old man involved in an automobile accident who, despite being placed on a respirator, went on to develop severe and progressive respiratory failure and died within 48 hours. Our failure, in what we felt should have been a salvageable case, stimulated us to look for additional cases. A few weeks after our first case, a 12-year-old boy was admitted with a severe crushing chest injury. He too, began to follow a similar downhill course despite a tracheotomy and being placed on our only volume respirator, an Engstrom. Even with large volumes of air and 100% oxygen he was doing poorly. In desperation it was decided to try adding *end expiratory pressure*, which happened to be a feature of that model of Engstrom respirator. Dramatic improvement occurred in the patient's condition and he eventually went on to make a very good recovery. Several additional patients were then seen and treated with varying results.

"As we collected our data it became evident that these patients shared many common clinical features and also responded in a similar way to treatment. Our initial paper, presented in *Lancet* in August of 1967,[3] suggested that CPPB might be effective. This paper was our follow-up to a much larger series with definite clinical, and by this time, laboratory evidence that continuous positive pressure breathing was beneficial in the treatment.

"Since that time many other authors and institutions have made important contributions to our understanding of the acute respiratory distress syndrome. Continuous positive pressure breathing or positive end expiratory pressure, however, remains a real cornerstone in the management of these patients."

1. **Ashbaugh D G & Petty T L.** Positive end expiratory pressure. *J. Thorac. Cardiovas. Surg.* **65**:165-70, 1973.
2. **Jenkins M T, Jones R F, Wilson B & Moyer C A.** Congestive atelectasis, complication of intravenous infusion of fluid. *Ann. Surg.* **132**:327-47, 1950.
3. **Ashbaugh D G, Bigelow D B, Petty T L & Levine B E.** Acute respiratory distress in adults. *Lancet* **2**:319-23, 1967.

CC/NUMBER 40
OCTOBER 1, 1984

This Week's Citation Classic™

Nash G, Blennerhassett J B & Pontoppidan H. Pulmonary lesions associated with oxygen therapy and artificial ventilation. *N. Engl. J. Med.* **276**:368-74, 1967.
[Depts. Pathology, James Homer Wright Labs., Anesthesia Labs., and Respiratory Unit, Harvard Med. Sch., Massachusetts Gen. Hosp., Boston, MA]

Characteristic pathological changes were found in the lungs of a group of patients who died after prolonged mechanical ventilation. The alterations did not correlate with duration of mechanical ventilation but appeared to be associated with prolonged inhalation of high concentrations of oxygen. Pulmonary oxygen toxicity was implicated as a possible cause of morbidity and mortality in patients treated with mechanical ventilators. [The *SCI*® indicates that this paper has been cited in over 380 publications since 1967.]

Gerald Nash
Divisions of Anatomic Pathology
and Pulmonary Medicine
Cedars-Sinai Medical Center
Los Angeles, CA 90048

July 19, 1984

"In 1965, as a first-year resident in pathology at the Massachusetts General Hospital, I became intrigued with a problem that was troubling my clinical colleagues who were caring for patients requiring mechanical ventilation. They were puzzled by the occasional development of a progressive deterioration of pulmonary function that was apparently unrelated to the patient's underlying disease. The patients typically did well for a few days, then developed a progressive reduction in pulmonary compliance and vital capacity. They could not be weaned from the ventilator, and they eventually died of respiratory failure. Some physicians at the Massachusetts General Hospital believed that the mechanical ventilator was somehow the culprit, and they referred to the problem as the 'respirator lung syndrome.' H. Pontoppidan, of the Respiratory Unit, thought that the ventilator was being accused unjustly, and he was keenly interested in unraveling the mystery.

"J.B. Blennerhassett and I, in the Department of Pathology, were struck by unusual gross and microscopic appearances of the lungs of patients who died of this syndrome. With the enthusiastic support of Pontoppidan, we decided to compare the morphological findings of a group of patients who died in the Respiratory Unit with a control autopsy population. We found three major differences that characterized the study group: heavy lungs, hyaline membranes, and early interstitial fibrosis. These changes did not correlate with duration of mechanical ventilation, but they appeared to be related to prolonged inhalation of high concentrations of oxygen. Moreover, a review of the literature revealed that the lesions of pulmonary oxygen toxicity as described in animals were similar to those seen in our patients. We concluded that some of our patients with the so-called respirator lung syndrome probably had succumbed to oxygen toxicity.

"At the time this study was performed, oxygen was routinely administered in this country without concern for its possible toxic effects on the lung, and many patients were undoubtedly given toxic levels unnecessarily. This paper warned the medical community that pulmonary oxygen toxicity could develop during therapy for acute respiratory failure. We also recommended that the inspired oxygen concentration should be monitored, and if toxic concentrations must be given to sustain life, the dose should be lowered as soon as possible.

"After publication of this paper and others on the same topic, there was general acceptance of the notion that oxygen is potentially dangerous and its administration should be closely monitored. The paper helped pave the way to a more judicious use of the gas, and in the process it became highly cited. The subject has been recently reviewed by Deneke and Fanburg.[1] Another reason the paper is so highly cited is that it contains the first description of the evolution of a common, nonspecific morphological reaction of the lung to a variety of deleterious agents in addition to oxygen. The lesion is now well recognized and is known as 'diffuse alveolar damage.' "[2]

1. **Deneke S M & Fanburg B L.** Normobaric oxygen toxicity of the lung. *N. Engl. J. Med.* **303**:76-86, 1980.
2. **Katzenstein A A, Bloor C M & Leibow A A.** Diffuse alveolar damage—the role of oxygen, shock, and related factors. *Amer. J. Pathol.* **85**:210-24, 1976. (Cited 105 times.)

CC/NUMBER 32
AUGUST 6, 1979

This Week's Citation Classic

Wagner J C, Sleggs C A & Marchand P. Diffuse pleural mesothelioma and asbestos exposure in the North Western Cape Province. *Brit. J. Indust. Med.* **17:**260-71, 1960.
[Pathol. Div., Pneumoconiosis Res. Unit Council for Scientific and Indust. Res., Johannesburg, West End Hosp., Kimberley, & Dept. Thoracic Surg., Univ. Witwatersrand & Johannesburg General Hosp., S. Africa]

Primary malignant tumours of the pleura are uncommon. Thirty-three cases of diffuse pleural mesothelioma are described; all but one have a probable exposure to crocidolite asbestos (Cape blue). Most of the cases were exposed on the Cape asbestos fields. The tumour has not been observed in the other asbestos mining areas in South Africa. This paper demonstrates a new occupational hazard. [The *SCI*® indicates that this paper has been cited over 240 times since 1961.]

J.C. Wagner
MRC Pneumoconiosis Unit
Llandough Hospital
Penarth, Glamorgan, Wales CF6 1XW

February 10, 1978

"As with so many 'Citation Classics' the events that led to our 1960 paper were based on a series of coincidences.

"At the end of my student career at the University of Witwatersrand, I worked for six months on chest surgery with Libero Fatti and his senior assistant, Paul Marchand.

"In 1957, I was appointed Asbestosis Research Fellow at the South African Institute for Medical Research. South Africa was the ideal place to investigate the asbestosis problem, as it was the only country which produced the three main types of asbestos: chrysotile, crocidolite, and amosite.

"In 1958, I examined a black mine worker thought to have died of tuberculous pleurisy. I was astonished to find a large gelatinous tumour occupying the whole of the right chest. Vaguely, I recalled reading about mesotheliomas of the pleura but had never seen one. Some authorities denied their existence. I asked Basil 'Bunny' Becker for advice. He came to the mortuary and supported the diagnosis, and we did a meticulous study to exclude any other possible source of tumour.

"Dennis Munday, who is still my chief assistant, and I carried out a detailed study to establish that the tumour was a mesothelioma. We presented our findings at the next monthly meeting in chest medicine. Munday observed that 'asbestos bodies' were present in the lung tissue indicating exposure to asbestos dust.

"The following day, Fatti went to Kimberley where he was approached by C.A. Sleggs, the superintendent of a new Tuberculosis Hospital. Tuberculosis was endemic and until 1952 when streptomycin became available, there was little effective treatment. By 1956, Sleggs had established some sort of control, but he observed that cases of tuberculous pleurisy from the east of Kimberley were responding to drugs, but those from the west were not. He asked Fatti to examine some patients and Fatti found features similar to those in the mesothelioma case I had presented in Johannesburg. He arranged for Marchand to take biopsies from the cases, and soon we had fifteen cases. Professor Paul Steiner from Chicago was visiting us and supported our diagnosis.

"We then considered the aetiology. Munday had found a few asbestos bodies in the first case, and also in two further cases. One hundred miles west of Kimberley were the Blue Asbestos Mountains, the world's principal source of the (blue) crocidolite asbestos. I suggested that crocidolite was implicated. Sleggs questioned the patients but none had worked on the asbestos mines. They included housewives, domestic servants, lawyers, a water bailiff, and road workers. It was Marchand who discovered that we had been asking the wrong question! Once we changed to asking whether they had lived in the vicinity of an asbestos mine, the situation became clear. Harold Stewart of the National Institutes of Health was visiting us and appreciated the international significance of the investigation, and encouraged the authorities to give us additional support. We were thus able to demonstrate that these tumours occurred only in those who had lived in the vicinity of the crocidolite mines and not in those associated with the chrysotile or amosite areas. When the paper was submitted for publication it was rejected, because eminent London pathologists stated that mesotheliomas did not exist. However, Professor Jethro Gough, at Cardiff, had seen the material and was able to persuade the editor to accept the paper."

This Week's Citation Classic

NUMBER 2
JANUARY 8, 1979

Avery M E & Mead J. Surface properties in relation to atelectasis and hyaline membrane disease. *Am. J. Dis. Child.* **97**: 517-23, 1959.

Low surface tension in the lining of the lung permits stability of the alveoli at end-expiration. Lacking such a material, the lung is predisposed to atelectasis. Measurements of the surface tension of lung extracts confirm the presence of a very surface-active substance in lungs of infants over 1,000-2,000 gm and in children and adults. In lung extracts of immature infants and infants dying with hyaline membrane disease, surface tension is higher than expected. This deficiency of surface-active material may be significant in the pathogenesis of hyaline membrane disease. [The *SCI*® indicates that this article was cited 376 times in the period 1961-1977.]

Mary Ellen Avery
Department of Pediatrics
Harvard Medical School
Boston, MA 02115

December 29, 1977

"Nearly twenty years have elapsed since we wrote on surface properties in relation to atelectasis and hyaline membrane disease. In retrospect, a more fitting title would have been 'Deficient alveolar surfactant in lungs of infants with hyaline membrane disease. The word surfactant had not been applied to the alveolar lining layer at that time; indeed the concept of surface tension was not widely appreciated by physicians, most of whom last heard of it in their high school physics course.

"As with most discoveries, the stage was set for this one by others. Peter Gruenwald, the pathologist, had written on abnormal patterns of expansion in lungs at autopsy and suggested that surface forces might be abnormal. Richard Pattlein England had described the stability of foam of pulmonary edema and wondered if abnormalities would promote atelectasis and transudation. Jere Mead at the Harvard School of Public Health had participated with Edward Radford and James Whittenberger in studies on surface forces in mammalian lungs, and John Clements had demonstrated the essential dependency of surface area and surface tension in lung extracts measured on a Wilhelmy surface balance.

"All that was needed was one person with an interest in lungs of infants, an awareness of the work of physiologists on surface forces, and the encouragement of a preceptor. Jere Mead was the preceptor who actually made the surface balance (out of a paraffin-lined slide box with a strain gauge) on which I carried out the first measurements.

"The results were clear-cut but they only established an association of surfactant deficiency with hyaline membrane disease. Much further work followed, but results came slowly at first. We pursued the morphological aspects; others embarked on biochemical studies. When different approaches gave concordant results, interest in the observation mounted. Only after clinical applicability with the use of the lecithin/sphingomyelin ratio to assess the amount of surfactant in amniotic fluid (shown by Gluck and colleagues) was the essential role of the surfactant widely appreciated and a part of standard textbook teaching.

"It is pleasant not to have to describe the behavior of bubbles on tubes or define surface tension to pediatric audiences in 1979. The message got through.

"Renewed interest in the metabolism of the lung followed, and abnormalities in synthesis and degradation of lung surfactants remain an important area of study. Hyaline membrane disease of the prematurely born infant remains the prototype of diffuse surfactant deficiency. Other causes can occur at other ages, and include fulminant pulmonary edema which washes out surface-active materials, paraquat poisoning, certain viral pneumonias and that group of disorders called adult respiratory distress syndromes. Little wonder that our demonstration of surfactant deficiency in human infants' lungs is widely cited."

Chapter

12

Psychiatry-Psychology-Neurology

Twenty-six "This Week's Citation Classic" (TWCC) commentaries describing publications on depression, pharmacotherapy of psychopathologic disease, sleep, and related subjects are united in this chapter. Here as in other chapters most of the original articles have been cited fewer than 300 times. Because of limitations in subject matter, author repetitions are not unexpected. Klerman appears as a co-author of three Citation Classics, and Schou, Paykel, and Weissman authored two each, thus accounting for nine of the 27 articles. Tremendous progress has been made in the neurosciences in the past few decades, and this is reflected by the number of these articles that have made Citation Classic status, despite the relatively few medical scientists in its specialties.

Naturally, a diagnostic rating scale is an essential aid for psychiatrists in the identification of specific psychoses and in the separation of these diseases from related conditions. From data on the emotional importance of the loss of life goal or companion (p. 323) or on stress (p. 324), it was possible to develop the needed rating scales (p. 325–328). The last Classic in this group written by Sheehan on imagery has application outside mental depression—to other neuroses and hypnosis, for example—and this accounts for Sheehan's receipt of letters about the paper over a period of 17 years. A companion to this group is the Classic by Carney that refers to a study of 129 patients with depression who were investigated and followed for 6 months. Ten factors were used to identify and discriminate depression due to different causes and to predict ECT (electroconvulsive therapy). ECT has more recently been reevaluated after many years of disfavor and demonstrated to have positive benefits and very few undesirable side effects.

The appropriate yet provocative title chosen by Weissman and Klerman for their article and the surge of interest in women's rights, while contributing to their article's popularity, probably masked the scientific merit of their study and may, as Weissman states, have been an erroneous citation for those (chauvinists) seeking to find a psychosocial basis for depression among our distaff associates. Weissman and Klerman are joined by several other co-authors in the next Classic on a study in which the combination of chemotherapy with psychotherapy was proved superior to the use of either alone.

As stated earlier, Schou is an author of two Classics (on one he served as a co-author), and both describe the status of lithium in the treatment and prophylaxis of manic depression. The first Classic originated from evidence that, over a 6½-year period in which 88 patients were observed, continuous lithium therapy reduced reacerbations of their illness. The status of lithium in psychiatric therapy, its effect on the normal mind, and its use as a drug formed the basis for the second, a review article.

Two other antidepressive studies described by Raskin and Knoll cited the effect of chlorpromazine and impramine (in one study) and inhibitors of monoamine oxidase. Raskin's TWCC contains an interesting—partly modest, partly humorous—paragraph on his reaction to mention of his scoring system at scientific meetings where he was in attendance. The paper by Knoll and Magyar described monamine oxidase inhibitors more from a pharmacologic-biochemical viewpoint than as psychiatric tools, and included the first description of deprenil, an inhibitor of monoamine oxidase B, as an antidepressant.

One of the two Classics in this chapter cited more than 700 times is the review by Schildkraut on the relationship of catecholamine metabolism and affective disorders. Although catecholamine metabolism cannot account for all such disorders, a deficiency of catecholamines results in depression and an excess causes mania. A continued search to prove this hypothesis has been a contributor to the popularity of this report.

Annual surveys have revealed that Valium has been among the five most used drugs in the United States. Now that generic formulations for this drug have been approved, it will undoubtedly remain a popular tranquilizer. A monograph published in 1961 summarized the clinical experience with this diazepam drug and its nearest competitor (p. 337). In view of the past 25 years of use of this drug, it is not surprising to read today that Valium and related diazepam compounds afforded many advantages. Chemotherapy of neuroses is not hazard-free, of course. Crane amply confirmed this in a survey of patients with tardive dyskinesia, many having this condition as a result of neuroleptic drug therapy. Fortunately, Crane's warning prompted an extensive study of neuroleptic drug safety as well as stimulating neurochemical research in kinetic disorders.

The most overt neuroses perhaps require little medical expertise to be diagnosed accurately, although such expertise is obviously required for a differential diagnosis from closely related illnesses and for the selection of proper therapy. Borderline patients present problems even to experienced psychiatrists, and a partial solution to the diagnostic problems they create was provided by Gunderson and Singer's report that identified six key diagnostic features. In some instances, these criteria are applicable to the hyperactive child as an example of a borderline personality disorder. Hyperactive children are often free of any brain dysfunction, and aging may reduce their spontaneous hyperactivity, but a 5-year follow-up indicated that most children retain behavioral or emotional problems. The TWCCs by Stewart and by Weiss address this problem.

Although aging may alleviate hyperactivity, it is a major associative factor with sleeplessness. The older we become, the less sleep we require. True insomniacs of any age actually do sleep less than other persons; they do not simply think their sleep pattern differs from others and that they sleep less. They have much less rapid eye movement and more complete awakenings than noticed in other disturbances. Electroencephalograms proved that different brain-sleep patterns can be charted for the poor sleeper versus the good sleeper regardless of the age group studied (p. 342 and 343).

EEGs are the basis of the next three Citation Classics, one on the topography of the electrical potentials as they relate to normal facial, hand, or foot movements, etc. (p. 344), one on EEG asymmetry in verbal as related to spatial tasks (p. 345), and the last on responses to patterned (checkerboard) sources of light (p. 346). These are essentially studies in brain electrophysiology. The next to last Classic in this chapter is on memory and auditory stimuli.

The closing of this chapter, or of this volume, could not be more effectively phrased than in the last sentence of Cravioto's TWCC.

It may be their very nature that has caused the behavioral sciences to generate so many review journals. Most medical libraries subscribe to at least half a dozen of them. These range from *Advances in Behavioral Biology, Advances in Biochemical Psychopharmacology, Advances in Psychosomatic Medicine, Advances in Neurochemistry,* and *Advances in the Study of Behavior* to *Progress in Behavior Modification, Psychiatric Clinics,* and *Seminars in Neurology.* But as the references listed here demonstrate, numerous other journals contain review articles that are related to the content of this chapter.

Breier A, Charney D S & Heninger G R. The diagnostic validity of anxiety disorders and their relationship to depressive illness. *Am. J. Psychiatr.* **142:**787–97, 1985.

Cantwell D P. Depressive disorders in children: validation of clinical syndromes. *Psychiatr. Clin.* **8:**779–92, 1985.

Cobb J. Behavioural psychotherapy for neurological illness. *Adv. Psychosomat. Med.* **13:**151–84, 1985.

Goldberg L I. Dopamine: receptors and clinical applications. *Clin. Physiol. Biochem.* **3:**120–26, 1985.

Horton, A J, Jr. & Miller W G. Neuropsychology and behavior therapy. *Prog. Behavior. Mod.* **19:**1–55, 1985.

Ingbar D H & Gee B. Pathophysiology and treatment of sleep apnea. *Annu. Rev. Med.* **36:**369–395, 1985.

Kupfer D J. A critical review of sleep and its disorders from a developmental perspective. *Psychiat. Dev.* **1:**367–86, 1983.

Luk S L. Direct observation studies of hyperactive behaviors. *J. Am. Acad. Child Psychiat.* **24:**338–44, 1985.

Reynolds E H & Trimble M R. Adverse neuropsychiatric effects of anticonvulsant drugs. *Drugs* **29:**570–81, 1985.

Ruehlman L S. Depression and evaluative schemata. *J. Pers.* **53:**46–92, 1985.

Salzman G. Geriatric psychopharmacology. *Annu. Rev. Med.* **36:**217–28, 1985.

Stricker E M & Zigmond M J. Brain catecholamines and the central control of food intake. *Int. J. Obes.* **8**(Suppl. 1):39–50, 1984.

Tarsy D & Baldessarini R J. Tardive dyskinesia. *Annu. Rev. Med.* **35:**605–24, 1984.

Willis G L & Smith G C. Amine accumulation in behavioral pathology. *Brain Res.* **356:**109–32, 1985.

Yung C Y. A review of clinical traits of lithium in medicine. *Pharmacol. Biochem. Behav.* **21**(Suppl. 1):51–5, 1984.

Schmale A H, Jr. Relationship of separation and depression to disease. I. A report on a hospitalized medical population. *Psychosom. Med.* **20**:259-77, 1958.
[Depts. Psychiatry and Medicine, Univ. Rochester Sch. Medicine and Dentistry, Strong Memorial and Rochester Municipal Hosps., Rochester, NY]

Feelings of helplessness or hopelessness were reported as a reaction to life events and change in relationships prior to the apparent onset of disease which led to hospitalization. These feelings indicated that a psychobiological giving up had occurred in relation to a perceived impasse in patients' lives. [The *Science Citation Index*® (*SCI*®) and the *Social Sciences Citation Index*® (*SSCI*®) indicate that this paper has been cited in over 210 publications since 1958.]

Arthur H. Schmale
Cancer Center
University of Rochester
Medical Center
Rochester, NY 14642

January 18, 1984

"The ideas for this work began at the University of Maryland under the tutelage of Greenhill, Finsinger, and Lisansky and were brought to fruition under the direction of Engel, Greene, and others at the University of Rochester. As a result of a number of opportunities to interview unselected medical patients in emergency room, clinic, and hospital settings soon after the onset of the symptoms which led to their seeking medical help, I began to appreciate there were similarities across disease, personality, and demographic differences. Up until this time, the research emphasis on the psychological setting of disease onset had been on one disease or one *versus* another.

"The response to the paper was predominantly favorable and fit with the observations of a number of investigators. (The observation that disease followed the loss of an important person or goal was not a new one and had been repeatedly mentioned down through the centuries.) Those less impressed with the paper said it was a blinding glimpse of the obvious, or just a retrospective distortion for those who needed an explanation for getting sick.

"Interest in proving or elaborating the process by which psychological state-environment interactions allow changes in health to occur has gone in spurts and followed many advances in theory and measurement in these areas. Life events, moods, engagement, and self-esteem have been the psychological variables considered most relevant to the model, while advances in measuring autonomic nervous system functioning, hormones, neurotransmitter substances, and, more recently, immune system functioning have led to studies trying to understand the biological changes associated with grief, depression, or learned helplessness.

"One of the interesting and important sides of this work to me has been the recognition that there is a basic biological homeostatic regulatory mechanism underlying giving up. Engel and Reichman, in their study of a psychologically deprived infant, Monica, with an esophageal atresia, labeled a behavioral triad of relative immobility, quiescence, and unresponsiveness to the sight of a stranger conservation-withdrawal.[1] Their observations were found to be consistent with what was being seen in relation to giving up in adults. Conservation-withdrawal is built in as part of the homeostatic controls of all organisms which protect them from environmental extremes of too much or too little stimulation.[2] Such a shutting down is seen most clearly in hibernation and tonic immobility in animals and sleep and fainting in man.

"As is true with much of science, what begins as a clinical observation which needs explanation becomes the elusive golden ring which provides the impetus for many other discoveries. The chase goes on."

1. **Engel G L & Reichman F.** Spontaneous and experimentally induced depression in an infant with a gastric fistula: a contribution to the problem of depression. *J. Amer. Psychoanal. Assn.* **4**:428-52, 1956. (Cited 65 times.)
2. **Engel G L & Schmale A H.** Conservation withdrawal: a primary regulatory process for organismic homeostasis. *Physiology, emotion and psychosomatic illness.* Amsterdam: Associated Scientific Publishers, 1972. p. 57-75.

CC/NUMBER 39
SEPTEMBER 28, 1981

This Week's Citation Classic

Paykel E S, Myers J K, Dienelt M N, Klerman G L, Lindenthal J J & Pepper M P. Life events and depression: a controlled study. *Arch. Gen. Psychiat.* **21**:753-60, 1969.
[Depts. Psychiatry and Sociology, Yale University, New Haven, CT]

Depressed patients were found to experience three times as many life events before onset as general population controls. The excess particularly involved undesirable events and exits from the social field. Findings indicated the general importance of life stress and of particular stresses in clinical depression. [The *SCI*® indicates that this paper has been cited over 155 times since 1969.]

E.S. Paykel
Department of Psychiatry
St. George's Hospital Medical School
University of London
London SW17 0RE
England

July 13, 1981

"The role of environmental stress in the development of psychiatric disorder has been a focus of vigorous debate in psychiatry. It polarises the two great schools of psychiatric orientation: on the one hand those who believe in the primacy of genetic, constitutional, and biological factors, and on the other those viewing all disorders as reactions to stress and earlier psychological conflicts. In 1966-1967, although life event inventories had been developed, there had been few empirical studies of the relation between clinical psychiatric disorder and recent life events, except for wartime stress and rare natural disasters. There had been no large-scale comparisons of the event experience of patients and matched controls from the general population.

"The study arose out of a collaboration between two research groups at Yale University. On the clinical side, led by Gerald Klerman, we were setting up the depression research unit within the department of psychiatry, with interests which included the role of life events. Early in 1967, I heard a presentation by Jerome Myers and his group in the department of sociology, of a projected epidemiological survey which would examine effects of life events on symptoms within the community. Impressed with the possibilities for collaboration, I went to see Myers, and we agreed a joint inventory covering the main life events was likely to be of importance. Ultimately this was administered to 185 depressed patients and to 938 subjects within the community from whom a closely matched control group could be selected. In analysing the data we grouped the life events into various categories and were excited to find that they behaved differently in their effects on depression.

"The study received considerable interest after publication partly, I think, because it was the first such comparison with general population controls, and partly because findings gave research confirmation to a clinically-derived belief in the importance for depression of loss experiences. However, the results also indicated that not all depressions were preceded by such experiences, suggesting that causation was often multifactorial.

"The study collaboration was a fruitful one which led to further studies[1] of life events in depression and in other psychiatric disorders, including suicide attempts and schizophrenia, together with other aspects of psychiatric epidemiology. The original investigators are now widely scattered, although the collaboration at Yale University between Myers and the depression research unit continues. I returned to England, but have continued with research related to depression, and to life events.[1] There have since been many studies into life events and psychiatric disorders with increasing sophistication of methods, leading to a solidly established corpus of knowledge, recently described in several reviews.[2,3] Much more is becoming apparent about the way in which life events interact with other causative factors to produce depression. The heat has gone from the argument, as in the other great controversies of psychiatry, as empirical knowledge has become established."

1. **Paykel E S.** Recent life events in the development of the depressive disorders. (Depue R A, ed.) *The psychobiology of the depressive disorders: implications for the effects of stress.* New York: Academic Press, 1979. p. 245-62.
2. **Lloyd C.** Life events and depressive disorder reviewed. *Arch. Gen. Psychiat.* **37**:541-8, 1980.
3. **Paykel E S.** Life events and early environment. (Paykel E S, ed.) *Handbook of affective disorders.* Edinburgh, Scotland: Churchill Livingstone. To be published, 1982.

This Week's Citation Classic

Hamilton M. A rating scale for depression.
J. Neurol. Neurosurg. Psychiat. **23**:56-62, 1960.
[Dept. Psychiatry, Univ. Leeds, England]

This scale was one of the first for measuring the severity of depressive illness. Based on psychometric theory, it was designed to be relevant, simple, and easy to use. [The *SCI*® indicates that this paper has been cited over 790 times since 1961.]

Max Hamilton
Department of Psychiatry
University of Leeds
Leeds LS2 9NZ
England

July 10, 1981

"I first became interested in psychiatry in a practical way in 1943, during my service in the Royal Air Force. My preparatory reading in modern psychology which, to my delight, included serious discussions on fundamental questions of scientific method, was a revelation to me and determined my future career. For the next 13 years I spent all the time I had to spare in studying psychometrics, statistics, and experimental design. My chiefs and colleagues regarded me at best as an amiable eccentric. My big chance came in 1956 when, as senior lecturer in the department of psychiatry in the University of Leeds, I organized a drug trial of a new anxiolytic drug. The outcome of this work was to turn my interest to the depressions. At this time, I was fortunate enough to obtain a research fellowship, but as I could not work half-time in the department, I gave up my university post.

"For my research, I devised a rating scale for the measurement of severity of illness, as there was nothing suitable at the time. During the next three or four years I showed the scale to many people but was met with nothing but apathy and indifference. By a happy coincidence, the first antidepressant drugs appeared soon after and the need to evaluate them then produced a demand for a suitable rating scale.

"The first consideration was that it should be applicable to all the subgroups of depressive illness, i.e., to cover all types of symptoms, though only common ones. It takes much time to inquire after rare symptoms and the information gained is meagre. The scale had to have a length of 12 to 20 items, because too short a scale is insufficiently reliable and when too long it is burdensome to fill in. Above all, it had to be clearly relevant and easy to use by clinicians working in their usual setting.

"The items selected covered the major symptoms of the depressions. The number of grades of severity chosen, for those present, was four: trivial, mild, moderate, and severe. Too many grades makes judgement very difficult and too few loses sensitivity. Four grades also ensured the elimination of the common bias to choose a midpoint. Preliminary tests showed that the patients could not provide sufficient information to make these fine distinctions for some of the symptoms, so they were reduced to two: doubtful or trivial, and clearly present. Experts are very dubious about two ranges of grading, but clinicians find them appropriate. This is the ultimate basis for the popularity of the scale. It is simple and easy to use in the routine of clinical practice, and it is meaningful and relevant. It is highly valid against clinical judgement and its reliability is equally high (far higher than many biochemical tests). All these account for its acceptance as a standard all over the world and its translation into many languages. Despite its deficiencies, it has lasted over 20 years and continues to flourish,[1,2] although doubtless it will be replaced in time."

1. **Hamilton M.** Development of a rating scale for primary depressive illness. *Brit. J. Soc. Clin. Psychol.* **6**:278-96, 1967.
2. **Hedlund J L & Viewig B W.** The Hamilton rating scale for depression: a comprehensive review. *J. Operat. Psychiat.* **10**:149-65, 1979.

This Week's Citation Classic

Zung W W K. A self-rating depression scale. *Arch. Gen. Psychiat.* **12**:63-70, 1965.
[Duke Univ. Med. Ctr., Dept. Psychiatry, Durham, NC]

The need for assessing depression as an emotional illness in order to document its presence qualitatively and quantitatively led to: (1) formulation of an operational definition of depression as a psychiatric disorder, (2) its application by the construction of a rating scale, (3) establishing its validity and reliability, and (4) use of the resulting measurement of depression in research and clinical settings. [The *Science Citation Index®* *(SCI®)* **and the** *Social Sciences Citation Index™ (SSCI™)* **indicate that this paper has been cited over 335 times since 1965.]**

William W. K. Zung
Department of Psychiatry
Duke University Medical Center
Durham, NC 27706

July 29, 1978

"My interests from the beginning as a research investigator focused on depression as an emotional disorder in terms of: (1) How do we diagnose this illness? (2) How can we best assess changes in the severity of the illness when various treatment methods are used? (3) Are there physiological changes that can characterize this disorder? and (4) Can we relate the behavioral dysfunctions of depression to brain structure?

"The first step in the research procedure was to identify and select patients with this disorder, using previously agreed upon diagnostic criteria. I found that this was not a simple task and that there were many ways of diagnosing presumably the same disorder. The first task was to solve the dialectical dilemma and to find an agreement among diverse opinions as to what is a depressive disorder. By using the approach that common characteristics are more commonly found, I reduced the hundreds of symptoms and signs to disturbances of four basic categories: (1) psychic-affective, (2) physiological, (3) psychomotor, and (4) psychological. In addition, within each of the categories, specific symptoms/signs were selected on the basis of their heuristic value as a potentially testable brain function-structure relationship. For example, sleep is a physiological function which is disturbed in patients with depressive disorders. Sleep as a physiological process can be understood in terms of the sleep-awake system regulated by specific systems of the CNS. Sleep can be researched in the psycho-physiology laboratory using all-night EEG, EOG, and EMG recordings. From this, specific characteristics of sleep disturbance were found for patients with depressive disorders, and which correlated highly with treatment intervention.

"Having decided as to the qualitative features of the diagnostic criteria, the next step was to apply this quantitatively. The goal was to construct a rating instrument based upon this operational definition that would fulfill the following: (1) be all-inclusive with respect to symptoms of the illness, (2) be short and simple, (3) quantitate in addition to qualitate, and (4) be self-rated and indicate the subject's own responses at the time the scale is completed.

The resulting Self-rating Depression Scale or SDS proved to be useful in providing a measurement of depression. It has proven to be useful for others for the same purpose, but in different settings outside of research, such as in family practice, out-patient medical clinics, and mental health clinics."

CC/NUMBER 4
JANUARY 24, 1983

This Week's Citation Classic

Crown S & Crisp A H. A short clinical diagnostic self-rating scale for psychoneurotic patients. The Middlesex Hospital Questionnaire (M.H.Q.). *Brit. J. Psychiat.* **112**:917-23, 1966.
[Academic Psychiatric Unit, Middlesex Hospital, London, England]

A personality rating was designed to measure clinically relevant dimensions of neuroses: free-floating, phobic, and somatic anxiety; obsessionality; and depression and hysteria (HYS). Neurotic outpatients were differentiated from normal controls. The sub-tests correlated low with each other, significantly with the external criterion. The need to further investigate the HYS scale was noted. [The *Science Citation Index®* **(***SCI®***) and the** *Social Sciences Citation Index®* **(***SSCI®***) indicate that this paper has been cited in over 165 publications since 1966.]**

Sidney Crown
Department of Psychiatry
London Hospital
Whitechapel, London E1 1BB
England

December 7, 1982

"Interested in psychosomatic problems, Crisp and I needed a brief, standardized measurement of mental status as routinely assessed by psychiatrists. The most widely used questionnaire in the UK, the Eysenck Personality Inventory (EPI), measures neuroticism and extraversion. Important and robust dimensions, certainly, but, for a clinician, neuroticism in particular needed further differentiation. Tests widely used in the US are either too long and forbidding for the psychologically unsophisticated British outpatient, the Minnesota Multiphasic Personality Inventory (MMPI) especially, or they are idiosyncratic in conception as with Cattell's 16-Personality Factor (16 PF).[1]

"Discussion with psychiatric and psychological colleagues suggested the sub-tests for a new test. The Middlesex Hospital Questionnaire has now been renamed the Crown-Crisp Experiential Index (CCEI). The sub-tests measure free-floating anxiety; phobic and somatic anxiety; obsessionality; and depression and hysterical traits. A preliminary form of the test was standardized, item-analyzed, shortened, and tested for reliability and validity as described in our original publication. Further standardization, data, and clinical and research applications up to the end of 1979 are summarised in *Manual of the Crown-Crisp Experiential Index.*[2] Three more recent independent validations are by Bagley[3] and Alderman[4] using factor analysis and a US validation by Mavissakalian and Michelson.[5] The CCEI has been translated into Italian, Hebrew, and Hindi.

"The CCEI has been used to investigate a variety of specific problems. These include study difficulty in students; parents of handicapped children; bereavement; deliberate self-harm; fire raisers; personality in Ménière's disease; stereotactic leucotomy; epilepsy; hypertension; rheumatoid arthritis; cigarette smoking; sickness absence in industry; ischaemic heart disease; anorexia nervosa; obesity; back pain; and sleep disturbance.

"There are two problem areas in relation to the test. First, the impossibility of measuring clinical hysteria: the HYS sub-scale correlates highly with EPI extraversion of which it is probably a measure especially of the sociability component. A second problem is that the CCEI sub-scale assesses both symptoms and personality traits. This has been clearly demonstrated with the obsessional (OBS) sub-scale. Factor analysis has revealed two short scales, one measuring obsessional neurotic symptoms, the other obsessionality as a personality trait.[2] It seems possible that the level of citation and the relative popularity of the CCEI relates to its genuine fulfillment of a need for a brief, easily administered and scored personality test with a psychiatric base, useful for testing clinically devised hypotheses particularly in the psychosomatic field."

1. **Cattell R B, Eber H W & Tsatsuoka M M.** *Handbook for the sixteen personality factor questionnaire.* Champaign, IL: Institute for Personality and Ability Testing, 1970. 388 p.
2. **Crown S & Crisp A H.** *Manual of the Crown-Crisp Experiential Index.* Kent, UK: Hodder & Stoughton, 1979.
3. **Bagley C.** The factorial reliability of the Middlesex Hospital Questionnaire in normal subjects. *Brit. J. Med. Psychol.* **53**:53-8, 1980.
4. **Alderman K J.** Factor analysis and reliability studies of the Crown-Crisp Experiential Index. *Brit. J. Med. Psychol.* In press, 1983.
5. **Mavissakalian M & Michelson L.** The Middlesex Hospital Questionnaire: a validity study with American psychiatric patients. *Brit. J. Psychiat.* **139**:336-40, 1981.

CC/NUMBER 37
SEPTEMBER 10, 1984

This Week's Citation Classic™

Sheehan P W. A shortened form of Betts' Questionnaire upon Mental Imagery. *J. Clin. Psychol.* **23**:386-9, 1967.
[Institute of Pennsylvania Hospital and University of Pennsylvania, Philadelphia, PA]

The cause of imagery within the *Zeitgeist* has continued to advance significantly since the 1960s, and measurement of imagery function is an essential part of the research endeavour. This paper reports on the measurement of imagery across different sensory modalities and offers a brief instrument which has good psychometric support. [The *Science Citation Index*® (*SCI*®) and the *Social Sciences Citation Index*® (*SSCI*®) indicate that this paper has been cited in over 165 publications, making it one of the most-cited papers for this journal.]

Peter W. Sheehan
Department of Psychology
University of Queensland
St. Lucia, Queensland 4067
Australia

July 20, 1984

"The research for this paper was part of work completed for my doctoral dissertation. It was supported by the National Institute of Mental Health (US) for study in Australia of the relationship between imagery, fantasy, and hypnosis. The project was a team effort, and this member of the team (under the direction of J.P. Sutcliffe) became very much interested in the function and nature of imagery. It was only later that I turned to research, just as energetically, on hypnosis. There were no real obstacles to the research, and cooperative effort obviously facilitated the work.

"The research can be placed relatively firmly within the *Zeitgeist* of the time. The cause of imagery was advancing. Francis Galton[1] began the emphasis in psychology on quantitative assessment of imagery and produced the first generally acknowledged method of measuring voluntary imagery ability. Galton's questionnaire was adapted by Betts,[2] but Betts' Questionnaire upon Mental Imagery was too long and so not particularly useful. The work reported in the above article aimed to provide a useful test that was brief, maintained measurement across sensory modalities (i.e., wasn't exclusively visual), and had good psychometric support.

"From a content analysis of citations that I have conducted, the major reason to emerge for the work being cited across time is clearly the perceived usefulness of the instrument for assessing individual differences in imagery ability. The most common fields of inquiry in which the work is cited for the purpose of measurement are imagery, hypnosis, experimental psychopathology, and clinical psychology (therapy). Not surprisingly, the earliest field where the work was cited was imagery. This extended into the fields of hypnosis and clinical abnormality in the early 1970s. The test began to be used heavily in the fields of special education and child psychology in the late 1970s, and interest broadened as far afield as art psychotherapy and parapsychology in the late 1970s. Currently, the scale is being used heavily in psychophysiological studies of conditioning and work investigating the effectiveness of cognitive therapy.

"With time, however, reasons for citation other than measurement emerged. The scale, for instance, has been studied extensively in its own right (e.g., what response sets affect performance on it?) and authors cite it because they are attempting to substantiate or refute original claims made about what the scale measures. The work is also cited frequently as relevant background material for the development of new scales and is used to train both subjects and practitioners in the employment of imagery skills. An update on the literature associated with measurement appears in a chapter by Ashton, White, and me.[3]

"While as a researcher I would not have chosen the work reported here as the most satisfying I have conducted, it is clearly the piece of research that has generated the most personal correspondence over the years. From postgraduate students to clinicians to established researchers, queries about the test have been steady over the 17 years since its construction. Psychology apparently needed a brief and easily administered test to tap individual differences in imagery ability, and perhaps it still does."

1. **Galton F.** *Inquiries into human faculty and its development.* London: Macmillan, 1883. 387 p.
2. **Betts G H.** *The distribution and functions of mental imagery.* New York: Teacher's College, Columbia University, 1909. 99 p.
3. **Sheehan P W, Ashton R S & White K D.** The assessment of mental imagery. (Sheikh A A, ed.) *Imagery: current theory, research and application.* New York: Wiley, 1983. p. 189-221.

CC/NUMBER 43
OCTOBER 26, 1981

This Week's Citation Classic

Carney M W P, Roth M & Garside R F. The diagnosis of depressive syndromes and the prediction of ECT response. *Brit. J. Psychiat.* **111**:659-74, 1965.
[Blackpool and Fylde Hosp. Group; Lancaster Moor Hosp.; and Depts. Psychol. Med. and Appl. Psychol., Univ. Newcastle upon Tyne, England]

One hundred twenty-nine depressives, admitted for ECT, were investigated and followed up for three to six months. A factor analysis supported the validity of the endogenous/neurotic distinction. Discriminate function analysis yielded lists of ten features for a) making the differentiation between endogenous and neurotic depressions and b) predicting response to ECT. [The ***Science Citation Index*® (*SCI*®)** **and the** ***Social Sciences Citation Index*® (*SSCI*®)** **indicate that this paper has been cited over 225 times since 1965.]**

M.W.P. Carney
Northwick Park Hospital and
Clinical Research Centre
Harrow, Middlesex HA1 3UJ
England

August 21, 1981

"I first became interested in classifying depressive disorders soon after I entered psychiatry. I have an orthodox medical background and regarded traditional medical ways of making a diagnosis and a prognosis as relevant to psychiatry. It soon struck me that, contrary to the view then prevailing in British psychiatry, depression was not just a unitary condition, varying only in severity, but a heterogeneous state comprising two or more varieties, each needing a different mode of management. One difference was that endogenous depressives tended to respond to ECT whereas reactive/neurotic depressives did not. The advent of the antidepressant drugs and, later, lithium carbonate seemed to heighten the need for a logical classification of predictive value. About this time I started to work with Sir Martin Roth in Newcastle. We were both impressed with the work of Wayne and his colleagues[1] in devising a diagnostic index for the separation of thyrotoxic from euthyroid patients. About this time I read Sir Cyril Burt's *The Factors of the Mind*[2] and profited from the experience of L.G. Kiloh and Roger Garside, also working in Newcastle, who were applying multivariate statistical methods to the problem of predicting imipramine responders from nonresponders. Roth suggested that I investigate the feasibility of dividing a large retrospective series of inpatients treated with ECT at Newcastle General Hospital over the previous three years by means of a list of weighted clinical features, the weights being derived from an intuitive appreciation of their importance in making the separation between endogenous and other forms of depression. On doing this, I found it possible to obtain a good separation between endogenous depressives who did well with ECT and neurotic-type depressives who did poorly. I was thus encouraged to start a prospective investigation of depressed patients admitted to all the major psychiatric units of Newcastle upon Tyne. From the statistical analyses of the results we were able to devise one series of weighted features for the diagnosis of endogenous and neurotic depressions and another for the prediction of response to ECT. The diagnosis index later came to be known as the Newcastle index.

"At that time, Roth's department was seething with research ideas, especially with respect to affective disorders, and a number of studies were proceeding in parallel conducted by (among others) Kiloh, D.W.K. Kay, Tom Fahy, Pamela Beamish, and Claire Gurney.

"I think the paper is so often cited because it applied statistical methods to aid the resolution of a problem of psychiatric taxonomy, produced a small number of weighted features to help the clinician and the researcher in making the differential diagnosis in depression and forecasting response to ECT, and generated a continuing controversy which now seems to be resulting in a consensus that there is an endogenous depression, symptomatically and aetiologically distinct from other depressive disorders. The topic is well reviewed by Matussek *et al.*"[3]

1. **Crooks J, Murray I P & Wayne E J.** Statistical methods applied to the clinical diagnosis of thyrotoxicosis. *Quart. J. Med.* **28**:211-34, 1959.
2. **Burt C L.** *The factors of the mind; an introduction to factor-analysis in psychology.* London: University of London Press, 1940. 509 p.
3. **Matussek P, Söldner M & Nagel D.** Identification of the endogenous depressive syndrome based on the symptoms and the characteristics of the course. *Brit. J. Psychiat.* **138**:361-72, 1981.

CC/NUMBER 5
JANUARY 30, 1984

This Week's Citation Classic™

Weissman M M & Klerman G L. Sex differences and the epidemiology of depression. *Arch. Gen. Psychiat.* **34**:98-111, 1977.
[Dept. Psychiat., Yale Univ. Sch. Med.; Depression Res. Unit, Conn. Mental Health Ctr., New Haven, CT; Dept. Psychiat., Harvard Med. Sch.; and Psychiat. Serv., Mass. Gen. Hosp., Boston, MA]

This article reviews the evidence for differing rates of depression between the sexes in the US and elsewhere during the last 40 years, and then critically analyzes the various explanations offered. These explanations include the possibility that the trends are spurious because of artifacts produced by methods of reporting symptoms, or that they are real because of biological susceptibility (possibly genetic or female endocrine), psychosocial factors such as social discrimination, or female-learned helplessness. [The *Science Citation Index*® (*SCI*®) and the *Social Sciences Citation Index*® (*SSCI*®) indicate that this paper has been cited in over 230 publications since 1977.]

Myrna M. Weissman
Depression Research Unit
Department of Psychiatry
Yale University School of Medicine
New Haven, CT 06519

November 27, 1983

"Although this paper was published in 1977, its writing was begun in 1974. In that year, I finished a PhD in epidemiology and published a book, *The Depressed Woman*,[1] with Eugene Paykel. These events had conflicting consequences. The provocative title of the book, a rather dry scientific study with statistics and tables, suddenly stimulated invitations to speak on oppression and depression in women. As a new PhD, I was uncomfortable giving offhand lectures on subjects that I really knew little about, and as a mother of four small children I didn't want to be traveling around the country. I asked Gerald Klerman the question frequently asked of me, 'Why are women more depressed than men?' and he answered, 'Are they?'

"We agreed we didn't know and decided to assess the evidence. Six months of collecting international epidemiologic data answered the first question. 'Yes, women are depressed more often than men.'

"That led to the next question, 'Why?' Over the next six months, we reviewed the possible explanations. It was an intellectual challenge to prepare as exhaustive a list as possible of all the reasons we could think of. Answering the last question, 'What is the available evidence for these various possibilities?' took another year. The organization of the paper follows our own sequence of questions. We concluded that depression is more common in women than men, that there were a number of possible explanations, and that the evidence for any one of them wasn't compelling but suggested many opportunities for investigation.

"This paper has been highly cited for several reasons. The article appeared at a time when there was scientific and public concern about the status of women. Moreover, even without this concern, a sex difference in rates of any disorder is an important epidemiologic clue which suggests a variety of possible etiologies. Whereas this subject is often the source of ideological dispute and polemic, we tried to avoid premature closure and ideology.

"The paper we originally submitted to the *Archives of General Psychiatry* was much more lengthy than the one published. We are amused that, although we didn't find strong evidence for any one explanation, the paper is often cited as evidence to support a psychosocial explanation for women's depression.

"We are pleased that the article stimulated others to systematically investigate this controversial issue. Over the last few years we have been examining some of the genetic hypotheses which may account for the differences, and we have been collecting more systematic epidemiologic data. We are planning to update the paper."

1. **Weissman M M & Paykel E S.** *The depressed woman: a study of social relationships.* Chicago, IL: University of Chicago Press, 1974. 289 p. (Cited 190 times.)

CC/NUMBER 34
AUGUST 22, 1983

This Week's Citation Classic

Klerman G L, DiMascio A, Weissman M, Prusoff B & Paykel E S. Treatment of depression by drugs and psychotherapy. *Amer. J. Psychiat.* **131**:186-91, 1974.
[Dept. Psychiat., Harvard Med. Sch., Dept. Mental Health, Commonwealth of Mass., Boston, MA; Dept. Psychiat., Yale Med. Sch., New Haven, CT; and St. George's Hosp., London, England]

The comparative efficacy of drugs and psychotherapy alone and in combination were compared in a randomized controlled trial using a 3 by 2 factorial design. The six treatment cells were psychotherapy alone, amitriptyline alone, amitriptyline plus psychotherapy, psychotherapy plus placebo, placebo alone, and low contact, no pill. The patients entered the study after having improved with open treatments with amitriptyline with an acute episode of depression. All patients were ambulatory females, non-psychotic and non-bipolar. Drug treatment prevented return of symptoms and relapse. Psychotherapy improved social functioning and interpersonal relations. The two treatments were additive. There was no placebo effect. [The *Science Citation Index*® (*SCI*®) and the *Social Sciences Citation Index*® (*SSCI*®) indicate that this paper has been cited in over 165 publications since 1974.]

Gerald L. Klerman
Stanley Cobb Psychiatric
Research Laboratories
Massachusetts General Hospital
Harvard Medical School
Boston, MA 02114

June 19, 1983

"During the late 1950s and early 1960s, the field of psychopharmacology expanded greatly and the randomized controlled trial became accepted as the standard technique for evaluating new drugs. Only slowly had this technique diffused into modes of evaluating other treatments in psychiatry, particularly psychotherapy. Based on early experience, mainly with drug treatment, when I moved to Yale University in 1964 I became interested in exploring the relationship between pharmacotherapy and psychotherapy, both in comparison with each other and in combination. Our research group at that time included Eugene Paykel, now at the University of London, St. George's Hospital; Myrna Weissman, now at Yale; Alberto DiMascio, since deceased; and Brig Prusoff, now at Yale. We designed a randomized trial comparing the efficacy of drugs alone, psychotherapy alone, the combination, and a controlled group in the maintenance treatment of depressives who had recovered from an acute episode and who were followed for nine months. This was part of a series of similar studies sponsored by the National Institute of Mental Health (NIMH), including a comparison of drug and group therapy undertaken at Johns Hopkins University,[1] and Friedman[2] *et al.* on marital therapy and medication in the Philadelphia Psychiatric Center, Pennsylvania.

"The field of psychotherapy research has gained continuing prominence. The interpersonal form of psychotherapy which was first described in its developmental stages in the 1974 paper has been subsequently modified and a manual has been developed and further control trials have been undertaken.[3,4] Along with cognitive therapy, interpersonal therapy is being evaluated in a large, multicenter collaborative study of the psychotherapy of depression being sponsored by NIMH. There are at least 15 controlled studies of brief therapy for depression now recorded and many more are under way.

"In our opinion, this paper has been highly cited because its appearance involved a happy confluence of the methodology of the randomized controlled clinical trial, interest in maintenance therapy of depressives treated with medication, and a growing interest in the efficacy of short-term forms of psychotherapy for depression."

1. **Covi L, Lipman R S, Derogatis L R, Smith J E & Pattison J H.** Drugs and group psychotherapy in neurotic depression. *Amer. J. Psychiat.* **131**:191-8, 1974.
2. **Friedman A S.** Interaction of drug therapy with marital therapy in depressive patients. *Arch. Gen. Psychiat.* **32**:619-37, 1975.
3. **Klerman G L & Weissman M M.** Interpersonal psychotherapy: theory and research. (Rush J, ed.) *Short-term psychotherapies for depression.* New York: Guilford Press, 1982. p. 88-104.
4. **Klerman G L, Weissman M M, Rounsaville B J & Chevron E.** *Short-term interpersonal psychotherapy (IPT) for depression.* New York: Basic Books. To be published, 1984.

CC/NUMBER 4
JANUARY 26, 1981

This Week's Citation Classic

Baastrup P C & Schou M. Lithium as a prophylactic agent: its effect against recurrent depressions and manic-depressive psychosis. *Arch. Gen. Psychiat.* **16**:162-72, 1967. [Psychiat. Hosp., Glostrup; Psychopharmacol. Res. Unit, Inst. **Psychiat., Risskov**; and Aarhus Univ. Sch. Med., Denmark]

Over a period of six and a half years 88 patients with frequent recurrences of mania or depression were observed before and during continuous lithium administration. Lithium treatment led to a marked fall of episode frequency and time ill. On discontinuation of lithium, episodes reappeared. [The ***Science Citation Index®*** ***(SCI®)*** **and the** ***Social Sciences Citation Index®*** ***(SSCI™)*** **indicate that this paper has been cited over 355 times since 1967.]**

Poul Christian Baastrup
Psychiatric Hospital
2600 Glostrup
Denmark
and
Mogens Schou
Aarhus University
Psychiatric Hospital
8240 Risskov
Denmark

October 13, 1980

"Our study originated in two clinical observations: the first, made by Cade[1] and confirmed in a systematic trial by Schou and associates,[2] that lithium exerts strong antimanic action; the second, made independently by Hartigan[3] and by Baastrup,[4] that continuous lithium administration may lower the frequency of not only manic but also depressive relapses.

"Collaboration took place across the country. Baastrup, in Glostrup, collected, treated, and observed the patients; Schou, in Risskov, attended to the systematic analysis of the data and to their presentation. The collaboration also involved interaction of different temperaments. Stubbornness crossed swords with impatience, and only friendship and a common goal kept the project going. Our strongest incentive to continue what at times seemed overwhelmingly difficult was that both of us had seen individual patients whose existence before lithium had been cruelly invalidated by frequent and severe relapses and who during lithium treatment returned miraculously to a normal life with reestablishment of family and working relations. It seemed most unlikely that such dramatic and long-lasting changes could have been spontaneous or accidental, but evidence must clearly be obtained from large numbers of patients treated and observed over long periods of time.

"The outcome of the trial was puzzling. Although of obvious therapeutic value in mania, lithium had not given promise of exerting antidepressive action. Nevertheless, continuous lithium administration significantly attenuated or prevented depressive as well as manic relapses, and a prophylactic action could be seen in unipolar patients, those with depressions only, as well as in bipolar cases. Such a double action, an effect on both clinical manifestations of manic-depressive illness, was, although well established for electric convulsive treatment, not shared by any other antimanic or antidepressive drug treatment, and there were those who found difficulty in accepting the data and the conclusions. A debate on methodological and ethical issues was followed by further trials, carried out by ourselves and by others, in which lithium was compared double-blind with placebo. These studies confirmed the conclusions of the original paper.

"This was the first study demonstrating clear-cut prophylactic drug action against relapses of one of the major psychoses, and it emphasized the importance of longitudinal intervention in diseases with a recurrent course. Continuing interest in our article presumably reflects continuing interest in lithium, which remains without any valid alternative. Maintenance treatment with antidepressant drugs may be of some prophylactic value in unipolar patients; in bipolar patients lithium is without peer."

1. **Cade J F J.** Lithium salts in the treatment of psychotic excitement. *Med. J. Australia* **36**:349-52, 1949.
2. **Schou M, Juel-Nielsen N, Strömgren E & Voldby H.** The treatment of manic psychoses by the administration of lithium salts. *J. Neurol. Neurosurg. Psychiat.* **17**:250-60, 1954.
3. **Hartigan G P.** The use of lithium salts in affective disorders. *Brit. J. Psychiat.* **109**:810-14, 1963.
4. **Baastrup P C.** The use of lithium in manic-depressive psychosis. *Compr. Psychiat.* **5**:398-408, 1964.

NUMBER 38
SEPTEMBER 17, 1979

This Week's Citation Classic

Schou M. Lithium in psychiatric therapy and prophylaxis. *J. Psychiat. Res.* **6**: 67-95, 1968. [Aarhus University Psychiatric Institute, Risskov, Denmark]

The paper reviews the evidence for a therapeutic effect of lithium in mania and a prophylactic effect against manic and depressive recurrences of manic-depressive disease. It further discusses lithium effects on the normal mind, the pharmacokinetics of lithium, side effects, poisoning, preparations, dosage, treatment control, and mode of action. [The *Science Citation Index®* *(SCI®)* **and the** *Social Sciences Citation Index™ (SSCI™)* **indicate that this paper has been cited over 260 times since 1969.]**

Mogens Schou
Aarhus University
Psychiatric Hospital
8240 Risskov, Denmark

July 31, 1979

"It is not clear why this particular review has reached the rank of 'Citation Classics.' I hope that quality played a role, but it has probably also been of significance that the paper appeared when it did.

"Although introduced into psychiatry in 1949 lithium had during the following eighteen years gained only limited acceptance as a psychotropic drug. It was recognized as having good therapeutic effect in mania, but its rather narrow therapeutic range and the slow onset of action made it a weak competitor of the less specific but more quickly acting neuroleptics. In 1967, however, a new and unexpected effect of lithium was discovered.[1] When the drug was given on a long-term basis, it could to a large extent attenuate or prevent recurrences of mania or depression or both. This was seen in unipolar as well as in bipolar patients.

"It was on this basis that the editor of *Journal of Psychiatric Research,* Dr. Seymour Kety, suggested that I review the lithium literature. A review from 1957 had dealt mainly with the biology and pharmacology of lithium.[2] In this new one, the emphasis was on use in psychiatry as well as on the relevant pharmacokinetics and toxicology. The review aimed at speaking the language of both psychiatrists and pharmacologists. For those about to start clinical or experimental work on this new/old drug, the review may have been a source of information and references.

"Controversy attracts attention, and it so happened that one of the main points of the review, the prophylactic action of lithium in manic-depressive disorder, became the object of heated scientific debate during the following years. Superficially the debate dealt with the methodology of prophylactic trials. Fundamentally, opinions differed about the nature and the course of recurrent manic-depressive disorder as understood by a group of British psychiatrists and a group of Danish psychiatrists. The discussion continued for some years until further studies, some of them double-blind, confirmed the conclusions drawn from the original trial.

"Lithium prophylaxis has served to focus attention on the longitudinal aspects of manic-depressive disorder and on the need for prophylactic or maintenance treatment. This important development started at about 1968, and the consequent colossal upswing of interest in the biology and clinical uses of lithium is reflected in the number of papers published before and after that time. During the five years preceding 1968 the number totalled 500; during the five years following 1968 it was 1,700. I would like to think that my review to some extent contributed to this development.

"Recent publications bring the topic of the 1968 paper up to date."[3,4]

1. **Baastrup P C & Schou M.** Lithium as prophylactic agent. Its effect against recurrent depressions and manic depressive psychosis. *Arch. Gen. Psychiat.* **16:**162-72, 1967.
2. **Schou M.** Biology and pharmacology of the lithium ion. *Pharmacol. Rev.* **9:** 17-58, 1957.
3. **Jefferson J W & Greist J H.** *Primer of lithium therapy.* Baltimore, MD: Williams & Wilkins, 1977. 211 p.
4. *Lithium in medical practice.* (Johnson F N & Johnson S, eds.) Lancaster: MTP Press, 1978. 459. p.

CC/NUMBER 49
DECEMBER 3, 1984

This Week's Citation Classic™

Raskin A, Schulterbrandt J G, Reatig N & McKeon J J. Differential response to chlorpromazine, imipramine, and placebo: a study of subgroups of hospitalized depressed patients. *Arch. Gen. Psychiat.* **23**:164-73, 1970.
[Natl. Inst. Mental Health, Psychopharmacology Res. Branch, Collaborative Depression Study Group, Chevy Chase, MD]

Imipramine was generally more efficacious than either chlorpromazine or a placebo in a double-blind study of 555 depressed patients from 10 collaborating hospitals. Imipramine was especially beneficial for the psychotic patients and where symptoms of depressed mood and anergia were prominent features of the clinical picture. [The *Science Citation Index*® (*SCI*®) and the *Social Sciences Citation Index*® (*SSCI*®) indicate that this paper has been cited in over 190 publications since 1970.]

Allen Raskin
Anxiety Disorders Section
Pharmacologic and Somatic Treatments Research Branch
Alcohol, Drug Abuse, and Mental Health Administration
Rockville, MD 20857

August 15, 1984

"When this study was conceived, many psychiatrists were reluctant to prescribe antidepressants for their patients. Evidence of clinical efficacy for these drugs was just beginning to emerge, and concerns were being voiced about their potential for adverse side effects. It was because of these widely held beliefs and attitudes that Jonathan Cole, who was then chief of the Psychopharmacology Research Branch at the National Institute of Mental Health, decided to launch a multicenter trial of drug treatment in depression. I was hired for the specific purpose of designing and coordinating this study. When I accepted this assignment, I envisioned a three- or four-year commitment. Instead, three studies were conducted with the same group of collaborators and over 30 publications emerged from these studies over a 15-year period. I am particularly proud of the fact that data from these studies formed the bases of three doctoral dissertations.

"I would like to think that the article that has become a *Citation Classic* achieved this distinction because it provided clinicians with convincing evidence that an antidepressant, imipramine (Tofranil), was an effective treatment for depression and that this drug was well tolerated by most patients. Both of these statements are true. On the other hand, I suspect that the frequency with which this article has been cited is due to the methodological innovations first described in it. Not the least of these is a simple three-item scale developed to screen candidates for the study to ensure that they met an empirically defined criterion of severity of depression. This screen, the Three-Area Severity of Depression Scale, was later dubbed by other investigators the 'Raskin Scale' and found its way into antidepressant drug trials in this country and abroad. This screen found particular favor with pharmaceutical manufacturers because of its simplicity and ease of administration and has been widely cited by them in their trials with new antidepressant drugs.

"To this day, I squirm when someone refers to this screen as the Raskin Scale. I have a vision of a mental health professional trying to match the expression on a patient's face to a series of photographs depicting me in varying stages of gloom and despair. When mention is made at a professional meeting of a patient or patients having a Raskin of seven or a Raskin of nine, all eyes turn to me, and I feel almost honor bound to graphically illustrate the meaning of these scores. I take some solace from the fact that I share this discomfort with others, most notably Max Hamilton, the developer of the Hamilton Depression Scale.[1] He, too, must endure references to a Hamilton of 13 or, worse yet, a Hamilton of 18.

"This article also provided the initial reference to a series of more expansive and detailed depression rating scales developed by my colleagues and me. These have also found some favor with investigators but, unfortunately, not to the extent of the three-item screen. Readers interested in current developments in this field are referred to a recent edition of the *Psychopharmacology Bulletin*,[2] guest edited by Robert Prien, that featured articles based on papers presented at a workshop entitled 'The Role of the New Antidepressants.'

"I would like to take this opportunity to acknowledge the efforts of my coauthors, Joy Schulterbrandt, Natalie Reatig, and James McKeon, who truly broke new ground in this field in the areas of scale development, data management, and innovative approaches to statistical analyses. I would also like to acknowledge the efforts of the psychiatrists, psychologists, nurses, and social workers at the 10 collaborating hospitals who were the backbone of this study and who are, unfortunately, too numerous to cite individually."

1. **Hamilton M.** A rating scale for depression. *J. Neurol. Neurosurg. Psychiat.* **23**:56-62, 1960.
[See also: **Hamilton M.** Citation Classic. *Current Contents/Clinical Practice* **9**(33):18, 17 August 1981.]
2. Workshop report—antidepressant drug therapy: the role of the new antidepressants. *Psychopharmacol. Bull.* **20**:209-302, 1984.

CC/NUMBER 28
JULY 12, 1982

This Week's Citation Classic

Knoll J & Magyar K. Some puzzling pharmacological effects of monoamine oxidase inhibitors. *Advan. Biochem. Psychopharmacol.* **5**:393-408, 1972.
[Dept. Pharmacology, Semmelweis University of Medicine, Budapest, Hungary]

No selective inhibitor for the B type of monoamine oxidase (MAO) was known until we demonstrated that (-) Deprenil, developed by us in 1964, is a preferential inhibitor of the metabolism of benzylamine and metaiodobenzylamine. Thus it was this paper which introduced (-) Deprenil, the first highly selective inhibitor of MAO-B. [The *SCI*® indicates that this paper has been cited in over 215 publications since 1972.]

J. Knoll
Department of Pharmacology
Semmelweis University of Medicine
Budapest 1445
Hungary

January 15, 1982

"Monoamine oxidase (MAO) inhibitors played an unforgettable role in the development of modern biological psychiatry. They were introduced into clinical practice as antidepressant agents, but because of the blockade of intestinal and liver MAO, the inhibited metabolism of pressor amines (mainly tyramine) in foodstuffs (e.g., cheeses) led in a number of cases to serious, sometimes fatal, hypertensive crises. The 'cheese effect' discredited the MAO inhibitors, the use of which became strictly limited.

"The discovery that two kinds of mitochondrial MAO, A and B type, exist started a new chapter in the history of MAO. Two studies, Johnston's[1] and ours, played the rate limiting role in the realization of the dual nature of mitochondrial MAO. Johnston developed a new MAO inhibitor, clorgyline, in 1968, and found that this substance inhibited the oxidative deamination of serotonin in low concentration and left the metabolism of benzylamine unchanged. He introduced the name MAO-A for the 'clorgyline-sensitive' form of the enzyme and MAO-B for the 'clorgyline-insensitive' one. This terminology is still in use.

"No selective inhibitor for MAO-B was known until, in 1971, we succeeded in demonstrating that Deprenil developed by us[2] inhibits in low concentrations the metabolism of benzylamine and metaiodobenzylamine leaving the oxidative deamination of serotonin unaffected.

"Deprenil and clorgyline became and are still indispensable tools for the mapping of the two forms of MAO in the brain and other tissues and were used in hundreds of papers during the last six to eight years. Our paper is regularly quoted because it introduced (-) Deprenil as the first, and still the best, highly selective inhibitor of MAO-B.

"As (-) Deprenil is the only MAO inhibitor without the 'cheese effect,' it is successfully combined with levodopa in the long-term chemotherapy of parkinsonism.[3]

"There is an age-related increase in the activity of MAO-B which might be in causal relationship with the decreased dopaminergic tone of the aging brain.

"The possibility of improving the quality of life in senescence by counteracting the consequences of this biochemical lesion by the long-term administration of (-) Deprenil which facilitates dopaminergic tone in the brain was recently suggested and is now open for careful clinical scrutiny. A review has recently been published."[4]

1. **Johnston J P.** Some observations upon a new inhibitor of monoamine oxidase in brain tissue. *Biochem. Pharmacol.* **17**:1285-97, 1968.
2. **Knoll J, Ecsery Z, Kelemen K, Nievel J & Knoll B.** Phenylisopropylmethylpropinylamine (E-250), a new spectrum energizer. *Arch. Int. Pharmacodyn. Ther.* **155**:154-64, 1965.
3. **Birkmayer W & Riederer P.** *Die Parkinson Krankheit (Biochemie, Klinik, Therapie).* Vienna: Springer-Verlag, 1980.
4. **Knoll J.** The pharmacology of selective MAO inhibitors. (Youdim M B H & Paykel E S, eds.) *Monoamine oxidase inhibitors—the state of the art.* New York: Wiley, 1981. p. 45-61.

CC/NUMBER 29
JULY 20, 1981

This Week's Citation Classic

Schildkraut J J. The catecholamine hypothesis of affective disorders: a review of supporting evidence. *Amer. J. Psychiat.* **122**:609-22, 1965.
[Sect. Psychiatry, Lab. Clinical Science, National Institute of Mental Health, Bethesda, MD]

Pharmacological findings suggesting that the clinical effects of various mood altering drugs might be related to their neuropharmacological effects on catecholamine metabolism led to the formulation of a hypothesis concerning the biochemical pathophysiology of the affective disorders. [The *SCI*® indicates that this paper has been cited over 735 times since 1965.]

Joseph J. Schildkraut
Department of Psychiatry
Harvard Medical School
Neuropsychopharmacology Laboratory
Massachusetts Mental Health Center
Boston, MA 02115

June 26, 1981

"This review was written in 1965, while I was a clinical associate in Seymour Kety's laboratory at the National Institute of Mental Health. At that time, basic neuropharmacological studies of the newly introduced clinically effective antidepressants and other mood altering drugs were beginning to suggest that the clinical effects of these drugs might be related to their effects on catecholamine metabolism. This, in turn, led to the formulation of the catecholamine hypothesis of affective disorders, which proposed that 'some, if not all, depressions are associated with an absolute or relative deficiency of catecholamines, particularly norepinephrine, at functionally important adrenergic receptor sites in the brain,' whereas manias might be associated with an excess of catecholamines.

"By focusing on the evidence supporting this hypothesis, I hoped that my review would stimulate this field of research at a critical point in its early development.

"While the catecholamine hypothesis of affective disorders remains to be verified, the expanding body of research on catecholamine metabolism in patients with affective disorders provides evidence of its heuristic value. Moreover, during the past decade, many studies[1] have explored the role of catecholaminergic neuronal systems in various aspects of animal behavior, and these studies have suggested that catecholaminergic neurons may be of importance in the mediation of many of the psychological functions that are altered in affective disorders, including arousal, motor activation, reinforcement, and reward. These factors may explain why this paper has been highly cited.

"However, even in 1965, it was clearly recognized that abnormalities in catecholamine metabolism alone could not conceivably account for all of the diverse clinical and biological phenomena in all types of affective disorders. Thus, in my review, I stressed that this hypothesis was 'at best a reductionistic oversimplification of a very complex biological state' that undoubtedly involved many other biochemical abnormalities (including alterations in the metabolism of indoleamines and other neurotransmitters, ionic changes, and endocrine disturbances), as well as physiological and psychological factors.

"The clinical and biological heterogeneity of the depressive disorders also was discussed in this review, since it seemed likely that the clinical heterogeneity of depressions might be related, in part, to differences in catecholamine metabolism, and that biochemical measures related to catecholamine metabolism might help to differentiate among subtypes of depressive disorders. While further investigation is still needed, many studies[1] already have provided evidence supporting this possibility, and we are now beginning to see the first practical clinical applications emerging from this line of research."

1. **Schildkraut J J.** The current status of the catecholamine hypothesis of affective disorders. (Lipton M A, DiMascio A & Killam K F, eds.) *Psychopharmacology: a generation of progress.* New York: Raven Press, 1978. p. 1223-34.

CC/NUMBER 47
NOVEMBER 24,1980

This Week's Citation Classic

Randall L O, Heise G A, Schallek W, Bagdon R E, Banziger R, Boris A, Moe R A & Abrams W B. Pharmacological and clinical studies on Valium™ a new psychotherapeutic agent of the benzodiazepine class.
Curr. Ther. Res. **3**:405-25, 1961. [Depts. Pharmacology and Clinical Pharmacology, Hoffmann-La Roche, Inc., Nutley, NJ]

This monograph first described the pharmacological properties of Valium. It was qualitatively similar to Librium but more potent in many pharmacological tests for taming, muscle relaxant, anticonvulsant, and sedative effects. It was well tolerated in rats, dogs, monkeys, and man. [The *SCI*® indicates that this paper has been cited over 260 times since 1961.]

Lowell O. Randall
Department of Pharmacology
University of California
Irvine, CA 92717

October 24, 1980

"This monograph summarized for the first time the pharmacological properties of Valium (diazepam) in comparison with Librium and tolerance testing in man. It reported the contributions of various members of the pharmacology and clinical pharmacology departments of Hoffmann-La Roche, Inc.

"The story of the chemical development of Librium and Valium was told by Sternbach.[1] The serendipity involved in the invention of this class of compounds was matched by the trials and errors of the pharmacologists in the discovery of the tranquilizing activity of the benzodiazepines. The discovery of Librium in 1957 was due largely to the dedicated work and observational ability of a gifted technician, Beryl Kappel. For some seven years she had been screening compounds by simple animal tests for muscle relaxant activity using myanesin as a standard and then meprobamate and chlorpromazine when they became available. All compounds submitted by the chemical staff for central nervous activity were screened. It was this battery of tests that picked out RO 5-0690 (Librium, chlordiazepoxide) as being similar but more potent than meprobamate. Within three months of receipt of the compound, we reported to management the muscle relaxant activity in mice and cats, blocking of spinal reflexes in cats, appetite stimulation and anti-inflammatory activity in rats, and only slight effects on blood pressure and autonomic responses in dogs and cats. By late fall sufficient pharmacological and toxicity data had been accumulated to recommend tolerance testing in man. This was authorized at a meeting of management in the Pocono mountains. It was perhaps coincidental that we rushed out of dinner one night to watch Sputnik cross the clear sky.

"In 1967, ten years after the discovery of Librium, a review by Zbinden and me[2] summarized the status of the benzodiazepines. Over 2,300 papers had been published on the clinical activity of these compounds. The laboratory and clinical work on 22 benzodiazepines that had been subjected to tolerance testing in man was summarized. It was reported that the best correlation of animal testing methods with clinical activity was observed with the early antimetrazol test in mice and the muscle relaxant test in cats. Ten animal screening tests reliably separated the highly active group from the intermediate and the low potency compounds. The excellent tolerance in man confirmed the high safety margins observed in animals between the effective pharmacological doses and the toxic dose. The selection of 22 new benzodiazepines from a long list of synthetic analogs, their tolerance testing in animals and man was done in those ten exciting years of drug development before the heavy hand of government bureaucracy throttled such work.

"This paper has been cited because (1) it was the first publication summarizing the pharmacological properties of Valium in comparison with Librium, (2) these compounds became the standard of reference for all work done in the Roche Laboratories and in other pharmaceutical companies on this class of compounds, (3) neuroscientists became interested in the mechanism of action of compounds having such a broad range of pharmacological and clinical activity, (4) samples of compounds were made freely available to all scientists who requested them for experimental work."

1. **Sternbach L L.** Pioneering in medical chemistry. *Chemist* **14**:5-8, 1979.
2. **Zbinden G & Randall L O.** Pharmacology of benzodiazepines: laboratory and clinical correlations. *Advan. Pharmacol.* **5**:213-91, 1967.

CC/NUMBER 11
MARCH 14, 1983

This Week's Citation Classic

Crane G E. Tardive dyskinesia in patients treated with major neuroleptics: a review of the literature. *Amer. J. Psychiat.* **124**(Suppl.):40-8, 1968.
[Psychopharmacology Research Branch, National Institute of Mental Health, National Institutes of Health, Chevy Chase, MD]

Between 1957 and 1966, 34 papers were published on tardive dyskinesia, an irreversible side effect of neuroleptic drugs used for psychoses. The cited publication reviews the literature on this disorder and attempts to bring to the attention of the medical profession the hazards of the long-term prescription of these chemicals. [The *Science Citation Index*® *(SCI*®) **and the** *Social Sciences Citation Index*® *(SSCI*®) **indicate that this paper has been cited in over 265 publications since 1968.]**

George E. Crane
639 Stratford Court 1
Del Mar, CA 92014

January 15, 1983

"Abnormal motility in patients receiving neuroleptic drugs had been reported since such agents were first introduced in psychiatry, but what most clinicians did not know was that motor disorder could be permanent and sometimes disabling. I became aware of this problem at a symposium in the Federal Republic of Germany in the winter of 1965 when Degkwitz[1] presented his observations on the condition later referred to as tardive dyskinesia. At that time, I was with the Psychopharmacology Research Branch of the National Institute of Mental Health (NIMH). I realized then that permanent damage of the central nervous system in drug-treated patients could become a major medical problem in view of the universal use of chemotherapy for psychoses. This was confirmed by a preliminary survey of patient populations I made in one of the hospitals collaborating with the NIMH and by studies I carried out throughout the 1970s.[2]

"The search of the literature for reports on tardive dyskinesia revealed that 34 papers had been published on this subject up to the end of 1966. While I was waiting for my investigations and those of others to be completed and published, I decided to devote a whole paper to a review of the literature. First, I wanted to give credit to all the authors who had made contributions in this area. This would not have been possible if I had attempted to cover all the work done by previous investigators in the introductory portions of my original papers. Editors of scientific journals do not allow enough space for this purpose. Second, the number of contributions on tardive dyskinesia was very manageable. Thus, I was in a position to provide a complete review of the literature of an important medical problem. Ordinarily, this is an impossible task even in the most specialized area of biomedical research. Third, it seemed to me that the psychiatric profession should have been informed without delay of the hazards of prescribing powerful chemicals for long periods of time. In my preliminary survey and in subsequent examinations of hospital populations, I detected tardive dyskinesia in hundreds of persons, yet it was not diagnosed in a single case. Fourth, a complete and detailed report on the literature was important, because the topic was likely to be controversial due to the belief that neuroleptics were both effective and perfectly safe. In fact, the editor of the *American Journal of Psychiatry* made my manuscript available to N.S. Kline whose comments appeared as an addendum to my presentation in the same issue of the journal.[3] This unusual editorial procedure clearly indicates how important it was not to alarm the profession.

"The fear that psychiatrists would refrain from using neuroleptics for their patients proved unfounded. In fact, their prescribing habits have changed little over the years. On the other hand, clinicians in academia realized that tardive dyskinesia could have a major impact on the practice of drug use in psychiatry, which explains why the number of papers on this unsuspected complication increased exponentially in the 1970s. Significantly, most of the observations by the early investigators were confirmed by more sophisticated and generously funded research. Furthermore, basic scientists became aware of the possibility that a study of tardive dyskinesia could clarify some aspects of drug action on the brain. Thus, the cited paper contributed to research, which increased our knowledge of neurochemistry."

1. **Degkwitz R, Wenzel W, Binsack K F, Herkert H & Luxenburger O.** Zum Problem der terminalen extrapyramidalen Hyperkinesen an Hand von 1600 langfristig mit Neuroleptica Behandelten. *Arzneim-Forsch.—Drug Res.* **16**:276-8, 1966.
2. **Crane G E.** Tardive dyskinesia and related neurologic disorders. (Iversen L L, Iversen S D & Snyder S H, eds.) *Handbook of psychopharmacology. Volume 10. Neuroleptics and schizophrenia.* New York: Plenum Press, 1978. p. 165-96.
3. **Kline N S.** On the rarity of irreversible oral dyskinesia following phenothiazines. *Amer. J. Psychiat.* **124**(Suppl.):48-54, 1968. [The *SCI* indicates that this paper has been cited in over 45 publications since 1968.]

CC/NUMBER 19
MAY 9, 1983

This Week's Citation Classic

Gunderson J G & Singer M T. Defining borderline patients: an overview. *Amer. J. Psychiat.* **132**:1-10, 1975.
[Harvard Medical School, Boston; McLean Hospital, Belmont, MA; and Univ. California, Berkeley, CA]

This review of an extensive clinical literature identified six converging features which could be used to identify patients with a borderline personality disorder. [The *Science Citation Index*® **(***SCI*®**) and the** *Social Sciences Citation Index*® **(***SSCI*®**) indicate that this paper has been cited in over 175 publications since 1975.]**

John G. Gunderson
Department of Psychiatry
McLean Hospital
Belmont, MA 02178

March 9, 1983

"I first became aware of the need to develop a more rational system for identifying patients who were clinically being called borderline while still a first-year resident in psychiatry. At that time, the term was used frequently and loosely—generally signifying that a patient had been creating problems for the members of the treatment staff. Thus, not only did it in fact have a disparaging connotation, but it also had no respectability within psychiatry as a part of its standard nosological system.

"The actual work on this project began during my residency and continued for two years afterward. At that time, I came in contact with Margaret Singer, who was much interested in this project and had independently planned to review the literature on psychological test characteristics of such patients. This coincidence led to our collaboration despite the fact that we rarely met and had only limited correspondence during the preparation of this report. Her credentials in an independent area of clinical and academic pursuit added greatly to the breadth of interest and readership which our review eventually attracted. It had been my expectation at the time this review was completed that it would largely serve as a springboard for future empirical studies which I intended to do. I had not anticipated how welcome our effort to clarify the diffuse and often contradictory prior literature would be.

"In the years since the publication of this work, there has been a remarkable proliferation of empirical work. In 1978, along with Jonathan Kolb,[1] I published results of an initial study which showed that, to a large extent, the characteristics of borderlines described in the literature could be used to identify a highly discriminable psychiatric syndrome. Since then, many different investigators using different patient populations and different methods of assessment have identified these same basic characteristics.[2] These studies provided the basis for identification of borderline personality disorder as a new diagnostic category in the new standard diagnostic manual of the American Psychiatric Association. Its more widespread adoption is foreshadowed by the roughly 25 foreign countries which are now undertaking studies on this patient group. In short, the borderline category has changed from being a 'wastebasket' diagnosis into a widely used and much studied category in the mainstream of psychiatric interest."

1. **Gunderson J G & Kolb J E.** Discriminating features of borderline patients. *Amer. J. Psychiat.* **135**:792-6, 1978.
2. **Gunderson J G.** Empirical studies of the borderline diagnosis. (Grinspoon L, ed.) *Psychiatry 1982, annual review.* Washington, DC: American Psychiatric Press, 1982. p. 415-36.

CC/NUMBER 24
JUNE 13, 1983

This Week's Citation Classic

Stewart M A, Pitts F N, Craig A G & Dieruf W. The hyperactive child syndrome. *Amer. J. Orthopsychiat.* **36**:861-7, 1966.
[Washington University School of Medicine, St. Louis, MO]

Thirty-seven hyperactive children, aged five to 11 and free of definite brain dysfunction, were compared with a like number of controls matched on demographics. Dependent variables included behavioral symptoms, development, school record, and age of onset. A clear picture of this presumed syndrome emerged. [The *Science Citation Index*® **(***SCI*®**) and the** *Social Sciences Citation Index*® **(***SSCI*®**) indicate that this paper has been cited in over 185 publications since 1966.]**

Mark A. Stewart
Department of Child Psychiatry
University of Iowa
Iowa City, IA 52242

March 3, 1983

"This paper was born of ignorance. In 1963, I was a postdoctoral fellow in pharmacology at Washington University and working on glucose metabolism in peripheral nerve. I had just finished a residency in psychiatry and, wanting to broaden my clinical experience, I volunteered to work in a pediatric neurology clinic. I hoped to see children who were retarded so that I might apply my neurochemical knowledge. Instead, almost all the children my two colleagues and I saw were hyperactive and apparently free from brain damage.

"None of us knew how the children came to be hyperactive or how to treat them, other than by giving stimulants. We had trained in the only program which was research oriented and nonpsychoanalytic at that time, so we put no stock in the anecdotal reports which made up the literature in child psychiatry. All we could find on the subject of hyperactivity consisted of two British papers[1,2] on epileptic and brain damaged children and a rather limited description of hyperkinetic child syndrome in the *Journal of Pediatrics.*[3] The impetus for the study was simple then. We had to construct our own account of these children.

"Luckily, I came from a department which prided itself on rediscovering the science of clinical psychiatry. Under Eli Robins, George Winokur, and Sam Guze, I had learned how to go about defining a syndrome through systematic study of the clinical picture, natural history, family background, and response to treatment. The study was my first amateurish attempt to put their teachings into practice. Looking back I am embarrassed at the uncritical way in which I assumed that hyperactive children were a reasonably homogeneous group and at my failure to include a control group of children with problems other than hyperactivity.

"The study was easily done. There was no trouble finding the subjects and little in finding the controls. I did most of the interviewing and was responsible for writing up the results. The work was naive, but it was the first systematic description of this broadly defined group of children. I can only think that this is the reason for its being cited.

"Since those days there has been an explosive growth in research on hyperactivity and its different facets. My own interest has shifted to aggressive conduct disorder, but I am still intrigued as to what the different kinds of hyperactivity are and what they mean in terms of brain dysfunction. In the past few years, I have been working on the relationship of hyperactivity to conduct disorder[4,5] and have helped Jerry August with a series of studies comparing hyperactive boys who have conduct disorder with those who do not."[6-8]

1. **Ounsted C.** The hyperkinetic syndrome in epileptic children. *Lancet* **2**:303-11, 1955.
2. **Ingram T T S.** A characteristic form of overactive behavior in brain damaged children. *J. Ment. Sci.* **102**:550-8, 1956.
3. **Laufer M W & Denhoff E.** Hyperkinetic behavior syndrome in children. *J. Pediatrics* **50**:463-74, 1957.
4. **Stewart M A, Cummings C, Singer S & deBlois C S.** The overlap between hyperactive and unsocialized aggressive children. *J. Child Psychol. Psychiat.* **22**:35-45, 1981.
5. **Stewart M A, deBlois C S & Cummings C.** Psychiatric disorder in parents of hyperactive boys and those with conduct disorder. *J. Child Psychol. Psychiat.* **21**:283-92, 1980.
6. **August G & Stewart M A.** Is there a syndrome of pure hyperactivity? *Brit. J. Psychiat.* **140**:305-11, 1982.
7. -------------------------------. Familial subtypes of hyperactivity. *J. Nerv. Ment. Dis.* In press, 1983.
8. -------------------------------. A 4-year follow-up of hyperactive boys with and without conduct disorder. *Brit. J. Psychiat.* In press, 1983.

CC/NUMBER 5
JANUARY 31, 1983

This Week's Citation Classic

Weiss G, Minde K, Werry J S, Douglas V & Nemeth E. Studies on the hyperactive child. VIII. Five-year follow-up. *Arch. Gen. Psychiat.* **24**:409-14, 1971. [McGill Univ., Montreal; Univ. Illinois, Urbana, IL; and Montreal Children's Hosp., Montreal, Canada]

Sixty-four severely handicapped hyperactive children, most of whom had associated handicaps of the minimal brain dysfunction syndrome, were restudied behaviourally, scholastically, and neurologically five years later at adolescence. While the hyperactivity had diminished, other handicaps, notably social and intrapsychic difficulties, and attentional and learning disorders, persisted. [The *Science Citation Index*® **(***SCI*®**) and the** *Social Sciences Citation Index*® **(***SSCI*®**) indicate that this paper has been cited in over 225 publications since 1971.]**

Gabrielle Weiss
Department of Psychiatry
Montreal Children's Hospital
Montreal, Quebec H3H 1P3
Canada

November 23, 1982

"In 1961, John S. Werry (presently professor of psychiatry, Auckland School of Medicine) and I began our residency training at the Montreal Children's Hospital and concurrently launched our first study with hyperactive children. In this, we were strongly encouraged and supported by the director of the department, Taylor Statten, who founded child psychiatry in Canada.

"We chose to study hyperactive children for several reasons. At the time, the etiology of this condition was thought to be brain damage, and we felt that this had never been clearly demonstrated. Children with symptoms of hyperactivity were common in our outpatient clinic and the clinical impression was that they did not benefit as much as did neurotic children from psychotherapy. We felt (naively) that we would be able to clearly define the syndrome operationally, and thus be able to study a fairly homogeneous population. Recognizing that the difficulties of hyperactive children lay not only in behaviour but sometimes also in cognitive functioning—we wanted to look at the effects of psychoactive medication on both of these aspects. Finally, we planned to follow our young patients to determine their outcome. It was one of those fortunate circumstances that Virginia Douglas was at that time senior psychologist at the Montreal Children's Hospital. She agreed to work with us at the onset of the studies and taught us much of what we learned and applied with respect to research methodology.

"The article cited above was the first publication of several on the follow-up of 100 hyperactive children who had met criteria for inclusion in our study. Before its publication, Klaus Minde had joined our team and participated with his special expertise in the work described in the paper.

"Several factors were probably responsible for the frequent citation of the paper. 1) At the end of the 1960s and the beginning of the 1970s, there was a great deal of interest on the part of parents, teachers, and professionals in 'hyperactivity' in children. Some of this interest resulted from well-designed, controlled studies demonstrating the short-term efficacy of stimulant drugs on this condition. 2) Follow-up studies of children who had behavioural or emotional problems (with the notable exception of the work of Lee N. Robins[1]) were rare. Our study was one of the first prospective follow-up studies of children with specific behavioural problems whose outcome was compared with, or matched against, a normal group of children. 3) The findings summarized above indicated that the prognosis of hyperactive children as they became adolescents was relatively poor. This came as somewhat of a surprise since the paediatric literature generally gave the impression that children outgrew problems of hyperactivity in adolescence.

"At different periods, Werry, Douglas, Minde, and Lily Hechtman have been a part of the research team which studied hyperactive children at the Montreal Children's Hospital. We have shared a very special camaraderie and there has been much mutual teaching and cooperation. An example is the paper cited. When first submitted, the journal's editor felt it was too long. As first author, I felt it would be impossible to cut and I sent it to Werry, who had been on our team, and who was at that time at the University of Illinois, for advice. He returned it shortened and better written and it was resubmitted. I learned from him how to distinguish the important from the less important, and he taught me to write scientific articles. I consider the article cited to be the joint creation of all of us on the team."

1. **Robins L N.** *Deviant children grown up*. Huntingdon, NY: Krieger, 1974. 351 p.

CC/NUMBER 23
JUNE 6, 1983

This Week's Citation Classic

Monroe L J. Psychological and physiological differences between good and poor sleepers. *J. Abnormal Psychol.* **72**:255-64, 1967.
[University of Chicago, IL]

Compared with good sleepers, poor sleepers (moderate insomniacs) had significantly less total sleep, a higher proportion of Stage 2 sleep, markedly less REM sleep, more awakenings, and greater sleep latencies. Insomniacs scored much higher on various measures of neuroticism and showed higher levels of physiological activity before and during sleep. [The *Science Citation Index*® (*SCI*®) and the *Social Sciences Citation Index*® (*SSCI*®) indicate that this paper has been cited in over 195 publications since 1967.]

Lawrence J. Monroe
Department of Psychiatry
Clinical Psychology
Ohio State University
Columbus, OH 43210

March 31, 1983

"This study was conceptualized in the early years of the 'golden era' of modern sleep research while I was a graduate student in clinical psychology at the University of Chicago. The concept of the relative 'depth' of the various sleep stages had emerged and was the impetus for a number of investigations pertaining to light and deep sleep; however, no studies had been reported on the differences, if any, between light sleepers and deep sleepers. In an attempt to identify light and deep sleepers through questionnaire procedures, I discovered that people had very definite impressions about whether they were good or poor sleepers and that these respondents were much more concerned with the quality of their sleep than they were with the depth of sleep. The somewhat unexpected results about the perceived importance of the presence or absence of good sleep, coupled with the prevailing paucity of scientific investigations into the quality of sleep, led to the development of a proposed study for my PhD dissertation. The specific question investigated was whether or not there were measurable differences between self-defined good and poor sleepers in electrophysiologically determined sleep patterns, in psychophysiological functions, and in personality patterns.

"There are several apparent reasons why this paper has become a classic in the field of sleep research. The timing was important in that this was the first study to report physiological, psychological, and EEG-defined sleep-pattern differences between people who sleep well and those who report considerable suffering. The study has been cited by numerous authors as being the first EEG investigation into the qualitative aspects of sleep; these findings established poor sleep or insomnia as a valid disorder, thus disproving the common notion that insomnia is just an unfounded hypochondriacal complaint. This research was also a major stimulant for subsequent studies of poor sleep, insomnia, and related sleep disturbances. One surprising aspect of this study was the robustness as well as the number of meaningful differences observed between the good and poor sleepers. Perhaps even more surprising is the frequency and consistency with which the major findings of this study have been confirmed by other investigators over the past 15 years. The originally suggested relationship between insomnia and heightened levels of physiological and emotional functioning has been verified and remains a significant factor in current theorizing about insomnia."[1,2]

1. **Kales A, Caldwell A B, Preston T A, Healey S & Kales J D.** Personality patterns in insomnia. *Arch. Gen. Psychiat.* **33**:1128-34, 1976.
2. **Johns M W, Gay T J A, Masterson J P & Bruce D W.** Relationship between sleep habits, adrenocortical activity and personality. *Psychosom. Med.* **33**:499-508, 1971.

CC/NUMBER 18
MAY 3, 1982

This Week's Citation Classic

Williams R L, Agnew H W, Jr. & Webb W B. Sleep patterns in young adults: an EEG study. *Electroencephalogr. Clin. Neuro.* **17**:376-81, 1964. [Dept. Psychiatry, Coll. Med., and Dept. Psychology, Coll. Arts and Sciences, Univ. Florida, Gainesville, FL]

A composite picture of a typical night's sleep showed that EEG sleep stages do not appear in any consistent temporal sequence from night to night. However, stages 3 and 4 predominate in the first third of the night while stage 1-REM is most prevalent in the last third. [The *Science Citation Index*® (*SCI*®) and the *Social Sciences Citation Index*® (*SSCI*®) indicate that this paper has been cited over 220 times since 1964.]

Robert L. Williams
Department of Psychiatry
Baylor College of Medicine
Texas Medical Center
Houston, TX 77030

March 5, 1982

"My initial interest in human sleep, which culminated in a book establishing EEG norms for the ontogeny of human sleep,[1] was kindled by Wilse Webb, one of the coauthors of this paper at the University of Florida. While exploring the relationship of sleep to mental disorders, we discovered that psychophysiologic norms for human sleep had not been established. Particularly lacking was an EEG composite of a typical night's sleep and evidence of whether sleep was consistent night after night. With Webb contributing the research design and Harman Agnew organizing a system for collecting and analyzing the data, we tackled these problems as a team.

"Our research in this pioneering field might never have 'gotten off the ground' (and into the bedroom) without the support of the aerospace industry. All scientific research had been sharply curtailed until the launching of *Sputnik*. In its wake came renewed support for scientific research having possible relevancy to space exploration. Whether astronauts could sleep in space was one of the questions to which the Air Force Office of Scientific Research was seeking quick answers. When astronauts subsequently reported difficulty sleeping on the *Gemini* and *Apollo* flights, the need for an objective way to measure and evaluate the sleep-wake cycle became crucial. In turn, the rapid technological advances spawned early in the space era—e.g., microelectronic devices, computer automation—made our work more accurate.

"Sampling the citations to our paper revealed several likely reasons why our paper has been highly cited. It was the first to quantify the composite features of a typical night's sleep: sequencing of EEG sleep stages, length of each sleep stage, number of sleep stage changes, prevalence of sleep stages, and their distribution over the course of the night. Often cited in subsequent papers was our revised method of analyzing EEG records, which provided criteria for marking an epoch as one of five sleep stages or the waking state. This not only helped establish the consistent methodology that is so critical on any research frontier, but also provided a standard against which to check the reliability of automated sleep analysis.

"Our discovery of the highest incidence of REM sleep in the last third of the night and of stages 3 and 4 in the first third was also mentioned frequently. These distribution data were applied clinically to diagnose and treat poorly understood sleep and arousal disorders as well as to identify symptoms of diseases that could be detected only during sleep.

"As a result of my early work on normal sleep, in 1970 I was awarded a special Public Health Service Research Fellowship from the National Institute of Mental Health, which partially supported a professional development leave from my administrative and academic duties. This award enabled me to devote full-time study to the EEG of human sleep at both the Florida laboratory and the University of Edinburgh.

"More recent advances in normal human sleep have been in the exploration of regional cerebral hemodynamics[2] and sleep-wake periodicity. For current research findings in the sleep field, see *Psychophysiological Aspects of Sleep*."[3]

1. **Williams R L, Karacan I & Hursch C J.** *Electroencephalography (EEG) of human sleep: clinical applications.* New York: Wiley, 1974. 169 p.
2. **Sakai F, Meyer J S, Karacan I, Derman S & Yamamoto M.** Normal human sleep: regional cerebral hemodynamics. *Ann. Neurol.* 7:471-8, 1980.
3. **Karacan I,** ed. *Psychophysiological aspects of sleep: proceedings of the Third International Congress of Sleep Research.* Park Ridge, NJ: Noyes, 1981. 225 p.

CC/NUMBER 10
MARCH 8, 1982

This Week's Citation Classic

Vaughan H G, Jr., Costa L D & Ritter W. Topography of the human motor potential. *Electroencephalogr. Clin. Neuro.* **25**:1-10, 1968.
[Dept. Neurology, Albert Einstein Coll. Med., Bronx, NY]

The scalp topography of cortical potentials associated with voluntary movements of the face, tongue, hand, and foot was maximum in amplitude over the contralateral precentral cortex and exhibited distributions consistent with the known arrangement of body parts within the motor cortex. [The *Science Citation Index*® (*SCI*®) **and the** *Social Sciences Citation Index*® (*SSCI*®) **indicate that this paper has been cited over 140 times since 1968.]**

Herbert G. Vaughan, Jr.
Rose Fitzgerald Kennedy Center for
Research in Mental Retardation
and Human Development
Albert Einstein College of Medicine
Bronx, NY 10461

January 11, 1982

"In 1961 our laboratory began a systematic study of the cortical electrical activity associated with human information processing, using computer averaging techniques to extract the tiny signals specifically related to sensorimotor processes from the random activity that predominates in the scalp-recorded electroencephalogram. Although cortical potentials elicited by external stimulation had begun to be widely studied, no brain activity related to the initiation of voluntary movements had been observed, either in man or in experimental animals. Such activity should, in principle, be detectable by signal averaging methods if the brain activity related to movement could be adequately synchronized.

"We initially observed movement-related potentials from scalp recordings overlying the motor cortex when brisk responses of the hand or foot were made in response to visual or auditory stimulation.[1] Similar 'motor potentials' were recorded when movements were self-initiated, but in contrast to the stimulus-triggered condition, activity preceded the movements by one second or more.[2] These 'readiness potentials,' concurrently reported by Kornhuber and Deecke,[3] provided evidence that preparatory neural mechanisms were volitionally activated long before the phasic discharge of corticospinal neurons reflected in the potentials that immediately preceded movement initiation. The next step in our investigation involved the detailed mapping of the motor potentials in an effort to identify the cortical regions that generated them. Our findings, reported in this paper, indicated a somatotopic distribution of potentials preceding face, hand, and foot movements consistent with the spatial organization of motor cortex which Penfield and Boldrey had demonstrated by direct electrical stimulation in the 1930s.[4] Subsequent work from several laboratories[5-7] has further examined the configuration and scalp topography of movement-related potentials in both normal subjects and in patients with motility disorders.

"Although some issues regarding the specific neural structures that generate the complex sequence of potentials associated with voluntary movement remain to be empirically resolved, the motor potentials provide a non-invasive index of cortical mechanisms involved in the initiation and control of human voluntary movement. Following the discovery of the scalp-recorded movement-related potentials in man, studies of single neurons in monkeys trained to perfo'm specific movements have contributed a substantial amount of information on the brain mechanisms underlying motor control. There is a close relationship between firing patterns of neurons within the motor cortex and the motor potentials of monkeys. Furthermore, the human and simian movement-related potentials closely resemble one another, both in waveform and topography.[8] Thus, these potentials provide a bridge between the analysis of motor mechanisms in experimental animals and the study of cerebral processes related to movement in man.

"This report has presumably been frequently cited because it was the first effort to relate the scalp distribution of human movement-related potentials to the underlying somatotopic organization of sensorimotor cortex."

1. **Vaughan H G, Jr., Costa L D, Gilden L & Schimmel H.** Identification of sensory and motor components of cerebral activity in simple reaction-time tasks. *Proceedings of the 73rd Annual Convention of the American Psychological Association, 1965.* Washington, DC: American Psychological Association, 1965. p. 179-80.
2. **Gilden L, Vaughan H G, Jr. & Costa L D.** Summated human EEG potentials with voluntary movement. *Electroencephalogr. Clin. Neuro.* **20**:433-8, 1966.
3. **Kornhuber H H & Deecke L.** Hirnpotentialänderungen bei Willkurbewegungen und passiven Bewegungen des Menschen: Bereitschaftspotential und reafferente Potentiale. *Pflügers Arch. Ges. Physiol.* **284**:1-17, 1965.
4. **Penfield W & Boldrey E.** Somatic motor and sensory representation in the cerebral cortex of man as studied by electrical stimulation. *Brain* **60**:389-443, 1937.
5. **Deecke L, Scheid P & Kornhuber H H.** Distribution of readiness potential pre-motion positivity, and motor potential of the human cerebral cortex preceding voluntary finger movements. *Exp. Brain Res.* **7**:158-68, 1969.
6. **Shibasaki H, Barrett G, Halliday E & Halliday A M.** Components of the movement-related cortical potential and their scalp topography. *Electroencephalogr. Clin. Neuro.* **49**:213-26, 1980.
7. **Deecke L, Englitz H G, Kornhuber H H & Schmitt G.** Cerebral potentials preceding voluntary movement in patients with bilateral or unilateral Parkinson akinesia. (Desmedt J E, ed.) *Attention, voluntary contraction, and event-related cerebral potentials.* Basel: Karger, 1977. p. 151-63.
8. **Arezzo J C & Vaughan H G, Jr.** Intracortical sources and surface topography of the motor potential and somatosensory evoked potential in the monkey. (Kornhuber H H & Deecke L, eds.) *Motivation, motor and sensory processes of the brain: electrical potentials, behaviour, and clinical use.* Amsterdam: Elsevier/North-Holland Biomedical Press, 1980. p. 77-83.

CC/NUMBER 49
DECEMBER 5, 1983

This Week's Citation Classic

Galin D & Ornstein R. Lateral specialization of cognitive mode: an EEG study. *Psychophysiology* 9:412-18, 1972.
[Langley Porter Neuropsychiatric Institute, San Francisco, CA]

EEG asymmetry in normal subjects was studied during verbal and spatial tasks. The right-over-left ratio of whole band EEG power from the temporal and the parietal regions was greater in the verbal tasks than in the spatial tasks. This measure provides a means to distinguish these cognitive modes as they occur in normal subjects using simple scalp recording. [The *Science Citation Index*® (*SCI*®) and the *Social Sciences Citation Index*® (*SSCI*®) indicate that this paper has been cited in over 200 publications since 1972.]

David Galin
Langley Porter Psychiatric Institute
University of California
San Francisco, CA 94143

September 12, 1983

"Interest in hemispheric specialization and integration had been stimulated greatly by the dramatic studies of commissurotomy ('split-brain') patients by Sperry and his colleagues.[1,2] However, most of what was known was inferred from deficits following damage to one hemisphere or the other, or to their interconnections. Our paper is cited because it showed that the intact brain does make use of lateral specialization, and demonstrated a simple noninvasive method with which to study brain mechanisms in cognition in normal people.

"The EEG could be used during complex, naturalistic behaviors like speaking and drawing, unlike the event-related potential (ERP) method which required repetitive, transient stimuli, greatly restricting the kind of activities which could be studied. (We have recently described a 'probe-ERP' approach with advantages of both EEG and ERP.[3,4])

"In spite of great hopes since the EEG was discovered in the 1920s, there had been little previous success in relating electrophysiological recordings to cognitive functions. Luckily, we had naively taken into account three factors which had been neglected in the past: 1. Recording while the subject is engaged in a task. 2. Selection of cognitive tasks known to depend more on one hemisphere than the other. 3. Selection of temporal and parietal leads, which should be the most functionally asymmetrical. Unfortunately, occipital leads had been used most often.

"We subsequently showed that task-dependent asymmetry depended on the alpha band and studied a wide variety of tasks and task difficulty, individual differences (between lawyers and artists, between the sexes, and among handedness groups), and dyslexic children.

"This work was made possible by my Research Career Award from the National Institute of Mental Health which, in those days, endorsed a particular scientist and the general directions he wanted to take, rather than a specific experiment. This is difficult in our current, mission-oriented, publication-oriented, short-term funding climate.

"The work was also facilitated by the atmosphere of interchange at the Langley Porter Institute, where Research Director Enoch Callaway had gathered scientists with differing perspectives. I had been studying attention in cats and would have continued if not for my colleague Ornstein, then a fellow of our Interdisciplinary Training Program. He persuaded me that since my underlying interest was human consciousness it would be better to study it directly. Together we began to study the subjective state associated with EEG alpha using the biofeedback approach pioneered by Joe Kamiya at Langley Porter. In those days it was usually done by recording from a single midline occipital electrode, taking this as representative of the whole brain's activity. We quickly found this 'high alpha' with many different states. To get more specificity we pursued the idea that since the two hemispheres were associated with different types of thought, perhaps alpha from each side had a different significance, and that led us to this series of experiments."

1. **Sperry R.** Some effects of disconnecting the cerebral hemispheres. *Science* **217**:1223-6, 1982.
2. **Bogen J E.** The callosal syndrome. (Heilman K & Valenstein E, eds.) *Clinical neuropsychology*. New York: Oxford University Press, 1979. p. 308-59.
3. **Galin D.** EEG studies of lateralization of verbal processes. *Neurological bases of language disorders in children.* Washington, DC: US Government Printing Office, 1979. National Institute of Neurological and Communicative Disorders and Stroke Monograph No. 22; National Institutes of Health Publ. No. 79-444.
4. **Johnstone J, Galin D, Fein G, Yingling C, Herron J & Marcus M.** Regional brain activity in dyslexics and control children during reading tasks. *Brain and Language*. To be published, 1984.

CC/NUMBER 42
OCTOBER 19, 1981

This Week's Citation Classic

Spehlmann R. The averaged electrical responses to diffuse and to patterned light in the human. *Electroencephalogr. Clin. Neuro.* **19**:560-9, 1965.
[Mayo Clinic and Mayo Foundation, Rochester, MN]

The electrical response of the human occipital cortex to patterned light differs from that to diffuse light and varies with the density of contrast borders between dark and light pattern elements. The pattern response represents the electrical correlate of the visual content of the stimulus. [The ***SCI*®** **indicates that this paper has been cited over 130 times since 1965.]**

Rainer Spehlmann
Neurology Service
Veterans Administration
Lakeside Medical Center
and
Department of Neurology
Northwestern University
Chicago, IL 60611

August 7, 1981

"In the early 1960s, neurophysiological investigation of the human visual system was helped by the appearance of averaging computers capable of extracting small electrical cerebral responses to sensory stimuli from scalp EEG recordings. Many investigators, using flashes of diffuse light, described basic features of the human visual evoked potential. When I started my training in clinical neurology at the Mayo Clinic in 1962, I was assigned to the EEG laboratory where Reginald Bickford had just acquired a new averaging computer. Looking for a research project, I remembered my fellowship at the Neurophysiological Institute of Richard Jung in Freiburg, Germany. My colleagues there had worked on the ramifications of recent microelectrode studies from animal visual systems which had indicated that the projection of a contrast border between light and darkness onto the retina changes the firing of neurons representing that part of the retina in a manner that may serve visual discrimination of contours. This made me wonder if the computer could be used to show that visual evoked potentials in man follow the same rules as neuronal responses in animals. If the retina were stimulated with densely spaced contrast borders, the resulting visual evoked potential, representing the summed activity of occipital neurons, should differ from the potential evoked by diffuse retinal illumination. I decided to test this idea by using checkerboard patterns, mainly because by decreasing the check size one can increase the density of contrast borders without changing the total luminance. So I drew the first set of checkerboard stimulus patterns at my kitchen table and used them on my fellow residents. I soon found that responses to diffuse and patterned light differed profoundly. The difference increased with interface density, was abolished by refractory errors, and persisted during fast stimulation causing steady state responses and during paired stimuli at various intervals. I used these pairs to plot excitability cycles in a few subjects willing to endure long hours of experimentation (the excitability cycles in figures 4 and 5 are from my wife).

"When I submitted the paper for publication, it was written so badly that it was saved from rejection only by an extremely kind reviewer who rewrote almost every one of my awful sentences. It has since been cited often perhaps because it showed that visual evoked potentials are not entirely determined by invariable, structural characteristics of the visual system but may contain correlates of the visual content of the stimulus and reflect important visual functions, notably discrimination. Checkerboard patterns were thereafter widely adopted for studies of human visual evoked potentials. Later, Halliday, McDonald, and Mushin[1] found that responses to patterned light are more sensitive to pathology than responses to diffuse light. Visual evoked potentials to checkerboard stimuli, now often generated by abrupt check reversal or shift, have become a useful clinical tool for the detection of conduction defects in the optic nerve and are finding their way into the diagnosis of cerebral lesions involving the posterior part of the visual path."

1. **Halliday A M, McDonald W I & Mushin J.** Delayed visual evoked response in optic neuritis. *Lancet* **1**:982-5, 1972.

CC/NUMBER 36
SEPTEMBER 3, 1984

This Week's Citation Classic™

Massaro D W. Preperceptual images, processing time, and perceptual units in auditory perception. *Psychol. Rev.* **79**:124-45, 1972.
[Department of Psychology, University of Wisconsin, Madison, WI]

A theoretical account of the auditory recognition process is given in terms of the information in a preperceptual image and the time it is available for perceptual processing. Necessary distinctions are drawn between auditory detection, recognition, and short-term memory. [The *Science Citation Index*® (*SCI*®) and the *Social Sciences Citation Index*® (*SSCI*®) indicate that this paper has been cited in over 140 publications since 1972.]

Dominic W. Massaro
Program in Experimental Psychology
University of California
Santa Cruz, CA 95064

July 18, 1984

"When I was notified that a publication of mine was identified as one of the most-cited items in its field, my first terrifying thought was that I was citing my own work too frequently. This is not the case for the paper in question, however, since most of my research areas after the cited paper have been 'something completely different,' to steal a phrase from Monty Python.

"As a graduate student and a postdoctoral fellow, I was impressed with the information-processing framework as a heuristic for psychological inquiry. Performance in any domain could be conceptualized as involving a set of processing stages, and it is important to isolate and define the nature of the information and the operations performed on it at each stage of processing. This paradigm has major implications for experiment and theory. The primary one in my mind was that it served as an organizational framework to relate disparate areas of investigation previously believed to be concerned with fundamentally different psychological questions.

"My interest in auditory perception evolved from my thesis research on memory for pitch, a situation chosen to eliminate the possibility of subvocal rehearsal during the forgetting interval. It became apparent that memory performance was as much dependent upon 'perception' as memory, and this realization clarified previous studies of verbal memory.[1] I pursued the study of auditory perception utilizing many of the concepts developed in the visual information-processing area[2] and quickly discovered the widely different approaches to the study of the problem. The approaches ranged from the highly sensory orientation of psychoacoustics to the study of the auditory modality in memory tasks. The goal of the cited paper was to review the relevant literature across these areas and to provide a single theoretical account of phenomena rarely related to one another.

"Why choose such a project for a Wisconsin summer after a long, cold winter's first year of teaching? Although we had a gigantic garden on our new country land, weeding wasn't a problem and there was much time for library research. (There seems to be less time for such endeavors today.) The project and its apparent success provided a model for employing a similar organization for a textbook.[3]

"The frequent citation of the publication is probably due to the value of the information-processing framework for clearly expressing psychological facts and to the paper capturing the state of the art for the following decade. Although some of the central themes have since been hotly debated, criticized, and supported, the endeavor has been healthy and progressive. The most encouraging outcome has been the general success of the theoretical framework even when extended beyond its original domain."[4-6]

1. **Massaro D W.** Perceptual processes and forgetting in memory tasks. *Psychol. Rev.* **77**:557-67, 1970. (Cited 35 times.)
2. ------------------. Preperceptual auditory images. *J. Exp. Psychol.* **85**:411-17, 1970. (Cited 65 times.)
3. ------------------. *Experimental psychology and information processing*. Chicago, IL: Rand McNally, 1975. 651 p. (Cited 115 times.)
4. **Cowan N, Suomi K & Morse P A.** Echoic storage in infant perception. *Child Develop.* **33**:984-90, 1982.
5. **Kallman H J & Massaro D W.** Backward masking, the suffix effect and preperceptual storage. *J. Exp. Psychol.—Learn. Mem. Cogn.* **9**:312-27, 1983.
6. **Watson C S & Kelly W J.** The role of stimulus uncertainty in the discrimination of auditory patterns. (Getty D J & Howard J H, Jr., eds.) *Auditory and visual pattern recognition.* Hillsdale, NJ: Erlbaum, 1981. p. 37-59.

CC/NUMBER 34
AUGUST 20, 1979

This Week's Citation Classic

Cravioto J, DeLicardie E R & Birch H G. Nutrition, growth and neurointegrative development: an experimental and ecologic study. *Pediatrics* **38**:319-72, 1966. [Hospital Infantil de Mexico, Mexico City, Mexico; Department of Pediatrics, Albert Einstein College of Medicine, Bronx, NY]

The paper presents the results of an ecologic study documenting that malnutrition in children influences the development of effective interrelations among the separate sense systems as it influences the child's physical size. With the exception of mother's education, none of the demographic factors present in the malnourished environment influenced neurointegrative development. [The *SCI*® indicates that this paper has been cited over 165 times since 1966.]

Joaquin Cravioto
Instituto Nacional de Ciencias y Technologia
de la Salud del Nino-DIF
Insurgentes Sur 3700
Mexico 22, D F Mexico

May 17, 1979

"In 1961 it was apparent that treatment based on our knowledge of the biochemical pathology of malnutrition had markedly increased the number of survivors. Since malnutrition could not only decelerate certain aspects of biochemical maturation but also was capable of producing retrogressions to earlier age-specific patterns, we became concerned with the possibility that significant lags in nervous system maturation might also have occurred. It was decided to first document if the reductions in body size characteristic of survivors of early malnutrition were associated with reduced mental development. This decision was based on the consideration that a negative finding would indicate that the lower performance found in malnutrition was a transient phenomenon which disappeared with nutrition rehabilitation. On the other hand, if children, years after the severe episode, still exhibit significant lags, the implications for policy making and national economic planning would be of such an importance that a systematic investigation of the intervening nutritional and non-nutritional factors ought to be carried on. On a personal basis this would mean leaving the laboratory of biochemistry to enter the realm of behavioral sciences, starting from scratch to learn psychology and social anthropology.

"At the end of 1962 it was clear that in survivors of early severe malnutrition, decreased body size was associated with lower intelligence test scores. The time was now ripe for the examination of some of the primary mechanisms underlying cognitive growth since the psychological tests used only partially suggest the manner in which the nervous system functioning is altered to result in lower levels of intelligence. While searching for a meaningful procedure for measuring brain function, Voronin and Guselnikov's paper on the phylogenesis of internal mechanisms of the analytic and synthetic activity of the brain[1] attracted our interest; the problem was how to make operational for the child an experimental study of phylogenesis. In deciding how to devise an appropriate test, Herbert G. Birch's monograph on intersensory development[2] answered our dilemma. Now we could ask if in humans, malnutrition influences neurointegrative development as it influences body size. But how to control for the non-nutritional variables that affect mental growth? Since our knowledge on relevant and irrelevant factors was not good enough to make a meaningful selection we opted for including a question on the role of the socio-economic deprivation generally present in the context of malnutrition.

"Birch was invited to review a draft of the paper and to join us as co-author. His positive response started a truly rewarding association with a most humane scientist whose untimely death deprived us of science and affection.

"Perhaps the many questions raised and left unanswered in the paper, its review of the literature available in English and other languages, a non-intervention research design, the first attempt to test for brain function without intelligence tests, and data documenting that in underprivileged societies bigger is better while in affluent societies bigger is irrelevant, are our guesses as to why this work is frequently cited. The paper motivated high caliber scientists to enter the field; this to us is its primary value."

1. **Voronin L G & Guselnikov V I.** On the phylogenesis of internal mechanisms of the analytic and synthetic activity of the brain. *Zh. Vyss. Nerv. Deyat. Pavl. SSSR* **13:** 193-202, 1963.
2. **Birch H G & Lefford A.** Intersensory development in children. *Monogr. Soc. Res. Child Develop.* **28:**5 Serial No. 89, 1963.

Chapter

13

Miscellaneous

Gathered here are 17 Citation Classics that defy classification in the other chapters and which are to a large extent unrelated to one another. This is not literally true since four were written on topics in anesthesiology and three on dermatologic conditions. Two are based on standard tables—one on life expectancy and one on growth. Another pair are based on studies of obesity. Thus, there are some patterns, but it has not been possible to do other than group these under the heading Miscellaneous, certainly an inglorious treatment for articles that became Citation Classics.

The first four Citation Classics, those dealing with anesthesiology, were published between 1953 and 1967. Consequently, the substance of these reports is well known to most scientists associated with anesthesiology. The neural basis of the activity of anesthetics (p. 352), the action of diethyl ether on the catecholamine neurotransmitting system (p. 353), the solubility of halothanes in blood and tissues (p. 354), and the first use of ketamine (p. 355) are the subjects of these Classics.

It is doubtful that many medical scientists would view an unexpected awakening at 5 a.m. by a roommate at a scientific meeting with much enthusiasm. Cutler does not state that Ederer did either, but the eventual result of this was an interpretation of the life table for analyzing patient survival that became a Citation Classic. Readers will surely agree with Cutler that the use of survival tables for the evaluation of the cancer reporting systems at the National Cancer Institute helped popularize their paper. The other "standard table" Classic is based on changes in the growth pattern of British children from birth to maturity. Tanner's remark that the editors accepted this two-part paper though they (the editors) didn't understand it is an observation that might receive universal sympathy among medical scientists. Tanner also points out a problem with the table that many parents have noticed, namely, some children mature early and others much later. Consequently, the growth table was later modified to incorporate this information.

Few dieters would deny the affirmation by Stunkard and McLaren-Hume that outpatient treatment for obesity is fruitless. A continuing successful application of will power is needed to lose weight initially and to prevent its regain if dieting is to be successful. Many commercial approaches to weight control have capitalized on these important aspects of dieting. The surgical ileal bypass for treatment of obesity (p. 359) passed through a phase of popularity that has now waned. Unforeseen complications not due to surgery were also encountered.

The first "This Week's Citation Classic" (TWCC) on dermatologic problems is based on a review on scleroderma (p. 360). Scleroderma is a mysterious disease indeed, sometimes highly damaging and at other times quite benign. The TWCCs on psoriasis and skin pigmentation focus respectively on the cellular and chemical nature of these two dermatologic problems. Psoriasis continues as an unsolved medical problem (p. 361), but it is alleviated temporarily by peritoneal dialysis. Melaninogenesis is interrupted in certain pigmentary or depigmentation conditions. Mishima identified the central role of tyrosine metabolism and melanosome function in these disorders by an analysis of electron micrographs.

The most cited article in this diverse collection is that by van Rossum on dose-response curves. The article contained a review on the molecular theory of drug action, and in the last paragraph of his TWCC, van Rossum states his view of how research on the popular topic of cell receptors should be conducted.

Marston's Citation Classic is important to the medical audience on two accounts. First, physicians must appreciate the difference in behavioral attitudes of patients from different social groups in terms of acceptance of and compliance with a therapeutic regimen. Second, physicians as a special social group must consider their own attitudes to this problem since the evidence indicates that physicians are among the patient groups most likely to abandon a treatment program before its recommended termination. It is perhaps well that knowledge of this is not widespread.

The next three TWCCs continue the diversity already seen in this chapter and are based on the radiologic study of bone disease, poisoning by polychlorinated biphenyl contaminants in cooking oil, and an XX individual as an intersex phenotype. The last TWCC, by Chappell, describes the crude understanding of membrane transport phenomena in mitochondra as it existed in 1965. Now the complexities of antiport, synport, the malate shuttle, and the carrier proteins necessary for these phenomena are among the most exciting topics on the regulation of cell metabolism.

One might expect to confront several dilemmas when attempting to append references to a chapter on miscellany. Since there is no thematic continuity in the chapter itself, it is obviously not possible to select references from a unified area of medicine. Moreover, since rarely do more than two TWCCs in the chapter touch on any one topic, how can the selection be made to extend a particular subject in the review bibliography? Lacking a focal point in the chapter, isn't it just as well to select the references by whimsy? Actually, it didn't "fall-out" that way at all. Several of the references listed apply directly to certain of the TWCCs in the chapter simply because obesity and drug therapy, for example, remain subjects of medical interest.

Bray G A. Hypothalmic and genetic obesity: an appraisal of the autonomic hypothesis and the endocrine hypothesis. *Int. J. Obes.* **8**(Suppl. 1):119–37, 1984.

Burton M E. Comparison of drug dosing methods. *Clin. Pharmacokinet.* **10**:1–37, 1985.

Caranasos G J, Stewart R B & Cluff L E. Clinically desirable drug interactions. *Annu. Rev. Pharmacol. Toxicol.* **25**:67–95, 1985.

Cooke J E. Drug interactions in anesthesia. *Clin. Plast. Surg.* **12**:83–9, 1985.

Epstein L H. The direct effects of compliance on health outcome. *Health Psychol.* **3**:385–93, 1984.

Greenland S. Tests for interaction in epidemiologic studies: a review and a study of power. *Stat. Med.* **2**:243–51, 1983.

Morley J E & Levine A S. The pharmacology of eating behavior. *Annu. Rev. Pharmacol. Toxicol.* **25**:127–46, 1985.

Sternberg E M. Pathogenesis of scleroderma: the interrelationship of the immune and the vascular hypotheses. *Surv. Immunol. Res.* **4**:69–80, 1985.

CC/NUMBER 22
JUNE 1, 1981

This Week's Citation Classic

French J D, Verzeano M & Magoun H W. A neural basis of the anesthetic state. *Arch. Neurol. Psychiat.* **69**:519-29, 1953.
[Veterans Administration Hosp., Long Beach, and Depts. Surgery and Anatomy, Univ. California Sch. Med., Los Angeles, CA]

Earlier studies had identified areas of the central core of the brain stem, differentiated from the primary motor and sensory pathways, which, when stimulated facilitated or inhibited motor activity and aroused sleeping animals. This paper found that the loss of wakefulness and motor activity, induced by anesthetic agents, resulted from their blockade of these central brain stem mechanisms. This observation provided an initial understanding of the physiological processes involved in the anesthetic state. [The *SCI*® indicates that this paper has been cited over 275 times since 1961.]

John D. French
Brain Research Institute
Center for the Health Sciences
University of California
Los Angeles, CA 90024

April 17, 1981

"H.W. Magoun published the fundamental information leading to this *Citation Classic*, which lists my name first, and must be recognized as an essential coinvestigator in the work. Magoun and I became friends in 1946 in Chicago. He was a member of Northwestern's Institute of Neurology; he had revived use of the Horsely-Clarke stereotaxic instrument, disregarded for decades by scientists. With the instrument, stimulating or recording electrodes could be inserted into deep centers of the brain. Magoun was also a regular visitor at the Illinois Neuropsychiatric Institute where Percival Bailey was my preceptor.

"In 1944, Magoun published the first of a notable series of research reports which were to identify functional capabilities exhibited by the central reticular formation of the brain stem.[1] Stimulation of one portion elicited facilitation of motor activity while excitation of another led to motor inhibition. In 1949, he and a visiting scientist from Italy, G. Moruzzi, discovered that ascending influences of the same general region induced EEG and behavioral arousal in sleeping animals.[2] Later, it was found that lesions of this region led to coma.

"In 1950, Magoun and I came together again at the Veterans Administration Hospital in Long Beach, California, where I was chief of neurosurgery. Jointly, a growing number of laboratories were established there to provide research facilities for the many neuroscientists attracted to UCLA's new school of medicine, then being built in Los Angeles. Marcel Verzeano, one of these investigators attracted to Long Beach, had a special competence in electronics, a valuable asset in this work.

"The Long Beach laboratories were a beehive of activity at that time. Many of us were interested in the reticular formation and its functions in wakefulness and sleep. The next logical step was to find out how anesthetic agents influenced these brain stem mechanisms for wakefulness and motor modulation. The experiments, which occupied the better part of a year, indicated that loss of wakefulness and accompanying muscular changes during the anesthetic state were the result of selective action of the agents administered upon the reticular formation. The high density of cellular junctions in the area, in contrast to the simpler structure of the primary motor and sensory pathways, appeared to provide it with a special sensitivity to the drug action.

"There were a number of reasons for the interest aroused by the paper. First, it appeared during the surge of research interrelating the reticular formation with behavioral states. In addition, the title suggested a clinical relevance of the work which may have attracted the attention of the medical profession. In this connection, perhaps the findings offered a prospect of attaining better control over anesthetic procedures.

"Unfortunately, the exciting days at Long Beach gradually came to an end for most of us. Magoun soon became tied up on the UCLA campus with pressing responsibilities in establishing a department of anatomy and a Brain Research Institute; somewhat later I followed him there as director of the Institute. Verzeano is now professor of psychobiology at the University of California, Irvine.

"It is 28 years since this paper was published and there is still much to be learned from further investigation of neural mechanisms involved in drug-induced states which will contribute substantially to the effectiveness and safety of anesthesia."

1. **Magoun H W.** Bulbar inhibition and facilitation of motor activity. *Science* **100**:549-50, 1955.
2. **Moruzzi G & Magoun H W.** Brain stem reticular formation and activation of the EEG. *Electroencephalogr. Clin. Neuro.* **1**:455-73, 1949.

NUMBER 30
JULY 23, 1979

This Week's Citation Classic

Price H L, Linde H W, Jones R E, Black G W & Price M L. Sympatho-adrenal responses to general anesthesia in man and their relation to hemodynamics. *Anesthesiology* **20**:563-78, 1959 [Dept. Anesthesiology, University of Pennsylvania School of Medicine, Philadelphia, PA]

The development of a sensitive, highly specific method for detecting catecholamines permitted us to determine, for the first time, whether or not certain general anesthetics caused sympathetic nervous excitation in man. We found that diethyl ether and cyclopropane did so, thus explaining the great safety of these anesthetic agents, since their directly depressant actions on myocardium are partially antagonized by sympathetic stimulation. [The ***SCI***® **indicates that this paper has been cited over 215 times since 1961.]**

Henry L. Price
Department of Anesthesiology
Hahnemann Medical College &
Hospital of Philadelphia
Philadelphia, PA 19102

March 3, 1978

"Shortly after the end of the Second World War, a new class of general anesthetics was introduced into clinical practice. These agents had in common extreme potency, halogen substitutions for hydrogen on the parent molecule, lack of explosion hazard, and severe circulatory depression in the recipient. It occurred to us that, since some of the older and safer anesthetics had been suspected of inducing sympathetic nervous activation (which could have counteracted the directly depressant actions of the anesthetics), the newer agents might simply fail to do so.

"Unfortunately, there was at this time no acceptable way of estimating the level of sympathetic nervous discharge in man. Attempts were soon to be made to measure concentrations of epinephrine and norepinephrine in plasma, but these were of limited specificity, since they involved condensation with ethylenediamine and therefore did not distinguish between simple catechol nuclei and the catecholamines which possessed biological activity. It was at this point that the trihydroxyindole method, developed in Scandinavia by Lund,[1] came to our attention. This method, while specific for catechol compounds possessing a B-OH grouping characteristic of the naturally-occurring biologically active sympathetic amines, was of limited sensitivity and not suitable for analyzing the low levels of epinephrine and norepinephrine which ordinarily occur in plasma.

"The principal impetus which made the cited study possible was the use of a two wave-length activation of the fluorescent trihydroxyindole compound produced, suggested by a colleague A. deT. Valk, and to further refinements by my wife, M.L. Price, without whose efforts this work would never have come to fruition.

"The basic finding was that the older, safer anesthetics are sympathetic excitants, while most halogenated agents and the barbiturates are either depressants or have no effect. This action appears to explain the relative safety of the older anesthetics such as cyclopropane and diethyl ether, which are both capable of increasing plasma levels of norepinephrine in man. Of course, it was recognized at the time that there would be difficulties in interpretation, and the bulk of the paper dealt with various considerations needed to put the data into perspective. Viewed in retrospect, the interpretations offered appear prescient and they seem to have withstood the test of time."

1. **Lund A.** Fluorimetric determination of adrenaline in blood; chemical constitution of adrenolutine (the fluorescent oxidation product of adrenaline). *Acta Pharmacol. Toxicol.* **5**:121-8, 1949.

CC/NUMBER 43
OCTOBER 22, 1984

This Week's Citation Classic™

Larson C P, Jr., Eger E I & Severinghaus J W. The solubility of halothane in blood and tissue homogenates. *Anesthesiology* **23**:349-55, 1962.
[Dept. Anesthesiology and Cardiovascular Res. Inst., Univ. California Med. Ctr., San Francisco, CA]

Partition coefficients of halothane in blood and body tissue homogenates of man and cattle were determined by equilibrating these substances with known volumes of liquid halothane in closed flasks and analyzing the halothane concentration of the overlying gas phase by infrared analysis. Whole blood coefficient was 2.3 and tissue coefficients ranged from 3.6 for kidney to 8.3 for cerebral white matter. [The *SCI*® indicates that this paper has been cited in over 150 publications since 1962.]

C. Philip Larson, Jr.
Department of Anesthesia
Stanford University School of Medicine
Stanford, CA 94305

July 20, 1984

"Shortly after I began my research fellowship in July 1960, my research advisers, John Severinghaus and Ted Eger, suggested that I attempt to determine the partition coefficient for halothane in blood and other tissues. They thought that it could be done by equilibrating halothane between liquid and gas phases and then measuring the concentration in the gas phase using the newly developed infrared halothane analyzer. From their clinical experience with halothane, they thought that the blood/gas value of 3.6 reported by Raventós[1] might be too high.

"The experiments were conducted in John's laboratory in the Cardiovascular Research Institute at the University of California at San Francisco. I added accurately measured volumes of liquid halothane to known volumes of outdated human blood in sealed flasks and measured the concentration of halothane in the gas phase using a calibrated infrared halothane analyzer. To my surprise, I obtained a consistent value of 2.3 ± 0.1 SD. Using the same experimental model, tissue/gas solubility coefficients were determined for homogenized specimens of whole brain, gray and white matter, liver, kidney, muscle, and fat. Halothane proved to be 1.5 to 3.5 times as soluble in tissues (excluding fat) as in blood, a finding that was at variance with the value of 1.0 that had consistently been found for all other anesthetics studied.

"Because the volume of human tissues from autopsy sources was limited, officials at the Swift and Co. meat-packing plant agreed to donate beef blood and other tissues. On several occasions, I made a 'tissue run' to the south San Francisco butchering plant where I collected buckets of fresh blood, brain, and other tissues immediately after the animal had been killed. An untimely automobile accident on a San Francisco street would certainly have caused an unwelcome sensation.

"Prior to publication of our results, I was invited to present them at a conference on uptake and distribution of anesthetic agents held in New York City under the auspices of the National Research Council and the New York Academy of Medicine. However, of even greater concern, William A.M. Duncan, a coauthor with Raventós of the first publication on the pharmacokinetics of halothane anesthesia,[2] was in attendance. I was certain that Duncan would challenge my findings and produce data to prove me wrong. My fears were unfounded. Duncan, a gentleman throughout, stated that he was able to confirm our findings using a somewhat different methodology.[3]

"In examining why this publication has become a *Citation Classic*, three explanations are possible. First, halothane holds a premier position as the most versatile anesthetic in anesthesia. It has been studied more extensively than any prior anesthetic. Since its physical properties, including solubility, determine its pharmacological actions, frequent reference is made to solubility coefficients. Second, accurate solubility values are essential to predict uptake and distribution characteristics of an anesthetic, so any studies of pharmacokinetics of halothane refer to our solubility studies. Third, and perhaps most important, the technique that we used for determining halothane solubility was a major departure from the traditional extraction methods that had been used for determining the solubility of halothane and other anesthetics. Virtually all studies of the solubility of volatile anesthetics developed after halothane was synthesized have used the technique that we introduced. Our technique has been used recently to determine the solubility of the reductive metabolites of halothane."[4]

1. **Raventós J.** The action of fluothane—a new volatile anaesthetic. *Brit. J. Pharmacol.* **11**:394-410, 1956. (Cited 300 times since 1956.)
2. **Duncan W A M & Raventós J.** The pharmacokinetics of halothane (fluothane) anaesthesia. *Brit. J. Anaesth.* **31**:302-15, 1959. (Cited 90 times since 1959.)
3. **Larson C P, Jr.** Solubility and partition coefficients. (Papper E M & Kitz R J, eds.) *Uptake and distribution of anesthetic agents.* New York: McGraw-Hill, 1963. p. 5-19.
4. **Denson D D & Ford D J.** How reactive are the reductive metabolites of halothane? *Anesthesiology* **51**:S243, 1979.

CC/NUMBER 26
JUNE 25, 1984

This Week's Citation Classic™

Virtue R W, Alanis J M, Mori M, Lafargue R T, Vogel J H K & Metcalf D R. An anesthetic agent: 2-orthochlorophenyl, 2-methylamino cyclohexanone HCl (CI-581). *Anesthesiology* **28**:823-33, 1967.
[Div. Anesthesiology, Cardiovascular Pulmonary Lab., and Electroencephalography Lab., Univ. Colorado Medical Ctr., Denver, CO]

Animal experiments indicated that CI-581 anesthesia does not sensitize a heart to epinephrine, and that it does not depress spontaneous respiration, while giving excellent analgesia. Human beings responded similarly in a variety of surgical circumstances. The drug failed to depress reflexes and afforded no relaxation. [The *SCI*® indicates that this paper has been cited in over 150 publications since 1967.]

Robert W. Virtue
Department of Anesthesiology
University of Colorado Medical Center
Denver, CO 80262

January 16, 1984

"Anesthesiologists are constantly looking for better and safer agents. When information came from the University of Michigan that a congener of Sernyl (Sernyl produced analgesia but was followed by extreme mental disturbance and excitement) appeared which had fewer undesirable qualities, it seemed valuable to observe firsthand what the drug would do. Gracious cooperation by Corssen, Domino, and McCarthy,[1-3] as well as support from the Parke Davis Co., led to observation in Ann Arbor of the effects of the drug on patients undergoing eye surgery. Recovery after use of the new congener (ketamine) was substantially different from that after the common anesthetics then in use. The drug did not depress respiration as other agents (except ether) did. It is the only anesthetic agent that can be intravenously administered that permits adequate spontaneous respiration. After preliminary animal experiments at the University of Colorado, the drug was given to several surgical patients in unusual circumstances, such as a man who was to have an anterior neck fixation because of a dislocation of vertebrae. It was deemed dangerous to move the neck (the patient was immobilized with tongs). Because of the impossibility of holding a mask while the surgeon operated, and the difficulty of inserting an endotracheal tube without moving the neck, normal anesthetic procedures were ruled out. With ketamine there was no problem because spontaneous respiration could continue. Our work extended the use of ketamine to various types of surgery and indicated that, when one realized the limitations of ketamine, it could be the safest agent available.

"Approximately ten percent of patients have vivid dreams during anesthesia with ketamine. Some are disagreeable, but not all. One woman, after three previous anesthetics, said, 'Everyone should have that anesthetic; it was so wonderful!' Analysis by Albin *et al.*[4] of the mental state of persons who had received ketamine showed that, compared to those who had other agents, dreams were not excessive.

"Due to commercial manipulations, distribution of ketamine was allocated to a second drug outlet, which in its effort to get the drug on the market quickly, sent samples to many anesthesiologists around the country without stressing the precautions necessary for its proper use. The drug soon came into disfavor because warnings that recovery needed a quiet environment (the drug gives no relaxation) and that the patient should be undisturbed during recovery were not given. Some years elapsed, therefore, before the drug could find its proper place in anesthesiology.

"After about 15 years, the position of ketamine in anesthesiology has been reasonably stabilized, as indicated in a 1982 review of its properties and uses.[5]

"Citations to the investigations of ketamine are probably due to the observations made at the University of Colorado which were the first to include its use in a variety of human surgical cases, and which provided EEG data along with usual physiological studies."

1. **McCarthy D A, Chen G, Kaump D H & Ensor C.** General anesthetic and other pharmacological properties of 2(o-chlor-phenyl)-2-methylamino cyclohexanone HCl (CI-581). *J. New Drugs* 5:21-33, 1965.
2. **Domino E F, Chodoff P & Corssen G.** Pharmacologic effects of CI-581, a new dissociative anesthetic, in man. *Clin. Pharmacol. Ther.* **6**:279-91, 1965.
3. **Domino E F.** Citation Classic. Commentary on *Clin. Pharmacol. Ther.* **6**:279-91, 1965. *Current Contents/Life Sciences* **27**(25):16, 18 June 1984.
4. **Albin M, Dresner J, Paolino A, Sweet R, Virtue R & Miller G.** Long term personality evaluation in patients subjected to ketamine hydrochloride and other anesthetic agents. (Abstract.) (American Society of Anesthesiologists) *Abstracts of scientific papers. 1970 ASA annual meeting.* Park Ridge, IL: ASA, 1970. p. 166-7.
5. **White P F, Way W L & Trevor A J.** Ketamine—its pharmacology and therapeutic use. *Anesthesiology* **56**:119-36, 1982.

NUMBER 16
APRIL 16, 1979

This Week's Citation Classic

Cutler S J & Ederer F. Maximum utilization of the life table method in analyzing survival. *J. Chronic Dis.* **8**:699-712, 1958
[Biometry Branch of the National Cancer Institute, Bethesda, MD]

The authors present the rationale and computational details of the life-table method. They describe the advantages of the method in terms of statistical reliability, i.e., the Standard Error of the survival rate, and an estimate of Effective Sample Size. [The *SCI*® indicates that this paper has been cited over 530 times since 1961.]

Sidney J. Cutler
Division of Biostatistics and Epidemiology
Gerogetown University School of Medicine
Washington, D.C. 20007

March 10, 1978

"My co-author, Fred Ederer, and I are gratified to learn that our 1958 paper is frequently cited and are delighted to describe the circumstances of its conception—at 5 a.m. in a hotel room in Cleveland, Ohio. We were involved in the development of a national program of cancer case reporting and evaluation of the results of therapy, sponsored by the National Cancer Institute. In describing patient survival, we utilized the actuarial or life-table method, which makes possible the use of all survival information accumulated up to the closing date of a study.

"In 1959 Fred and I were sharing a hotel room at a scientific meeting. I awoke early one morning with a question on my mind: 'Why is it advantageous to utilize all information at hand; how can the advantage be demonstrated?' The fact that it was 5 a.m. did not stop me from calling out, 'Fred, are you sleeping? I have a question.'

"Our paper was not a methodological breakthrough. The application of the life-table method to the description of patient survival had been used for a good many years, and had been described by Pearl in 1923[1] and Greenwood in 1926.[2] Several papers describing and applying the method had been published during the 1950s. It is therefore interesting to conjecture on the reasons for the popularity of our paper. Perhaps it is because we set out to convince ourselves that the life-table method would in fact help extract the maximum amount of information from the data being collected in the newly organized cancer-reporting system. In convincing ourselves, we apparently convinced others.

"The national cancer-reporting system resulted in the publication of a steady stream of papers utilizing the life-table method for describing patient survival. My associates and I published a number of methodological extensions of the life-table procedure. A number of alternative approaches were proposed by others. These varied publications served to bring readers' attention to the basic paper that was published in 1958. In addition, the paper has been used as a teaching tool in schools of medicine and public health. The paper may be cited frequently because many workers in the field learned the methodology through our paper."

REFERENCES

1. **Pearl R.** *Introduction to medical biometry and statistics.* Philadelphia and London: W.B. Saunders Company, 1923, 379p.
2. **Greenwood M.** The "errors of sampling" of the survivorship tables. *Reports on public health and medical subjects,* No. 33, Appendix 1. London: H.M. Stationery Office, 1926.

NUMBER 43
OCTOBER 22, 1979

This Week's Citation Classic

Tanner J M, Whitehouse R M & Takaishi M. Standards from birth to maturity for height, weight, height velocity, and weight velocity: British children, 1965. I & II. *Arch. Dis. Child.* **41**:454-71; 613-35, 1966. [Department of Growth and Development, Institute of Child Health, University of London, London, England]

The paper introduces standards for children's rate of growth in addition to the conventional standards for size attained. It emphasises the difference in construction between 'longitudinal' standards suitable for following individuals as they grow, and 'cross-sectional' standards suitable for once-off surveys, and presents both types. [The *SCI®* indicates that part one was cited over 310 times and part two over 240 times since 1966.]

J.M. Tanner
Institute of Child Health
Department of Growth
and Development
University of London
London WC1N 1EH
England

August 15, 1979

"I am delighted, of course, that this long and not particularly easy paper should have been cited so often. I suppose this is chiefly because, like so many other 'Citation Classics,' it is a paper introducing a method—or rather two. The standard growth curve is itself a method which clinicians, nutritionists, and others may use to estimate the degree of health of a child, or of progress under treatment. Much more important, however, the paper discusses the methodology of the construction of such standards and it is in this respect that it may lay claim to some originality. I suspect that most of the citations simply refer to the use of the paper's standard curves, just as many of the citations of biochemical papers simply refer to the use of a method in a given research study. However, I hope I am wrong, and that other researchers and clinicians find the methodology of standards interesting. The evidence is somewhat contrary, for so far relatively few papers have appeared in which the new things in our paper—the velocity standards and the longitudinal-type approach—have been used.

"As usual, the paper represents a long-continued preoccupation with its subject. In 1948 Reg Whitehouse, then academically innocent and fresh from nine years of administrative duties in the Royal Army Medical Corps, joined me and we began the Harpenden Growth Study, a longitudinal study of individual children from early childhood to maturity. While we were waiting for results, we embarked on a theoretical analysis of growth patterns. In 1952 this resulted in a paper on the construction of standards for height and weight which I sent to the editor of the *Archives of Disease in Childhood*, since it was aimed at pediatricians, who were at that time woefully ignorant of anything concerning growth.[1] To my surprise the editor replied that though neither he nor his referees could understand the paper, he thought the subject very important and would publish the paper in full.

"Thus encouraged, and with the help of Michael Healy, now professor of statistics at the London School of Hygiene, and in 1963-65 of Masahiro Takaishi, now in charge of the department of maternal and child health of the Tokyo Institute of Public Health, we carried the analysis further, and used our longitudinal data to devise standards which truly represented the growth of individuals. This the current standards failed to do (now as then) because they averaged out children who matured early and those who matured later. The problem had been pointed out by Boas long ago and again by Shuttleworth in the 1930s but nobody had ever provided a very practical solution.[2-4] I hope the citation record shows that we have succeeded in doing so."

1. **Tanner J M.** The assessment of growth and development in children. *Arch. Dis. Child.* **27**:10-33, 1952.
2. **Boas F.** The growth of children. *Science* **19**:256-7, 1892.
3. **Boas F.** The growth of children. *Science* **20**:351-2, 1892.
4. **Shuttleworth F K.** *Sexual maturation and the physical growth of girls age 6-19.* Chicago, IL: Society for Research in Child Development, 1937. 253 p.

CC/NUMBER 47
NOVEMBER 21, 1983

This Week's Citation Classic

Stunkard A & McLaren-Hume M. The results of treatment for obesity: a review of the literature and report of a series. *Arch. Intern. Med.* **103**:79-85, 1959. [Depts. Psychiatry and Medicine, Univ. Pennsylvania Sch. Medicine, Philadelphia, PA and Dept. Nutrition, New York Hosp., NY]

This paper was the first to document the ineffectiveness of outpatient treatment for obesity, thereby leading to a more realistic assessment of the problem. A literature review revealed that only 25 percent of patients lost more than 20 pounds and clinic patients fared even less well. [The *Science Citation Index*® (*SCI*®) and the *Social Sciences Citation Index*® (*SSCI*®) indicate that this paper has been cited in over 305 publications since 1961.]

Albert Stunkard
Department of Psychiatry
University of Pennsylvania
Philadelphia, PA 19104

August 3, 1983

"This study grew out of an attempt to resolve a paradox—the contrast between my difficulties in treating obesity and the widespread assumption that such treatment was easy and effective. At the time, I was working in Harold Wolff's Psychosomatic Research Group at New York Hospital and at first attributed my difficulties to problems of patient selection. Growing doubts, however, led me to review the literature on outpatient treatment of obesity to see if other people really were doing as well as the current optimism implied. This review revealed serious problems in the reporting of data, including the omission of data on patients who had dropped out of treatment (and who presumably had not done well) and grouping of data so as to obscure the outcome of treatment of individual patients. When subjected to even minimal criteria, the vast literature (even in 1959) on the treatment of obesity shrunk to just eight reports. Alvan Feinstein, who was then working on obesity at the Rockefeller Institute, suggested assessing outcome by listing the percent of patients in each report who lost 20 and 40 pounds. When this was done, it became clear that the results of outpatient treatment were remarkably similar and remarkably poor. With the exception of Feinstein's own series, only 25 percent of patients lost more than 20 pounds and only five percent lost more than 40 pounds. Furthermore, these reports were all by experts. It seemed likely that patients of the average practitioner fared even less well.

"To find out whether this was, in fact, the case, I enlisted the help of a dietician, Mavis McLaren-Hume, in following the course of 100 consecutive patients referred to the Nutrition Clinic of New York Hospital. This clinic was an ideal resource, since all patients who were treated for obesity in any clinic in the hospital were referred here for a diet, and since their records in these clinics were available for follow-up. These results were, as I had suspected, even worse than those in the literature. Instead of 25 percent, only 12 percent of patients lost 20 pounds, and instead of five percent, only one percent lost 40 pounds. Furthermore, two years later, only two percent of patients had maintained their 20-pound weight loss.

"I believe that this paper has been cited frequently because it documented for the first time the ineffectiveness of outpatient treatment for obesity, and thereby led to a more realistic assessment of the problem and of the means for coping with it. These means are still limited, as Wing and Jeffery have shown in their recent review.[1]

"Soon after the publication of this paper, I received the Annual Award for Research of the American Psychiatric Association.

"*Citation Classics* are particularly valuable in opening a window on the personal origins of research, a topic that is as important as it is poorly understood. Those interested in this area might enjoy *The Pain of Obesity*,[2] which describes similar, more detailed accounts of seven other research efforts. Interestingly, the present study had not seemed worth including."

1. **Wing R R & Jeffery R W.** Outpatient treatment of obesity: a comparison of methodology and clinical results. *Int. J. Obesity* 3:261-79, 1979.
2. **Stunkard A J.** *The pain of obesity.* Palo Alto, CA: Bull Publishing, 1976. 236 p.

CC/NUMBER 48
NOVEMBER 30, 1981

This Week's Citation Classic

Payne J H & DeWind L T. Surgical treatment of obesity.
Amer. J. Surg. **118**:141-7, 1969.
[Hosp. Good Samaritan Medical Ctr., and Dept. Medicine and Surgery, Univ. Southern California, Sch. Medicine, Los Angeles, CA]

The jejuno ileal intestinal bypass (Payne procedure) is a technique to induce significant weight reduction in the malnourished, morbidly obese patient. Our clinical study began in 1956. To this date, some type of surgical procedure has proven to be the only successful therapy for uncontrolled obesity. [The *SCI*® indicates that this paper has been cited over 265 times since 1969.]

J. Howard Payne
1245 Wilshire Boulevard
Los Angeles, CA 90017

September 3, 1981

"Loren DeWind and I are honored to have our manuscript included in this publication.

"Why do we think our paper has been so highly cited? It is our opinion that the surgeons, internists, and research workers in the problems of human hyperobesity were ready for this report. There had been no report from our departments since the report on jejunocolic intestinal bypass in 1963.[1] Our conclusions were that jejunocolic bypass resulted in metabolic disaster and this operation should be abandoned.

"The 1969 report was a new approach and was the first article written since 1963 about a significant number of carefully selected, controlled, and diligently followed group of malnourished, morbidly obese subjects.

"We received no awards or honors except the respect and gratitude of our patients; a synopsis of the article was published and reviewed in the 1970 *Year Book of General Surgery*.[2] In 1978, R.B. Phillips referred to our work[3] providing widespread attention and coverage.

"As for problems—we had our share. Many obstacles were thrown in our path during our early efforts to continue the work and have it accepted for presentation or publication at a major surgical meeting, the Pacific Coast Surgical Association, and eventually the American Surgical Association.

"There were long discussions with the Hospital of the Good Samaritan research committee, but very little difficulty with the University of Southern California School of Medicine, department of surgery. At times some of our friends and foes thought we 'didn't have all our oars in the water.' Eventually we were granted full permission by the appropriate committees to continue the work.

"A major difficulty was dealing with the patients' medical insurance companies. It was their contention that this was a cosmetic operation. After considerable discussion and exchange of correspondence, we were able to convince the carriers that we were operating on malnourished, morbidly obese subjects. Thus the diagnosis, 'malnutrition morbid obesity,' was defined, coined, and accepted.

"All too often the important personnel around you are not given credit for their contribution. The surgical personnel were always understanding, flexible, and many were excellent. They had special instruments made when necessary. The residents, physicians, and ICU and floor personnel learned to understand these huge patients and to treat them as desperately ill patients and not as 'fat slobs.' They provided a friendly atmosphere in which to recover in dignity.

"Most of our obese patients were anesthetized by the same doctor. Without his skill, tenacity, and intelligence, I do not think we could have safely done this type of surgery on these giant patients. There was only one death attributable to anesthesia. Most patients left the operating room extubated and awake. Ironically, I enticed the anesthesiologist to submit a manuscript for publication relating his very successful methods of how to safely anesthetize the hyperobese patient; it was rejected with a letter indicating what he was doing wrong!

"All surgeries were done by the same surgeon.

"If our work has proven nothing else, there is evidence that the hyperobese patient can be safely anesthetized to undergo major intraabdominal surgery!"

1. **Payne J H, DeWind L T & Commons R R.** Metabolic observations in patients with jejunocolic shunts. *Amer. J. Surg.* **106**:273-89, 1963.
2. **Payne J H & DeWind L T.** Surgical treatment of obesity. (DeBakey M E, ed.) *Year book of general surgery.* Chicago, IL: Year Book Medical Publishers, Inc., 1970. p. 20-1.
3. **Phillips R B.** Small intestinal bypass for the treatment of morbid obesity. *Surg. Gynecol. Obstet.* **146**:455-68, 1978.

CC/NUMBER 42
OCTOBER 17, 1983

This Week's Citation Classic

Tuffanelli D L & Winkelmann R K. Systemic scleroderma: a clinical study of 727 cases. *Arch. Dermatol.* **84**:359-71, 1961.
[Mayo Clinic and Mayo Foundation, Rochester, MN]

Seven hundred twenty-seven patients with systemic scleroderma seen at the Mayo Clinic in the period from 1935 through 1958 were studied. The usual course and findings of the disease were determined and the unusual features were stressed. The prognosis of scleroderma was determined. [The *SCI*® indicates that this paper has been cited in over 275 publications since 1961.]

Denny L. Tuffanelli
450 Sutter Street
Suite 1306
San Francisco, CA 94108

July 28, 1983

"The cited article was largely a product of the Mayo Clinic system of medicine and biostatistics. Richard Winkelmann, an enthusiastic staff member, suggested that a clinical review of the Mayo Clinic experience with scleroderma patients would be valuable as a basis for future evaluations and study of the disease. Because of the clinic's status as a tertiary referral care center, and the specific interests of Paul O'Leary of the dermatology department, a vast clinical experience with scleroderma had accumulated. The prospect of doing a scholarly, in-depth study of a single, chronic, catastrophic illness appeared promising to me, and I accepted the project.

"The study was quite time-consuming, and occupied most of my spare time over the next two years. Current patients were examined, and all available charts were reviewed from cover to cover, in the precomputer era. The clinical and laboratory data on 727 patients with systemic scleroderma observed at the Mayo Clinic from 1935 through 1958 were correlated. Scleroderma is a capricious disease. Some patients had a fulminating course with death in a year or two. Others had a chronic, extremely debilitating illness. Rare patients improved spontaneously. Many of the charts were poignant short stories. The tragedy overwhelming many of the patients was amply documented in the records. I enjoyed library research and read over 400 references on scleroderma. The superb Mayo Clinic library was a pleasant place to spend the cold Minnesota evenings.

"Finally, the literature review and clinical data were presented as a master's thesis, and with Winkelmann's collaboration three published papers resulted,[1,2] the major one being the *Archives of Dermatology* article.

"The article was, and remains, a review of the largest number of patients with scleroderma. The incidence of Raynaud's phenomenon, and cutaneous features including sclerosis, telangiectasia, calcinosis, cutaneous ulcerations, and pigmentary changes, were documented. Similarly, the incidence of systemic features, particularly gastrointestinal, pulmonary, and renal, was determined. Prognostic studies furnished the valuable information that 29.7 percent of the patients died in less than five years (from time of diagnosis at Mayo) while 70.3 percent of patients survived five years without benefit of a specific therapy. The ten-year survival rate of 58.9 percent indicated that the prognosis was not as bleak as previously thought.

"The study focused my academic interest on connective tissue diseases and following dermatology residency I decided to further study this fascinating group of diseases. For the past 20 years, I have conducted a connective tissue disease clinic and immunopathology laboratory at the University of California in San Francisco. Over 150 publications have been generated by this experience.[3]

"The small coterie of physicians interested in scleroderma has provided international friendships and meetings.[4] Medical directorship of the United Scleroderma Foundation, a national group of scleroderma patients, has provided further personal experience with the disease.

"So the paper has certainly been a personal hallmark. The paper is perhaps cited because it is a simply presented, statistically relevant documentation of the clinical features of a fascinating medical problem."

1. **Tuffanelli D L & Winkelmann R K.** Scleroderma and its relationship to the "collagenoses": dermatomyositis, lupus erythematosus, rheumatoid arthritis and Sjogren's syndrome. *Amer. J. Med. Sci.* **243**:133-46, 1962.
2. --. Diffuse systemic scleroderma: a comparison with acrosclerosis. *Ann. Intern. Med.* **57**:198-203, 1962.
3. **Tuffanelli D L.** Connective tissue diseases. (Malkinson F D & Pearson R W, eds.) *The year book of dermatology.* Chicago: Year Book Medical Publishers, 1978. p. 9-36.
4. **Tan E M, Rodnan G P, Garcia I, Moroi Y, Fritzler M J & Peebles C.** Diversity of antinuclear antibodies in progressive systemic sclerosis: anti-centromere antibody and its relationship to CREST syndrome. *Arthritis Rheum.* **23**:617-25, 1980.

This Week's Citation Classic

NUMBER 41
OCTOBER 8, 1979

Van Scott E J & Ekel T M. Kinetics of hyperplasia in psoriasis.
Arch. Dermatol. **88**:373-81, 1963.
[Dermatology Branch, National Cancer Institute, NIH, Bethesda, MD]

Mitotic counts and planimetric measurements on skin specimens from persons with psoriasis reveal lesions to have a 9-fold increase in replicating epidermal cells and a 9-fold increase in volume of dermal papillae. Epidermal hyperplasis is found to be primarily due to expansion of the germinative cell population, less so to increased mitotic rates. Expansion of the germinative cell population may be initiated by proliferation of supporting connective tissue. [The *SCI*® indicates that this paper has been cited over 155 times since 1963.]

Eugene J. Van Scott
Health Sciences Center
School of Medicine
Temple University
Philadelphia, PA 19140

February 8, 1978

"I appreciate the opportunity to provide a commentary on this article and am pleased and gratified that it has been so often cited. I am doubly fortunate because of your request for the above abstract, since the publishing journal in 1963 somehow omitted printing the abstract provided with the paper at the time of its submission—the only time it has ever happened to me.

"The work reported, performed while I was at the National Cancer Institute in the Dermatology Branch, was undertaken because of the need for more information on determinants of hyperplasis in benign and cancerous processes. More particularly, it was started to understand better the events causing the immense degree of epidermal cell exfoliation in psoriasis, a disease that still plagues over a million Americans today.

"The techniques available then were tedious and time consuming, requiring resolute counting of mitoses, planimetric measurements, and arithmetic computing. These were doggedly carried out by Thomas Ekel, who, because he was also an accomplished semiprofessional bridge player, must have been by nature exceptionally exacting and deliberate.

"The reasons for the article having been cited so much, in my judgment, are: (1) It represented one of the early works relevant to later work that aimed to define cell cycles, and cycling and noncycling cell compartments of various epithelia; (2) The conclusions drawn by us from data obtained by those now-antiquated methods have retained their validity over time; and (3) Our findings in regard to the epidermal-dermal relationships were pertinent to the general phenomena of epithelial-mesenchymal interrelationships, in that they suggested that an epithelial event (hyperplasia) was secondary to connective tissue proliferation.

"A consequence of our findings, and those of others that called attention to excessive epidermal cell replication in psoriasis, has been a wide search for and trial of antimitotic agents, other than methotrexate, for treating the disease. Unfortunately the search has not yet proven fruitful, and many of us are prepared to consider that further search may be futile. As our paper in 1963 suggested, epidermal hyperplasia probably is consequent to events and changes in the underlying connective tissue. Therefore, to treat psoriasis with drugs that restrain epidermal replication without diminishing the dermal determinants may be somewhat like bailing out a leaking boat without attempting to seal the leak. While retrospectively this may seem elementary, to assume such apparent logic at an earlier time would have required a kind of clairvoyance that few would dare to admit to or attempt to defend."

CC/NUMBER 23
JUNE 4, 1984

This Week's Citation Classic™

Mishima Y. Macromolecular changes in pigmentary disorders.
Arch. Dermatol. **91**:519-57, 1965.
[Dept. Dermatology, Wayne State Univ. Sch. Medicine, Detroit, and Veterans Admin. Hosp., Dearborn, MI]

This was the first full study to delineate changes occurring in functioning macromolecules, such as melanosomes, within melanogenic compartments of pigment cells in their dysfunctional and neoplastic disease status. The evidence presented in the paper covered the following three subjects: 1) melanosome polymorphism; 2) intracellular localization of tyrosinase in disturbed melanogenesis-albinism; and 3) cellular nevi: subcellular and cytochemical characteristics with reference to their origin. [The *SCI*® indicates that this paper has been cited in over 135 publications, making it one of the ten most-cited papers for this journal.]

Yutaka Mishima
Department of Dermatology
Kobe University School of Medicine
Chuo-ku, Kobe 650
Japan

February 9, 1984

"Shortly after my arrival in the US in the summer of 1958, following my clinical training in dermatology at the University of Tokyo Hospital, I met Hermann Pinkus who, through his perception and gentle brilliance, inspired me to venture into a new era of macromolecular pathology.

"The era of electron microscopy in biomedical sciences had just begun. The level of precision and reliability of this newly developed, highly sensitive technique became good enough to apply intricate, complex problems of biological and clinical changes occurring in human cell systems.

"The melanocyte is a cell which has distinct biological characteristics, specific enzyme systems, unique subcellular organization, location, and functions. The melanocyte undergoes numerous and diverse pathological changes which can profitably be classified into three categories of pigmentary disorders. The first and largest group is neoplasia of the pigment cell; the second group includes those disorders caused by hypofunctional melanocytes; and the third group of pigmentary disorders is characterized by the hyperfunction of melanocytes.

"In these disorders, production, excretion, and degradation of melanosomes results in characteristic pathological skin color changes. To delineate pathogenesis and cause of pigmentary disorders, basic knowledge of melanogenesis is essential.

"Fortunately, around that time, melanogenesis at the macromolecular level became increasingly clarified. Before that time, melanin was considered to be synthesized within the mitochondria which disagreed with the newly discovered melanosome concept. However, based on electron microscopic as well as biochemical evidence, this dispute was soon resolved, the melanosome concept was accepted, and it was found that melanin biosynthesis proceeds in specific cytoplasmic organelles, melanosomes, which are considered to be formed in the Golgi apparatus or smooth ER under genetic control.

"Thus, I began investigation on the basis of this new melanosome concept of melanogenesis. First, we found specific melanosome polymorphism occurring in all three types of pigmentary disorders. These findings can be used as criteria in the diagnosis of pigmentary disorders and also for the further investigation of their pathogenesis.

"Secondly, active tyrosinase was found to be present within melanosomes of human and certain animal albino melanocytes, in which melanization could be induced *in vitro* with the addition of the appropriate substrate and/or hormonal stimuli.

"Thirdly, subcellular and enzymic characteristics of various cellular nevi and resulting malignant melanoma, as well as other melanotic tumors, were disclosed with reference to their pathogenesis and developmental ontogeny.

"These discoveries resulted in my receiving the first prize in the Annual Essay Contest of the American Dermatological Association in the summer of 1964.

"I believe this paper has been highly cited because it was the first to throw light on the macromolecular changes within pigment cells which lead to their disorders.

"This has further led us to clarify various regulatory mechanisms[1-3] of melanogenesis at the macromolecular level. One of our recent findings is the integral role of glycosylation[4,5] for maturation of tyrosinase and its accepting function by premelanosomes."

1. **Mishima Y, Imokawa G & Ogura H.** Functional and three-dimensional differentiation of smooth membrane structures in melanogenesis. (Klaus S N, ed.) *Biologic basis of pigmentation.* Basel: S. Karger, 1980. p. 277-90.
2. **Imokawa G & Mishima Y.** Isolation and biochemical characterization of tyrosinase-rich GERL and coated vesicle in the melanin synthesizing cells. *Brit. J. Dermatol.* **104**:160-78, 1981.
3. **Mojamder M, Ichihashi M & Mishima Y.** Effect of DOPA-loading on glutathione-dependent 5-S cysteinyldopa genesis in melanoma cells *in vitro*. *J. Invest. Dermatol.* **78**:224-6, 1982.
4. **Imokawa G & Mishima Y.** Loss of melanogenic properties in tyrosinases induced by glycosylation inhibitors within malignant melanoma cells. *Cancer Res.* **42**:1994-2002, 1982.
5. **Mishima Y & Imokawa G.** Selective aberration and pigment loss in melanosomes of malignant melanoma cells *in vitro* by glycosylation inhibitors: premelanosomes as glycoprotein. *J. Invest. Dermatol.* **81**:106-14, 1983.

CC/NUMBER 30
JULY 26, 1982

This Week's Citation Classic

van Rossum J M. Cumulative dose-response curves. II. Technique for the making of dose-response curves in isolated organs and the evaluation of drug parameters. *Arch. Int. Pharmacodyn.* **143**:299-330, 1963.
[Dept. Pharmacol., Roman Catholic Univ. Med. Sch., Nijmegen, The Netherlands]

The importance of the study of dose-response curves for the analysis of the mechanism of action is stressed. A detailed description is given of the technique of making cumulative dose-response curves in various isolated organs. A brief review of the molecular theory of drug action is presented. Methods are derived to calculate relevant drug parameters. [The *SCI*® indicates that this paper has been cited in over 700 publications since 1963. Based on an analysis of *SCI* data 1961-80, this paper is the most cited published in the journal.]

J.M. van Rossum
Department of Pharmacology
Catholic University of Nijmegen
6500 HB Nijmegen
The Netherlands

April 26, 1982

"The study of dose-response curves of drugs in isolated organs has been the main topic of research during the first decades of the newly established department of pharmacology at the Catholic University of Nijmegen Medical School. Shortly after Ariëns was appointed chairman of the department, I moved with him in 1954 from the Rudolf Magnus Institute in Utrecht to Nijmegen.

"Nijmegen University, where the medical school had to find its course among the existing faculties of the humanities, was not used to the budgets necessary to do research in medical science, so the funds were meager. Dose-response curves and especially cumulative dose-response curves were made with relatively primitive means but nevertheless provided a wealth of information on the mechanism of action of drugs, receptor pharmacology, classification of drugs, and the relationships between chemical structure and pharmacological activity. Based on the tradition of quantitative pharmacology inherited from the Rudolf Magnus Institute it still took a good deal of pioneering and combined effort of an excellent team to reach our goals.

"The results, starting with the first series of papers by Ariëns and de Groot,[1] followed by studies by Ariëns, myself, and Simonis,[2] and by myself and Ariëns,[3] finally culminated in the monograph *Molecular Pharmacology*, edited by Ariëns in 1964.[4]

"Although we are not sure who first used the cumulative dose-response technique, it certainly was demonstrated in the paper by Ariëns and de Groot,[1] using the rectus abdominis muscle of the frog. The method, being practical and economical, was soon applied to other isolated organs in a number of PhD theses.

"From lectures presented at various departments and discussions with many colleagues, it became evident that there was a need for a paper covering the theory of drug receptor interaction combined with a detailed instruction on the technique of cumulative dose-response curves, of which we had years of experience. Frans van den Brink and I wrote an introduction,[5] while Coby Hurkmans used her expertise by carefully carrying out the many experiments used in the classical paper.

"I was surprised that this paper became a *Citation Classic*, although this type of research contributed to the S.E. de Jongh award, which I received in 1966. Probably the combination of presenting a theoretical basis underlying drug-receptor interaction and a clear experimental design greatly added to the impact of this paper. The continued interest in drug-receptor studies probably stimulates graduate students to use this paper as a starting point for their research.

"Receptor research should not merely rely on binding experiments, but should be in harmony with studies in intact tissues responding to drug receptor interaction. Pharmacology dealing with extremely complex systems such as the human body needs to study well-defined subsystems such as isolated tissues, but finally aims at understanding the interaction of drugs with the total system. It is this dynamic systems approach that is the topic of our current research. Recent work in the field has been published."[6-8]

1. **Ariëns E J & de Groot W M.** Affinity and intrinsic-activity in the theory of competitive inhibition. Part III. Homologous decamethonium-derivatives and succinyl-choline-esters. *Arch. Int. Pharmacodyn.* **99**:193-205, 1954.
2. **Ariëns E J, van Rossum J M & Simonis A M.** A theoretical basis of molecular pharmacology. I. Interactions of one or two compounds with one receptor system. *Arzneim.-Forsch.* **6**:282-93, 1956.
3. **van Rossum J M & Ariëns E J.** Pharmacodynamics of parasympathetic drugs. *Arch. Int. Pharmacodyn.* **118**:418-46, 1959.
4. **Ariëns E J**, ed. *Molecular pharmacology: the mode of action of biologically active compounds.* New York: Academic Press, 1964. Vol. 1. 503 p.
5. **van Rossum J M & van den Brink F G.** Cumulative dose-response curves. I. Introduction to the technique. *Arch. Int. Pharmacodyn.* **143**:240-7, 1963.
6. **Cools A R & van Rossum J M.** Excitation-mediating and inhibition-mediating dopamine receptors: a new concept towards a better understanding of electrophysiological, biochemical, pharmacological, functional and clinical data. *Psychopharmacologia* (Berlin) **45**:243-54, 1976.
7. **van Rossum J M**, ed. *Handbook of experimental pharmacology. Vol. 47. Kinetics of drug action.* Berlin: Springer-Verlag, 1977. 436 p.
8. **Bozler G & van Rossum J M.** *Pharmacokinetics during drug development: data analysis and evaluation techniques.* Stuttgart: Gustav Fischer Verlag, 1982.

CC/NUMBER 4
JANUARY 23, 1984

This Week's Citation Classic™

Marston M 'V. Compliance with medical regimens: a review of the literature. *Nurs. Res.* **19**:312-23, 1970.
[Frances Payne Bolton School of Nursing, Case Western Reserve University, Cleveland, OH]

This was the first comprehensive review of research on compliance with medical regimens. It addressed problems of comparing compliance rates across studies which utilized dissimilar criteria; summarized demographic, illness, and social-psychological variables used to predict compliance; and suggested directions for future research, especially aspects of the patient-provider relationship. [The *Science Citation Index*® (*SCI*®) and the *Social Sciences Citation Index*® (*SSCI*®) indicate that this paper has been cited in over 185 publications since 1970.]

**Mary-'Vesta Marston-Scott
School of Nursing
Boston University
Boston, MA 02215**

December 11, 1983

"Beginning in the 1950s, the US Public Health Service made fellowships available to nurses which enabled them to undertake doctoral preparation in the behavioral and biological sciences on which professional nursing rests so heavily. I was the first nurse to be admitted to the social and personality program in the psychology department at Boston University.

"My nursing experiences had raised many questions as to why people fail to adopt healthy life-styles, take advantage of screening procedures for early detection of disease, and follow well-authenticated treatment regimens. Doctoral study in social psychology provided me with exciting ideas as to research which needed to be done and how one might go about helping people improve their health and prevent complications following untreated chronic illness.

"This review paper was an outgrowth of my doctoral dissertation research and represented my attempt to outline the parameters of what I considered to be a large and important problem which needed to be addressed by behavioral scientists, by health care professionals, and especially by nurses.

"Interest in health behavior and compliance was advanced by two international conferences, held at McMaster University in Hamilton, Ontario, Canada, which culminated in two monographs; a series of conferences sponsored by the Public Health Service; official documents such as *Healthy People: The Surgeon General's Report on Health Promotion and Disease Prevention* **and** *Promoting Health/Preventing Disease: Objectives for the Nation*; **and, most recently, formal recognition of health psychology by establishment of Division 38 of the American Psychological Association.**

"I am frequently told that my paper played a large part in providing a succinct statement concerning what was known about determinants of compliance and promising directions for future research. In the period of time since my paper was published, the important topical areas which have emerged as being important in predicting health behavior and compliance are the Health Belief Model, the Locus of Control construct, social support, aspects of the patient-provider relationship, Fishbein's theory of reasoned action, attribution theory, and behavior modification and contracting. A more recent review of the implications of the research on health behavior and compliance for nursing practice is found in Hardy and Conway.[1] (A revision of this paper, and book, are in process.)

"I developed and direct a health behavior cognate within our doctor of nursing science program at Boston University. This program is the first of its kind in a school of nursing. The focus is on developing research to advance knowledge of the determinants of health behavior and compliance, and students are encouraged to conduct intervention studies. I believe my major contributions have been through the papers and research of my doctoral and master's students (see, e.g., references 2-5)."

1. **Marston M 'V.** The use of knowledge. (Hardy M E & Conway M E, eds.) *Role theory: perspectives for health professionals*. New York: Appleton-Century-Crofts, 1978. p. 211-30.
2. **Arakelian M.** An assessment and nursing application of the concept of Locus of Control. *Advan. Nurs. Sci.* **3**:25-42, 1980.
3. **Kulbok P A.** A concept analysis of preventive health behavior. (Chinn P L, ed.) *Advances in nursing theory development*. Rockville, MD: Aspen Systems Corporation, 1983. p. 125-51.
4. **Mikhaiel B.** The Health Belief Model: a review and critical evaluation of the model, research and practice. *Advan. Nurs. Sci.* **4**:65-82, 1982.
5. **McLaughlin J S.** Toward a theoretical model for community health programs. *Advan. Nurs. Sci.* **5**:7-28, 1982.

Jowsey J, Kelly P J, Riggs B L, Bianco A J, Jr., Scholz D A & Gershon-Cohen J. Quantitative microradiographic studies of normal and osteoporotic bone. *J. Bone Joint Surg.-Amer. Vol.* **47-A**:785-806, 1965. [Mayo Clin. and Mayo Found., Rochester, MN & Albert Einstein Med. Ctr., Philadelphia, PA]

Quantitative microadiography permits comparison of stained sections of bone with a microradiograph depicting mineral distribution. Bone formation, resorption, abnormalities of mineralization, and differences in remodeling can be quantitated in metabolic bone diseases, and the early effects of therapy in bone disease can be evaluated. [The *SCI*® indicates that this paper has been cited over 220 times since 1965.]

Jenifer Jowsey
421 B. March Avenue
Healdsberg, CA 95448

March 20, 1978

"Twenty-five years ago there was much interest in radioactive isotopes that were produced by atomic fission. Many of the long-lived radioisotopes are concentrated in the skeleton, and some of the most hazardous, such as strontium and yttrium, are associated with the mineral phase of bone. It therefore became necessary to use a method of looking at bone that did not involve demineralization; microradiography was used. At that time I was working with a MRC (Medial Research Council) team in Oxford under the guidance of Dame Janet Vaughan. I later developed the method of quantitative microradiography. Bone formation and resorption can be recognized on the microradiograph, and if the corresponding stained section has good cellular detail, there is a correlation between the presence of bone cells and the appearance of the surface of mineralized bone on the microradiograph. The percentage of bone surface that is undergoing formation or resorption yields numerical values that are representative of bone remodeling.

"The first use of the method was to characterize the different metabolic bone diseases in terms of bone remodeling. Almost without exception, metabolic bone disease shows loss of bone. However, in hypercortisolism, for example, bone resorption is increased and bone formation is decreased, while in osteoporosis bone resorption is increased but bone formation is normal. Almost no metabolic bone disease shows exactly the same bone remodeling features. This information has been useful in understanding some of the hormonal relationships in bone disease. It thus became possible for the first time to investigate the mechanism of bone loss and to evaluate deficiencies in mineralization. This, in essence, is what the paper describes.

"After developing the method, I became particularly interested in osteoporosis. I came to the Mayo Clinic fifteen years ago largely in order to collaborate with physicians in studies of this disorder. It is probably true to say that the major use of the method has been to quantitate the effects of the treatment of bone disease. By taking bone biopsies of patients before and after treatment with various substances that have promise in this disease, we can predict whether bone mass will increase or decrease more rapidly or less rapidly than in untreated patients. These changes can be seen many years before any change is evident by the more conventional techniques of x-ray or before there is symptomatic relief of pain. It is with the use of the technique of quantitative microradiography that the successful treatment of osteoporosis with fluoride and calcium was first documented, later to be confirmed by x-ray changes of increased density.

"I am now leaving the Mayo Clinic and, with my husband, an ophthalmologist, and two children, moving west to Healdsburg, CA. Having recently collected the long-term fluoride and calcium data for publication in the near future[1] a study that reconfirms our earlier work published in the same journal in 1972,[2] and having written two books, *Metabolic Diseases of Bone*[3] and *The Bone Biopsy*[4] which sum up my experience in these two fields, the time to leave is perhaps ripe. My time there has been very fruitful, and for patients with the miseries of bone-losing diseases, a successful form of treatment has been established.

1. **Jowsey J, Arnaud C D & Johnson K A.** Effect of combined treatment with flouride, calcium, vitamin D and estrogen on osteoporosis. Unpublished paper.
2. **Jowsey J, Riggs B L, Kelly P J & Hoffman D L.** Effect of combined therapy with sodium fluoride, vitamin D and calcium in osteoporosis. *Amer. J. Med.* **53**: 43-9, 1972.
3. **Jowsey J.** *Metabolic diseases of bone.* (Sledge C B, consulting editor.) W. B. Saunders, Philadelphia, PA: 1977. 312 p.
4. **Jowsey J.** *The bone biopsy.* (Aviolo L B, series editor). New York, NY: Plenum Medical Book Co. 1977, 158 p.

This Week's Citation Classic

CC/NUMBER 6
FEBRUARY 8, 1982

Kuratsune M, Yoshimura T, Matsuzaka J & Yamaguchi A. Epidemiologic study on Yusho, a poisoning caused by ingestion of rice oil contaminated with a commercial brand of polychlorinated biphenyls.
Environ. Health Perspect. **1**:119-28, 1972.
[Dept. Public Health, Fac. Med., Kyushu Univ., Fukuoka, Japan]

In 1968, an epidemic of a peculiar disease similar to chloracne occurred in Japan. This paper presents the epidemiological evidence indicating that it was caused by ingestion of rice oil contaminated with polychlorinated biphenyls (PCBs). It also briefly refers to clinical aspects of this unique food poisoning, probably the first one ever experienced by man. [The *SCI*® indicates that this paper has been cited over 120 times since 1972.]

Masanori Kuratsune
Department of Public Health
Faculty of Medicine
Kyushu University
Fukuoka 812
Japan

December 8, 1981

"Early in June 1968, an American jet fighter crashed on our campus, causing utter chaos in the whole university which had already been suffering from a serious student riot. Later, in October 1968, an extensive epidemic of severe acne-like eruptions was reported in our prefecture and we were obliged to clarify its cause by organizing a research team in the school.

"Shibanosuke Katsuki, professor of internal medicine and chief of the team, was wise enough to organize the team with not only physicians, but also the staff of the faculties of pharmaceutical sciences, agriculture, and engineering. This multidisciplinary approach facilitated the study very much. Furthermore, strangely enough, the crisis at the school seemed to stimulate and firmly unite all these divergent professionals to achieve the goal.

"Katsuki, epidemiologically well minded, asked me to develop epidemiological investigations. Although I had not professionally been trained in epidemiology, I complied with his request and immediately designed and started extensive surveys with my associates and the staff of the local health departments, simply following the principles and methods of epidemiology which I had already understood by reading a book.[1]

"About ten days after the research team was organized, the chemical group discovered a large amount of PCBs (KC-400 produced by a company) in the rice oil used by patients as well as in their subcutaneous tissue. Thus, the chemical demonstration of toxic agents was very quick, but we continued the surveys for another four months trying to collect all the epidemiological evidence necessary for unequivocal proof of the cause. All the epidemiological evidence thus obtained fully agreed with the clinical and chemical features of the epidemic. Without the epidemiological approach and knowledge and without the devoted cooperation of my associates and many others, I am sure that this success would not have materialized.

"There was one thing, however, which I could not be very sure of, that is, the acnegenicity of pure PCBs in man. Oral administrations of KC-400 (pure PCB) did not yield acne in animals and a thorough check of the literature reporting occupational cases of chloracne as caused by PCBs revealed that the PCBs used were not pure at all, containing a large amount of chlorinated naphthalenes. Thus, there was no definite evidence for the acnegenicity of pure PCBs in man. Fortunately, I heard that Ichiro Hara at the Osaka Prefectural Institute of Public Health observed chloracnes among workers handling pure PCBs. I asked him to publish his observations and he did.[2] Thus, I finally became fully convinced of the cause of the epidemic.

"I cannot be completely sure of the reasons why our paper has been highly cited. I suppose that the good epidemiological evidence collected by us, the uniqueness of the poisoning, and the general serious concern about PCB pollution may be the main reasons. Recent work in this field has been published."[3,4]

1. **MacMahon B, Pugh T F & Ipsen J.** *Epidemiologic methods.* Boston: Little, Brown, 1960. 302 p.
2. **Hara I.** Health supervision of workers exposed to chlorodiphenyl in an electric condenser factory. *Proc. Osaka Prefect. Inst. Public Health Educ. Ind. Health* 7:26-31, 1960.
3. **Masuda Y & Kuratsune M.** Toxic compounds in the rice oil which caused Yusho. *Fukuoka Acta Med.* **70**:149-57, 1979.
4. **Kuratsune M.** Yusho. (Kimbrough R, ed.) *Halogenated biphenyls, terphenyls, naphthalenes, dibenzodioxins, and related products.* Amsterdam: Elsevier/North-Holland Biomedical Press, 1980. p. 287-302.

This Week's Citation Classic

CC/NUMBER 28
JULY 14, 1980

Hungerford D A, Donnelly A J, Nowell P C & Beck S. The chromosome constitution of a human phenotypic intersex.
Amer. J. Hum. Genet. **11**:215-36, 1959.
[Inst. Cancer Res., Amer. Oncologic Hosp., and Dept. Pathol., Sch. Med., Univ. Pennsylvania, Philadelphia, PA]

An individual of outwardly male appearance, clinically diagnosed a 'true hermaphrodite,' was found to have an XX sex chromosome complement. The first full description appears here of our adaptation to cytogenetic use of a method for culturing human leukocytes. [The *SCI*® indicates that this paper has been cited over 370 times since 1961.]

David A. Hungerford
Institute for Cancer Research
Fox Chase Cancer Center
Philadelphia, PA 19111

June 16, 1980

"The case was ascertained by Andy Donnelly, late pathologist to the American Oncologic Hospital, with whom I shared a lab at the Institute for Cancer Research. He suggested this study and contributed the clinical and histopathological findings. The subject was male in appearance, except for gynecomastia of recent origin. The initial diagnosis was supported by biopsy of an intra-scrotal ovotestis and confirmed by examination of internal structures later removed surgically by Sidney Beck. Leukocytes from circulating blood were cultured by Peter Nowell of the University of Pennsylvania School of Medicine. Squash preparation and the metaphase chromosome studies were my responsibility. A normal chromosome number and XX sex chromosome constitution, without evidence of a Y, were demonstrated. Periodic examination of the subject continued thereafter, and skin biopsies were obtained from a number of sites. Cells cultured from these provided cytogenetic results which confirmed and augmented our original findings.[1] The subject's enlistment in the armed forces precluded further study.

"This report briefly interrupted a collaborative project that Pete and I had initiated late in 1957, soon after he had found mitosis in human leukemic cells cultured according to Osgood's 'gradient' method. This observation prompted him to inquire whether anyone in the Philadelphia area was then active in human chromosome studies. At the time, I was apparently the only one who answered that description. Our investigation of chromosomes in cultured leukemic leukocytes followed, and it was soon clear that normal leukocytes could also divide in this system. Within a short time Pete was to make the classic discovery that phytohemagglutinin (PHA), used to agglutinate erythrocytes and facilitate their removal from the inoculum, was also a mitogen, a finding that made this investigation possible. Within a short time, a major technical improvement was made by Paul Moorhead, who substituted the air-drying method for squashing.[2] Leukocyte culture quickly became the method of choice in human cytogenetics, remaining so to the present. My introduction of KCl as an agent for hypotonic treatment accomplished further significant improvement,[3] gradually becoming standard in preparing mitotic cells from other sources.

"I suspect that the methods described in this early paper have had more to do with its frequent citation than have our findings, even though they are the first published on an intersex of this kind. The proliferation of lymphocytes *in vitro* is accompanied by their retention of specific functional capacities, and for this reason the method has profoundly influenced many other fields.

"The paper is also particularly memorable to me as the basis on which I was to participate in the 1960 Denver conference, at which the initial proposals were formulated for a standard nomenclature of human mitotic chromosomes. These recommendations, since revised and greatly expanded, remain a foundation of international agreement."

1. **Hungerford D A, Donnelly A J & Nowell P C.** The chromosome constitution of a human phenotypic intersex: reconfirmation of a 46-chromosome, XX, apparently non-mosaic "true hermaphrodite." *Hereditas* **52**:379-86, 1965.
2. **Moorhead P S, Nowell P C, Mellman W J, Battips D M & Hungerford D A.** Chromosome preparations of leukocytes cultured from human peripheral blood. *Exp. Cell Res.* **20**:613-16, 1960.
3. **Hungerford D A.** Leukocytes cultured from small inocula of whole blood and the preparation of chromosomes by treatment with hypotonic KCl. *Stain Technol.* **40**:333-8, 1965.

This Week's Citation Classic

NUMBER 3
JANUARY 15, 1979

Chappell J B. Systems used for the transport of substrates into mitochondria. *Brit. Med. Bull.* **24**: 150-7, 1968.

This short review describes the evidence for the existence of specific substrate transporting systems in mitochondrial membranes. A discussion of the probable metabolic role of these carriers is given. [The *SCI®* indicates that this paper was cited 256 times in the period 1968-1977.]

J. B. Chappell
Department of Biochemistry
University of Bristol
Bristol, BS8 1TD, United Kingdom

January 23, 1978

"This paper, which is a short review, represented some of the thoughts which were in my colleagues' and my minds at that time. The realization of the existence of the mitochondrial substrate translocators came from experiments performed as a consequence of two sets of observations. One was the catalytic effect of malate on the oxidation of isocitrate by substrate-depleted liver mitochondria; the other some work by Tony Crofts and me on the permeability of mitochondria to phosphate, inferred from studies on cation transport. I had never been happy with my (mis) interpretation of the catalytic effect of malate, and the work with Crofts indicated that, apart from phosphate, small anions were unable to permeate mitochondria. Older work with Guy Greville on the 'latency' of mitochondrial rhodanese (thiosulfate transulfurase) also indicated that small anions may not be able to penetrate mitochondria. Since it was known that most of the dehydrogenases and other enzymes dealing with the metabolism of anions were located in the mitochondrial matrix, this impermeability posed a real problem.

"The major part of the new experimental material referred to in the paper was known at the end of one day's work by a graduate student, Keith Haarhoff, and myself. The morning of that day was spent in making up iso-osmotic solutions of the ammonium salts of various anions. Mitochondrial swelling was followed with a crude but effective home-made light-scattering apparatus. The first experiments were disappointing; mitochondria swelled very well in phosphate (which we already knew) but not in malate or citrate. Was the failure to swell in malate due to some effect of large amounts of malate? Was the phosphate carrier inhibited in the presence of malate? Addition of even small amounts of phosphate to mitochondria suspended in iso-osmotic ammonium malate produced an unexpectedly large amount of swelling. Phosphate appeared to be necessary for malate permeation. It was a short step to show that malate allowed citrate entry (when phosphate was present). The groundwork was laid.

"The discovery that glutamate was necessary for aspartate permeation into liver mitochondria was made by Angelo Azzi while he was working in Bristol, and was due to an error! Repeated attempts to oxidise intramitochondrial NAD(P) which had been reduced by oxoglutarate (in the presence of malonate) by addition of aspartate had failed; the oxidation was expected since oxaloacetate would be generated intramitochondrially by transamination. On one occasion the experiment 'worked'; however, glutamate had been added after aspartate instead of more aspartate as was intended. The two tubes stood in ice side by side, and in the gloom required for the proper running of the spectrophotometer, Azzi erred."

Index of Authors

All authors of Citation Classics are listed. An asterisk after a page number indicates that a commentary by the author appears on that page.

Index of Subjects

Index of Institutions

The institutions listed are those at which the work reported in the Citation Classic was done.